KU-301-968

Postgraduate Orthopaedics

ity Hospital – Staff Library

Postgraduate Orthopaedics

The Candidate's Guide to the FRCS (Tr & Orth) Examination

Edited by

Paul A. Banaszkiewicz

FRCS (Glas) FRCS (Ed) FRCS (Eng)
FRCS (Tr & Orth) Cert Clin Ed
Consultant Orthopaedic surgeon
Queen Elizabeth Hospital and North East Surgery Centre
Gateshead, UK

Associate Editors

Deiary F. Kader

FRCS (Tr & Orth) MFSEM (UK)
Consultant Orthopaedic Surgeon
Queen Elizabeth Hospital and North East Surgical Centre
Gateshead, UK
Visiting Professor, Sports Science
Northumbria University
Newcastle upon Tyne, UK

Nicola Maffulli

MD MS PhD FRCS (Orth)
Professor of Trauma and Orthopaedic Surgery
Keele University School of Medicine
Stoke on Trent
Staffordshire, UK

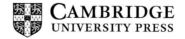

CAMBRIDGE UNIVERSITY PRESS

CAMBRIDGE UNIVERSITY PRESS
Cambridge, New York, Melbourne, Madrid, Cape Town, Singapore, São Paulo, Delhi

Cambridge University Press
The Edinburgh Building, Cambridge CB2 8RU, UK

Published in the United States of America by Cambridge University Press, New York

www.cambridge.org
Information on this title: www.cambridge.org/9780521674638

© Cambridge University Press 2009

This publication is in copyright. Subject to statutory exception
and to the provisions of relevant collective licensing agreements,
no reproduction of any part may take place without
the written permission of Cambridge University Press.

First published 2009
Reprinted 2009

Printed in the United Kingdom at the University Press, Cambridge

A catalogue record for this publication is available from the British Library

ISBN 978-0-521-67463-8 paperback

Cambridge University Press has no responsibility for the persistence or
accuracy of URLs for external or third-party internet websites referred to
in this publication, and does not guarantee that any content on such
websites is, or will remain, accurate or appropriate.

Every effort has been made in preparing this publication to provide accurate and up-to-date information which is in
accord with accepted standards and practice at the time of publication. Although case histories are drawn from actual
cases, every effort has been made to disguise the identities of the individuals involved. Nevertheless, the authors,
editors and publishers can make no warranties that the information contained herein is totally free from error, not least
because clinical standards are constantly changing through research and regulation. The authors, editors and publishers
therefore disclaim all liability for direct or consequential damages resulting from the use of material contained in this
publication. Readers are strongly advised to pay careful attention to information provided by the manufacturer of any
drugs or equipment that they plan to use.

Contents

List of contributors   vii

Foreword by Mr Peter Gibson   ix

Preface   xi

Glossary   xiii

Section 1   The FRCS (Tr & Orth) examination   **1**

1.   General guidance   3
Paul A. Banaszkiewicz and
Simon Barker

Section 2   The written paper   **7**

2.   Written paper guidance   9
Paul A. Banaszkiewicz

Section 3   The clinicals   **11**

3.   The short cases   13
Paul A. Banaszkiewicz

4.   Short case list   15
Paul A. Banaszkiewicz

5.   The long cases   17
Paul A. Banaszkiewicz

6.   Long case list   19
Paul A. Banaszkiewicz

7.   Hand and wrist clinical cases   20
Paul A. Banaszkiewicz and
John W. K. Harrison

8.   Shoulder and elbow clinical cases   51
Paul A. Banaszkiewicz

9.   Spine clinical cases   64
      Paul A. Banaszkiewicz

10.   Hip clinical cases   71
      Paul A. Banaszkiewicz

11.   Knee clinical cases   105
      Deiary F. Kader and Leo Pinczewski

12.   Foot and ankle clinical cases   110
      Paul A. Banaszkiewicz

13.   Paediatric clinical cases   126
      Paul A. Banaszkiewicz

**Section 4   Adult elective
orthopaedics oral   133**

14.   General oral guidance   135
      Paul A. Banaszkiewicz

15.   Shoulder and elbow oral core topics   138
      Niall Munro

16.   Hip oral core topics   155
      Paul A. Banaszkiewicz

17.   Knee oral core topics   194
      Deiary F. Kader and Leo Pinczewski

18.   Foot and ankle oral core topics   215
      Paul A. Banaszkiewicz

19.   Spine oral core topics   237
      Niall Craig

Section 5   The hand oral   271

20.   Syllabus and general guidance   273
      Paul A. Banaszkiewicz

21.   Hand oral core topics   276
      Paul A. Banaszkiewicz and
      John W. K. Harrison

Section 6   The paediatric oral   357

22.   Paediatric oral topics   359
      Joseph Alsousou and
      Paul A. Banaszkiewicz

Section 7   The trauma oral   401

23.   Trauma oral topics   403
      Abayomi Animashawun and
      Paul A. Banaszkiewicz

Section 8   The basic science oral   459

24.   Basic science oral core topics   461
      Simon Barker and
      Paul A. Banaszkiewicz

Section 9   Miscellaneous topics   567

25.   Candidates' accounts of the
      examination   569
      Paul A. Banaszkiewicz and Niall Munro

26.   Examination failure   587
      Paul A. Banaszkiewicz

Index   591

Contributors

Mr. Abayomi Animashawun BSc (Hons) MRCS (Ed)
Queen Elizabeth Hospital
Gateshead, UK

Mr. Joseph Alsousou LMSSA (Lon) MRCS (Ed)
Queen Elizabeth Hospital
Gateshead, UK

Mr. Simon Barker BSc (Hons) MD FRCS (Tr & Orth)
Royal Aberdeen Children's Hospital
Aberdeen, UK

**Mr. Paul A. Banaszkiewicz FRCS (Glas) FRCS (Ed)
FRCS (Eng) FRCS (Tr & Orth) Cert Clin Ed**
Queen Elizabeth Hospital
Gateshead, UK

Mr. Niall Craig FRCS (Ed) FRCS (Tr & Orth)
Aberdeen Royal Infirmary
Aberdeen, UK

**Mr. John W. K. Harrison MSc FRCSEd (Tr & Orth)
MFSEM (UK)**
Queen Elizabeth Hospital
Gateshead, UK

Mr. Deiary F. Kader FRCS (Tr & Orth) MFSEM (UK)
Queen Elizabeth Hospital
Gateshead, UK
Visiting Professor, Sport Science
Northumbria University
Newcastle upon Tyne, UK

Mr. Niall Munro MD FRCS (Tr & Orth)
Golden Jubilee Hospital
Glasgow, UK

Mr. Leo Pinczewski MBBS FRACS
North Sydney Orthopaedic and Sports Medicine
Centre
Sydney, NSW
Australia

Foreword

The aim of this book is to allow candidates to orientate themselves towards the intercollegiate speciality examination in orthopaedics leading to the FRCS (Tr & Orth) award. It affords guidance on the appropriate examination skills and approaches, which hopefully will lead to success in this examination.

The FRCS (Tr & Orth) continues to evolve with significant changes in both the written part of the exam, which must now be successfully completed prior to entry into the clinical, and to the oral.

This book has been written by those who have recently successfully completed the examination. It is written from the candidate's point of view and experience in the way the examination is conducted.

While no single book can be a substitute for wide clinical experience and knowledge of the orthopaedic literature, I believe that this text will be of value to candidates preparing to sit the examination. There is no doubt that presentation in the examination setting is important in ensuring success.

Peter Gibson
Consultant Orthopaedic Surgeon
Head of Training North East of Scotland Rotation
Ex Examiner for the FRCS (Tr & Orth)

Preface

This book has been written specifically for candidates preparing for the Intercollegiate Board Examination in Trauma and Orthopaedic Surgery. It is an attempt to guide the orthopaedic trainee better in his or her preparation before they are thrown into the lion's den. It is not intended to replace or be a substitute for the numerous orthopaedic textbooks available. I make no claim for the originality of the material contained within this text. The core material originated from notes made whilst preparing for the FRCS Orth examination from a wide variety of differing sources. We are not trying to re-invent the wheel!

The curriculum for this examination is vast and therefore we have asked a variety of colleagues to contribute to various sections. Our aim was to put forth differing views and opinions regarding the key essentials for success in this examination and to give as broad a prospective as possible to candidates preparing to sit the examination. There is no doubt that the FRCS Orth is a stressful experience even for the most well prepared candidate. There is nothing more frustrating than a good candidate with good knowledge failing the examination because of lack of orientation and technique in the examination.

We have broken the book down into various sections to make revision easier. The first section covers the written paper. We give general advice about preparation. The "clinicals" – long and short cases – are crucial because if this aspect is failed, doing well in the orals does not allow redemption. In this section we cover a series of the most likely orthopaedic long and short cases that regularly appear in the exam.

The general orthopaedics and pathology oral covers a great breadth of orthopaedics, with a large number of subjects dealt with. To simplify matters we have broken the oral down into five core subspecialties; namely, shoulder/elbow, hip, knee, foot/ankle and spine. Within each core subspecialty we have dealt with various topics by way of a series of key points that guide the candidate through important details of the subject. At the end of each topic we have tried to re-emphasize important aspects of the subject by giving specific examples of how in reality questions tend to be asked. We have called this section "Examination corner" for obvious reasons. This is an important part of the book as candidates may know the subject well but fail to appreciate how the questions are going to "run" during an oral.

The next four sections cover the remaining orals; namely, Basic science, Trauma, Hands and Paediatrics.

In the candidates' accounts of the exam section we have give several candidates' blow-by-blow accounts of their whole examination performance. This gives candidates a prospective of the whole picture of their potential examination.

We hope that this is an enjoyable book to read and provides you with sound guidance in your preparation for the examination, in which we wish you every success. Finally, Paul Banaszkiewicz would like to acknowledge his special thanks to David Jaffrey for his help and guidance in the past.

Glossary

ABC	airway, breathing, circulation
ACJ	acromioclavicular joint
ACL	anterior cruciate ligament
AD	autosomal dominant
ADL	activities of daily living
ADM	abductor digiti minimi
AER	apical ectodermal ridge
AFO	ankle-foot orthosis
AIIS	anterior inferior iliac spine
AIN	anterior interosseous nerve
ALL	anterior longitudinal ligament
ALVAR	aseptic lymphocyte-dominated vasculitis-associated lesions
AP	anterior–posterior
APB	abductor pollicis brevis
APL	abductor pollicis longus
ARDS	adult respiratory distress syndrome
AS	ankylosing spondylitis
ASB	anatomical snuffbox
ASIS	anterior superior iliac spine
ATFL	anterior talofibular ligament
ATLS	Advanced Trauma Life Support
ATP	adenosine triphosphate
AVN	avascular necrosis
BDGF	bone-derived growth factor
BMG	bone matrix gelatin
BMP	bone morphogenetic protein
BMUs	basic multicellular units
BOA	British Orthopaedics Association
BPTB	bone patella tendon-bone
CAP	Clubfoot Assessment Protocol
CCL	coracoclavicular ligament
CFL	calcaneofibular ligament

CIA	carpal injury adaptive		EPL	extensor pollicis longus
CIC	carpal instability complex		ESR	erythrocyte sedimentation rate
CID	carpal instability dissociative		EUA	examination under anaesthesia
CIND	carpal instability non-dissociative		FBC	full blood count
CJD	Creutzfeldt–Jakob disease		FCR	flexor carpi radialis
CL	capitolunate		FCU	flexor carpi ulnaris
CMAP	compound muscle action potential		FDB	flexor digitorum brevis
CMC	carpometacarpal		FDL	flexor digitorum longus
CMV	cytomegalovirus		FDP	flexor digitorum profundus
CP	cerebral palsy		FDQ	flexor digiti quinti
CPM	continued passive motion		FDS	flexor digitorum superficialis
CPN	common peroneal nerve		FGF	fibroblast growth factor
CR	cruciate retaining		FHL	flexor hallucis longus
CRP	C-reactive protein		FPA	foot progression angle
CRPS	complex regional pain syndrome		FPB	flexor pollicis brevis
CSF	cerebrospinal fluid		FPL	flexor pollicis longus
CTEV	congenital talipes equinovarus		FTA	foot thigh angle
CVP	central venous pressure		GA	general anaesthetic
DCP	dynamic compression plate		GAGs	glycosaminoglycans
DCS	dynamic condylar screw		GI	gastrointestinal
DD	Dupuytren's disease		HEA	Hilgenreiner's epiphyseal angle
DDH	developmental dysplasia of the hip		HMSN	hereditary motor sensory neuropathies
DHS	dynamic hip screw		HNP	herniated nucleus pulposus
DI	dorsal interosseous		HO	heterotopic ossification
DIP	distal interphalangeal		HPT	hyperparathyroidism
DIPJ	distal interphalangeal joint		HTO	high tibial osteotomy
DISH	diffuse idiopathic skeletal hyperostosis		HU	Hounsfield units
DISI	dorsal intercalated segmental instability		HVA	hallux valgus angle
DP	distal phalanx		IDGF	insulin-derived growth factor
DRUJ	distal radioulnar joint		II	image intensifier
DV	dorsoventral		ILs	interleukins
DVT	deep vein thrombosis		IMT	intermetatarsal
ECRB	extensor carpi radialis brevis		IP	interphalangeal
ECRL	extensor carpi radialis longus		IPJ	interphalangeal joint
ECU	extensor carpi ulnaris		ISB	Intercollegiate Specialty Boards
EDC	extensor digitorum communis		IVC	inferior vena cava
EDL	extensor digitorum longus		JCA	juvenile chronic arthritis
EDM	extensor digiti minimi		JRF	joint reaction force
EDQ	extensor digiti quinti		KAFOs	knee-ankle-foot orthoses
EGF	epidermal growth factor		LCDCP	low-contact dynamic compression plates
EHL	extensor hallucis longus			
EIP	extensor indicis proprius		LCL	lateral collateral ligament
EMG	electromyograph		LCP	low compression plates
EMIs	extended matching items		LHB	long head of biceps
EPB	extensor pollicis brevis		LISS	less invasive stabilization system

LRTI	ligament reconstruction tendon interposition
LTL	lunotriquetral ligament
MCL	medial collateral ligament
MCP	metacarpophalangeal
MCQs	multiple choice questions
MDP	methylene diphosphonate
MEN	multiple endocrine neoplasia
MEPs	motor-evoked potentials
MFC	medial femoral condyle
MFH	malignant fibrous histiocytoma
MMP	metalloproteinase
MS	multiple sclerosis
MSU	monosodium urate
MUA	manipulation under anaesthetic
NCS	nerve condition studies
Nf-1	neurofibromatosis type 1
Nf-2	neurofibromatosis type 2
NICE	National Institute for Health and Clinical Excellence
NSAIDs	non-steroidal anti-inflammatory drugs
OA	osteoarthritis
OCD	osteochondritis dissecans
ODF	osteoclast differentiation factor (aka RANK ligand)
OPG	osteoprotegerin
OPLL	ossification of the posterior longitudinal ligament
ORIF	open reduction with internal fixation
ORL	oblique retinacular ligament
PCL	posterior cruciate ligament
PD	proximodistal
PDGF	platelet-derived growth factor
PE	pulmonary embolism
PEEK	polyetheretherketone
PET	positron emission tomography
PFFD	proximal focal femoral deficiency
PFJ	patellofemoral joint
PGE_2	prostaglandin E_2
PICU	paediatric intensive care unit
PIN	posterior interosseous nerve
PIP	proximal interphalangeal
PIPJ	proximal interphalangeal joint
PL	palmaris longus
PLAD	posterior lip augmentation device

PLIF	posterior interbody lumbar fusion
PLL	posterior longitudinal ligament
PMMA	polymethyl methacrylate
POP	plaster of Paris
PP	proximal phalanx
PQ	pronator quadratus
PS	posterior-stabilized
PT	pronator teres
PTFL	posterior talofibular ligament
PTH	parathyroid hormone
PVNS	pigmented villonodular synovitis
RA	rheumatoid arthritis
RHK	rotating-hinge knee
RLT	radiolunotriquetral
ROM	range of movement
RSD	reflex sympathetic dystrophy
RSWP	radial side wrist pain
RTA	road traffic accident
RVAD	rib vertebral angle difference
SACH	solid ankle cushion heel
SBA	single best answer
SCIWORA	spinal cord injury without radiological abnormality
SCJ	sternoclavicular joint
SEPs	sensory-evoked potentials
SHH	sonic hedgehog
SI	sacroiliac
SL	scapholunate
SLAC	scapholunate advanced collapse wrist
SLAP	superior labrum anterior to posterior
SLL	scapholunate ligament
SLR	straight leg raise
SNAC	scaphoid non-union advanced collapse wrist
SNAP	sensory nerve action potential
SOMI	Sternal Occipital Mandibular Immobilizer
SSEPs	somatosensory evoked potentials
STAR	Scandinavian total ankle replacement
STR	soft-tissue realignment
STT	scaphotrapeziotrapezoid
SUFE	slipped upper femoral epiphysis

TAR	total ankle arthroplasty	TORCH	**t**oxoplasmosis, **o**ther, **r**ubella, **c**ytomegalovirus, **h**erpes simplex
TBW	tension band wiring		
TENS	transcutaneous electrical nerve stimulation	TT	tibial tubercle
		UCL	ulnar collateral ligament
TFA	tibiofemoral angle	UHMWPE	ultra high molecular weight polyethylene
TFCC	triangular fibrocartilage complex		
TGF	transforming growth factor	UKA	unilateral knee arthroplasty
THA	total hip arthroplasty	UKR	unilateral knee replacement
TIMPs	tissue inhibitory metalloproteinases	US	ultrasound
		USS	ultrasound scan
TKA	total knee arthroplasty	USWP	ulnar side wrist pain
TKR	total knee replacement	VIP	vasoactive intestinal polypeptide
TLHKAFO	thoraco-lumbar-hip-knee-ankle-foot orthosis	VISI	volar intercalated segment instability
TLIF	transforaminal lumbar interbody fusion	VMO	vastus medialis obliquus
		VP	ventriculoperitoneal
TLSO	thoracolumbar spinal orthosis	VVC	varus-valgus constrained
TMJ	temporomandibular joint	WCC	white cell count
TNF	tumour necrosis factor	ZPA	zone of polarizing activity

SECTION 1

The FRCS (Tr & Orth) examination

1. General guidance   3
Paul A. Banaszkiewicz and Simon Barker

General guidance

Paul A. Banaszkiewicz and Simon Barker

The FRCS Orth examination is generally considered to be fair although very searching and stressful. It is a major obstacle and hurdle to negotiate during higher specialist orthopaedic training. The syllabus is very broad and so the examiners can ask anything they really want to. About 6–12 months of hard work will be required beforehand if you wish to face the examiners with some degree of confidence over the green baize table.

The aims of the examination are to see if you have sufficient knowledge to become a consultant orthopaedic surgeon and be able to practise safely. Much of the examination can be passed with the knowledge and skills acquired during everyday training, unfortunately it does have to be backed up with a broad knowledge base. The written paper is now referred to as section I and the clinicals and orals as section II. The written paper is now a separate examination held several weeks before the clinicals and orals. The written paper format has been changed to multiple choice questions (MCQs) and extended matching item questions (EMIs) and has to be successfully passed before a candidate is allowed to sit the clinicals and orals. The MCQ/EMI paper is regarded as more difficult to pass than the old style written paper as it tests a much larger breadth and depth of orthopaedics.

It is important to polish up on examination technique before sitting the actual exam; it is an expensive way to practise if you fail it first time! Practise techniques of history taking and clinical examination in front of colleagues, for this can be a humbling experience better shared with friends before formal examinations. Providing you have had sufficient clinical experience, have read the books properly and practised your examination and oral techniques – just keep your head and think before you speak (making sure your answers conform to safe practice) – you should hopefully pass.

Do not compromise your examination performance by being a cheapskate and staying in low-priced accommodation to save money. Book into a decent hotel as you have already spent over £2,000 in exam fees so what is the point in worrying about a little extra money? Ask for a room in the quietest part of the hotel. You will spend a lot of time there, especially if you have a day off between the clinicals and the orals. Make sure you look after yourself. Be careful about staying up too late the night before as this can give you a cloudy head the following day – you want to think straight in the examination and be at peak performance. Although a small amount of work is needed every night, try to limit it to a couple of hours, eat well and try to get enough sleep. Be careful with both coffee and alcohol.

Some candidates talk about the "hype" generated by 100 or so 30-something candidates whose lives are on hold during the examination with everything hinging on the result of the next few days as being "something else". These comments are not particularly helpful as the examination is very important to most if not all candidates. Often the candidates who make these remarks are the worst offenders.

Postgraduate Orthopaedics: The Candidate's Guide to the FRCS (Tr & Orth) Examination, Ed. Paul A. Banaszkiewicz, Deiary F. Kader, Nicola Maffulli. Published by Cambridge University Press. © Cambridge University Press 2009.

Table 1.1 Suggested marking framework

	Possible marks for:	
Orals	Long case	Short cases
8 – Exceptional Pass	8 – Exceptional pass	8 – Exceptional Pass
7– Good pass	7 – Good pass	7 – Good pass
6– Pass	6 – Pass	6 – Pass
5 – Fail	5 – Fail	5 – Fail
4 – Complete fail	4 – Complete fail	4 – Complete fail
No of orals = 4		No of sections to short cases[2] = 2
No sections to each oral = 2	No of sections to long case[1] = 3	No of cases each section = 3
No examiners to each oral = 2	No examiners to each long case = 2	No of examiners each short case = 2
Bare pass 64	Bare pass 24	Bare pass 48
Maximum marks 128 (8×4×2×2)	Maximum marks 48 (8×3×2)	Maximum marks 96 (8 × 2 × 3 × 2)

[1] History, examination and discussion.
[2] Upper and lower limb sections.

Marking

The clinical short cases are divided into upper limb and lower limb sections with a minimum of three cases in each section. There are two separate pairs of examiners for the upper and lower limb cases. Each case is scored from 4 to 8 by each examiner to give a maximum total score of 24 from one examiner, 48 from one pair of examiners and a combined maximum total score of 96 from both pairs of examiners.

The long case is divided into three sections, which are history, examination and discussion. Each section is marked from 4 to 8 by each examiner to give a maximum total score of 24 from one examiner and a combined maximum score of 48 from both examiners. Orals are scored 4–8 with 6 a pass mark and 8 an exceptional pass and therefore extremely rare. Each oral is divided into two parts and each examiner marks each part separately. Therefore the maximum score for the four orals is 128 (8 × 4 × 2 × 2). Sections are "close" or "tightly marked" with most candidates obtaining a score around the pass mark unless exceptionally good or bad (Table 1.1). The aim should be for a steady consistent 6 all the way along. A score of 4 is

a complete fail but I am not aware of it being a veto against allowing a candidate to pass the exam; in theory one can still compensate for this poor mark elsewhere.

It is now possible to still pass the exam if you fail your long case or short cases or even both provided that your overall score is a pass and has been compensated for elsewhere. In reality this scenario is very unlikely to occur, as it would be extremely difficult to make up additional marks elsewhere in the orals. The old examination marking system was easier to understand. It was not possible to pass the exam if you failed the long case. A marginal fail in the short cases could be compensated for elsewhere in the examination but not a poor fail. A fail in one oral could be compensated for elsewhere but not two oral failures.

Most candidates find the short cases difficult and so try to obtain a basic pass in this one. Likewise the children's orthopaedics and hand surgery orals and applied basic science orals can be tricky so play it safe and attempt to obtain a basic pass in each rather than go for the gold medal.

Candidates will have up to three attempts to pass section II, after which candidates would be required to re-enter section I.

Table 1.2 Old versus new exam

OLD		NEW	
One written paper	Five short answer questions MCQ interpretation of a paper	Two written papers	SBA paper[1] EMI[2] paper
Orals	Adult/pathology Trauma Paediatric/Hands Basic science	Structured interviews (four 30-min orals)	Adult elective orthopaedics Trauma Children's orthopaedics and hand surgery Applied basic sciences related to orthopaedics
Orals	Long case Short cases	Clinicals with patients	Clinical long case (30 min) Clinical short cases (2×15 min)

[1] Note: the first 12 questions in this paper will relate to the published paper.

[2] Extended Matching Item questions (EMI) involve a list of possible answers from which the candidate must choose the most appropriate answer to a series of questions.

The new exam

The final sitting of the current exam format took place in November 2006. The new format exam from 2007 has de-coupled the written examination from the clinicals (Table 1.2).

Eligibility to sit the new examination will be determined by three structured references, one of which *must* be from your programme director.

Written papers will take place twice a year and must be passed before attempting the clinicals on a later date.

Although the *format* is changing the *standard* and *content* are **not**. The techniques and information you need to pass the examination are therefore virtually unaltered. The content of this book is equally applicable to old and new format examinations.

NOTE:

These details should be checked by candidates with the Intercollegiate Specialty Boards (ISB) website since details may be subject to change during/following publication: http://www.intercollegiate.org.uk.

The ISB issued the following guidance for SHORT CLINICAL CASES in May 2005:

The purpose of the Short Clinical Case Examination is for you to demonstrate that your observational and clinical examination skills, and your knowledge, are sufficiently well developed to make a relatively quick and accurate diagnosis for conditions that have typical clinical signs. For complex problems you may not necessarily come to a diagnosis but you should be able to list an appropriate differential diagnosis. The examination is rather like seeing a patient in the out-patient clinic and making a provisional diagnosis. Because of time limitations, the normal pleasantries of shaking hands on meeting the patient, taking a conventional history and carrying out a general examination of the patient are not expected of the candidate. Instead the examiner will give clear instructions about the part to be examined such as "Please examine this patient's right hand and tell me what you observe". There is no intention during this examination to trick the candidate and candidates are strongly encouraged to do exactly what is asked of them by the examiner. You should of course show respect for the patient and attempt to avoid inflicting unnecessary pain during the examination. The examiner will expect an answer like "I see a diffuse swelling over the dorsum of the hand and wrist which is soft on palpation and may be a synovitis of the extensor tendons". The examiner may then ask the probable diagnosis.

Radiographs may be available for a number of the cases and these may form part of the examination if they are clinically relevant. The Short Case Clinical Examination will involve two separate 15-min examinations with two separate pairs of examiners. Although it is possible for one patient to have more than one clinical problem you will generally meet at least three patients during each 15-min part of the examination.

Marking: The examiners will allocate two marks – one for each of the two 15-min sections of the examination.

The written paper

2. Written paper guidance   9

Paul A. Banaszkiewicz

Written paper guidance

Paul A. Banaszkiewicz

In 2006 the written paper underwent a significant change in format. Previously it was two hours long and consisted of 5 short answers or notes (60% marks) and 20 multiple choice questions (MCQs) based on the statistical analysis of a journal paper negatively marked (40% marks).

As of November 2006 the written test was composed of a combination of MCQs (single best answer, 1 from 5) and extended matching item (EMI) questions with no negative marking.

Candidates had to sit two papers. Paper 1 consisted of 120 single best answer (SBA) MCQs (2 hours) in the morning. Paper 2, sat in the afternoon, consisted of 120 EMIs and 15 MCQs relating to a published paper section (2 hours). Most candidates found that the time allowed was just about right for paper 1 but were rushed with paper 2 due to the additional time needed to read the published paper section.

The written paper continues to evolve and develop in direct response to feedback from candidates.

Paper 1 now consists of 120 MCQs (2 hours plus 15 minutes additional reading time for the published paper). The first 12 questions in the paper relate to the published paper. Paper 2 consists of 120 EMIs (2 hours).

Apparently the papers are reviewed after each sitting by the examiners and any ambiguous or inappropriate questions are removed and not scored.

Early feedback from the new trial (guinea pig[1]) candidates is that the new format is harder to pass

than the old written paper. By the time this book is in press the format may have changed again.

Each paper has been carefully prepared to cover the curriculum content so that there is a much wider testing of a candidate's knowledge base than was previously the case. More ground is covered so that passing the written paper now requires a much greater breath and depth of orthopaedic knowledge than before. The examiners set the pass mark for the paper, which is around the 60% mark.

The short notes section of the old exam did have its moments but most reasonably well prepared candidates could easily answer three questions from just basic reading. Everything in the orthopaedic syllabus is now covered with a particularly strong emphasis on anatomy.

Periodically the value of the statistical analysis paper is called into question. For better or worse it has been kept in place for the new written exam albeit with a reduced number of questions (12 instead of 20). The paper and journal chosen vary greatly from exam to exam. Reading last year's *Journal of Bone and Joint Surgery* in order to paper spot is a waste of time. If by some miracle you do spot the intended paper it is of questionable value as you will not be able to accurately predict the questions that will follow on from the paper. Be careful with educated guesses in the statistical analysis questions as they invariably have a habit of tempting you with the incorrect answer. There are a lot of double negative questions designed to catch you out.

Previously candidates sat the written paper on the Sunday morning continuing on with the clinical

---

[1] New candidate's quote; not mine!

Postgraduate Orthopaedics: The Candidate's Guide to the FRCS (Tr & Orth) Examination, Ed. Paul A. Banaszkiewicz, Deiary F. Kader, Nicola Maffulli. Published by Cambridge University Press. © Cambridge University Press 2009.

examinations the following day. For operational reasons there is now an interval of around 12–16 weeks between the written and clinical sections.

At present there are the beginnings of various MCQ books aimed specifically at the FRCS Orth arriving on the market to mixed reviews. The main concerns are that they do not reflect the type of question that will appear in the real exam and that the questions may be too easy and lull the candidate into a false sense of security. There have been concerns raised that some candidates may use these types of books as a major tool for learning the material for the examination. This will not get you through the examination as at best these types of books are really only useful for quick revision near the end of your preparations, a sort of confidence boost.

The other thing which may be useful is that the structure and question style are really quite different from the American Academy of Orthopaedic Surgeons (AAOS) MCQs and many feel it is not necessarily fruitful to spend time going through large numbers of questions from the AAOS.

Finally several regional training programmes are now running annual MCQ exams for trainees based on the FRCS Orth exam format. It is anticipated that this may be taken a step further and introduced nationally across the UK. This is being piloted at present by elogbook using the UK and Ireland in Training Examination (UKITE) for educational purposes. It is run on a voluntary basis but it will be interesting to see if this becomes compulsory for trainees to sit and part of the record of in-training assessment (RITA) and appraisal process.

The clinicals

3. **The short cases** 13
   Paul A. Banaszkiewicz

4. **Short case list** 15
   Paul A. Banaszkiewicz

5. **The long cases** 17
   Paul A. Banaszkiewicz

6. **Long case list** 19
   Paul A. Banaszkiewicz

7. **Hand and wrist clinical cases** 20
   Paul A. Banaszkiewicz and
   John W. K. Harrison

8. **Shoulder and elbow clinical cases** 51
   Paul A. Banaszkiewicz

9. **Spine clinical cases** 64
   Paul A. Banaszkiewicz

10. **Hip clinical cases** 71
    Paul A. Banaszkiewicz

11. **Knee clinical cases** 105
    Deiary F. Kader and Leo Pinczewski

12. **Foot and ankle clinical cases** 110
    Paul A. Banaszkiewicz

13. **Paediatric clinical cases** 126
    Paul A. Banaszkiewicz

The short cases

Paul A. Banaszkiewicz

Many candidates regard the short cases as the most difficult part of the FRCS Orth examination. The aim is for a safe comfortable pass. Often examiners say that there are very few surprises in the short cases as for sure a "Rheumatoid" or "Dupuytren's" hand is certain to be present in the examination hall. However, there are also rare or more complex cases and these can catch you out if you are not familiar with them.

A recent major change in the format of the short cases exam was to divide it into upper and lower limb sections. These last 15 minutes each but with the same pair of examiners. Previously there was a more random allocation of short cases although in fairness there was usually a balanced mix of both upper and lower limb cases.

When unsure of something we can all say stupid things to the examiners in the heat of the moment. Easy cases can be ruined and failed if things are going badly. Some candidates would claim that the key to the short cases is a good start with the opening first two cases. A poor start can easily deteriorate into a fail if you are unable to turn it around. Avoid the downward spiral. Try not to become demoralized, take a deep breath and attack the next case anew. Allowances are usually made for first-case nervousness but if this continues into the second or third case examiners will quickly lose patience and fail you.

The usual advice – "Be smart and look the part". This is so obvious that it does not warrant any further discussion. It is important to remember that you are trying to join a club and as such appearing like the other members is a good way to get started.

It is not traditional to wear a white coat for the examination. Wear a smart neutral coloured suit. For the men it is probably sensible to avoid loud or novelty ties although some candidates will wear them and pull off a comfortable pass. Have a clean handkerchief available to wipe away the sweat as it pours off your forehead down into your face at the most inopportune time.

Previously a big issue was sometimes made of trying to see as many cases as possible in order to score more marks. In practice candidates varied enormously in how many patients they saw. The average candidate saw about 7 cases but this varied from 3–4 to 12. Some cases were a spot diagnosis and took only a few seconds to complete whilst others took a lot longer. Some examiners preferred you to spend a while with each patient and examine them more thoroughly and so invariably you saw fewer patients. The change in short case format means that candidates have a much more even and uniform short case clinical examination than previously. Candidate feedback suggests it is now very uncommon to deviate from seeing any more than three patients in either the lower and upper limb sections. The following hints may seem a bit tired and cliché ridden but you may find some of them useful:

- A lack of polish and fluidity may make the examiners reflect on the clinical competence of a candidate
- Look the examiners in the eye
- Imagine that you are seeing cases in the clinic and presenting your findings to your boss

Postgraduate Orthopaedics: The Candidate's Guide to the FRCS (Tr & Orth) Examination, Ed. Paul A. Banaszkiewicz, Deiary F. Kader, Nicola Maffulli. Published by Cambridge University Press. © Cambridge University Press 2009.

- The most important part is to look professional as though you have done it a hundred times
- Go to wards to see as many short cases as possible in the 6 weeks before the exam
- Do not run around wildly trying to see as many cases as possible to score maximum marks if you cannot elicit the relevant clinical signs properly or are unsure of their significance
- The more you practise at short cases the better you will become
- The short cases are easy and you have seen them all before; there are no tricks, really there are none, we want to pass everybody!
- I am sure they assess you very quickly as to whether they would let you fix their grandmother's fractured hip or not
- Certain favourite topics always appear in the short cases. Make sure you know these extremely well
- Listen to the instructions
- Look fascinated if the examiners make a point
- Take note of the examiners' guiding comments; they are trying to help you
- Smile, be pleasant with patients
- Act like a doctor
- Always stick to the look, feel, move, neurovascular then special tests routine
- Do not fumble about examining the patient in silence; the examiners want to hear you say something even if it is only half sensible. Talk through your examination confidently
- Be friendly, courteous and polite to patients and professional, but moreover relax and be yourself during the examination
- The short cases are very artificial but you have to feel comfortable with your technique. If you feel embarrassed or lack confidence in your approach you will flounder
- Get down to eye level with children and try to make them feel at ease
- It is where you need your wits about you. The questions are straightforward but it is just an unnatural situation
- Always thank the patient afterwards just before you move on

- No amount of bookwork can prepare you for the short cases. As much experience as possible beforehand under examination conditions is the best preparation
- Although candidates should be fully prepared for an Apley approach this may not be what the examiners want, so be flexible
- I had two totally different examiners in terms of their approach and line of questioning, which made it very difficult for me to determine how well I had done
- Keep your head and think before you speak
- In my experience, the examiners seemed to vary in terms of their expectations from candidates for the short cases. Some examiners wanted the candidate to literally see patients for a spot diagnosis and then discuss the case whilst walking to the next patient, whereas other examiners wanted a more formal look, feel and move approach
- Make sure your answers conform to safe practice
- The right tone to strike is friendly, efficient and businesslike
- The short cases seem to fly by – remember the obvious things such as be nice to your patients and introduce yourself. If you don't know something, say so and do not waffle – the examiners don't like people who waste time on things they know nothing about
- You need to work out how quickly your examiner wants you to go but if you are not sure go through the look, feel and move plan
- At the end of your short cases try not to dwell too much on your own performance even if it has fallen short of expectations. Refocus and move on to the next part of the examination
- Do not assume you have failed and not turn up for the remaining part of the examination. There are legendary tales of candidates not bothering to turn up to the orals thinking they had failed the clinicals only to have subsequently found out they had comfortably passed the clinicals.

Short case list

Paul A. Banaszkiewicz

Not an exhaustive list but big enough to stir up uncomfortable feelings of hard work ahead. Try to imagine the typical scenario of each case, the likely positive clinical findings and possible questions the examiners will ask afterwards.

Shoulder

- Acromioclavicular joint (ACJ) dislocation
- ACJ pain
- Brachial plexus muscle power testing
- Clavicular non-union
- Erb's palsy
- Frozen shoulder
- Impingement tests
- Instability of the shoulder post trauma
- Instability testing – unidirectional and multi-directional
- Klippel–Feil syndrome
- Long head of biceps rupture
- Osteoarthritis of the shoulder
- Pseudoarthrosis of the clavicle
- Pseudoparalysis of the shoulder (septic arthritis) – destruction of the humeral head as an infant
- Rotator cuff pathology and testing of muscle strength
- Voluntary posterior dislocation of the shoulder

Elbow

- Bilateral congenital radial head dislocation
- Unilateral congenital dislocation of the radial head
- Congenital absence of forearm
- Cubitus valgus
- Cubitus varus
- Madelung's deformity plus multiple osteochondromas
- Osteoarthritis of the elbow post trauma
- Radioulnar synostosis
- Rheumatoid elbow
- Rheumatoid nodules
- Tennis elbow – demonstration of tests

Wrist and hand

- Any congenital abnormality – cleft hand, syndactyly, polydactyly, etc.
- Bilateral Dupuytren's
- Bilateral Dupuytren's plus peripheral neuropathy
- Carpometacarpal osteoarthritis
- Combined nerve lesions
- Deformed hands due to Ollier's disease
- Demonstration of Allen's test
- EPL rupture
- Ganglion right middle finger
- Kienböck's disease
- Madelung's disease
- Non-union of radius and ulna
- Quadriga effect
- Rheumatoid hand
- RSD post ulnar fracture
- Severe carpal tunnel syndrome
- SLAC and SNAC wrist
- Spaghetti wrists

Postgraduate Orthopaedics: The Candidate's Guide to the FRCS (Tr & Orth) Examination, Ed. Paul A. Banaszkiewicz, Deiary F. Kader, Nicola Maffulli. Published by Cambridge University Press. © Cambridge University Press 2009.

- Ulnar claw hand
- Wrist drop

Hip

- Osteoarthritis of the hip secondary to AVN post ORIF acetabular fracture
- Perthes with secondary osteoarthritic changes
- Untreated developmental dysplasia of the hip
- Osteoarthritis of the hip

Knee

- ACL plus posterolateral instability
- ACL rupture
- Blount's disease
- General examination including checking for effusion/synovial thickening
- Lateral meniscal cyst
- MCL/ACL laxity post knee dislocation
- Osteochondral defect of the knee
- Patellectomy
- Post surgery for HTO
- Post compartment syndrome release of the leg
- PVNS knee
- Semimembranosus bursa
- Testing for ACL and PCL injury

Ankle and foot

- Ankle arthrodesis
- Calcaneal fracture with compartment syndrome and clawed toes

- Drop foot
- Gout ankle
- Growth arrest after physeal injury
- Haglund's deformity
- Hallux rigidus
- Hallux valgus
- HMSN/bilateral foot drop
- Osteoarthritis ankle
- Pes cavus due to any cause: HMSN, spinal dysraphism
- Polio
- Rheumatoid foot
- Synostosis of tibia/fibula and degenerative ankle
- Tarsal coalition
- Tibialis posterior tendon rupture

Spine

- Neurofibromatosis and scoliosis

Paediatrics

- Cerebral palsy with foot and knee problems
- Curly toes
- Erb's palsy
- Foot abnormalities in arthrogryposis multiplex congenital (post fusion)
- Genu varum/valgus
- Osteogenesis imperfecta
- Overriding fifth toe
- Proximal femoral focal deficiency
- Surgically treated club feet

The long cases

Paul A. Banaszkiewicz

Old versus new

There has been a major change in the way the long case is now conducted. Up until 2006 candidates were allowed 30 minutes alone with a patient to take a history, perform a clinical examination and collect their thoughts together before the examiners would arrive. Candidates would then present the history and demonstrate appropriate positive clinical signs to the examiners before being led away for the discussion part of the long case. The long case history and examination are now conducted in front of the examiners.

This has provoked a mixed response from candidates. Most candidates believe it works in their favour, as examiners are more able to appreciate difficulties encountered in obtaining a history from a poor or difficult historian, which they would not otherwise have directly observed. Other candidates suggest it is one go only with the examination with no room for rechecking clinical signs.

Pass the long case

Failing the long case used to be absolute disaster; there was no coming back or rallying around and the whole examination was failed. For better or worse this has now changed so that you can fail the long case and still pass the exam. There seems to be more emphasis on dividing it into the three sections of history, examination and discussion than previously. One can score a 5 in one section and make it up in the other sections and pass the long case overall. One could marginally fail the long case overall and make the marks up elsewhere and still pass the examination. In theory one could have a bad fail in the long case and make up the marks elsewhere and therefore still pass the exam. This is probably unlikely as the aim is to pass with a steady consistent 6 all the way through, and to score above 6 to make up for deficiencies elsewhere is difficult.

Some candidates can seriously underestimate the long case. Paradoxically a few candidates may proceed to pass this effortlessly with what seems like minimal preparation.

The myths

Unfortunately failing the long case does happen to even well prepared and good candidates. This is a senior, exit, long-case clinical examination and must be treated with the respect it deserves. There is no room for complacency. Rehearse, prepare and practise for it long beforehand.

The long case

A good positive start to the history, with name, age, occupation (dominance) and presenting complaint, sets the tone for the rest of the examination. Make the history interesting for the examiners. Try to develop a rapport between yourself, the examiners

Postgraduate Orthopaedics: The Candidate's Guide to the FRCS (Tr & Orth) Examination, Ed. Paul A. Banaszkiewicz, Deiary F. Kader, Nicola Maffulli. Published by Cambridge University Press. © Cambridge University Press 2009.

and the patient. One may need to ask leading questions. Try not to get dragged into obtaining irrelevant detail; keep to sharp, focused and direct questions. History taking is an art, which must be practised to perfection.

It has been suggested that the examiners automatically expect you to obtain a decent history, that they are not really interested in it, are usually bored and are waiting to see how well you examine the patient to decide if they are going to pass you or not. This is a rather extreme view but there is probably an element of truth to it. Whilst obtaining a good history from a patient may count for little with the examiners, if it is poorly done with important details missed out this will immediately put a candidate on the back foot even if their factual knowledge is good. A lot of ground will then need to be made up and a candidate may never recover.

Likewise an over nervous manner by and large goes down poorly with the examiners. One-dimensional examiners, instead of trying to put a candidate at ease, will quickly lose patience. Most candidates are perceptive and will sense this, such that their performance nose-dives. Other examiners are more careful and measured in their approach but will still fail candidates who are too tense and edgy.

Candidates are usually led away to a room where the long case is discussed. Discussion usually begins with a review of radiographs and moves on to management of that particular patient. Thereafter you can be asked almost anything. Surgical approaches are well known to crop up. With a long case of osteo-arthritis of the hip or knee, almost everything on the subject can be covered. With a rheumatoid case half of the discussion may be spent concentrating on neck or medical problems.

Long case list

Paul A. Banaszkiewicz

General

- Ankylosing spondylitis
- Diaphyseal aclasia
- Juvenile chronic arthritis
- Ollier's disease
- Polyarticular rheumatoid arthritis

Lower limb

- Avascular necrosis of the hip
- Bilateral avascular necrosis of the hips post steroid treatment
- Bilateral developmental dysplasia of the hip with pain 10 years post shelf procedure
- Bilateral idiopathic avascular necrosis of the hip
- Bilateral osteoarthritis of the knees with varus deformities
- Coxa vara
- Mal-united femoral fracture
- Mal-united SUFE
- Old arthrodesis hip with contralateral symptoms
- Unilateral old developmental dysplasia of the hip
- Osteoarthritis of the hip
- Osteoarthritis of the hip post acetabular fracture
- Paget's disease with arthritis of the knee and hip
- Painful total hip arthroplasty: loosening, infection
- Painful total knee arthroplasty: check hip, spine and vessels
- Periprosthetic fracture after total hip arthroplasty
- Periprosthetic fracture after total knee arthroplasty

- Polyarticular osteoarthritis: bilateral total hip and total knee arthroplasty
- Rheumatoid: bilateral THA/shoulders
- Rheumatoid: bilateral THA/TKA/elbows, etc.
- Rheumatoid: bilateral TKA/hands
- Surgically treated club feet
- Tuberculosis hip

Spine

- Idiopathic scoliosis
- Spondylolisthesis
- Lumbar disc prolapse
- Cervical myopathy

Tumours

- Osteogenic sarcoma, right femur
- Ewing's sarcoma

Upper limb

- Brachial plexus injury
- Polyarticular rheumatoid arthritis: elbow, shoulder and hand

Paediatric

- Neurofibromatoses with pseudoarthrosis of the tibia

Postgraduate Orthopaedics: The Candidate's Guide to the FRCS (Tr & Orth) Examination, Ed. Paul A. Banaszkiewicz, Deiary F. Kader, Nicola Maffulli. Published by Cambridge University Press. © Cambridge University Press 2009.

Hand and wrist clinical cases

Paul A. Banaszkiewicz and John W. K. Harrison

Introduction

The FRCS (Orth) is essentially a clinical exam. The majority of candidates who fail do not do so because of a lack of knowledge. The clinicals are an artificial situation where you are required to demonstrate physical signs on a patient with generally a pain-free condition and not an acute one. The cases can be predicted with some certainty and a polished examination should be practised repeatedly, so that when you are nervous in the exam it will not be forgotten. Time is short and the examiners tend to be quite focused towards the signs they want demonstrated. Suggested equipment required includes a goniometer, key, paper clip and torch.

Common cases

The following upper limb cases are likely to appear (not in order of frequency):
- Rheumatoid hand
- Ulnar nerve lesion
- Dupuytren's
- Shoulder
  - Think AGE:
    - Young: instability
    - Middle age: calcific tendonitis, frozen shoulder, impingement
    - Older: rotator cuff tear/arthropathy, osteoarthritis
- Swelling (e.g. ganglion)
- Brachial plexus lesion
- Carpal tunnel
- Arthrogryposis
  - No skin creases (!), stiff joints, pectoralis major transfer/Steindler flexorplasty for elbow flexion
- Elbow
  - Radial head fracture, radioulnar synostosis, congenital radial head dislocation

Examination of the wrist

- Four articulations (DRUJ, radiocarpal, midcarpal, carpometacarpal)

Radial side wrist pain (RSWP)

- De Quervain's (Finklestein's)
- First carpometacarpal joint OA (grind test)
- Scaphoid non-union
- STT joint (pronate wrist against resistance)
- Intersection syndrome
- Wartenberg's neuritis (superficial branch of the radial nerve deep to brachioradialis)

Ulnar side wrist pain (USWP)

- DRUJ
- TFCC
- Ulnar impaction
- Lunotriquetral instability
- Pisotriquetral OA
- (Kienböck's can be either RSWP or USWP)

Postgraduate Orthopaedics: The Candidate's Guide to the FRCS (Tr & Orth) Examination, Ed. Paul A. Banaszkiewicz, Deiary F. Kader, Nicola Maffulli. Published by Cambridge University Press. © Cambridge University Press 2009.

Look

- Nails (clubbing, pitting)
- Swellings (ganglion, ulnar head, synovitis)
- Scars
  - Wrist – dorsal midline/transverse/arthroscopy/first dorsal extensor compartment
  - Hand – transverse MCP joints/thumb IP joints/CTD/Brunner's/midlateral to digits
- Deformity (distal radial fracture, base of thumb)
- Muscle wasting (FCU/hypothenar/interossei/thenar)

Feel

- Base of the thumb metacarpal/ASB/first extensor compartment/SLL (distal to Lister's tubercle)/lunate/ulna head/TFCC/DRUJ/pisiform/hook of hamate/median nerve

Move

- Wrist – flexion/extension (75°)/ulnar deviation (35°)/radial (20°)/pronation–supination (80°–75°) – holding pen

Special tests (SLL/LTL/DRUJ/TFCC)

- Midcarpal instability – pseudostability test – hold forearm and hand, feel AP laxity
- Scapholunate instability – ballottement
- Kirk Watson's test
  - Arm wrestling position (patient's elbow on table and flexed); examiner's thumb over scaphoid tubercle, index finger over SLL dorsally, examiner's other hand around metacarpals. Move patient's hand from ulnar to radial deviation. Exert pressure with the thumb to prevent scaphoid flexing as radially deviate. Positive test if click or pain. Compare to opposite (20% positive is normal)
- DRUJ – compress midshaft radius and ulna and rotate forearm (piano keys test)
- LTL (VISI) – Reagan's ballottement
- Pisotriquetral joint – press radial side of pisiform

- TFCC – ulna deviate wrist and compress and rotate hand

Examination of the hand

Grip (6) – power, simian, chuck, tripod, key (thumb to side index), fine (tip to tip)

Short cases – Dupuytren's, carpal tunnel syndrome, rheumatoid hand, mucous cyst, ganglion, trigger finger, tumour, tendon rupture, tenosynovitis, ulnar nerve

Tumours – giant cell tumour, glomus, PVNS, neurilemmoma, epidermoid inclusion, intramuscular lipoma, sarcoma, infection (tuberculosis, fungi)

Look

Forearm – cubitus valgus, rheumatoid nodules, FCU

Fingers – clawing, boutonnière, swan-neck mallet deformities, Wartenberg's disease

Nails – clubbing, pitting

Muscle wasting – hypothenar, thenar, interossei, FCU

Swellings – ganglia, Dupuytren's, rheumatoid nodules

Congenital – polydactyly, syndactyly

Feel

Ask where it is tender

Feel for swellings

Feel palm for nodules

Move

Mass movement (make fist)

Digits – MCP joint 90°, PIP joint 100°, DIP joint 70°, tip-to-palm distance

Thumb – opposition, flexion, abduction, adduction, retropulsion (palm on table)

EDC – extend MCP joints

Interossei – DAB PAD (mnemonic for Dorsal ABducts, Palmar ADducts)

Quadriga effect – FDP have common muscle belly; flexion of all digits is limited by the shortest FDP

Neurology

Sensation – median (index finger pulp = palm), ulnar (little finger), radial (dorsum first web space) and dermatomes (C7 – middle finger)
Motor – Median (APB)
      – Ulnar (Froment's test for adductor pollicis, first DI, interossei, ADM)
      – AIN: FDP, FPL, PQ (fine pinch)
PIN – nine muscles (radial deviation with wrist extension/weak extension MCP joints)

Pulses

(Allen's test = intact palmar arch, see page 26)

Special tests

Flexor tendons

FDP – test each individually, resisted DIPJ flexion with PIPJ held extended
FDS – isolate by holding other digits extended (to exclude FDP). Index finger has a separate FDP so keep DIPJ extended while testing FDS. FDS to little finger is absent in 10% of people
FPL – resist IPJ flexion of the thumb with the MCP joint held extended

Tenodesis test (for intact extrinsics)

Passive flexion wrist and MCP joints extend, extend wrist and MCP joints flex

Intrinsics (lumbricals and interossei)

Plus – MCP joints flexed, IP joints extended
Minus – MCP joints hyperextended, IP joints flexed
1. Bunnell–Littler test – extend MCP joint, if cannot flex IP joint = intrinsic tightness or tight capsule, so flex MCP joint; if still tight = contracture

2. Intrinsic versus extrinsic flexor tightness – flex wrist (this relaxes long flexors); if you can flex IP joints = tight intrinsics

Lumbrical plus finger

IP joints extend on attempted finger flexion due to laceration of FDP distal to the origin of the lumbrical

Bouvier's test (PIP joint capsule and extensor mechanism)

Prevention hyperextension MCP joints = extension of IP joints by EDC.

Central slip extensor tendon

Elson's test – flex PIP joint over the table edge; weak extension of the middle phalanx and hyperextension of the DIP joint = rupture of the central slip (DIP joint extends due to pull of lateral bands)
Boyes' test – hold PIP joint hyperextended, there is failure of DIP joint flexion if the central slip is retracted and adherent

Rheumatoid hand and wrist

This is almost a guaranteed case. These patients have pain and the exam is passed by description mainly, so know how to describe the deformities. Listen to the examiner – if they specifically say the hand, just examine the hand. Rheumatoid arthritis can also be a long case.

History

- Pain – site, severity, night pain
- Weakness
- Paraesthesia
- Neck symptoms – neck pain, radicular pain, myelopathy
- Previous surgery
- Function

- ADLs
  - Shop independently
  - Stairs
  - Dressing (buttons)
  - Washing (face, hair)
  - Eating
- Previous medical history (and DVT)
- Medications (and allergies)
- Social – smoking, alcohol, job, hobbies, partner, stairs
- Family history

Examination

"I would normally examine the neck and joints more proximal."

Look

Swelling over the dorsum of the wrist (tenosynovitis ±caput ulnae), carpus volar subluxed and supinated, metacarpals radially angulated, swellings over MCP joints, volar-ulnar subluxation of MCP joints, dropped fingers, swan-neck boutonnière deformities of the digits, Z-thumb, palmar erythema, muscle wasting

Feel

Tenosynovitis; feel the digits to gauge whether they are floppy (arthritis mutilans), and the subcutaneous border ulnar for nodules

Move

Mass movement – ask the patient to make a fist

Specific lesions

Dropped fingers (NB IP joint extension due to lumbricals)

Causes
- Vaughan–Jackson – ruptured EDM/EDC, tenodesis test

- Ulnar subluxed extensor tendons – test with MCP joints extended
- PIN palsy – tenodesis test, radial deviation (ECRL) on wrist extension
- Dislocated MCP joints – reduce and take radiographs
- Locked trigger finger

Mannerfelt lesion

Ruptured FPL due to tenosynovitis in carpal tunnel. Tenodesis test and rule out anterior interosseous nerve palsy (treatment: graft or fuse IP joint)

Inspection

The most important part of the examination. An initial general description of the hand is often a good opening line.

"This patient has features of a symmetrical polyarthropathy of the small joints of the hand probably rheumatoid arthritis. There are swellings over the dorsum of both wrists and the MCP joint. There is spindling of the fingers due to soft-tissue swelling at the PIP joints and MCP joints but the DIP joints are spared."

"On closer inspection I can see ulnar deviation of the fingers at the MCP joints, volar subluxation of the MCP joints, radial deviation of the wrists and prominent distal ulnar heads. There is a Z-deformity of the thumb, swan-neck deformity of the left little and ring fingers."

"There is drooping of the right little and ring fingers suggestive of possible long extensor tendon rupture.[1] I can see scars of previous surgery over the wrist,[2] thumb,[3] and fingers.[4] There are boutonnière deformities of the index and main fingers. There are firm subcutaneous nodules at the elbow, over the extensor tendons and in the palm. The flexor aspects of the fingers appear bulky due to chronic synovitis. There is wasting of the small muscles of the hand. There is thin bruised skin; pale nail beds and nail

---

[1] Dropped finger suggests tendon rupture but remember dropped fingers may also be a result of tendon subluxation, joint subluxation or dislocation, PIN palsy or flexor contracture produced by intrinsic tightness.
[2] Usually arthrodesis of the wrist for strength and stability.
[3] Usually arthrodesis of the MCP joint for strength and stability.
[4] Usually Swanson Silastic® joint replacements for movement and pain relief.

fold infarcts are present. There is no nail pitting or scaly rash seen.[5] On the palms I am looking for pallor in the palmar creases indicating anaemia[6] and palmar erythema."[7]

Examiner questions

- Can you explain the reasons for the ulna deviation, subluxation and boutonnière deformity?
- Why is the wrist like this?
- What are the important functions of the hand?
- What is a boutonnière deformity?
- What is a rheumatoid nodule?

Feel

Feel each joint gently and quickly. Care is required when palpating the hand, as several conditions can be fairly painful. Remember the rule "Do not hurt the patient".

"Are your hands painful?"

"I would now like to palpate the hands feeling for any areas of tenderness or boggy swellings.[8] There is evidence of bony destruction of the PIP and MCP joints with sparing of the DIP joints. I cannot feel any rheumatoid nodules or Heberden's nodules in the hand. None of the joints is tender or warm at present."

Feel for triggering and tenosynovitis in both flexor and extensor tendons.

Move

Mass screening test – "*Can you make a fist and now straighten your fingers and thumb?*"[9] Is a full range

of movement present? Is any deformity fixed or correctable? Note any extensor lag-tendon rupture or subluxation. Compare both sides.

Try to reduce the MCP joints (passive correctability of deformed joints). Correct the ulnar deviation and extend the fingers ("*Can you keep your fingers straight?*") – feel the extensor tendons contract. No sensory loss does not exclude PIN palsy. Extend the MCP joint of the affected finger: improvement in the deformity indicates shortening of EDC; if deformity becomes worse this indicates tight interossei. Hold all fingers in the extended position, leaving the affected finger free. Ask the patient to flex the finger – if they cannot, the most likely cause is a ruptured FDS. Assess the movement of the PIP joint – a stiff immobile joint will detract from the results of MCP joint replacement. Perform the Bunnell–Littler test for intrinsic tightness in both the deformed and corrected positions.[10]

Sensation

Quick test for sensory deficit in the median (thumb–index finger pulp), ulnar (ulnar border of the little finger) and radial nerve territory (dorsum first web space). It is usually better to assess nerves by sensation rather than power since the hand may be too weak to assess motor function accurately.

Other possible features

- **Carpal tunnel syndrome**
  - Caused by flexor synovitis. Check for thenar muscle wasting and test the power of APB
- **Triggering of digits**
  - Secondary to tenosynovitis
- **Palmar erythema**
  - Non-specific change indicative of a hyperdynamic circulation

---

[5] Psoriatic arthropathy is an asymmetrical arthropathy involving mainly the DIP joints with pitting of the finger nails and hyperkeratosis. There is a red, scaly rash over extensor surfaces.

[6] There are five main causes of anaemia in rheumatoid arthritis: anaemia of chronic disease, GI bleed, bone marrow suppression, associated with pernicious anaemia, Felty's syndrome.

[7] Redness around the palm sparing the central area is associated with rheumatoid arthritis, pregnancy, liver disease.

[8] Talk to the examiners – tell them what you are doing as you go along. Do not let the examiners assume/think that because you are not saying anything you know nothing. It is useful to communicate your findings to the examiners at each stage.

[9] Try not to get bogged down in describing one abnormality in the hand; work through problems systematically and be

guided by the examiner as to what they specifically want you to concentrate on, particularly with special tests.

[10] Use simple, clear language when asking patients to perform various movements during any hand examination. It is often simpler if, in addition, you demonstrate each movement yourself. Most of all it is very important not to dry up in the actual exam and forget this language interaction (patter) such that the patient is not able to understand what you want from them.

- **Arterial pulses**
  - And do Allen's test
- **PIN palsy**
  - Can occur at the elbow in patients with rheumatoid disease. The patient will present with the inability to extend the fingers and thumb although the wrist can be extended, albeit into radial deviation. The differential diagnosis is rupture of the extensor tendons at the wrist. The two conditions can be differentiated by observing the tenodesis effect upon either active or passive flexion of the wrist. If the extensor tendons are intact the fingers will passively extend upon wrist flexion. If the extensor tendons are ruptured the fingers will not extend

"This patient has severe rheumatoid disease affecting both hands. I would like to now assess function of the hands and review radiographs of the hand. To complete my examination I would like to examine the cervical spine and look for extra-articular manifestations of rheumatoid arthritis."

Examination corner

Short case 1

Florid rheumatoid hands, elderly female

Over 5 min spent discussing clinical features, assessment, management, etc.

Short case 2

Rheumatoid hand

General discussion on the classic deformities seen

Short case 3

After rapid progression through the first two warm-up cases the candidate was asked to examine a lady's hand. Clinical features were of rheumatoid hands. The examiners did not want a description, only the spot diagnosis. The examiner then asked the candidate: "Why is she wearing a cervical collar?"

The candidate, who had noticed it but not mentioned it, said it could be due to atlanto-axial subluxation

---

Short case 4

Rheumatoid hand – mild deformities

Describe and examine

Short case 5

Rheumatoid hand – severe deformities

Describe and examine

Short case 6

Extensor tenosynovitis in the rheumatoid hand

- Diagnosis
- Differential diagnosis
- Complications
- Tendon rupture and caput ulnae
- Principles of tendon reconstruction in a rheumatoid hand

Short case 7

Rheumatoid hand after a Swanson MCP joint replacement operation

"How would you perform the operation?"

Short case 8

Young rheumatoid female. Right wrist fused. Left wrist replaced – discuss

Performing bilateral wrist arthrodeses in patients with inflammatory arthritis is controversial. Patients with bilateral wrist fusions are believed to have less dexterity and greater functional compromise than those with one wrist fused and arthroplasty of the other. There is disagreement as to which wrist should be fused. Arthrodesis of the non-dominant hand and arthroplasty of the dominant hand is generally recommended

Dupuytren's disease (DD)

An absolute A-list topic for the short cases and hand oral. Pattern recognition is important – a Dupuytren's hand can easily be summarized in a few lines.

Differential diagnosis of Dupuytren's

- Locked trigger finger
- Camptodactyly
- Skin contractures (secondary to burns or scarring)
- Tendon contracture (thickened cord moves on passive flexion of the finger)

History

- Age, hand dominance
- Age of onset of the disease
- Rate of progression of the disease
- Functional deficit: difficulty putting hand in pocket, washing face, wearing gloves, etc.
- Foot or penile involvement
- Family history
- Previous medical history: diabetes, epilepsy, alcohol, smoking, trauma
- Occupation, hobbies
- Previous hand surgery

Inspection

Look

Ask patient to straighten out fingers, palms up.

"The hand is held with a flexed posture to the little and ring fingers at the MCP and PIP joints. There are skin pits (Dupuytren's inserting vertically into the skin) and nodules present in the palm."

Feel

"There is a cord to the little and ring fingers causing a contracture at the MCP/PIP joint. There are no obvious scars suggestive of previous surgery present in either the palm or

fingers. There are no Garrod's pads present (dorsum proximal interphalangeal joints)."[11]

Ask the patient to flex their fingers fully.

Measure

As the cords cross more than one joint, flex the PIP joint fully to measure an MCP joint contracture (place a goniometer on the back of the digit), then flex the MCP joint fully to measure a PIP joint contracture.

Sensation

It is very important to test for sensation distal to any proposed site of surgery especially if there are scars from previous surgery present (1.5% risk of digital nerve injury). Assess the circulation with digital Allen's test. (Press either side of the fingertip and milk the blood out proximally to the base. Release pressure on one side and observe if the finger perfuses. Repeat for other digital artery.)

Examiner: What else would you like to examine?
Candidate: The soles of the feet,[12] the dorsal knuckle pads.[11] DD is also associated with Peyronie's disease.[13]
Examiner: How would you decide on management?
Candidate: I would perform a Hueston's tabletop test. More precisely I would offer surgery for an MCP joint contracture >30°, or for any significant PIP joint contracture, in practice again 30°.
Examiner: Consent me for a partial fasciectomy.
Candidate: The aim is to excise diseased tissue and restore movement through a zigzag incision. It is performed under general anaesthetic. You will wake up with your hand in a bulky dressing and go home on the same day. Therapist will see you at 48 hours and remove the dressing and commence splinting. Your sutures are taken out at 10 days, then you have wound management to soften the skin and splinting at night for 6 months. Surgery is

---

[11] The knuckle pads (Garrod's pads) can often be thickened.
[12] Can affect the plantar aponeurosis.
[13] Fibrosis of the corpus cavernosum causing curvature of the penis. The examiners are unlikely to expect you to confirm this association!

not curative; recurrence in 50%. Complications include: wound infection, haematoma, digital nerve injury (1.5%), stiff hand, RSD and amputation.

Examiner: Why may a PIP joint contracture not correct fully?

Candidate: The question relates to the position of safety for splinting the hand (wrist extended 20°, MCP joints flexed 90°, IP joints extended fully). Flexion contracture of the PIP joint leads to shortening of the volar plate. An extensive release (check-rein ligaments, sheath, accessory collaterals, ±volar plate) may be needed for a marked contracture (>70°) and this is controversial as it can lead to further scarring, even limiting flexion. In the MCP joint a 90° flexion contracture does not shorten the collaterals and the joint will always straighten after excision of the Dupuytren's.

Examiner: What is the incidence of nerve injury at recurrent surgery?

Examination corner

Short case 1

Elderly man, bilateral DD

Spot diagnosis

Asked to examine hands and comment on typical features of DD. A few minutes general discussion about DD

What are the various cords and what are the bands that contribute to each? ("Band" is normal, "cord" is diseased)

Various finger incisions

Role of open palm technique

Diathesis

Recurrence rate

Short case 2

Elderly gentleman, DD right hand

Examiner: Would you examine this gentleman's hands please.

Candidate: On inspection there is a flexed attitude of the little and ring fingers of the right hand. Looking at the palm there appear to be cord-like structures beneath the skin extending into the little and ring fingers. There are no obvious surgical scars present. Can you turn your hands around for me sir?

On inspecting the dorsal surface of the hand there are thickenings of skin over the PIP joint knuckles suggestive

of Garrod's pads. This gentleman has DD and I would like to access the degree of flexor contracture of the little and ring fingers.

I took out a goniometer and made a show of measuring angles. He has a 30° flexor contracture of his little finger MCP joint and 20° PIP joint. In the ring finger there is a 20° MCP joint contracture and the PIP joint is minimally affected. There also appears to be a cord running between the thumb and index finger, which I hadn't noticed.

Examiner: What do you call that cord?

Candidate: Commissural cord. Can you put your hand down flat on the table please sir? The patient is unable to put his hand down flat on the table, the so-called tabletop test of Hueston, indicating that we may need to consider surgery in this gentleman's case. Can you feel me touching the side of your finger, does that feel normal?

The candidate continued to test digital nerves of each finger whilst the examiners in background were heard to mutter, "Yes good".

Candidate: There is normal sensation present in each digit.

Examiner: What are the various bands in the hand?

Candidate: The normal bands in the hand are the longitudinal peritendinous bands, spiral bands, natatory ligaments, Cleland's ligaments, Grayson's ligaments and the lateral digital sheath.

Examiner: And what are the diseased cords?

Candidate: Central cord, spiral cord, lateral cord, retrovascular cord and abductor digiti minimi cord.

Examiner: Yes the abductor digiti minimi cord; a lot of people forget about this cord and as you can see this gentleman has an abductor digiti minimi cord that should be excised at surgery or else you will not get full correction of the digit. How are you going to manage this gentleman?

Candidate: I would perform a partial fasciectomy using a Brunner's zigzag incision.

Examiner: This patient is listed for surgery next week. What would you be concerned about from an anaesthetic point of view?

Candidate: There is a higher incidence of ischaemic heart disease, chronic pulmonary tuberculosis, chronic lung disease, diabetes and excessive alcohol intake in patients with DD.

Examiner: How would you obtain informed consent of the patient?

Candidate: I would mention surgery is not curative; there may be a recurrence. We are unlikely to get full correction of the finger and there is a small possibility of loss of sensation of the digit due to digital nerve contusion or division. There is also the possibility that the blood supply to the finger can be compromised due to stretching, spasm or division and very occasionally the finger may have to be amputated if the circulation does not recover. The wound can look very alarming postoperatively but this is normal. The hand can become stiff and take several weeks to recover. There is the possibility of a wound haematoma and infection developing in the hand. I would also mention that the hand would need to be splinted at night for several months afterwards in order to lessen the chance of the deformity reoccurring.

The candidate was stopped at this stage, the examiners were bored and wanted to move on to the next case.

Short case 3

Elderly man bilateral DD

Asked to examine hands. Inspection only and then discussion about aetiological factors (bell went).

Short case 4

Bilateral DD contracture

Examination

Management

Short case 5

Young male with bilateral DD

Describe the condition

What questions would you ask in the history in order to evaluate in this particular patient for aetiology, prognosis and management?

Logic of treatment

Indication for surgery

Short case 6

A gentleman with bilateral DD

One side had been operated on and he was pleased with the outcome from surgery. The other side had a 50° flexion deformity of the MCP joint of the little and ring fingers with no PIP joint contracture. I gave a spot diagnosis and had

a quick look at the rest of the hand for Garrod's pads and checked the sensation of the digits.

The examiner asked me to explain the options for management and I said I would go for a partial fasciotomy; I was then asked what other procedures could be performed. I explained that I could perform a percutaneous fasciotomy, which is normally the first of a two-stage procedure or, in the elderly, a definite single procedure.

Further questions included where to make the incision for a percutaneous fasciotomy, risk factors and criteria for surgery. My impression was that it was a fairly straightforward case with no hidden traps or tricks to catch you out. The examiner scoring me did not seem to really take much interest and I thought at this stage he had decided whether I had passed or failed.

Short case 7

DD palm

- Spiral cord components
- Surgical importance of the band
- Management options including open palm technique
- How long does it take for the wound to heal in the open palm technique?
- What is Dupuytren's diathesis?

Short case 8

A patient with DD

- Spot diagnosis
- Questions on conditions associated with DD
- Operative management options

Short case 9

Discussed bands, cords, management, surgical approaches

Short case 10

Examiner: Look at this hand and tell me what you find.

Candidate: DD of all the fingers except thumb with 90° contraction of the PIP of the little and ring fingers.

Examiner: Talk to the patient about his condition and treatment you are going to do.
   What are the complications of surgery?

Short case 11

Young male with recurrent Dupuytren's contracture of the left hand

- Examine this man's hands
- Management
- How will you consent him?
- What is Dupuytrens' diathesis?

Short case 12

Elderly man with bilateral DD

Candidate: On examination there is DD of both hands with a severe fixed flexion deformity at the PIP joints of the little and ring fingers.
Examiner: What do you think?
Candidate:
   • No Garrod's pads
   • Positive family history
   • No ectopic disease
   • Neglected DD or diathesis
Examiner: What treatment would you offer this patient?
Candidate: My preferred option would be a partial palmar fasciectomy. A useful procedure in this particular case would be application of an external fixator (joint jack) and then palmar fasciectomy at a later date. Amputation of the involved digits should certainly be considered although this may be a bit drastic and wouldn't be my first option.

Ulnar nerve lesion

Memorandum 1

"On inspection there is a well-healed longitudinal surgical scar over the volar ulna aspect of the wrist. There is abduction of the little finger[14] and hypothenar muscle

[14] Due to denervation of ADM.

wasting.[15] The attitude of the hand is suggestive of ulna claw hand with flexion of the ring and little finger PIP joints. The distal IP joints are also flexed suggesting the FDP is intact.[16] There is also hyperextension of the MCP joints of the little and ring fingers. There was no obvious skin ulceration,[17] brittleness of the nails[18] or tropic changes. The nerve was tender when palpated just lateral to the FCU tendon at the wrist, however Tinel's test at the wrist for ulnar nerve irritation was negative. There is decreased sensation at the ulnar border of the little finger but normal sensation on the dorsum of the hand."[19]

   "*Can you stretch both arms out please?*"

   "On inspection there is no obvious deformity such as cubitus valgus or varus suggestive of an old elbow fracture.[20] There are no obvious scars around the elbow, forearm and wrist."

Memorandum 2

"Would you roll up your sleeves and place your hands palm down on your lap/this table please?"

   "On inspecting the dorsal surface of the hand there is marked interosseous muscle wasting, particularly of the first dorsal interosseous muscle with hollowing of the skin on the dorsal aspect of the first web space. There is marked muscle wasting on the medial side of the forearm and a cubitus valgus deformity at the elbow. There are no obvious scars on the medial side of the elbow suggesting previous ulnar nerve decompression or other scars of note."

Palpation of the nerve

"I would now like to go on and palpate the nerve at the elbow."

   "*Can you straighten and bend your elbow please?*"

Flex and extend the elbow looking and feeling for abnormal mobility of the nerve behind the medial

[15] Due to denervation of the hypothenar muscles.
[16] Ulnar paradox: clawing of the hand is more obvious in low ulnar nerve lesions because the FDP is intact and less obvious in high lesions.
[17] Due to unnoticed trauma on the desensitized medial skin of the dorsum and palm and the medial (ulnar) 1½ digits.
[18] Due to denervation.
[19] Indicates that the lesion is distal to the wrist joint and the dorsal branch of the ulnar nerve is spared.
[20] Cubitus varus deformity occurs most often with supracondylar fractures whilst cubitus valgus deformity is more suggestive of an old mal-united lateral condyle fracture.

epicondyle.[21] Roll the nerve under your fingers above the medial epicondyle and follow it until it disappears under the FCU.

"Is it tender? Do you feel any numbness or tingling in your hand when I feel the nerve?"

"There was obvious tenderness and thickening of the nerve when palpated behind the medial epicondyle of the elbow. Tinel's test at the elbow was negative as was the ulnar nerve hyper-flexion test at the elbow."

Sensation

"I would now like to test for sensation."

"*Can you feel me touch you here* (little finger pulp), *here* (index finger) *and here* (ulnar and radial sides of the ring finger)? *Does it feel the same as here on the other hand?*"

Motor function

"I would now like to move on to test for motor power."

Practise the patter and a get a rhythm for the exam.

Palmar interossei

Card test

"Hold your hand out. Palm down, fingers together please. I'm just going to slide this card between your fingers (middle and index). Keep your fingers straight. Can you grip the card between your fingers and stop me pulling it out? Now between your middle and ring fingers and finally ring finger and little finger."

In the case of weak palmar interossei it is easy to pull the card out.

Dorsal interossei

"Can you spread your fingers and please stop me pushing them together?"

---

[21] The nerve is palpable in the groove behind the medial epicondyle. If it snaps over the medial epicondyle when the joint is flexed and extended it may indicate a traumatic ulnar neuritis caused by a deficiency in the tissues that normally anchor it. This would be one definite indication for anterior transposition of the nerve if decompressive surgery was required.

First dorsal interosseous muscle

Press your thumb into the patient's first web space with the patient resisting index finger abduction abduction. Feel for the muscle bulk and contracture. Or

"Can you push your index finger against my finger?"

"I'm testing abduction of the index finger, which relies on the first dorsal interosseous."

Abductor digiti minimi

"Now push your little finger out against my finger."

Or

"Can you push your little fingers together?" (More sensitive test.)

FDP little finger[22]

Nerve abnormality at Guyon's canal or at the elbow (low or high nerve lesion).

Froment's test (book test)

"Finally I would like to perform Froment's test for adductor pollicis."

"*Could you grab hold of this sheet of paper with your thumb on top of it holding it against the side of your index finger? Now stop me pulling the paper away."*

Look for flexion of the IP joint of the thumb. This indicates that FPL (supplied by median nerve) is compensating for a weakened adductor pollicis. This becomes more pronounced if the examiner tries to pull out the sheet while the patient tries to hold it.

Flexor carpi ulnaris

Resistance is felt in the tendon when attempting to extend the wrist (with the wrist flexed and ulna deviated).

"The patient demonstrates signs of ulnar nerve palsy. It appears to be caused by … because …"

---

[22] Differentiates a high from a low nerve lesion.

Differential diagnosis

- Cervical radiculopathy
- Thoracic outlet syndrome
- Cervical rib
- Cervical spondylosis
- Pancoast's tumour
- Benediction hand versus claw hand[23]

Sites of compression neuropathy

Arcade of Struthers – formed by superficial muscle fibres of the medial head of triceps attaching to the medial epicondylar ridge by a thickened condensation of fascia

Olecranon (epicondylar) groove – the nerve lies within the epicondylar groove on the dorsal aspect of the medial epicondyle with the canal completed by a fibrous aponeurotic arch

Cubital tunnel – formed by fascia from the medial epicondyle to the olecranon (thickened Osborne's ligament)

Fascia of FCU – fascial bands connecting the two heads of FCU

Deep flexor-pronator aponeurosis – exit of the ulnar nerve from FCU

Causes of ulnar nerve palsy (proximal–distal)

Brachial plexus

- Trauma

At the elbow

- Bony abnormalities: osteophytes, bony spurs, cubitus valgus
- Scarring

[23] In a claw hand due to a high ulnar nerve palsy, the little and ring fingers are clawed-flexed at the IP joints and hyperextended at the MCP joints. The Benediction hand (sign) is the extended index finger (like that of a Benedictine monk giving a blessing) caused in high lesions of the median nerve. This is due to paralysis of FDP, which normally holds the index finger partially flexed at rest. I have also come across a claw hand due to a high ulnar nerve palsy called a Benediction hand but I do not think this is correct.

- Anomalous muscles (anconeus epitrochlearis muscle)
- Tumours
- Ganglia
- Trauma: old fractures (medial epicondyle nonunion), lacerations

At the wrist

- Lacerations
- Ganglia

Ulnar tunnel syndrome

Ulnar nerve compression in Guyon's canal.

Signs distal ulnar nerve lesion (low lesion)

- Sensation of the ulna side of the dorsum of the hand intact
- FCU intact
- No muscle wasting of forearm
- Ulna half of FDP intact (ulnar paradox), clawing
- Wartenberg's sign (loss P3), wasting hypothenar eminence-guttering-dorsal interosseous, scar cubital or Guyon's canal
- Tender over Guyon's canal
- Decreased sensation in ulnar 1½ digits (sensation of the dorsum of the hand preserved)

Functional loss low ulnar nerve lesion

Loss of stable pinch between thumb and index finger with hyperextension deformities at the MCP joints and compensatory flexion deformity of the IP joints causing finger clawing.

Tendon transfers low ulnar nerve

1. For weak pinch between the thumb and index finger (thumb adduction and index finger abduction)
   - Split insertion of middle finger FDS to adductor pollicis
   - EIP to first DI muscle

2. For loss of the interossei and ulnar two lumbricals (clawing hand)
   - Zancolli capsulodesis to stabilize the MCP joint, in which the superficialis tendon is looped volar to the A1 pulley and sutured through itself to produce 20° flexion MCP joints
   - Or split tendon transfers of FDS ±EIP to the radial dorsal extensor apparatus. Carried out to restore MCP joint flexion and interphalangeal joint extension

---

Examination corner

Short case 1

Ulnar claw hand, low lesion with pathology at Guyon's canal, no sensory change

Examiner: Would you care to examine this man's right hand and tell me what you see?

Candidate: There were various well-healed traumatic and surgical scars over the dorsal surface of the wrist. The volar ulnar border of the wrist had a recent longitudinal surgical scar over Guyon's canal. Gross interosseous muscle wasting and gross clawing of the hand were evident. I examined for sensory deficit, however none was present.

Examiner: What difference would you expect to find in sensation between a high and low ulnar nerve lesion?

Candidate: There would be decreased sensation at the ulnar border little finger but normal sensation on the dorsum hand if the lesion is low as the dorsal branch of the ulnar nerve is spared.

Examiner: What is ulnar paradox?

Candidate: Less clawing hand with more proximal nerve lesions. A more proximal lesion will paralyse FDP little and ring fingers reducing the amount of clawing of the hand.

Examiner: Would you care to examine the motor function of the ulnar nerve?

Candidate: Examination included Froment's test (positive), first dorsal interosseous muscle, ADM, etc. FDP little finger working. I therefore explained that it was a low ulnar nerve lesion affecting motor function but not sensory function.

Examiner: I will buy that, let us move on to another case.

[Pass]

Short case 2

Isolated ulnar nerve palsy with no scars present over limb

What is the commonest cause of an ulnar nerve palsy?
Common sites of nerve compression
Clinical tests
Management (conservative and surgical)

Short case 3

Examiner: Examine these hands.

Candidate: Mild clawing hand; intrinsic muscle wasting; FDP weakness little finger; ulnar nerve compression at the elbow.

Short case 4

Ulnar claw hand

Examiner:
   Describe the appearance
   Examine the nerves
   What is the differential diagnosis and why?
   Level and why
   What is a Martin–Gruber anastomosis?

Candidate: The Martin–Gruber anastomosis occurs when motor fibres normally carried entirely by the ulnar nerve enter the ulnar nerve from the median nerve via branches in the forearm. Disruption of the ulnar nerve above the level of anastomosis may not necessarily result in motor loss of ulnar-innervated muscles.

Brachial plexus lesion

Roots 5 (between scalenus anterior/medius), trunks, divisions 6 (behind clavicle), cords 3 (behind pectoralis minor, around axillary artery)

Radial nerve palsy

Radial nerve palsy, a classic short case.

Pre-	Horner's syndrome/all 5 roots involved/bruising root neck/paraesthesia above clavicle C4/loss of rhomboids and serratus anterior/Tinel's/fracture transverse process/raised hemidiaphragm
	Sensation – C7 middle finger
	Muscle power – trapezius, rhomboids, serratus anterior, deltoid, SS/IS, biceps, triceps
	If pre-ganglionic, dorsal root ganglion cell intact so SNAP intact
	EMGs show fibrillations and positive sharp waves at 2 weeks
Beware	Nerve grafts – accessory, intercostals, contralateral LPn
	Muscle grafts – latissimus dorsi to biceps, brachioradialis to triceps (C6)
Peripheral nerve injuries (Seddon)	Neurapraxia	Physiological, demyelination
	Axonotmesis	Endoneural tubes in continuity, Wallerian degeneration
	Neurotmesis	Epineurium divided, surgery
	Sunderland	grade I–V (III – scarring endoneurium, IV – complete scarring)
Myotome	Muscle mass supplied by a spinal nerve
Dermatome	Skin area supplied by a spinal nerve
Erb's palsy	Long-standing traction palsy to upper trunk C5/6
	Arm IR (suprascapular nerve)/elbow extended/forearm pronated/wrist – digits flexed
Klumpke's palsy	Claw hand, decreased sensation medial arm (C8, T1)
Claw hand	Combined median/ulnar nerve palsy, RA, Volkmann's contracture

Memorandum

"Would you roll up your sleeves and stretch your arms out in front of you please?"

"On inspection there is an obvious left wrist drop.[24] There is gross wasting of the left forearm muscles.[25] There does not appear to be any gross wasting of the triceps muscle.[26] There are no obvious scars or swellings visible. I would now like to test the motor function of the radial nerve."

Extensors of the wrist

Place patient's wrist in extension.

"Don't let me pull it down."

"I am testing the extensor muscles of the wrist. He has weakness of wrist extension MRC grade 4 minus."

Extensors of the fingers

"Can you bend your elbow into your side and give me your hand facing down (palm down)? I will support your wrist.

Can you try and straighten your fingers please? Straighten them. Don't let me push them down."

"He is able to extend his IP joints due to the action of his interossei and lumbrical muscles. He is however unable to straighten his MCP joints."

Test EPL

"Please place your palm flat on the table. Can you lift up your thumb?"

Tests retropulsion.

Test supinator

Elbow must be extended (nerve compression against middle third of humerus).[27]

"Now straighten your elbow. Can you turn your hand over (against me)? Don't let me stop you."

"I am testing the supinator muscle. There is a definite weakness of the supinator muscle."

---

[24] Due to loss of extensor muscles.
[25] Due to loss of extensors, the muscle bulk of which is in the forearm.
[26] In high lesions.

[27] Straighten the elbow to exclude the action of biceps, which also supinates the forearm. Loss of supinator suggests a lesion proximal to the supinator tunnel.

Test brachioradialis

Flex the elbow in the midprone position (nerve compressed against middle third of humerus).

"*Can you bend your elbow?*"

   "I am now testing brachioradialis muscle. There is a definite weakness of the brachioradialis muscle."

Test triceps[28]

Extend the shoulder.

"*Can you straighten your elbow?*" (Gravity excluded)

Then test resistance. Test triceps reflex.

"He has normal triceps power and no loss of his triceps reflex. Weakness of the supinator and brachioradialis muscle suggests a lesion above the supinator tunnel. Weakness of the triceps suggests a lesion at or above the midhumerus."

Sensation

"I would now like to test sensation."[29]

   "*Can you feel me touch you here? Here? Here? Does it feel the same as here on the other hand?*"[30]

   "There is sensory loss over the first dorsal interosseous muscle (anatomical snuff box).[31] This patient has features suggestive of low/high radial nerve palsy. There is evidence that this may have been caused by ..."

Radial nerve versus PIN palsy

Radial nerve
- Inability to extend elbow, supinate forearm, wrist drop

[28] Triceps weakness suggests a lesion at the midhumeral level. Loss of all triceps activity suggests a high (plexus) lesion.
[29] Use a pin, otherwise touch lightly with your fingers. Do not stroke over a large area and do not poke too hard.
[30] This is a bit obvious but it is amazing how in the stress of the exam one can forget things.
[31] Although the cutaneous supply of the radial nerve is more extensive than that of the first dorsal interosseous an overlap in supply of both the median and ulnar nerves means that only this small area will have impaired sensation. Loss of sensation along the back of the forearm suggests a higher lesion. When testing motor function be able to discuss the difference between power versus strength.

- Diminished sensation over first dorsal interosseous muscle (just over the anatomical snuff box)
PIN
- Nerve supply to ECRL and brachioradialis intact
- Able to supinate and extend wrist (with radial deviation)
- Unable to extend MCP joints
- No sensory loss

Causes of a radial nerve palsy

Axilla

- Saturday night palsy: neurapraxia from prolonged local pressure
- Ill-fitting crutches

Midhumerus

- Fracture of the shaft of the humerus
- Tourniquet palsies
- Lacerations, gun shot wounds

At and below the elbow

- Entrapment syndromes (FREAS; a mnemonic for **F**ibrous tissue bands, **R**adial **R**ecurrent vessels, fibrous **E**dge of ECRB, **A**rcade of Frohse, **S**upinator)
- Rheumatoid elbow
- Dislocated elbow
- Monteggia fracture
- Surgical resection of the head of the radius
- Mass lesions (ganglions)

Tendon transfer (Jones transfer)

- Wrist extension: pronator teres to ECRB
- MCP joint extension: FCR or FCU to EDC (through interosseous membrane)
- Extension and abduction thumb: palmaris longus to EPL

Supinator tunnel

The fibres of the supinator muscle are arranged in two planes, between which the deep branch of the radial nerve lies (PIN). The supinator arises from the lateral epicondyle of the humerus, the elbow joint and superior radial ulnar joint and the supinator crest and fossa of the ulna. It inserts into the posterior, lateral and anterior aspects of the neck and shaft of the radius as far as the oblique line.

Examination corner

Short case 1

- Humeral shaft fracture in a brace with associated radial nerve palsy
- Demonstration of clinical signs
- When do you operate on humeral fractures?
- What method?
- What approach?
- What size of plate do you use?

Short case 2

Radial nerve palsy

Candidate: A nerve lesion will often produce a specific resting position. If you prefer to be cautious describe the pattern of deformity and give a provisional diagnosis. If you are the gambling type straight out with the spot diagnosis and hope you are correct. The examiner in any case is likely to ask you to confirm your suspicions.

Carpal tunnel syndrome

Practise being put under pressure and getting harassed. Get some mock examiners to put you under stress. Nervousness gets no credit. The examiner is more likely to think that in the stress of an operation not going smoothly you would not rise to the challenge.

History

- Age
- Occupation
- Hand dominance
- Hobbies
- Numbness
- Pins and needles
- Clumsiness
- Morning stiffness
- General questioning to exclude any aetiology
- Lives alone

Examination

- Routine hand examination with particular attention to:
  - Sensory deficit
  - Muscle wasting
  - Motor deficit
  - Median nerve sudomotor deficit
  - Ulnar nerve signs
- Provocative tests: Tinel's sign, Phalen's sign, median nerve compression test

Memorandum

Check that the patient is adequately exposed before starting your examination. Make sure their shirt is rolled above their elbows.

"In normal clinical practice I would start by examining the cervical spine, shoulders and elbows but for the moment I will just concentrate on the hands."[32]

"This (middle-aged) lady complains of pain, numbness and paraesthesia in the palm and fingers. This is particularly severe at night and causes her to get up and shake her hands to relieve symptoms. There is thenar muscle wasting and sensory loss over her radial three and a half digits.

---

[32] In any examination of the hand at some stage you have to come out with this statement or something comparable. It is somewhat artificial especially when said at the beginning of a hand examination. It may produce either the retort, "Just do as you've been told and examine the hands only" or a loud moan and the reply, "Just concentrate on the hands".

I usually left this declaration until after inspection and palpation and would mention that "I would now like to go on and test for movements of the hand and wrist but before I do so I would like to perform some quick screening tests for movement of the cervical spine, shoulders and elbows". In general the examiner would say that it was not necessary and to just continue examining the wrist and hand.

There is definite weakness of abductor pollicis brevis compared to the opposite side."

"Can you pull your thumb into your palm and now push your thumb up to the ceiling?"

Resist this movement with a finger of one hand whilst simultaneously feeling for the contraction of abductor pollicis brevis with the fingers of the other hand.[33]

"There is also weakness of opposition of the thumb. The presence of the long flexor and variability of the nerve supply makes testing for flexor pollicis brevis of doubtful value."

"Tinel's sign is positive for median nerve irritation and likewise Phalen's sign is also positive at 20 seconds."

Look and be seen to be looking at your watch and test for at least a minute before saying it is negative.

"The median nerve compression test was positive.[34] The flexor muscles of the forearm are not involved suggesting a distal median nerve lesion."

Or

"The symptoms the patient describes are suggestive of carpal tunnel syndrome. There is normal sensation in the palm particularly over the thenar eminence. Tinel's and Phalen's tests were positive for median nerve compression but the nerve itself showed no motor deficit."

Signs

- Wasting thenar eminence (LOAF: mnemonic for **L**ateral two **L**umbricals, **O**pponens pollicis, **A**bductor pollicis brevis, **F**lexor pollicis brevis)
- Decreased sweating and increased temperature at the thenar eminence
- Decreased sensation in the radial 3½ digits (palmar branch proximal to tunnel)
- Power APB
- Carpal compression (Durkin's test) – most sensitive

---

[33] Don't forget to do this. Some examiners will pick you up on this if you omit it.

[34] Regarded as the most accurate test for median nerve irritation. Elbow extended, forearm supinated, wrist flexed to 60°, digital pressure applied with one thumb over the carpal tunnel. Test positive if paraesthesia or numbness within 30 seconds (again time it using your watch).

Test	Sensitivity (%)	Specificity (%)
Tinel's	74	91
Phalen's	61	83

Causes

Can be congenital or acquired. Majority of cases are idiopathic.

Congenital

- Persistent median artery (thrombosis of such an artery can cause an acute onset of carpal tunnel syndrome)
- High origin of lumbrical muscles

Acquired

- Inflammatory: synovitis, rheumatoid arthritis, gout
- Traumatic: Colles' fracture
- Fluid retention: pregnancy, renal failure, myxoedema, diabetes, congestive cardiac failure, steroids
- Space-occupying lesion: lipoma, ganglion

Differential diagnosis

- Cervical radiculopathy
- Collagen vascular disorders
- Thoracic outlet syndrome
- Reynolds disease
- RSD
- Spinal cord lesions – tumour, syrinx
- Peripheral neuropathy: alcohol, diabetes

Examination corner

Short case 1

A 60-year-old lady

I was directed to her left hand, which had marked APB muscle wasting, and was told she had had some tingling/

pain in her index/middle fingers. I said I would like to commence the examination proximally from the neck but was told to concentrate on the hand. Comparing both hands I commented on unilateral thenar eminence wasting with no DI wasting.

The examiners asked what I thought the diagnosis could be. I answered carpal tunnel syndrome and was asked what I would want to examine – I mentioned sensation, motor power and provocation tests.

I was then asked to examine motor power: APB was very weak but (ulnar) intrinsic power normal, which I commented on.

I then tested FDP to index, which appeared to be a little weaker than in the opposite hand. Challenged I said that non-dominance plus relative disuse may make it weaker although the possibility of proximal median nerve compression should be considered.

I was then asked to demonstrate the carpal tunnel syndrome provocation tests, which were all strongly positive.

Whilst walking to the next patient I was asked about management. I mentioned that conservative measures were unlikely to help given the marked wasting suggesting chronicity – therefore carpal tunnel decompression would be indicated. Asked what I would advise her about the outcome, I mentioned that there was a good likelihood of early night-pain relief but numbness could take up to 1 year to settle and the wasting would be permanent.

Short case 2

Bilateral carpal tunnel syndrome

History/exam

Short case 3

A 35-year-old lady with carpal tunnel syndrome

Short history
Examination starting with the neck
Provocative tests
Tests for proximal sites of compression of median nerve

Median nerve

Make sure that during the examination of the patient you let the examiner see that you are doing the correct things – as one does in a driving test (which in many ways is similar to the short case examination).

Memorandum 1

"On inspection of the left hand there is obvious thenar muscle wasting. The thumb appears to be lying in the plane of the palm – a simian thumb (ape-thumb deformity).[35] There is atrophy of the pulp of the index and main fingers,[36] dystrophic nail changes present, generalized nicotine-stained fingers and possibly a cigarette burn over the radial border of the distal phalanx of the index finger.[37] There is no obvious ulceration seen in the hand or fingers and no visible scars are present."

"The thumb cannot be apposed to the fingertips to produce useful function.[38] Testing for APB revealed MRC power grade 4 minus compared to the opposite normal side with reduced muscle bulk and tone present. However, testing for FPL revealed normal power."

Memorandum 2 (higher lesion)

"In addition, there is wasting of the lateral aspect of the left forearm.[39] The index finger is held in a position of extension – Benediction attitude.[40] On asking the patient to

---

[35] Due to wasting of the thenar eminence. Simian means "like a monkey". In this deformity the thumb lies in the same plane as the hand/wrist instead of at right angles to it. It occurs due to paralysis of the opponens pollicis muscle.

[36] Due to denervation of the lateral 3½ digits.

[37] Due to denervation.

[38] This tests opponens pollicis muscle. The function of this muscle is to appose the tip of the thumb to the other fingers. Apposition is a swing movement of the thumb across the palm and not a simple adduction. Adduction occurs with adductor pollicis (ulnar nerve).

[39] In high lesions (differentiates between high and low lesions).

[40] The Benediction sign is the extended index finger (like that of a Benedictine monk giving a blessing) caused in high lesions of the median nerve. This is due to paralysis of FDP, which normally holds the index finger partially flexed at rest.

make a fist the index finger remains pointed – finger pointing sign."[41]

"*I would now like to test for sensation. Can you feel me
touch you here? Here? Does it feel the same as here on the
other hand?*"

"There is sensory loss over the palmar aspects of the lateral 3½ digits and thenar eminence."[42]

"I would now like to test for power."

"*Lay your hand on the table, palm up please.*"

Abductor pollicis brevis

"*I am going to hold your wrist so you don't move your hand.
Now lift your thumb up off the table to touch my finger.
Push against it.*"[43]

"There is weakness of APB."[44]

Flexor pollicis longus

"*Now can I hold your thumb and ask you just to wiggle the
tip of it?*"[45]

Proximal phalanx is kept steady by the examiner.

"There is weakness of FPL."

Flexor digitorum superficialis

"There is also loss of flexion at the index and middle fingers."

---

[41] This is due to paralysis of the FDS and of the lateral half
of FDP (to the index finger) in a high (proximal to the elbow)
median nerve lesion. The available medial half of the FDP
(supplied by the ulnar nerve) makes flexion of the other
fingers possible.

[42] Sensory loss over the thenar eminence differentiates
between high and low nerve lesions.

[43] This tests for APB that is invariably and exclusively supplied
by the median nerve. The action of this muscle is to draw the
thumb forwards at right angles to the palm. If you only do one
test for the median nerve this is it. As the patient resists, it is
very important to feel for the muscle in the thenar eminence
and let the examiner know that this is what you are doing.
Compare muscle bulk with the opposite side.

[44] I think the "Pen Test" for APB is a better way to demonstrate
motor power. A pen is held above the thumb and the patient is
asked to touch the pen with the tip of their thumb.

[45] This tests for FPL, which is affected in lesions proximal to
the wrist or in injuries to the anterior interosseous branch.
Immobilize the proximal phalanx of the thumb and ask the
patient to flex the DIP joint.

Pronator teres[46]

"*I am going to hold your hand like a handshake. Now can
you twist against my hand while I feel your forearm?*"

Hold the patient's hand and resist as they try to pronate the forearm.

Low nerve lesion

- Loss of APB and variable loss of FPB (and opponens pollicis)
- Weakness of thumb abduction and opposition

High nerve lesion

Low lesion plus:
- Loss of flexion IP joint thumb (FPL)
- Loss of flexion index and middle fingers (FDS,
  FDP)
- FCR

Tendon transfers for low lesion

For thumb opposition (loss of APB)

- Ring finger FDS transfer to APB or EIP to APB
- MCP ±IP joint fusion

Tendon transfer for high lesion

For index and middle finger flexion

- FDP index and middle fingers sutured side-to-side
  (tenodesed) to the neighbouring intact FDP of the
  ring and little fingers (FDS cannot be used, as it is
  supplied by the median nerve)

For flexion IP joint thumb

Brachioradialis to FPL

---

[46] The patient extends the elbow, hand supine. Feel for a
contraction medially and just distal to the elbow. Testing
with the elbow fully extended puts the pronator quadratus
at a disadvantage and thus is a way of relatively isolating the
pronator teres.

For thumb opposition

- EIP to APB

Causes of a median nerve palsy

At the elbow

- Fractures
- Elbow dislocations

Distal to the elbow

- Pronator entrapment syndromes

In the forearm

- Lacerations
- Gun shot wounds
- Forearm bone fractures

Wrist

- Especially lacerations
- Colles' fractures
- Carpal tunnel syndrome

Pronator teres syndrome

Entrapment of the median nerve around the elbow.

History

- Ache or discomfort of the forearm after heavy use
- Weakness or clumsiness of the hand
- Paraesthesia in all or part of the median nerve

Examination

- Local tenderness to deep compression with reproduction of symptoms
- Tinel's sign is negative at the wrist but may be positive at the proximal anterior aspect of the forearm

- Negative Phalen's
- Weakness of thenar muscles but sparing of AIN-innervated muscles

Provocation tests

- Resist elbow flexion with forearm supinated (bicipital aponeurosis)
- Resist forearm pronation with elbow extended (two heads of pronator teres)
- Isolate long finger PIP joint flexion (FDS origin)

Sites of compression (four sites)

- Supracondylar process humerus (ligament of Struthers)
- Bicipital aponeurosis
- Between heads of pronator teres
- Proximal arch of FDS

EPL rupture

Classic short case: either a rheumatoid patient or a patient post Colles' fracture while a traumatic laceration is unlikely.

Memorandum

"On inspection we have a middle-aged woman with a generalized soft-tissue swelling over the right wrist joint. There is also a deformed appearance of the wrist suggestive of a recent fracture. The attitude of the right thumb is one of flexion at the IP joint. Active dorsiflexion of the wrist is reduced to 30° compared to almost 80° on the opposite normal side. Similarly palmar flexion of the wrist was to 50° compared to 70° on the opposite side. Pronation and supination are essentially normal. There was no active extension of the right thumb suggestive of EPL rupture. I was not able to feel any contracture of the EPL tendon. There was some mild swelling and tenderness around the dorsal radial surface of the wrist in the line of the EPL tendon and a suggestion of a gap present along this tendon."

Management

EIP to EPL tendon transfer. Requires a general anaesthetic and the patient will need a thumb outrigger splint for 4 weeks postoperatively.

Three incisions

- Transverse over metacarpal head index finger (EIP ulnar to EDC)
- Transverse incision just proximal to extensor retinaculum
- Oblique incision at the base of the thumb to identify EPL distal to rupture

---

Short case 1

Examiner: What tendon is used to replace the function of EPL?
Candidate: EIP.
Examiner: Where do you find EIP in the wrist?
Candidate: It is ulnar to the EDC.
Examiner: How many incisions do you do in this tendon transfer?
Candidate: Three.
Examiner: Show me where exactly on my hand you would place these incisions and what you are trying to achieve with each.
Candidate: At this stage the oral deteriorated rapidly as I got mixed up with the reason for the various skin incisions.

[Fail]

Hand oral 1

- What tendon rupture can you get after distal radius fracture?
- How would you manage it?
- Which tendon would you transfer?
- Show me the incisions.

Quadriga effect

This is short case material. Active flexion deficit in uninjured fingers. Normal passive range of movement. Due to failure of full excursion of the tethered tendon.

Memorandum

Scar over a finger extending into palm. Reduced active flexion of all the unaffected (uninjured) digits when affected digit is flexed and demonstration of normal flexion of unaffected digits when tested in isolation. Reduced excursion of all the profundus tendons and impairment of finger flexion. Involves an active flexion lag in the fingers adjacent to a digit with an injured, adhered or improperly repaired FDP tendon. It is due to the tethering of the normal FDP tendons by the injured or repaired FDP tendon because they all share a common muscle belly. As the injured tendon reaches its maximum flexion, the FDP tendons in adjacent digits have no further proximal excursion as all forces of the common muscle belly are being expended on the injured and tethered digit.

Management

Corrected by releasing the profundus tendon to allow proximal retraction.

Claw hand (intrinsic minus)

This is the intrinsic minus hand – hyperextension at the MCP joints and flexion at the IP joints. In ulnar claw hand these changes are seen in the ulnar two digits, as the radial two lumbricals are intact.

Differential diagnosis

- Brachial plexus injury – especially of the lower roots (Klumpke's paralysis)
- Peripheral nerve injury – ulnar nerve palsy, combined ulnar and median nerve palsy
- Spinal cord – polio, syringomyelia, amyotrophic lateral sclerosis
- Volkmann's ischaemic contracture

Memorandum

Weakness, paralysis or tightness of the intrinsic muscles results in overaction of the long flexors and long extensors conjointly. This results in MCP joint extension or hyperextension and partial flexion of the IP joints of the fingers and thumb.

The deformity is due to paralysis of the interossei and lumbricals, which cause flexion at the MCP joints and extension at the IP joints. The flexors of the finger are unaffected. The extensor digitorum is concerned mainly with extension at the MCP joint and has little action in extension of the IP joints. The extensor digitori act unopposed by the interossei at the MCP joint and the flexors of the fingers act unopposed by the action of the interossei at the IP joints. This causes the deformity.

Finger abduction and adduction are impossible. If all the intrinsics are affected, the thumb lies flat at the side of the hand and cannot be opposed. There is a loss of the ability to perform prehensile grasp and diminished grip and pinch strength.

Benediction hand versus claw hand

In the claw hand the little and ring fingers are claw shaped with hyperextension at the MCP joints. The Benediction hand (sign) is an extended index finger (like that of a Benedictine monk giving a blessing) caused by high lesions of the median nerve. This is due to paralysis of FDP, which normally holds the index finger partially flexed at rest.

Examination corner

Short case 1

Claw hand (main-en-griffe)

Describe

Short case 2

Wasting of the small muscles of the hand

On examination there is bilateral and marked wasting of the small muscles of the hand. There is wasting and weakness of the thenar and hypothenar eminences and of the other small muscles such that dorsal guttering is seen.

There is a claw deformity of the hand with hyperextension at MCP joints and flexion at the IP joints.

There is no evidence of a sensory impairment.

No fasciculations are seen.

Diagnosis

- Motor neurone disease
- Intrinsic minus hand
- No sensory signs
- Wasted fibrillating tongue
- Spastic paraparesis

Volkmann's ischaemic contracture

Background

This is ischaemic contracture of the muscles of the flexor compartment of the forearm. The affected muscles fibrose and are replaced by scar tissue, which contracts and draws the wrist and fingers into flexion. If the peripheral nerves are also affected there will be sensory loss and motor paralysis in the forearm and hand.

This condition is usually the end result of untreated compartment syndrome of the forearm or may follow arterial injury (brachial artery) secondary to a supracondylar fracture.

The muscles supplied by the anterior interosseous artery are most susceptible to ischaemic damage because this is an end artery. The most commonly affected muscles are FPL and FDP (ulnar half). Nerves injured by ischaemia sometimes partially recover and so numbness can be an inconsistent finding.

The condition classically produces an intrinsic positive hand (due to loss of function of the long tendons) but in some textbooks it is described as producing an intrinsic minus hand. This may be because of the secondary effects of peripheral nerve injury causing intrinsic paralysis. The intrinsic positive hand itself does not typically produce a claw hand deformity but invariably Volkmann's ischaemic contracture is described as producing a claw-hand type of deformity.

Memorandum

"On inspection there is clawing of the left thumb and fingers. There is marked wasting/atrophy of the muscles of the left forearm and hand. There is marked atrophy of the forearm with a flexion deformity of the wrist and fingers. The skin over the forearm and hand is dry and scaly and the nails show trophic changes. There is a claw hand secondary to ulnar/median nerve palsy or Volkmann's ischaemic contracture. The deformity is reduced (or abolished) by flexing the wrist. Volkmann's sign is positive; the patient is able to fully extend his or her fingers at the IP joints only if the wrist is flexed.[47] There is generalized hypoaesthesia of the hand. The thumb is adducted across the palm. Bunnell's test for intrinsic tightness is positive."[48]

Classification according to severity (Tsuge's classification)

Mild

- Flexor contractures of two or three fingers (usually middle and ring fingers)
- No sensory disturbance
- Common flexor origin release

Moderate

- FDP, FPL ±superficial flexors, ±wrist flexors
- Flexor contractures of all the fingers and thumb develop
- Wrist adopts a flexed position
- Claw hand
- Sensory disturbance of the median and ulnar nerves
- Radical release of flexor muscles including FPL and tendon transfers (brachioradialis and ECRL, attaching them to distal FDP stumps and FPL stumps)

---

[47] This is because when the wrist is extended, the shortened flexor muscle–tendon unit is stretched over the front of the wrist resulting in flexion of the fingers (constant length phenomenon).
[48] The intrinsic hand muscles fibrose and shorten, pulling the fingers into flexion at the MCP joints but the IP joints remain straight.

Severe

- Marked contracture of both the flexor and extensor compartments. Free muscle neurovascular transplantation

---

Examination corner

Trauma oral 1

Clinical photograph of Volkmann's ischaemic contracture forearm

Spot diagnosis
- Describe the photograph
- Causes
- Management

Short notes

How to decompress a forearm with compartment syndrome

Osteoarthritis of the base of the thumb

Definitely a short case FRCS Orth spot diagnosis – inspection and examination along with discussion of the management of the condition.

Memorandum

"Mrs Smith is a 56-year-old, right-handed retired schoolteacher. Her presenting complaint is of pain present at the base of her right thumb. This is a dull constant pain aggravated by activities such as turning a door key, holding a teacup or sewing (forceful pinch grip). This pain has been present for a number of years but has become much more severe in the last 6 months. She has now started dropping objects and is aware of a prominence at the base of the thumb. The pain is present every day and keeps her awake most nights. She takes regular painkillers and nonsteroidal anti-inflammatory medication. She is otherwise fit and healthy."

Functional assessment: knitting, undoing screw top jars, writing, using tin openers and turning latch door keys. A history of a Bennett's fracture subluxation or Rolando-type fracture should be sought.

"On inspection there are features of a mild generalized arthritis in the right hand with Heberden's nodes present at the bases of the distal phalanges. There is a shoulder sign present, which is a radial prominence at the base of the thumb from dorsal subluxation of the metacarpal on the trapezium. There is a web-space contracture of the right thumb with metacarpal adduction reducing the thumb index web angle. There is also a secondary flexion deformity at the IP joint. On palpation tenderness and swelling are felt, localized to the base of the right thumb. There is a positive grind test, which reproduces the normal pain she experiences, along with crepitus. The crank test was also positive, reproducing pain and crepitus and a palpable subluxation of the metacarpal. There was no evidence of co-existent carpal tunnel syndrome (43%), trigger finger or de Quervain's syndrome."

Special radiographs of the first carpometacarpal joint such as a Robert's view may be requested to confirm the diagnosis.

Differential diagnosis

- De Quervain's disease
- Non-union scaphoid fracture
- FCR tendonitis
- Scaphotrapezoidal osteoarthritis
- Referred pain from carpal tunnel

Classification: Eaton and Littler (Stages 1–4)

Based on the degree of degeneration and subluxation of the joint.

Management

Conservative

- Always non-operative management initially: splinting, physiotherapy to strengthen thenar muscles, steroid injections into joint possibly under an image intensifier, NSAIDs, etc.

Surgery

Stages 1 and 2 (early)
- Symptoms mainly due to instability

- Ligament reconstruction or extension abduction osteotomy

Stages 3 and 4 (late)
- Excision arthroplasty alone (trapeziectomy)
- Excision and ligament reconstruction – Burton and Pellegrini (ligament reconstruction tendon interposition (LRTI))
- Excision and soft-tissue interposition
- Silastic® interposition arthroplasty
- Osteotomy
- Arthrodesis

"There are several surgical options available and the choice should take into account the patient's age, degree of joint degeneration, level of activity. My own preference would be ... because ..."

Examination corner

Short case 1

Osteoarthritis CMC joint both thumbs

- Examine the hands
- Discuss management

Short case 2

Generalized OA hands

- Describe the condition
- DIP joints, CMC joints
- Demonstration of wrist movements
- Management
- Classification of OA of the CMC joint and treatment of the condition
- Management of this specific patient

Short case 3

Bilateral osteoarthritic hands

- Heberden's nodes
- CMC joint OA– management

Osteoarthritis of the hands

Memorandum

History

- Finger stiffness and pain
- Clumsiness and weakness

Examination

"There are Heberden's nodes present at the bases of the distal phalanges and Bouchard's nodes at the PIP joints. There is a square hand deformity due to subluxation of the base of the first metacarpal. The IP joints are tender to palpation with small, hard, bony swelling at the joint margin suggestive of osteophytes. The IP joints are painful when rocked from side to side. There is a reduced range of flexion of the ring, main and index fingers with a pulp to palm deficit of 2 cm."

"Individual movements for the ring/main fingers are: MCP joint 0°–90° (0°–90°); PIP joint 0°–80° (0°–110°); and DIP joint 0°–50° (0°–80°). Interphalangeal extension was preserved. Crepitus was felt during movement of the involved fingers. No mucous cysts are seen on the dorsal surface of the DIP joint or nail ridges."

Management

Conservative

Rest, analgesia, physiotherapy, etc.

Surgery

- IP joint arthrodesis
- PIP joint arthroplasty

DIP joint arthrodesis

Standard treatment for osteoarthritis. Best cosmetic result achieved in extension whilst functionally slight flexion is better. Some surgeons recommend fusing all the joints in 25° of flexion. Others recommend that the index joint is fused in 15° flexion and the angle of fusion is increased in a stepwise fashion for the middle (20°), ring (25°) and little fingers (30°).[49]

---

[49] Aside from the exam, in practice how accurate can you be with this?! I would be happy if I got the joint to fuse in a half decent position without any pain.

PIP joint arthrodesis

Some surgeons fuse all joints in 40° of flexion. Others recommend 30° flexion for the index finger, increasing to 45° flexion for the little finger.

Methods include tension band wire (Carroll method), lag screw, Herbert screw. Arthrodesis is usually stabilized by a K-wire.

PIP joint arthroplasty

PIP joint arthrodesis can cause significant disability. A Silastic® implant is reported to preserve a 50° arc of movement. This should be used with caution in young patients who place heavy demands on their hands, for whom fusion may be a better option.

Examination corner

Short case 1

Osteoarthritic hands

- Describe the appearance
- Typical DIP joint and CMC joint deformities
- Demonstration of wrist movements
- Classification of CMC osteoarthritis and treatment options
- Management of this particular patient

Kienböck's disease

The clinical examination is based on the traditional format of long cases and short cases but the emphasis is on the candidate's ability to make a competent assessment of the patient and mature judgement of how the patient should be managed.

Memorandum

"There may be few clinical signs. On inspection of the dorsal surface of the wrists and hands there appears to be a suggestion of some localized swelling centred over the dorsum of the radiolunate joint. On palpation there is tenderness over the lunate dorsally. Examination of wrist movements revealed restricted palmar flexion and particularly dorsiflexion when compared to the opposite, normal side. Radial and ulnar deviation was reduced but to a lesser extent. Supination and pronation were however unrestricted."

If OA develops findings tend to become more generalized. Swelling and tenderness are located to the mid dorsal area. Wrist movements are restricted but forearm rotation is unaffected. Grip strength is diminished. Passive dorsiflexion of the middle finger produces pain. Pain may also be exacerbated by percussion on the middle finger metacarpal head down the longitudinal axis.

SLAC wrist

Occasionally a SLAC wrist pitches up in the short cases. It is a fair bet that you would be asked to demonstrate and explain Kirk Watson's test. It is a progressive arthritis of the wrist due to chronic scapholunate ligament disruption, which leads to a disruption of normal wrist biomechanics.

Memorandum

History

- Pain
- Swelling
- Clicking
- Snapping
- Stiffness
- Hand weakness
- Interference with ADL

Examination

"On initial inspection of the hands the most obvious feature is a diffusely swollen left wrist, which is particularly marked dorsally. The wrist is deformed on the lateral aspect. The skin overlying this swelling appears normal, there is no skin discoloration and no scars are present. Palpation reveals bony swellings suggestive of osteophytes over the dorsal radiocarpal joint and radial styloid."

"All movements at the wrist joint are restricted and painful at their extremes. In particular, dorsiflexion is markedly reduced, being only 40° compared to 80° on the opposite side." (Get the goniometer out – it looks much more professional than guesstimating!)

Loud audible crepitus is heard on movements of the wrist. The Kirk Watson's test is positive. Thumb pressure over the scaphoid tubercle whilst the wrist was moved from ulnar deviation to radial deviation caused both pain and an audible click.

Radiographs

The proximal part of the scaphoid and distal radius becomes osteoarthritic. However, the radiolunate joint is well preserved.

Carpal height ratio

Carpal height ratio equals the carpal height divided by the length of the third metacarpal, and is usually between 0.46 and 0.6.

SNAC

With non-union of the scaphoid, the proximal pole behaves like a lunate. Osteoarthritis develops between the radial styloid process and the distal fragment of the scaphoid.

Management of a SLAC wrist

This is based on the time since injury, the amount of carpal instability and the presence of secondary changes in the carpus:
- Scaphoid excision and four-corner fusion (lunate–capitate/triqueteral–hamate) (transverse dorsal incision) or wrist fusion
- Other options include[50]:
  - Proximal row carpectomy (provided no luno-capitate arthritis exists)

[50] I personally would not mention these in the exam unless pressed – keep things simple and uncontroversial.

- Radial styloidectomy (makes the radioscaphoid joint more congruent)
- Wrist denervation (division of the anterior and posterior interosseous nerves at the wrist)

Management of a SLAC wrist would usually be with either a scaphoid excision and four-corner fusion or more definitively a wrist fusion. Other more controversial options would include …

Gout

Spot diagnosis or examine these hands.

Memorandum

"There is asymmetrical swelling affecting the small joints of the hands with tophi formation in the periarticular tissue. The joints are deformed. There are tophi on the helix of the ear and the olecranon bursa and Achilles tendon. There are no areas of skin ulceration or areas of necrotic skin overlying the tophi with exuding chalky material."

Examination corner

Short case 1

Gouty tophi of left big toe

Candidates were asked to describe what they saw and to give a differential diagnosis.

Examiner: It was amazing how many candidates got the diagnosis wrong. One candidate tried to be clever but we caught him out. He had obviously been talking to other candidates who had gone in before him and they had mentioned gout as one of the short cases. When he was asked to examine the big toe he mentioned straight away that the diagnosis was gout without even looking at the feet. We asked him a few questions and soon sorted him out and ended up failing him.

Madelung's deformity

Be ready for the onslaught.

Background

Abnormal growth of the distal radial epiphysis with premature fusion of the ulnar half of the distal radial epiphysis. The idiopathic variety is thought to be a congenital disorder but is seldom obvious until late childhood or adolescence. Incidence is greater in females than in males; frequently bilateral and can be a positive family history. It is a rare deformity that usually worsens with growth. It may present with median nerve irritation and may cause wrist pain although this is not a prominent feature.

Memorandum

"A spot diagnosis in a short case, which should be apparent on inspection. On inspection of the dorsal surfaces of both the hands and wrists there is an obviously prominent left distal ulna. The shape of the wrist is abnormal, with volar subluxation present. There is volar and ulnar angulation of the distal radius. The forearm is relatively shortened. Supination is restricted to 40°. There is volar ulnar deviation at the distal radial articular surface. Check wrist movements, as there is often limited movement."

Radiographs[51]

Cystic changes often present in the distal radial epiphysis, which appears triangular in shape due to growth failure in the volar and ulnar aspects of the epiphysis. There is dorsal radial bowing of the distal radius, as well as volar ulnar angulation of the distal radial articular surface. Premature fusion of the volar and ulnar aspects of the distal radial growth plate occurs. The ulna is subluxed dorsally and the ulnar head is enlarged. Depending on aetiology the ulnar can be longer or shorter than normal. The proximal carpal row appears to have subluxed in the ulnar direction and towards the palmar aspect into the distal radioulnar joint. The carpus appears wedge shaped with the lunate at its apex.

---

[51] Aim to describe the relevant radiographs slickly in the exam.

Aetiology[52]

- Idiopathic
- Other Madelung-like deformities occur with:
  - Trauma
  - Hereditary multiple exostosis
  - Various syndromes, e.g. Turner's syndrome
  - Skeletal dysplasia, e.g. achondroplasia
  - Ollier's disease
  - Infection

Management

Assess the patient fully. The severity of the deformity is variable. There are various management options, which depends on the following:
- Whether the growth plate of the radius is open or closed
- The degree of deformity
- The length of the radius

Conservative (do nothing)

Some authors have suggested that it is almost negligent to treat this surgically especially if the boat has been missed for the growth plate.[53]

Surgery

Epiphysiodesis of the distal ulnar growth plate – To prevent overgrowth of the ulna. Closing wedge osteotomy of the radius. Carried out to correct the deformity.

Epiphysiolysis of the fused growth plate of the radius – If there is premature fusion and the patient is very young.

Epiphysiodesis of the distal radius growth plate – To prevent progression of the deformity.

Wrist arthrodesis – In those with a mature skeleton, for severe pain and instability (salvage procedure).

---

[52] Likewise try not to struggle to remember the cause of Madelung's deformity in the exam – it doesn't look good. (We may be stating the obvious but this is the practical reality of the exam.)

[53] Controversial view – don't mention in the exam.

Excision distal ulna – In patients with a mature skeleton if they have ulnar prominence or pain from carpal instability.

In general, **fuse the radial growth plate** if it is still **open** and correct the deformity with an **osteotomy**. Plus carry out a **fusion** of the distal **ulnar growth plate** if it is still **open** and **ulnar shortening** if it is unduly long, or **ulnar lengthening** if it is too short.

Examination corner

Oral questions

Madelung's deformity

- What do patients usually present with?
- How are you going to treat this condition?
- Are there any other options?
- Is the physis open or closed?

Examination corner

Hand or Paediatrics oral 1

Radiograph of Madelung's deformity (Figure 7.1)

General advice

I have seen both sides of the coin with this particular oral. A couple of candidates stumbled along with their answers – the examiners having to point out various radiographic features that they omitted to mention. The examiners also had to prompt them with the causes of the deformity.

Another candidate launched effortlessly into the most detailed of radiographic descriptions possible – I was unsure whether he wanted to specialize in radiology rather than orthopaedics. Go through a dry run of describing the typical radiographic appearances of the Madelung type of deformity. In addition go through the various treatment options for the condition, as it is easy to come out with an answer that appears disjointed and all over the place if not previously rehearsed.

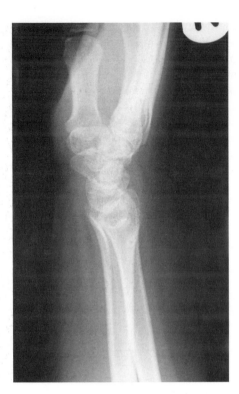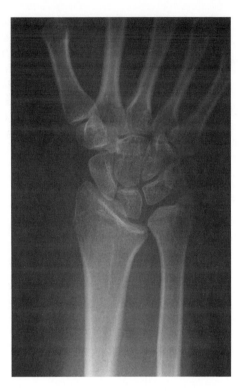

Figure 7.1a, b. Madelung's deformity. Premature fusion of the volar–ulnar half of the distal radial physis

Hand or Paediatrics oral 2

Clinical photograph of Madelung's deformity

Spot diagnosis
- What causes this deformity?
- How are you going to manage it?

Short case 1

- Examine this lady's hands
- Dwarf with caput ulnae syndrome and destroyed proximal carpal row

Trigger finger

The examiners more often than not are rushing you or hinting that you should be quick,

i.e. "a quick spot diagnosis" or "one last quick one before the bell". Describe what you see; it is unlikely that you will get as far as palpation or movement before the examiners will start asking you questions.

"Trigger finger has occasionally come up in the short cases. I would hesitate to call it a spot diagnosis unless the examiner is giving it away. This lady is complaining of catching of her finger – would you like to examine her hands? Do not assume anything – examine as you would do normally."

Memorandum

"On general inspection of the hands the patient's right middle (or ring) finger appears flexed. The finger remains flexed when he/she tries to open this hand from a fist. On further effort and with help from the opposite hand it suddenly straightens with a snap. The finger clicks when it is bent. A tender nodule is felt at the A1 pulley in the palm. The diagnosis is trigger finger."

Medical conditions such as RA, diabetes, gout, carpal tunnel syndrome, de Quervain's tenosynovitis and Dupuytren's contracture may be associated with triggering.

Management

Mild triggering may resolve spontaneously and need no treatment apart from reassurance.

Night splintage of the IP joints in extension improves locking on waking and may be sufficient in mild cases. Steroid/local anaesthetic injection into the tendon sheath. Open release of the A1 pulley.

Examination corner

Short case 1

Trigger finger in a rheumatoid patient

Management – synovectomy and not division of A1 pulley
How successful is steroid injection?

Ganglion

Basically an examination of a swelling in the hand.

Inspection

- Site (define exactly)
- Size
- Colour
- Shape: spherical, ovoid, pear-shaped, irregular
- Scars
- Effect of active movement
- Moves in the axis of the extensor tendons

Palpation

- Tenderness
- Consistency: stony hard, firm, rubbery, soft, jelly-like

- Edge: clearly defined, indistinct
- Relationship to superficial and deep structures
- Mobile or attached to skin, muscle or bone
- Temperature
- Fluctuation
- Signs of emptying
- Pulsatile
- Thrills
- Bruits
- Compressibility

Other features

- Distal neurovascular status
- Regional lymph nodes
- State of the surrounding skin

"A smooth surface, spherical and feels fluctuant. Usually not reducible, feels as though it slips away from my hand. The swelling is not attached to skin, and is freely mobile."

"Can you tense your muscles please?"

"The swelling does not appear to be attached to any surrounding muscles; I can move it freely in any plane with the underlying muscles contracted."

Definition

A mucin-filled cyst, which is attached to the synovial cavity of a joint or tendon; the wall consists of compressed collagen with no epithelial or synovial lining. It contains mucin, which is a mixture of glucosamine, albumin, globulin and hyaluronic acid.

Types of ganglion

- Dorsal wrist
- Volar radial
- Flexor sheath

Management

- Reassurance
- Aspiration
- Excision

Mention recurrence.

Differential diagnosis

My differential diagnosis would include:
- Pigmented villonodular synovitis (giant cell tumour tendon sheath)
- Epidermal inclusion cyst
- Neurilemmona
- Fibroma of tendon sheath
- Foreign body granuloma
- Xanthoma tuberosum
- Digital lipoma

Examiner questions

- What is a ganglion?
- What does it contain?
- How do you manage it?

8

Shoulder and elbow clinical cases

Paul A. Banaszkiewicz

Acromioclavicular joint arthritis

The AC joint may be prominent due to osteophytes or a type III or V ACJ dislocation. The patient will point to the joint if it is the cause of the pain. Direct palpation can reveal well localized tenderness and crepitus over the AC joint. Shoulder movement is rarely restricted although in long-standing cases mild restriction of internal rotation and/or cross body adduction may occur. Provocative tests such as reaching across to touch the opposite shoulder or placing the hand behind the back may cause discomfort.

Cross body (horizontal) adduction test. The patient's arm on the affected side is elevated to 90° and the examiner grasps the elbow and adducts the arm across the body. Simultaneously the examiner's thumb pushes the lateral end of the clavicle anteriorly. Reproduction of pain over the AC joint is suggestive of AC joint OA but not specific. The test may be positive in patients with subacromial impingement.

When full movement of the shoulder is possible a terminal impingement pain (pain above 120°) can be demonstrated on both active and passive movement. Differential diagnosis would include calcific tendinitis, early adhesive capsulitis and glenohumeral arthritis. Discussion may include description of the radiographic findings and management of the condition. Surgery would usually be arthroscopic distal clavicle resection either by a subacromial (indirect) approach or a superior (direct) approach.

Subacromial impingement

The clinical picture can be confused if co-existent shoulder pathology exists, such as restricted range of shoulder movement with muscle wasting and loss of power.

Memorandum

History

- Onset, duration, location and quality of pain
- Weakness, loss of motion (especially elevation), inability to sleep on the affected side, night pain, catching, crepitus
- Interference with ADL

Clinical examination

"On inspection of the shoulder from the front there is a shoulder strap incision/cleavage line scar over the ACJ."

There is minimal rotator cuff wasting, and occasionally marked shoulder muscle wasting especially in chronic cases.

"From behind there is a suggestion of muscle wasting at the postero-inferior aspect of the shoulder" (an important sign to describe if present). "I will now go on to palpation looking for areas of tenderness or swelling."

"Can you point to any painful areas?"

The acromion is palpated along its posterior, lateral and anterior margins. In impingement syndrome often there is tenderness at the anterolateral corner of the acromion. Tenderness of the ACJ is quite

Postgraduate Orthopaedics: The Candidate's Guide to the FRCS (Tr & Orth) Examination, Ed. Paul A. Banaszkiewicz, Deiary F. Kader, Nicola Maffulli. Published by Cambridge University Press. © Cambridge University Press 2009.

specific for pathology arising from this joint. There may be mild tenderness over the greater tuberosity, which is best demonstrated by extending and internally rotating the arm. The greater tubero-sity is brought anteriorly from under the acromion. It and the inserting supraspinatus tendon can be palpated. Tenderness is present with tears or tendonitis.

From behind check active abduction and forward flexion and assess scapula rhythm. Ideally there will be a mirror in front of the patient so any pain on active movement can be seen. On elevation the initial 60° is glenohumeral, 60°–120° is both glenohumeral joint and scapulothoracic, and above 120° is scapulothoracic.

To check for capsular tightness, stabilize the scapula with a hand on the acromion and abduct then forward flex the arm.

Now ask the patient to place their hand behind their back (extension and internal rotation) and compare with the other side. Then from the front check external rotation.

With impingement, there is classically a painful arc of movement between 70° and 120°. There may be an alteration of scapular rhythm. There may be soft crepitus when the arm passes through this arc. The pain is usually localized to the anterior region of the shoulder but may often radiate down to the deltoid insertion.

"The patient has a painful arc of motion between 70° and 120° but if I go past 120° it is not painful."

Test for the power of the rotator cuff muscles: you will see either normal power or a minor weakness on resisted movements of the rotator cuff. If a co-existent large cuff tear is present significant weakness of abduction and external rotation can be demonstrated.

Do not forget to mention examination of the cervical spine at some point during your shoulder examination.

Discussion

- Definition of impingement
- Difference between Neer's sign and test
- Impingement tests

Definition of impingement
Pain emanating from the subacromial space and due to either narrowing caused by a subacromial bony spur and thickening of the coracoacromial ligament, or a thickened bursa and tendonitis.

Difference between Neer's sign and Neer's test
Neer's sign – reproduction of the patient's symptomatic pain at maximal forward flexion whilst stabilizing the scapula.
Neer's test – local anaesthetic injection into the subacromial space eliminates pain.

Impingement tests
- Neer's sign[1]
  - Passive forward elevation in the plane of the scapula with slight internal rotation
- Hawkins' impingement reinforcement test
  - Passive internal rotation in 90° flexion
  - External rotation: unlimited
  - Internal rotation: limited, exhibits painful end point
  - Need to have full passive movement of the shoulder to be able to demonstrate impingement
- Abduction test
  - Classically painful between 70° and 120°, a painful arc as the rotator cuff is placed under maximum tension

Rotator cuff tears

- Take a short history (any trauma, site and provoking factors for pain)
- Examine
- Investigation and management options
- Comment on radiographs

Memorandum

Typical patient is likely to be middle-aged or elderly.

---

[1] Be careful to make the distinction between impingement sign and impingement test.

Examination

Look

Look at the shoulder posture, notably for the presence of any shoulder asymmetry, alterations in position and muscle wasting. Prominence of the AC joint indicates possible AC joint osteoarthritis. Look at the shoulder movements whilst undressing. If the injury is acute there is unlikely to be significant muscle wasting unless there is a pre-existing shoulder problem. In the exam you are more likely to be given a chronic (possibly massive) tear in which there will be obvious muscle wasting.

Inspect the shoulder girdle particularly the deltoid muscle, the supraspinatus fossa and the infraspinatus fossa. A combined supraspinatus/infraspinatus tear leads to prominence of the scapular spine and indicates a large tear. A ruptured long head of biceps gives a characteristic bulge (the "Popeye" sign).

Feel

Compress the lateral end of the clavicle to identify symptomatic arthritic change in the AC joint. There may be co-existent subacromial impingement caused in part by AC joint osteophytes.

In thin individuals defects in the cuff may be palpated. This is controversial as there are some shoulder surgeons who believe that the presence and extent of rotator cuff tears cannot reliably be elicited by palpation.

Move

There may be loss of active elevation and a disparity between active and passive ranges of movement. You may find abnormal scapular rhythm especially on lowering the arm due to eccentric contracture. Which tendon is torn? Assess rotator cuff strength and integrity.

Supraspinatus

Carry out Jobe's ("empty can") test – resisted elevation with the arm abducted to 20° in the plane of the scapula with the arm internally rotated and the thumb pointing down.

Subscapularis

Gerber's lift-off test – place the patient's hand behind their back and ask them to push backwards against the examiner's hand.

Belly press test (if the patient cannot place their hand behind the back) – both hands placed on their abdomen and asked to push elbows forward.

Infraspinatus/teres minor

Resisted external rotation with the arms at the side will test the muscle power of infraspinatus/teres minor. Hornblower's sign[2] demonstrates the difficulty in raising the hand to the mouth in the absence of external rotation of the shoulder. Positive test if the patient is unable to do so without abducting the shoulder. Drop-arm test performed with the patient's arm abducted to 90°; ask the patient to slowly lower the arm. If they are unable to lower their arm slowly and smoothly, this indicates a large/massive tear of infraspinatus. A positive Hornblower's sign/drop-arm test is a warning to the surgeon considering rotator cuff repair.

Three lag sign tests have been described to assess the integrity of the rotator cuff:

1. External rotation lag sign (infraspinatus): with the arm adducted and the elbow flexed 90°, the arm is placed in full external rotation, and then the patient is asked to actively maintain this position.
2. Drop-arm lag sign (supraspinatus tear): the arm is held in 90° of forward flexion, and the patient is asked to actively maintain this position.
3. Internal rotation lag sign (subscapularis): the patient is unable to hold their hand away from their back in near full internal rotation.

Investigations

• Radiographs. Three standard projections: true anteroposterior, supraspinatus outlet, axillary view

---

[2] Walch G, Boulahia A, Calderone S, Robinson AH (1998) The "dropping" and "hornblower's" signs in evaluation of rotator-cuff tears. *J Bone Joint Surg Br* 80(4): 624–8.

- Ultrasound. Cheap and non-invasive but operator dependent
- MRI. Most sensitive and allows assessment of muscle quality in large/massive full-thickness tears
- Arthroscopy. More specific for impingement and partial tears

Management

Conservative
- Small tears or irreparable tears in the elderly
- Physiotherapy (strengthening exercises for the rotator cuff and shoulder girdle), steroid injections, etc.

Surgery
- Open repair
- Arthroscopic repair

Postoperative management includes physiotherapy.

Examination corner

Short case 1

Massive rotator cuff tear in an elderly gentleman

Ask a short history: age, dominance, pain, stiffness and weakness. Shoulder examination included range of movement and testing of rotator cuff power. I was then shown radiographs and an ultrasound scan and asked about management.

Short case 2

Chronic rotator cuff tear shoulder in a middle-aged lady approximately 45 sitting in chair

Examiner: This lady is complaining of right shoulder pain. Just examine her shoulder and tell us what you're doing.
Candidate: Is your shoulder painful?
Patient: Yes.
Candidate: I'll try not to cause you any pain. Please let me know if it's sore and I will stop.

On inspection of the shoulder from the front there are no obvious scars, muscle wasting, or asymmetry. The shoulders are of symmetrical height. There are no other obvious features of note. From behind there is some wasting of supraspinatus and infraspinatus (mild but definite wasting).

Examiner: Whereabouts is this wasting?
Candidate: There is wasting over the right supraspinatus and infraspinatus muscles compared to the left side. (Demonstrating the wasting. An important physical sign to pick up if present.)
Where is your shoulder painful?
Patient: Over here (points to greater tuberosity).
Candidate: I am palpating the shoulder from a medial to lateral direction feeling for any areas of tenderness or crepitus. There is no pain over the sternoclavicular joint, clavicle or AC joint. She is sore over the supraspinatus tendon and also the greater tuberosity, to which she pointed previously. The anterior and posterior joint line is non-tender. There appears to be a gap in the supraspinatus tendon laterally (feeling for a rotator cuff tear laterally while rotating arm is controversial; some shoulder surgeons do not think a tear can be appreciated accurately), but I'm not entirely sure as the deltoid bulk is reasonably large.
Examiner: A gap laterally is very suggestive of a rotator cuff tear; you should be able to feel it – the deltoid bulk is not that large. (Controversial – see above.)
Candidate: I would now like to test this lady's range of movement at the shoulder. *Can you swing your arms out by your side and then upward into the air (abduction)?* The patient only has 80° of active abduction and it is painful with loss of normal scapulothoracic rhythm. Passively there is very little extra movement and this provokes more pain. *Can you swing your arms forward now (flexion)?*
Examiner: You need to stabilize the scapula when there is a discrepancy between active and passive movements of the shoulder (examiner is getting a bit annoyed).
Candidate: I usually test active and passive movements of the shoulder first and then go back and stabilize the scapula if there is limitation of movement in order to differentiate between scapulothoracic and glenohumeral movement. There is a restricted range of active forward flexion to 90° that I can't improve passively, and most of this movement is scapulothoracic (hand stabilizing the scapula when the movement is performed). *Can you swing your arms backwards?*
Again active extension is limited to 20° and painful.
Likewise external rotation is painful and only about 30° compared to the opposite side. I'd like to go on to test her rotator cuff muscles for power, testing supraspinatus, infraspinatus,

teres minor and subscapularis in both the normal and the abnormal shoulder. She has a marked loss of power in her right rotator cuff muscles compared to the left side.

Examiner: What do you think the diagnosis is?

Candidate: I think she may have an impingement syndrome.

I have no idea why I said this, as she certainly did not demonstrate any impingement signs and I did not specifically test for them. I chose to ignore the fact we had alluded to the diagnosis of a rotator cuff tear during the examination. I just felt she was the wrong age for a rotator cuff tear and that I had not clinically demonstrated a significant difference between active and passive movements of the shoulder typical of a large rotator cuff tear.

Examiner: You palpated a rotator cuff tear and also demonstrated a loss of power in her rotator cuff muscles. These findings would suggest a rotator cuff tear. What investigations would you perform to confirm the diagnosis?

Candidate: I would get some X-rays of her shoulder.

Examiner: What would you expect to find?

Candidate: There would be degenerative changes in the acromioclavicular joint, a decreased coracohumoral interval, a break in Shenton's line with superior migration of the humeral head and possibly cystic changes in the greater tuberosity.

Examiner: What is the investigation of choice?

Candidate: An MRI.

Examiner: OK. How are you going to operate on this lady's cuff tear?

Candidate: We need much more information than this. I need to know how large the tear is, whether it is full thickness or partial thickness and the state of the surrounding muscles.

Examiner: It is 4 cm and full thickness. (Not happy with the answer.)

Candidate: Then I would refer her on to an experienced shoulder surgeon who repairs these cuff tears on a regular basis.

With this we moved onto the next case.

The examiner was heckling me through out this case, trying to quicken the pace of the examination. It is important to take the hint and get on with it as swiftly as possible but not at the expense of appearing rushed or hurried. Try to remain professional and composed at all times during your clinicals. Defend yourself if you are being challenged but be sensible about it and try not to be too aggressive in your reply. To this day I am still unsure exactly what was wrong with this patient's shoulder. On clinical examination she did not present with the classic findings of a rotator cuff tear. I am still not entirely convinced that she had a rotator cuff tear. We went down the path of assuming it was a tear and discussed further management of it.

Frozen shoulder

Memorandum

A typical patient is middle aged and usually female. Adhesive capsulitis and calcific tendinitis are the cause of the most severe shoulder pain in the absence of trauma or any signs of infection.

"On examination there is a normal shoulder contour, except perhaps slight deltoid wasting. There is often no tenderness present to palpation."

"The patient demonstrates marked restriction of both active and passive movements of the shoulder. In particular there is passive restriction of shoulder elevation to less than 100° and marked restriction of external rotation when compared with the opposite normal side.[3] Examining shoulder movements again with my left hand stabilizing the scapula demonstrates that most of this shoulder movement is scapulothoracic with very little glenohumeral contribution. There was no palpable crepitus on movement of the shoulder. On testing power there was no obvious gross weakness of the rotator cuff muscles (normal power). It can be difficult to test power because of the restriction in shoulder movement."

"These features are suggestive of adhesive capsulitis. Because of the marked restriction of external rotation my differential diagnosis would include a locked posterior dislocation of the shoulder and gross osteoarthritis of the glenohumeral joint. Radiographs would exclude these two conditions."

Glenohumeral osteoarthritis

History

- Pain, stiffness, loss of motion
- Objective assessment of the patient's functional impairment:
  - Difficulty getting dressed
  - Brushing teeth
  - Reaching the top or the back of the head
  - Reaching the opposite axilla
  - Washing the perineum
  - Washing the face

[3] Pathognomonic of the condition. Limitation of external rotation to less than 50% of normal is often used as a diagnostic criterion.

- Combing the hair
- Writing or turning a key

Examination

"On inspection from the front the most obvious feature is gross generalized muscle wasting. There are no obvious scars but there is loss of the normal shoulder contour. The anterior shoulder appears swollen due to an effusion."

Asymmetry of the shoulder is due to gross muscle wasting and distortion of the bony anatomy. The displacement of the humeral head and severe erosion of the head or of the glenoid can markedly distort the contour of the shoulder.

"The posterior joint line is tender to palpation. There is gross painful restriction of shoulder movement with crepitus on glenohumeral joint movement."

There will be a slight difference between active and passive movements of the shoulder because of pain, but this difference is never as distinct as in the case of a rotator cuff tear.

With progression of the disease shoulder movement becomes restricted to scapulothoracic movement, which does not allow much rotation. Therefore, external and internal rotation are limited the most.

Power could be difficult to test smoothly because of the marked restriction of shoulder movement and pain (do not hurt the patient). The strength of the rotators and of the deltoid within the limited range may be surprisingly good. Pain rather than muscle wasting may cause some of the weakness.

Management options

- Physiotherapy, intra-articular steroid injections
- Synovectomy (open or arthroscopic in rheumatoid)
- Arthroscopic debridement
- Resurfacing arthroplasty
- Hemi-arthroplasty
- Total shoulder arthroplasty
- Resection arthroplasty
- Arthrodesis

> **Examination corner**
>
> ## Short case 1
>
> ### Glenohumeral right shoulder osteoarthritis
>
> - Examine shoulder movements
> - Describe the radiographs
> - Management
> - Arguments for and against hemiarthroplasty of the shoulder versus total shoulder replacement

Shoulder instability

Memorandum

"On inspection the patient is a well-built young man who favours his left arm while undressing. He has no scars/ two arthroscopic portal scars – one anterolateral and one posteriorly/an anterior deltopectoral scar consistent with previous shoulder surgery. There is no visible muscle wastage.[4] His neck and shoulder contours are normal. Palpation reveals no specific areas of tenderness or deformity. A full range of pain-free shoulder movements is present."

The power in all muscle groups was normal, as were sensation and the peripheral circulation. There were no signs of generalized hyperlaxity (Beighton score >7). The inferior sulcus sign was negative. Anterior drawer test was positive grade 2 compared to the opposite side. He demonstrated a positive apprehensive sign and positive Jobe's relocation test. The load and shift test was positive. Tests for posterior instability were normal.

> **Examination corner**
>
> Possibly a long case, much more likely a short case. Young male, with normal musculature, and normal movement and power of the shoulder. Diagnosis rests on demonstrating instability tests. You may be asked to just demonstrate instability tests rather than examine the whole shoulder.
>
> *Examiner*: What are the signs of instability and how do you elicit them? Do you know any instability tests?

---

[4] The patient is most likely to have normal musculature or at worst minimal shoulder wasting.

Short case 1

A short case of voluntary posterior dislocation of the shoulder.

Short case 2

Recurrent anterior dislocation shoulder

- Examination of the shoulder
- Apprehension test
- Arthroscopy portals and the role of arthroscopy
- Bankart and Hill–Sachs lesions
- Bankart repair

Rupture of the long head of biceps

Usually male, elderly. Large bulge in the arm; typically appears when the elbow is flexed. There is a large mass 4 cm by 3 cm in the anterior flexor compartment of the arm/anterior aspect of the distal upper arm suggestive of rupture of the long head of biceps. Test for power of flexion/extension. During flexion the biceps retracts proximally producing the classic deformity of the biceps contour. It is often associated with rotator cuff impingement or tears. Examine the region of the bicipital groove, which may show indentation or hollowing when the tendon is absent following a rupture. Carry out Speed's and Boyd's tests.

Proximal rupture repair

The management is usually non-operative.

Distal rupture repair[5]

One- or two-incision repair.

[5] I had a proximal long head of biceps rupture turned around on me in the short cases and was asked about the bony attachments, nerve supply and action of the short head of biceps tendon which I struggled through. To make matters worse I was then asked about distal biceps tendon repair, about which I knew nothing.

One incision: the modified Henry approach. Make a curvilinear incision over the anterior aspect of the elbow. Locate the ruptured distal biceps tendon. Insert bone suture anchors into the radial tuberosity and reattach the tendon.

Two-incision approach of Boyd and Anderson: Make a 3-cm transverse incision over the distal biceps tendon sheath. Insert a core tendon suture through the end of the tendon. Make a second incision on the posterolateral aspect of the elbow. Locate the tunnel between the radius and the ulna through which tendon originally passed. Make drill holes through the radial tuberosity in order to allow anchoring of the tendon. Retrieve the biceps through the distal incision; then pass sutures through the tuberosity drill holes and tie them down.

Examination corner

Short case 1

60-year-old man with large rotator cuff tear and coexisting biceps rupture

Examiner: What do you see?
Candidate: The biceps has increased in size, the popeye sign suggestive of biceps rupture.
Examiner: Can you confirm weakness of the biceps muscle?
Examiner: What else do you want to do?
Candidate: I would like to examine the shoulder to check for a possible rotator cuff tear. I was then asked about management of both the rotator cuff tear and biceps rupture

Shoulder arthrodesis

Examination corner

Short case 1

Candidate: On inspection there is a large scar extending from the spine of the scapula over the top of the shoulder down the arm. There is gross distortion of the normal shoulder contour with gross muscle wasting. Examination of shoulder movements revealed elevation to 100° although rotation was grossly restricted. In particular when stabilizing the scapula it was apparent that all movement was scapulothoracic, no glenohumeral movement was appreciated.

Examiner: What operation do you think he has had?

Candidate: I haven't seen this before but the length of the scar would suggest a shoulder arthrodesis. I'd like to confirm this clinically. To do this I stabilize the scapula with one hand and move the shoulder with my other hand: I see gross restriction of abduction, forward flexion, etc.

Indications

- Infection unresponsive to conservative treatment
- Stabilization of painful, paralytic disorders of the shoulder
- Post traumatic brachial plexus injury
- Salvage for a failed shoulder arthroplasty
- Stabilization after resection of a neoplasm
- Recurrent dislocations

Position of fusion

- 25°–40° abduction
- 20°–30° flexion
- 25°–30° internal rotation
- Or 30°, 30°, 30°

Method

- Extra-articular
- Intra-articular
- Combined

Brachial plexus

The prospect of getting a brachial plexus patient as the long case can fill candidates with a certain amount of fear and trepidation. The ultimate goal is to examine a brachial plexus patient well in the FRCS (Tr & Orth) exam and it will take a bit of time and practice to get your examination technique to a standard that flows well and is second nature to you. The aim of examination is to identify a pattern of injury that relates to an anatomical level within the brachial plexus (Table 8.1). To achieve this target it is necessary to be familiar with the anatomy of the brachial plexus and to have an examination routine that is both logical and methodical. In practice this localization is used to deduce whether the injury is supraclavicular or infraclavicular and how many roots are affected.

History

Pertinent points in the history include:
- Mechanism of injury
- Velocity of impact – high-velocity injuries suggest root avulsion
- Pre-morbid state
- Associated injuries
- Open/closed
- Vascular compromise (axillary or subclavian vessels)
- Concomitant bony injuries around the forearm or shoulder

Table 8.1 Motor and sensory loss by root level

Root level	Motor loss	Sensory loss
C5	Shoulder: loss of abduction	Lateral aspect of the deltoid muscle
C5 C6	Shoulder: external rotation, flexion and abduction Elbow: flexion Wrist: extension	Thumb and index finger
C5 C6 C7	As above but with: extension of the elbow, wrist, fingers and thumb	Thumb, index and middle fingers
C8 T1	Finger and thumb flexion; all intrinsics	Little and ring fingers Inner border of the forearm

• Pain – location, frequency, duration, quality and intensity as well as medication requirements and changes in the characteristics of the pain since the accident

Examination

Inspection

Ideally the patient should be stripped to the waist to allow visualization of both upper limbs and the torso's musculature. A typical case is as follows:
• Young man with a wasted limb
• Look at the eyes: Horner's ptosis (root avulsion T1)
• Look for old scars, both traumatic and surgical
• Are the shoulders level or is the shoulder subluxed and dangling inferiorly (weak abductor muscles)?
• Is there a prominent proximal humerus?
• Is there a mal-united clavicular fracture?
• Look for muscle wastage: shoulder, scapula, forearm and back
• Look for neurotrophic vasomotor changes

The resting position of the limb should be noted and any fixed deformity commented on, e.g. clawing of the hands, internal rotation of the shoulder, etc.

The upper limb is then inspected from the shoulders to the fingertips beginning with the deltoid and passing down the arm to the forearm and then into the hand, looking for:
• Deltoid wasting
• Supraspinatus/infraspinatus wasting
• Forearm wasting of the mobile wad, extensor and flexor compartments
• Inspect the hands looking for intrinsic muscle wasting between the metacarpals as well as the thenar and hypothenar eminences

Look for any evidence of other injuries in the upper limbs such as surgical scars from elbow fractures or forearm plating. Surgical procedures may have been performed if the plexus lesion is chronic, and muscle transfer scars, joint fusions and amputations should be noted. What is the pattern of muscle wastage?

Palpation

The chest, back and upper limb musculature are felt to assess muscle bulk.

Sensation

Move on to sensation. First ask the patient about sensation.

"Have you any areas of numbness, loss of sensation or pins and needles?"[6]

Ask about pain. *"Can you show me where it does not feel normal, is the limb painful?"* Objective assessment is then carried out testing for light touch with gentle digital pressure and pinprick with a neurological pin. Sensation above the clavicles and acromion is generally C4. The ninhydrin sweat test reveals damage to the sympathetic chain and is an indicator of lower root avulsion.

Assess for fixed contractures

It is important to assess the passive range of movement of both the upper limbs, as far as is practicable, to check for any fixed contractures. If this is not done it is not possible to accurately grade the power of the muscle groups according to the MRC grading system.
• Shoulder: *"Can you swing your arms forward?"* (Active and then passive)
• Elbow
• Wrist
• Hand

Test for muscle power[7]

Look and feel for muscle contracture. When assessing motor power, the MRC grading system is used. For a grade to be given, the joint being examined must have a full range of passive movement.[8]

---

[6] A recognized sensory dermatome can bail you out if you are unsure of the pattern of motor wasting.

[7] A full description of muscle testing can be found in the MRC publication on examination of peripheral nerve injuries. Medical Research Council (1976) *Aids to Examination of the Peripheral Nervous System.* Memorandum No. 45. London: HMSO.

[8] Occasionally one will come across a candidate who mentions an MRC power grading in a joint without a full passive range of movement. This may be commented on as an incorrect statement by a hawkish examiner out to get you.

Table 8.2 Upper limb motor testing

C5	C6	
Deltoid	Supinator	
Infraspinatus	Biceps	
	Pectoralis major	
C7	C8	T1
Wrist and finger extensors	Wrist flexors	Intrinsic muscles
Triceps	Finger and thumb flexors	

When active movement of the joint is possible the muscle must be able to pull the joint through a full range of movement otherwise a lower grade should be given. One should assess the power of each muscle in the upper limbs individually as far as is practical. This is best conducted in a systematized manner in the proximal to distal direction.

A system based on anatomical knowledge of the brachial plexus is necessary to avoid missing any lesions and to fully assess the extent of involvement at each level of the plexus. Each test is designed to isolate that muscle function only. Start with the patient facing away from the examiner (Table 8.2).

From behind the patient

Trapezius (spinal accessory nerve C3 C4) (XI cranial nerve)
"*Can you shrug your shoulders up?*" The contraction of trapezius superiorly can be seen and felt. The trapezius is an important muscle of the shoulder girdle; it may be used for tendon transfers, e.g. to the deltoid.

Serratus anterior (long thoracic nerve C5 C6 C7)
The patient is asked to push into a wall.

Rhomboids (dorsal scapular nerve C5)
Three tests are described for rhomboid function. However, keep it simple and stick to one method only.
1. "*Can you squeeze your shoulder blades together?*" The contraction of the rhomboids medial to the scapula can be seen and felt.

2. Gerber type test (as used for the subscapular muscle) as described in the MRC book.[7]
3. Or patient's hands on hips, stop me pushing your arms forwards.

Supraspinatus (suprascapular nerve C5 C6)
With the examiner behind the patient, the patient's shoulder is placed in internal rotation with the thumb pointing medially and is abducted 30° in the line of the scapula. Further abduction in the same plane is restricted. Alternatively Jobe's supraspinatus isolation test can be used.

Infraspinatus (suprascapular nerve C5 C6)
The shoulder is adducted and in neutral rotation with the elbow flexed to 90°. Instruct the patient to push their hands outwards, away from each other. External rotation is restricted at the forearm whilst the elbow is prevented from abducting with the other hand.

Deltoid (axillary nerve C5 C6 posterior cord)
Feel and test for the three parts of the muscle. The shoulder is abducted to 90° with the elbow flexed. Both sides are usually tested together.

From in front of the patient

Biceps (musculocutaneous nerve C5 C6 lateral cord)
Tested with the patient's shoulder adducted, the forearm supinated and the elbow flexed against resistance. The examiner stabilizes the patient's arm by grasping it at the posterior elbow and holds the patient's forearm just proximal to the wrist.

Triceps (radial nerve C6 C7 C8 posterior cord)
The patient's forearm is pronated, the shoulder flexed 45° and the elbow extended. The examiner stabilizes the patient's arm at the elbow and provides resistance against the forearm as the patient is instructed to "*push me away*".

ECRL (radial nerve C5 C6)
The patient's elbow is flexed 90°. With your hand, exert pressure over the dorsum of the index finger

MCP joint. *"Cock your wrist up, keep it there, and stop me pushing it down."*

Supinator (radial nerve C6 C7)

Extend the elbow to eliminate biceps. With the forearm pronated the patient's hand is grasped as though for a handshake and they are asked to supinate against resistance. *"Try to turn your hand over."*

Extensor digitorum communis (posterior interosseous nerve C7 C8)

To eliminate the effects of gravity, the palm of the patient's hand is supported and pressure is applied across the dorsum of the extended proximal phalanges of the fingers. *"Keep your fingers out straight."*

Oral questions

Outline the current views on management of brachial plexus injuries

---

Examination corner

Short case 1

Young male with closed brachial plexus injury following a motorbike accident

Examiner: Examine the brachial plexus and identify the level of injury.

Candidate: The injury is in the upper trunk, distal to the dorsal scapula nerve but proximal to the suprascapular nerve as the rhomboids are working but supraspinatus and infraspinatus are wasted.

Stiff elbow

Examiner: Examine this man's elbow.

Candidate: On inspection of the elbow there are no skin contractures or subcutaneous scarring. I can see scars present from previous surgery over both the medial and lateral aspects of the elbow. There is a reduced range of elbow movement. There is a "soft/hard" end point to movement. Active and passive range of elbow movement should be tested. A complete neurovascular examination should be performed especially if there is a history of previous surgery or trauma. Flexion contractures greater than 45° will significantly limit this patient's activities of daily living.

Surgical management

Ninety percent of ADLs can be carried out with movement of 30°–130° flexion. Radiographs should be taken to look for arthritic changes, previous fractures, deformity or heterotopic ossification.

Arthroscopic soft-tissue release

An arthroscopic elbow release allows possibly earlier recovery but no proven better long-term results. It should only be performed by an experienced arthroscopist due to the close proximity of radial and ulnar nerves.

Open soft-tissue release

The lateral column procedure is probably the procedure of choice but may need to be combined with a medial approach in resistant cases.

Open massive soft-tissue release

Capsular and collateral release with excision of any bony obstruction. The patient may develop an unstable elbow post-operatively as the procedure has the potential to injure the collateral ligaments. Protect against ectopic bone formation with radiotherapy or NSAIDs. There is always a concern for the ulnar nerve. Postoperative CPM is helpful in some patients but usually does not enhance end-range stretching. Occasionally an external fixator may be needed if the elbow is unstable at the end of the soft-tissue release.

Cubitus valgus

Memorandum 1

"*Can you show me your elbows please?*" (Demonstrate what you want the patient to do.)

A spot diagnosis. This patient demonstrates a cubitus valgus deformity of the elbow. There is also a suggestion of loss of full extension. There are no scars present over the lateral epicondyle.

Go now straight to the hand to look for ulnar nerve signs (wasting of the interossei, hypothenar muscle wastage, sensory changes, etc.).

"*Is there any weakness of your hand or numbness and tingling of your fingers?*"

The most common cause is a lateral condylar mass non-union from childhood leading to a valgus deformity of the elbow (Milch type 2 fracture). There is usually marked prominence of the medial epicondyle.

Memorandum 2

- Cubitus valgus elbow in a 65-year-old male
- Milch type 2 fracture of the lateral condyle missed at the age of 6 years
- Features of tardy ulnar nerve palsy

Examiner: Would you examine this gentleman's elbows and describe what you are doing as you go along?

Candidate: Can you show me your elbows please sir? On examination there is an obvious left cubitus valgus of the elbow present with a suggestion of loss of full extension.

Examiner (very quickly, heckling candidate): Come on where else do you want to look? (Not waiting for answer.) You look at his hands. Does he have evidence of ulnar nerve dysfunction?

Candidate: Looking at his hands there appears to be hypothenar muscle wasting.

Examiner (interrupting): Come on where else do you have wasting? What about the back of his hands? You should be jumping to examine it. What about his interosseous muscles?

Candidate: There is wasting of his dorsal interossei particularly the first dorsal interosseous. Can you feel me touching your little finger? Does it feel normal? He has reduced sensation over his ulnar 1½ digits and also over the ulnar, dorsal aspect of his wrist.

Examiner: Do you need nerve conduction studies to confirm your clinical findings?

Candidate: No.

Examiner: Good. What do you think of his X-rays?

Candidate: These are AP and lateral radiographs of the left elbow. They demonstrate an old lateral condylar fracture, which has gone onto a non-union. There are severe secondary arthritic changes present in the radiocapitellar and humeroulnar joints.

In view of his sensory and motor ulnar nerve symptoms and non-union present with secondary degenerative changes, I would offer him ulnar nerve decompression with medial condylectomy and anterior transposition of the nerve. I do not think a simple decompression is adequate management for this gentleman.

Rheumatoid elbow

Memorandum

"On examination the patient has features of a generalized polyarthropathy probably rheumatoid arthritis. There is an old well-healed scar over the lateral aspect of the elbow suggestive of previous surgery to the radial head. There are large rheumatoid nodules overlying the olecranon bursa. There are no features of either PIN or ulnar nerve neuropathy."

Mention co-existent assessment of shoulder and hand function.

Management

- Medical
- Open or arthroscopic synovectomy
- Radial head excision
- Total elbow arthroplasty
- Interposition arthroplasty

Tennis elbow (lateral epicondylitis)

Typically a short case in which the candidate would be asked to demonstrate provocation tests for tennis elbow.

Memorandum

Examiner: Would you like to examine this lady's elbow?

Candidate: On inspection the elbow looks normal. Flexion is full from 0° to 140° and painless. Full extension at its extreme point is however painful. There is definite point tenderness over the lateral epicondyle of the humerus and possibly weakness of grip strength.

Pain with the resisted wrist extension test

With their elbow extended, ask the patient, *"Could you make a fist please, can you cock your wrist backwards* (getting the patient to extend their wrist) *and resist me now?"* (Try to flex the wrist against resistance, feeling the lateral epicondyle at the same time.)

This should reproduce the patient's symptoms.

Middle finger extension test

Extending the middle finger against resistance reproduces pain by stressing ECRB.

Radiographs

Radiographs of the elbow are usually normal.

Lateral epicondylitis (tennis elbow)

This is a syndrome/symptom complex characterized by the following:

1. Pain over the lateral epicondyle and proximal forearm exacerbated by movements involving a combination of a gripping hand and a forearm rotation.
2. Tenderness on palpation of the extensor muscle origin at the lateral epicondyle.

3. Reproduction of pain when the forearm and wrist extensor muscles are actively extended or passively flexed.

Pathology

Uncertain; there are several theories:
- A vascular degenerative process
- Humeroradial bursitis
- Inflammation of the annular ligament of the radius
- Secondary trauma
- Or, it may present as part of a "generalized mesenchymal syndrome"

Clinical features

- Gradual onset of pain over the lateral epicondyle with radiation down the proximal forearm in line with the extensor muscles.

Differential diagnosis

- Radial tunnel syndrome

Management

Conservative
- Always initially conservative as 90% cases settle by 12 months
- Rest, modification of activities, NSAIDs, physiotherapy, Epi Clasp, steroid injection

Surgery
- Either open or arthroscopic release of ECRB
- Extensor origin may or may not be repaired
- On average 85% of patients will get complete relief of their symptoms with surgery, 5% will see no benefit and 10% will have residual symptoms

9

Spine clinical cases

Paul A. Banaszkiewicz

Ankylosing spondylitis

Introduction

This is classic long case material. There are good clinical signs present with a lot to talk about and discuss afterwards with the examiners.

Memorandum

On general inspection we have a male patient who is somewhat stooped as he walks into the room. On examination from behind the shoulders are of equal height, there is loss of normal lumbar lordosis, a fixed kyphosis of his thoracic spine and a forward thrust of his cervical spine. From the front his head appears to be translated forwards but his visual axis is just about horizontal. His pelvis is level but he tends to stand with a slightly flexed attitude of his hips and knees.

On examination of his neck movements there was very limited flexion and extension present. There is almost no lateral movement of his cervical spine. Examining his lumbar spine reveals a gross restriction of all movements. In particular he tends to flex his hips when bending forwards to compensate for a stiff spine.

The patient has a classic question mark posture with pronounced thoracolumbar kyphosis and flexion deformities of the hip.

Schober's test for lumbar forward flexion was 3 cm (normal=5 cm or more), which is markedly reduced. The wall test unmasks a flexion deformity of the spine. He is unable to stand with his back flush against the wall. Forced flexion, abduction and external rotation of the hip joint (Faber test) produces severe pain of the sacroiliac joints.

Maximum chest expansion from full expiration to full inspiration measured at the level of the nipples is reduced to 3 cm compared to a normal expansion of 7 cm. The patient is breathing predominantly by diaphragmatic excursion, which is the cause of his protuberant abdomen.

Discussion

Occasionally vertebral osteotomy is required for the correction of very severe spinal deformities. Patients are at high risk for cord injury during management of cervical trauma. There is a potential for massive epidural haemorrhage due to pre-existing fusion of the cervical vertebrae and secondary tearing of epidural veins.

Patients with ankylosing spondylitis may present problems with anaesthesia. Neck stiffness makes intubation difficult, reduced chest expansion affects lung capacity, cardiac involvement requires care and ossified spinal ligaments may make spinal or epidural anaesthesia impossible.

Other points to discuss include:
- Medical management of ankylosing spondylitis
- Order of preference for surgery; the hips or spine first?
- Indications and consent issues for spinal surgery
- Surgical approaches to the spine

Short case 1

This man is complaining of back pain. Please ask him a few questions and then examine his spine.

Postgraduate Orthopaedics: The Candidate's Guide to the FRCS (Tr & Orth) Examination, Ed. Paul A. Banaszkiewicz,
Deiary F. Kader, Nicola Maffulli. Published by Cambridge University Press. © Cambridge University Press 2009.

Brief history (how long, where, progression, radicular symptoms, night pain, etc.). Examination of spinal movements including Schober's test. Description of radiographs that demonstrated classic features of ankylosing spondylitis.

Drop foot gait (steppage gait)

There is wasting of the left anterior tibial and peroneal group of muscles. The patient cannot dorsiflex or evert the left foot, and there is impairment of sensation over the outer side of the left calf. The patient walks in equinus and on the lateral border of the foot. The toes of the affected leg hit the ground before the heel or sole of the foot, and the heel tends to strike the ground with a characteristic slapping sound. There is a loud clop of the foot as they walk.

The patient walks with weak or paralysed ankle dorsiflexors. The left knee and hip are raised higher than normal (increased flexion) to avoid dragging the toes on the ground, otherwise the foot slides along the ground. Ulceration may be present over the metatarsal heads or the lateral border of the foot.

Causes of drop foot gait

- Lumbar radiculopathy: posterolateral disc at L4/L5; rarely from far lateral or foraminal L5/S1 disc prolapse
- Trauma
- Peroneal nerve palsy
- Achilles tendon rupture
- Nerve root irritation from spondylolysis
- Lateral recess stenosis
- Space-occupying lesions (spinal neoplasm)
- Neurofibroma
- Ganglion
- Ischaemia
- Neurological disorders

Injury to the nerve usually occurs at the head of the fibula, where it can be involved in fractures or compressed by splints, tourniquets or bandages. The nerve has two branches – superficial and deep. The superficial branch supplies sensation to the lateral calf and dorsum of the foot and motor innervation to peroneus longus and brevis. The deep branch supplies sensation to the first web space and motor innervation to tibialis anterior, long extensors of the toes and the peroneus tertius muscle.

Management

- Ankle foot orthotic splint
- Anterior transfer of tibialis posterior tendon to the dorsum of the foot

---

Short case 1

Young boy with bilateral drop foot gait following Guillain–Barré infection

Examiner: This is a difficult case but I would like you to observe his gait and comment on any abnormality seen.

Candidate: Abnormal gait but nothing particularly obvious and I couldn't spot the diagnosis. I started to say that the gait wasn't Trendelenburg, antalgic, short leg, etc. I mentioned it could be a myopathic type of gait. The examiner mentioned the diagnosis and was happy enough for us to move on to another case.

I probably failed this particular short case but overall got a good pass – I had done a blitzkrieg job on the previous short cases.

Polio

Memorandum

On general inspection there is a below-knee calliper. On examination the right leg appears shorter with equinus of the ankle. There is a flexion deformity at the knee produced by muscle imbalance between the hamstrings and the quadriceps.[1] (There is genu recurvatum/genu valgum present.[2]) There is gross generalized muscle wasting of the lower limb. There is pelvic obliquity and a scoliotic deformity of the thoracolumbar spine, which is fixed. There is an

---

[1] The common deformities at the knee are flexion, hyperextension (recurvatum) and genu valgum.
[2] Genu valgum occurs when tensor fascia lata is active and the medial hamstrings and quadriceps are paralysed.

abduction external rotation deformity at the hip due to iliotibial band contracture. The hip is in joint; there is no paralytic hip dislocation.[3] In polio the foot and ankle can be variously affected. Depending upon the pattern of muscle groups paralysed, deformities such as equinus, calcaneus, varus or valgus, individually or in combination, develop.

Possible presentations encountered in the exam:

- Valgus deformity of the ankle joint and clawing of the lesser toes
- Severe equinocavus deformity of the foot
- Calcaneocavovarus deformity with clawing of the toes
- Isolated paralysis of tibialis posterior producing a paralytic pes planus (flat foot)

He demonstrates an unstable Trendelenburg gait due to abductor muscle paralysis. During walking there is a lack of flexion at the hip and hyperextension of the knee.

As mentioned previously the right leg is wasted, weak and flaccid with absent reflexes. The plantar response is normal. There is no sensory deficit. Look for leg length discrepancy as it is almost always present (97%) in polio. There will usually be obvious gross muscle wastage of the whole leg. The patient may have had some type of surgery such as subtalar fusion (look for obvious scars).

Short case 1

Polio affecting the quadriceps and tibialis anterior muscles

Scoliosis

Most likely to be a long case. Most likely to be idiopathic. One may be unlucky and get a congenital or neurofibromatosis type.

History (what are you going to ask in the history?)

- Age
- Occupation

---

[3] If pelvic obliquity is present the higher hip may dislocate. An abduction deformity can predispose to dislocation of the contralateral hip joint, as the pelvic obliquity causes the opposite hip to adopt an adducted posture.

- Is there a family history of spinal deformity (if brother has problems consider Duchenne's muscular dystrophy)
- Is it painful? If it is, this means pathology (a warning sign) that needs full evaluation
- Congenital problems: ask the patient whether their birth was normal and about their developmental milestones
- Any respiratory problems?
- Any neurological symptoms such as paraesthesia or numbness?
- What was the age of onset, and when was the deformity noticed?
- Progression
- Management
- Menarcheal history, growth spurts
- How did it present and who noticed the deformity?

Memorandum (what are you going to find on examination?)

Working from behind the patient, in the standing position. Look at the level of their shoulders and hips, waistline asymmetry and plumb-line measurements. Are the shoulders and ASIS level or is there asymmetry of the ASIS pelvic obliquity?

Where is the curve and is it balanced? Drop a plumb line from the head to the natal cleft. Deviations from this should be recorded, with the distance measured in centimetres (trunk shift). Describe the curve as apex-left or apex-right.

If there is a rib hump, does it become more prominent on bending forward? A rib hump may be more politically described as a scapula prominence.

How stiff is the spine in forward bending? Carry out Adams' forward bending test. If, when the patient is bending forwards, the curve disappears, it is a mobile curve – a so-called postural scoliosis. Check for lumbar lordosis, thoracic kyphosis and cervical lordosis in the sagittal plane. Does the curve correct on sitting down? If sitting down leads to full or partial correction, this indicates that the curve is not entirely rigid and that there is a flexible component to it. A scoliosis may be mobile secondary to a leg length inequality.

Are there café-au-lait spots present? If so how many? If it is neurofibromatosis type 1, what are the other features of the condition?

Check for hairy patches, naevi and dimples in the midline over the spine (present in spinal dysraphism).

How does the patient walk – is the gait spastic (cerebral palsy), flaccid (polio) or short leg (neurofibromatosis)? A good neurological examination is essential, paying particular attention to lower limb reflexes. If neurology is present it is absolutely essential you can define the level correctly.[4]

Check the patient's chest expansion, hamstring tightness and true/apparent leg length measurements.

Standing radiographs

Know how to calculate Cobb's angle. How do you delineate the most superior and inferior end vertebrae? Use the vertebra that is inclined most into the curve, and use either the disc or the pedicle.

Rotation is indicated if the pedicles are not seen end on. Look for any congenital anomalies of the vertebrae.

Bending films allows you to assess how stiff the spine is, and gives you some indication of what type of surgery to opt for: whether to fuse the front or back only or both the front and back.

Motor and sensory testing of the lower legs

A slick and confident neurological examination of the lower limbs only comes with time and practice.

---

[4] If you get levels mixed up for neurology, i.e. whether it is the S1 or L5 nerve root being compressed or you are unable to give the typical motor or sensory findings for a particular level, you are in trouble. In this instance, it does not matter whether you know the most up-to-date and fancy surgery for scoliosis, as you have just demonstrated to the examiners a lack of understanding of the basic principles and you are heading for a fail.

Motor

Flexion hip (iliopsoas) L2 L3

"Can you lift your leg up and stop me pushing it down?"

Extension of the hip: gluteus maximus

"I'm going to place my hand under your knee, and I want you to stop me from lifting your leg up."

Hip abduction L5 S1

"Can you open your legs and stop me pushing them together?"

Hip adduction L2 L3

"And can you now stop me pushing your legs apart?"

Extension of the knee (quadriceps) L3 L4

"I'm going to place my hand under your knee and I'd like you to straighten it. Now, stop me from bending your knee."

Flexion of the knee (hamstrings) L5 S1

"Please bend your knee, and then stop me from straightening it."

Dorsiflexion L4 L5

"Pull your foot up and stop me from pushing your foot down."

  "Cock your foot up and point your toes at the ceiling."

Plantar flexion S1 S2

"Push your foot down."

Inversion L4

"Push your foot in the way."

Eversion L5 S1

"Pull your foot out of the way, and stop me from pushing it in."

Test with the foot in a static functional position.

Sensory

Sensation can be rapidly assessed by gentle stroking of the skin and asking the patient to compare sides. Test individual dermatomes with a very clear dermatome map in mind. Using cotton wool and a sterile pinprick can further define decreased sensation:

L1: Groin
L2: Outer thigh
L3: Knee
L4: Inner calf
L5: Big toe, crosses lateral to medial
S1: Lateral border foot

Short case 1

Examiner: Watch this patient walk. What do you think the diagnosis is?

Candidate: Foot drop and high steppage gait. I confirmed this with a quick focused neurological examination including muscle testing, sensation and reflexes. The foot drop mainly affected the common peroneal nerve branch.

Various surgical scars over the left hip suggest a previous fracture/injury around the hip that required surgery with residual injury to the sciatic nerve.

Short case 2

Bilateral pes cavus deformity due to diastematomyelia

I performed a thorough neurological examination of motor power, sensation and reflexes to locate the level of the lesion.

Candidate: The examiners had just one thing on their mind – they wanted to see how slickly I could perform a neurological examination of the lower legs. I had practised this well and the examiners clearly thought that anything less was unacceptable in an exit exam.

Cervical radiculopathy and myelopathy

This is classic long case material. This topic could very easily catch you out if you are not familiar clinically with either examination of the neck or specifically the clinical findings you would look for in cervical myelopathy.

Be careful to distinguish between cervical radiculopathy and cervical spondylotic myelopathy. Most patients with cervical radiculopathy will present with symptoms and signs of monoradiculopathy but occasionally multiple roots are involved. Cervical radiculopathies are usually described as sharp or lancinating, precipitated or exacerbated by Valsalva manoeuvres.

The symptoms of cervical spondylotic myelopathy may include gait difficulties, decreased manual dexterity, paraesthesia or numbness of the extremities, urinary frequency or urgency, generalized and extremity weakness. In the upper limbs lower motor signs will be present whilst in the lower limbs upper motor neuron signs will be picked up.

History

- Can you write?
- Do you drop things?
- Can you dress yourself?
- Has there been any change in passing urine (urinary frequency or urgency)?
- Has there been any disturbance in bowel function (sphincter disturbance)?
- Have you got neck pain?
- Is there an increase in neck pain with Valsalva activities (increased thoracic pressure)?

Memorandum

Look for a cervical collar.

On examination the patient demonstrates a long stance phase of gait, the reverse of an antalgic gait. Cervical myelopathy presents with early gait disturbance, usually an insidious and slowly progressive stumbling or generalized gait disturbance. The patient may have an awkward or shuffling gait or suffer frequent falls. They have a characteristic, stooped, wide-based gait.

There is moderate restriction of neck movement particularly lateral flexion. Spurling's sign is positive, with arm pain reproduced by hyperextension and lateral rotation towards the symptomatic side (radiculopathy), and then gentle axial compression. This causes the foramina on the concave side to be compressed and increases any pain experienced in a dermatome pattern.

The shoulder abduction relief sign was positive, with abduction of the shoulder lessening the arm pain (radiculopathy). There is intrinsic muscle wasting of the small muscles of the hands.

Hoffman's reflex was positive (reflex finger and thumb extension with sudden long-finger DIP joint extension), which suggests cervical cord impingement.

The scapulohumeral reflex was positive – tapping the spine of the scapula elicits a brisk scapular elevation and abduction of the humerus.

There is a reverse asymmetrical inversion of the biceps and supinator jerks. The triceps jerk was brisk, suggestive of hyperreflexia. The patient exhibited a paradoxical brachioradialis reflex (inverted radial reflex), whereby tapping the distal brachioradialis tendon elicits a reciprocal spastic contracture of the fingers.

Lhermitte's sign was positive, as neck flexion or extension elicited burning electric shock sensations involving the upper and lower extremities and the trunk. The finger escape sign was positive, with the two ulnar digits drifting out. In the grip and release test the patient was unable to repeatedly form a fist and release all digits within a 10-second period. There are no sensory changes in the hands.

The legs in this elderly patient show spastic weakness – the tone is increased and the knee and ankle reflexes are brisk bilaterally.

There is an up-going plantar response (Babinski extensor plantar response). Clonus is present when the foot is rapidly brought up into dorsiflexion from a plantar position. Vibration sense is lost in the lower legs but joint position sense is maintained.

These features are suggestive of cervical myelopathy.

I would like to proceed with AP and lateral radiographs of the cervical spine as well as an MRI scan of the neuroaxis.

Discussion

- Differential diagnosis (intrinsic neoplasm (tumours of spinal cord parenchyma), extrinsic neoplasm (metastatic disease), syringomyelia, amyotrophic lateral sclerosis, vitamin B deficiency, subacute degeneration of the cord, spinal cord infarction, multiple sclerosis)
- Imaging: MRI and CT findings (spinal stenosis and spinal cord compression)
- Consent issues
- Posterior or anterior approach to the cervical spine
- Surgery (removal of osteophytes, disc material, instability, instrument or interposition of bone graft to promote fusion)
- Results of surgery (improvement or at least stabilization of symptoms)

Spondylolisthesis

History

The onset of symptoms is often spontaneous. In young patients there is often a history of trauma. The main symptom is low back pain during physical activity while standing and/or sitting. The pain radiates to the buttocks, to the posterior or lateral aspect of the thigh and occasionally more distally to the ankle or foot.

In severe slips symptoms may include:
- Gait disturbance
- Numbness
- Muscle weakness
- Symptoms of cauda equina compression

Memorandum 1

There is a global reduction in spinal movements to approximately 50% of normal, due to pain, paraspinal muscular spasm and hamstring tightness. There is localized tenderness around the fifth lumbar vertebra and a step can be felt between vertebrae L5 and S1. Hamstrings are tight, however SLR was unrestricted. Tone, power, reflex and sensation of the lower limbs were normal.

Memorandum 2 (severe slip)

The sacrum is in the vertical position due to retroversion of the pelvis and therefore there are prominent buttocks.

There is a short kyphosis at the lumbar sacral junction and a compensatory hyperlordosis of the lumbar spine. There is a lumbar spine scoliotic deformity that is secondary to pain and muscle spasm (it usually disappears after relief of symptoms). The patient is unable to extend their hips or knees fully during standing and they walk with a pelvic waddle. The hamstrings are extremely tight. Straight leg raising was reduced to 60° bilaterally due to pain but there were no true root tension signs. There is global muscle weakness of the lower legs at MRC grade 4+.

Discussion

- Investigations (MRI, CT)
- Meyerding classification
- Radiographs: slip angle, "Scottie dog" sign
- Conservative management
- Indications for surgery

Cervical rib

The cervical rib may be presented as a hand case or a neck examination so be careful. Do not miss a scar in the neck whilst focusing solely on examination of the hand.[5] The cervical rib is usually unilateral and is more common on the right side.

The majority of patients (90%) are asymptomatic. A patient may present with neurological, vascular and local symptoms.

---

[5] A recent downfall in an upper limb short case was not examining the neck in a hand case and missing a scar from cervical rib surgery.

Neurological symptoms

A cervical rib may present with tingling and numbness of the lower part of the brachial plexus (T1) along the medial border of the forearm and hand. There may be weakness and clumsiness of the intrinsic hand muscles.

Vascular symptoms

Compression of the subclavian artery may result in an aneurysm distal to the constriction. This is a potential source of microemboli to the hand and may cause gangrene of the fingertips. There may be a history of pain in the upper limb on using the arm or elevating the hand (claudication).

Local symptoms

Tender supraclavicular lump (anterior end of the cervical rib) that, on palpation, is bony, hard and fixed.

In more advanced cases there will be unilateral vascular changes in the hand: cold, white, mottled or blue, chronic changes or trophic ulcers, atrophy of the finger pulps. There is often thenar muscle wasting.

Feel the radial pulse, apply gentle traction to the arm and see if the pulse's character, volume or signal is altered. Compare both sides.

Hold the arm across the body and feel for the radial pulse. Ask the patient to look towards you and take a deep breath, again assessing both sides, and compare for any differences.

Listen for any bruit with a stethoscope in the supraclavicular fossa.

10

Hip clinical cases

Paul A. Banaszkiewicz

Ankylosing spondylitis

Introduction

Seronegative inflammatory disease of unknown aetiology primarily affecting younger men. Peripheral joint involvement is less common than spinal disease. The hip joint is involved in 30%–50% patients and is usually bilateral (50%–90%). Typical age of onset is 15–25 years. The younger the age at onset the more severe the disease is likely to be and the more likely the need for THA.

History

As for any inflammatory joint disease, the onset is often insidious and patients typically cannot give a precise time of onset or even pinpoint the initially affected side.

Clinical features

Early on the patient has a "hang-dog posture" (rounding of the shoulders and slight dorsal kyphosis). There is a loss of lumbar lordosis and limited spinal movements in all planes. Later, an advanced stoop develops, with limitation of forward vision (question mark posture). The chin brow angle, occiput to wall distance and gaze angle are used to evaluate functional deformity involving the cervical spine. There is severe loss of motion at the hip joint, a fixed flexion deformity or ankylosis. There is also reduced chest expansion.

Radiographs

Radiographs show ossification of the ligamentous origins and insertions about the trochanters, iliac crest and ischial tuberosities. Later on radiographs become similar to those for end-stage primary osteoarthritis.

Management options

If there is any uncertainty about whether the pain is arising from the hip joint or the spine then a local anaesthetic injection into the hip joint may be useful. Hip involvement ranges from flexion contractures to complete ankylosis, often in a disabling flexed position. Generally speaking THA is considered before spinal osteotomy because an improvement in the hip's range of movement and pain relief may obviate the need for a spinal osteotomy in patients with severe hip flexion deformity.

Indications for THA[1]

Indications include severe disabling debilitating pain and correction of severe hip flexion deformities.

Consider bilateral surgery for bilateral fixed flexion deformities. The patient will not be able to stand up straight until both hips have been operated

[1] The pseudoarthrosis test: the absolute indication for performing a total hip arthroplasty would be if the patient would be better off with a Girdlestone excision arthroplasty. The rationale is that if the THA failed and you had to remove it the patient would still be better off than they are at the moment.

Postgraduate Orthopaedics: The Candidate's Guide to the FRCS (Tr & Orth) Examination, Ed. Paul A. Banaszkiewicz, Deiary F. Kader, Nicola Maffulli. Published by Cambridge University Press. © Cambridge University Press 2009.

upon and if more than a few months is left between operating on the two sides the deformity will recur. Another relative indication for bilateral surgery is if there are risks and difficulties associated with the anaesthetic, e.g. need for fibre optic awake intubation. THA consistently improves the range of movement, function and pain.

Technical difficulties

Many surgeons consider THA in patients with ankylosing spondylitis to be a particularly demanding procedure. The correction of longstanding contractures and the accurate placement of the acetabular component in the presence of pelvic obliquity are technically challenging. There is a relatively high incidence of ectopic bone formation after THA, leading to a reduction in the postoperative range of movement.[2] It is more common when trochanteric osteotomy is performed. There are concerns over the young age of the patients, in that they place greater demands on the prosthesis compared to older patients, resulting in increased rates of wear and loosening. In addition ankylosing spondylitis tends to spare upper limbs, resulting in relatively high demands on hip prostheses because overall function is better.

Old DDH

Memorandum

"On examination the left leg appears shortened. The muscle bulk of the left thigh is markedly reduced. There is a compensatory pelvic obliquity/scoliosis/lordosis because of a leg length discrepancy/fixed flexion deformity. The attitude of the leg is one of external rotation compared to the opposite side. The patella is not facing forward suggesting that the rotation is occurring in the femur. I can only partially correct the pelvic obliquity with wooden blocks."

"Examination of gait demonstrates a short-leg antalgic/ waddling gait. There is increased lordosis of the spine and

***

[2] Controversial. Recent reviews of the literature suggest that HO rates may not be dramatically higher compared to age- and sex-matched counterparts.

the body is swaying from side to side on a wide base. The patient lurches on both sides whilst walking and is delayed Trendelenburg positive. When sitting on the bed the scoliosis of the spine only partially corrects, which means that there is an element of both a flexible and a fixed deformity of the spine."

When examining the patient supine on the couch attempt to straighten the pelvis if possible. Comment to the examiners if you can or cannot do this. Measure true and apparent shortening with a tape measure.

If the patient has a fixed pelvic obliquity then the apparent leg length (as measured from the umbilicus to the medial malleolus) should be used to determine the amount of lengthening that is necessary with total hip arthroplasty. Galeazzi's test and Bryant's triangle should be performed if there is any suggestion of true shortening. It is important to differentiate between true and apparent shortening and to be able to explain this to the examiners if asked. Check for a difference in rotation of the hip when flexed or extended due to discrepancy in the shape of the femoral head in the acetabulum.

"The peripheral pulses are palpable with good capillary refill of the toes. Straight leg raising did not produce any low back pain or root tension signs."

Technical considerations

Can be technically very difficult surgery depending on the severity of the DDH. The patient should be forewarned that the operation might be abandoned if either abductor musculature is poor or the bone of the pelvis is inadequate.

There is a possibility of fracturing the femur whilst attempting to reduce the THA, especially if reduction is tight because of leg lengthening. The level of the true acetabulum needs to be defined for placement of the cup (the surgical landmark is the obturator foramen). A drill hole may be used to perforate the medial part of the acetabulum and a depth gauge may be used to decide how far to ream the acetabulum. Be aware of the possibility of sciatic nerve injury from excessive lengthening.

In the discussion section of the long case you may be asked about:

- Advantages and disadvantages of anatomic versus non-anatomic reconstruction
- Whether to use an uncemented or cemented implant
- The need for bone graft (bone graft is a large and important topic and the examiners can take you anywhere with it)
- A classification system for DDH

Discussion

Surgery is only indicated if there is disabling pain and all conservative managements options have been exhausted. Subluxation or significant adduction deformity can cause functional shortening of the leg and secondary long leg arthritis in the opposite knee (due to walking on a flexed knee to compensate for a leg length discrepancy or indeed a valgus deformity of the ipsilateral knee due to severe adduction deformity of the ipsilateral hip).

Progressive knee arthritis may become a relative indication for joint replacement. Attempts to correct limb length discrepancy should be viewed with great caution. Is the hip subluxed (acetabular dysplasia) or dislocated?

Long case 1

17-year-old girl, bilateral DDH

Principal complaints are pain and shortening.

On examination

Bilateral Smith-Peterson scars (well healed) and a lateral proximal femoral scar. (Why would a young adult have a well-healed scar from an anterior approach to the hip?)

There is a right hip coxa vara deformity; the greater trochanter is very prominent.

The pelvis is not level: there is a leg length discrepancy with the right leg 1 cm short.

There is a compensatory scoliosis, apex-left; it is a combination of both structural and postural elements. The patient has a short-leg gait, Trendelenburg negative.

Sit patient on the edge of the couch to check the scoliosis deformity.

Ask the patient to lie supine: positive lump sign on the left (dislocated femoral head).

Straighten the pelvis: 1 cm shortening, Galeazzi's sign.

Carry out the Thomas test to test patient's range of movement.

Check internal and external rotation in extension (prone) (rotational profile).

When surgery has been performed through an anterior approach, it may be important to free up the anterior capsule and structures from the overlying femoral neurovascular bundle to prevent accidental damage either by dissection or retraction.

Long case 2

45-year-old lady with bilateral DDH

The patient had undergone open reduction and pelvic osteotomies when 2 years old. She had a right THA at the age of 35 years that is now painful. Her left hip is arthritic and painful; she is awaiting THA.

Take a detailed history of the DDH.

Demonstrate various signs: Thomas test, Trendelenburg test, hip range of movement.

Explain the management of a painful right THA and painful left hip.

Describe the technical difficulties in performing THA in DDH, explaining the role of the CT scan in planning the operation.

Describe the effect of anteversion on THA (component malalignment, dislocation).

Describe correction of leg length inequality in DDH (decide preoperatively, sciatic nerve function). Explain the use of bone grafts when performing THA. Describe the long-term results of THA in patients with prior DDH (when properly performed, THA for DDH can result in good long-term results. McKenzie reported 85% survival at 15 years).[1]

Revision of patients who have undergone THA for DDH is extremely difficult, particularly when the acetabulum has been placed high and revision has been delayed. There is often no anterior wall, little posterior wall and only the remnants of a medial plate. Femoral revision can be difficult, as the prosthesis may have been inserted with an uncorrected deformity. If a trochanteric osteotomy has gone on to develop a non-union, trochanteric drift is difficult to correct. Soft-tissue balance in these patients is extremely difficult and therefore dislocation rates are high.

[1] MacKenzie JR, Kelley SS, Johnston RC (1996) Total hip replacement for coxarthrosis secondary to congenital dysplasia and dislocation of the hip. Long-term results. *J Bone Joint Surg Am* **78**(1): 55–61.

Perthes disease

Memorandum

"On general examination the patient is of average height and build. He looks well for his age."

Standing

"On examination standing there are no scars present/a well-healed lateral proximal thigh scar/an anterior Smith-Peterson scar from a previous hip surgery (femoral osteotomy/acetabular osteotomy)."

Carefully look for mild/moderate thigh or gluteal muscle wastage and comment on this finding to the examiners. The thigh musculature may be normal if the individual is bulky with minimal disease. It is unlikely that a significant leg length discrepancy will be present; at worst there will possibly be some mild shortening of the affected leg by 1–2 cm. If by chance the shortening is >2 cm look for a flexed attitude of the uninvolved limb or equinus posture of the involved foot. There may be a mild external-rotation deformity of the affected leg. The patient may have a mild or moderate antalgic gait (with a short leg component – if shortening is present and clinically significant). The patient may have a Trendelenburg-positive or delayed Trendelenburg-positive test.

Supine

Comment on any additional features not apparent on initial inspection of the leg when standing.

Re-comment on any feature already mentioned particularly if it is more apparent supine. Comment on the attitude of the leg, especially if it lies in external rotation.

Look at the relative position of the heels as a rough guide to shortening (make sure the pelvis is level). Measure leg lengths and if shortening is present continue on and perform Galeazzi's test and digital Bryant's test, etc. Flex the hips to 45° and the knees up to 90° and place the heels together. Femoral shortening is apparent as a decreased prominence of the tibial tubercle. Tibial shortening shows similarly at the superior pole of the patella.

For the sake of completeness then go on to palpation of the hip. "Palpation of the hip revealed no specific areas of tenderness. Thomas test demonstrates a fixed flexion deformity of 50°."

Measure the range of movement of the hip and compare it to that of the opposite, normal side. Comment if it is painful and be careful not to hurt the patient. "There is a mild/moderate/gross painful restriction of all ranges of movement in the hip." Go on to perform a neurovascular examination of the lower leg. "Examination of the spine was normal with good forward flexion, extension and lateral flexion demonstrated." Similarly examination of both knees was unremarkable.

Radiographs

AP radiographs may demonstrate old features of Perthes disease: elongated, deformed and flattened femoral head with subluxation or a sagging rope sign (classic radiographic feature of Perthes disease). Mention the radiographic differential diagnosis for Perthes disease and if possible Stulberg's radiographic classification of residue deformity and degenerative joint disease (but be sensible; if you are only vaguely familiar with it, don't go there).

Management options

Conservative

Supervised neglect: analgesia, physiotherapy, hospital admissions for acute exacerbations and regular outpatient physiotherapy.

Ambulation abduction brace

This is controversial, as several studies have concluded that bracing does not alter the natural history of the disease.[3, 4]

Operative containment

- Proximal femoral varus osteotomy. This shortens the limb and aggravates the Trendelenburg limp. May require the removal of metalwork.
- Innominate osteotomy. May lengthen the affected leg by 1 cm.

Salvage

- Valgus osteotomy (abduction–extension). If hinged abduction is present. The patient should have at least 15° of passive adduction and should be comfortable in the adducted position. The limb is inevitably lengthened to a certain extent. Lateral displacement of the shaft is carried out to align the mechanical axis of the limb through the centre of the knee.
- Chiari osteotomy/shelf procedure. This is used for head coverage if a hinged abduction is seen in the proximal femur.
- Trochanteric advancement is occasionally required for trochanteric overgrowth when the disease causes premature closure of the capital femoral epiphysis. Elevation (overgrowth) of the greater trochanter decreases tension as well as the mechanical efficiency of the pelvis and trochanteric muscles.

Technical difficulties with THA in Perthes disease

An anteverted femoral neck may mislead the surgeon during stem insertion and lead to component mal-positioning. A previous femoral osteotomy may cause difficulties in reaming the femoral canal. If prior hip surgery has been performed, there is an increased risk of HO, infection, scarring, distorted anatomy, contracted musculature, etc.

Long case 1

History

Candidate: This is Mr. White. He is a 39-year-old male who works as a railway engineer and is married with three children who all live at home. His presenting complaint is of a painful right hip following Perthes disease as a child. Specifically in the last 3–4 years he has developed increasingly severe pain in this hip. The pain is felt mostly in the groin but can radiate down the anterior aspect of his thigh to the knee. His walking distance is reduced to 2 miles. He has occasional sleep disturbance. He is able to put his shoes and socks on, and get in and out of a bath and car. He sometimes has difficulty getting up and down stairs at home. He is taking analgesia intermittently when his hip is particularly painful. When he needs analgesics he usually takes paracetamol but occasionally needs dihydrocodeine. He is just about managing his job as a railway engineer but has been put on light duties in the last 6 months and is unsure whether he will be allowed to continue with this. He does not use any walking aids. He has a shoe rise in his right shoe, which he continues to use, but says he doesn't find it particularly useful.

    As regards the Perthes disease, in childhood it was managed conservatively without any operations.[1] It was first diagnosed when he was 7 years old. He did spend about 6 months in hospital at one stage when he was 11 years old because of severe pain but treatment was bed rest, traction and physiotherapy.

    He wore walking callipers for 2 years during his illness. He was followed up by his local hospital until he was 18 years old and then discharged. He was seen 6 years ago by the orthopaedic surgeons at his local hospital because of increasing pain in the right hip and I believe an arthrogram was performed and osteotomy of the hip considered at the time but decided against as symptoms were manageable. He has been seen regularly in the orthopaedic clinic at 6-monthly intervals for the past 2 years. He is otherwise well with an unremarkable past medical history: he has had no operations or any other specific medical conditions. He has no known allergies. He is a non-smoker and takes about 4 units of alcohol a week on a Saturday night.

[3] Meehan PL, Angel D, Nelson JM (1992) The Scottish Rite abduction orthosis for the treatment of Legg-Perthes disease. A radiographic analysis. *J Bone Joint Surg Am* 74(1):2–12.
[4] Martinez AG, Weinstein SL, Dietz FR (1992) The weight-bearing abduction brace for the treatment of Legg-Perthes disease. *J Bone Joint Surg Am* 74(1):12–21.

Examination

Examiner: We would like you to examine his hip and talk us through it as you go along.

Candidate: On examination we have a patient of muscular build, average height. Turning towards his right hip he has mild, right, proximal thigh muscle wasting but from the back his gluteal muscles seem reasonably well preserved.[2]

Examiner: If you look very closely there is in fact a small amount of gluteal wasting which is apparent when you compare it to the opposite side.

Candidate: I didn't look closely enough and missed this subtle clinical finding.

Candidate: Examining his gait he walks reasonably comfortably without any obvious abnormality present.

Examiner: I don't think that's quite the case. *Could you just walk for us again sir, away from us and then towards us?* He demonstrates a mild antalgic right gait (not particularly obvious).

Candidate: I will go on now and perform a Trendelenburg test. He is Trendelenburg positive on the right; I can feel his right hand push down on my left hand and his pelvis descends down to the right indicating abductor muscle dysfunction.

Examiner: That's a good demonstration of the Trendelenburg test except that you have tested the wrong leg.[3]

Candidate: I would like now to examine the hip supine. *Could you lie down on the couch for me now sir?* His pelvis is level, the anterior superior iliac spines are at the same level and the legs are square with the pelvis and straight. The right leg is shorter than the left. I'd like to confirm this by measuring leg lengths formally. I'm measuring from the anterior superior iliac spine to the medial malleolus; on the right side the leg measures 91 cm; the left, 92 cm. Thomas test reveals no fixed flexion deformity of either hip. There is a restricted range of movement of the right hip compared to the left. Flexion 70°, abduction 20°, adduction 10°, almost no internal or external rotation in flexion. Movements of the hip were painful especially at the extremes of movement.

Examiner: Did you examine anywhere else to exclude referred pain to the hip?

Candidate: I examined the spine. In particular I tested his spinal movements, which were unrestricted, and pain free.

Examiner: Are there any other causes of referred pain to the hip?

Candidate: The pain is arising from the hip joint. I have checked his spinal movements and these are normal. Forward flexion, extension, lateral rotation and lateral flexion are all full and pain free and straight leg raising was normal. These tests would seem to exclude the spine as a source of referred pain.

The limb was neurovascularly intact with good peripheral pulses palpated and normal capillary refill.

Examiner: Is there anything else that could be causing his pain?

Candidate: Examination of the right knee was unremarkable. I can't think of anything else in particular that could be a cause of his pain.

Examiner: You have excluded the main causes of referred pain to the hip. Can you think of anything else?

Candidate: No sir.

Examiner: Have you heard of the piriformis syndrome?

Candidate: No sir, sorry I have not.

Examiner: Well let me demonstrate it to you.

The examiner then proceeded to demonstrate this test on the patient describing to the candidate what he was doing as he went along. The test was negative. The examiner seemed to enjoy himself when demonstrating this test and it served as a useful learning point for the candidate.

Piriformis test

The piriformis test is performed with the patient in the lateral decubitus position with the side to be examined facing up. The patient's hip is flexed 45° with the knee flexed about 90°. The examiner stabilizes the patient's pelvis with one hand to prevent rocking. The other hand then pushes the flexed hip towards the floor. This manoeuvre stretches the piriformis muscle and elicits pain when the muscle is tight or involved with tendonitis. If the pain is not localized to the piriformis tendon but radiates in a manner suggestive of sciatica, a piriformis syndrome should be suspected. The piriformis syndrome is an uncommon cause of sciatica in which the radiation of pain along the course of the sciatic nerve is caused by entrapment within the piriformis muscle instead of lumbar disc disease.

Overview of clinical case

- Detailed history of the management of Perthes disease as a child
- Demonstration of full hip examination
- Discussion about causes of referred pain to the hip (did you check his spinal movements?)
- Piriformis syndrome and how to test for it (irritation of the sciatic nerve by the edge of the piriformis muscle)

Discussion

- General discussion about the radiographs of the right hip: moderate osteoarthritis, features of old Perthes disease, sagging rope sign, etc. Shown arthrogram pictures and asked to comment on them, which led on to a general discussion about the principles of arthrograms.
- Full discussion on the classification of Perthes disease (Catterall, Salter and Herring). I went through each one in turn and then mentioned which one I preferred and why. Discussion of Stulberg's[4] rating system of the femoral head at maturity and Herring treatment guidelines for Perthes disease.[5]
- Management: the patient's hip arthritis was too good for a THA so continue with conservative management for the time being. There is a possible role for osteotomy in the arthritic hip. Discuss the figures for survival of total hip arthroplasty in the young arthritic male (results from Wrightington, Swedish hip register[6]).[7]
- Clarify what type of THA you would perform and why.

Candidate: I was the last candidate of the day and the examiners began to get bored half way through the discussion. Presumably by that time they had decided to pass me. They seemed to run out of steam and struggled a bit to spin the discussion out to the bell. The patient was very helpful as he knew his history inside out by this stage and was very clear and concise with it. He even suggested I should be aware of the differences between real and apparent shortening.[8] The last candidate had been grilled on it for some time and the examiners were not entirely happy that they had explained it correctly.[9] The patient also suggested I might want to perform Galeazzi's test which I had forgotten to do.[10]

Long case 2[11]

Candidate: My long case was a 39-year-old man with an arthritic hip after having had Perthes disease as a child. He had no other problems.

I was clearly very lucky, because I had finished everything by about 20 minutes and even had time to go back and recheck my examination findings. Others had people with multiple joint problems and found they were a bit pushed for time.

The examiners came in and we spent 15 minutes going through the history and examination. They were both very pleasant and took things very gently.

Examinations carried out included:
- Trendelenburg test
- Thomas test
- Leg length discrepancy: real and apparent
- Galeazzi's test
- Tests for abduction, adduction and rotation

We then left and spent 15 minutes going through his X-rays, Perthes disease and the management options.

[1] It is important in the history for the sake of completeness to go into as much detail as possible about how the Perthes disease was managed as a child. (However, be quick about it and be careful with your time!) Did the patient have surgery, were they admitted to hospital at any time, did they use an ambulation abduction brace, etc.? The examiner may jump over this part of the history and not be interested in a long dialogue but could possibly probe you, especially if he or she thinks you have not been thorough enough in your history.

[2] Do not miss obvious muscle wasting!

[3] I got left and right mixed up but luckily the examiners let me off.

[4] Stulberg SD, Cooperman DR, Wallensten R (1981) The natural history of Legg-Calvé-Perthes disease. *J Bone Joint Surg Am* **63-A**: 1095–108.

[5] Herring JA (1994) The treatment of Legg-Calvé-Perthes disease. A critical review of the literature. *J Bone Joint Surg Am* 76(3): 448–58.

[6] Wroblewski BM, Siney PD, Fleming PA (2004) Wear of the cup in the Charnley LFA in the young patient. *J Bone Joint Surg Br* 86(4): 498–503.

[7] Know the prerequisites for an innominate osteotomy as the examiners could easily lead into this with follow-up questions.

[8] Old-style long case in which the candidate was left to take the history and exam without the examiners being there. The exam has changed format since then.

[9] There is a thin line between ungentlemanly conduct and opportunism.

[10] I hesitate to suggest that it would have been a glaring omission but it meant the examination proceeded much more comfortably than might otherwise have been the case.

[11] This is the same patient as in long case 1. It is included here as it gives a different candidate's account of the same long-case patient. It is rather like two paintings of the same scene by two different artists.

The hip needing revision surgery

History

Pain

Most patients complain of an aching type of pain, which is mechanical in nature. It is typically provoked by activity and relieved by rest. The intensity is usually variable although not often great. Failure of the acetabular component may cause groin and/or buttock pain. Femoral component failure more often causes thigh pain. Aseptic loosening is often associated with an initial marked exacerbation of discomfort when the patient first stands up, which reaches a steady state over the next few minutes and thereafter the pain may reduce. It is characterized by a pain-free interval following the initially successful arthroplasty surgery.

Patients with septic loosening may give a history of pain that has persisted since the time of the original operation. Alternatively there may be a sudden onset of pain following the spread of infection from some distant septic focus. The pain itself is typically insidious in onset and both gradually and relentlessly progressive.

Ambulation capacity

Patients may complain of a limp and a progressive reduction in walking distance. They have difficulty in climbing stairs.

Shortening

Progressive shortening may be noticed by the patient. This may be caused by proximal and medial migration of the acetabular component with or without subsidence of the femoral component.

Stiffness

Difficulty in donning shoes, putting on socks, cutting toenails, bending down to pick objects off the floor, etc.

Instability

Recurrent episodes of subluxation or dislocation. Instability can cause pain from capsular stretch and soft-tissue impingement. Symptoms can usually be reproduced by placing the limb in a certain position and usually recur each time that position is re-created.

Sepsis

Enquire about any delays in wound healing, haematoma formation, excessive wound drainage and antibiotic usage at the time of primary surgery. Is there any history of urinary catheterization following surgery? Has the hip always been painful or just in the last year or so? Have there been any recent chest or urine infections or generalized systemic upset?

Referred pain

Lumbar spondylosis, spinal stenosis and sciatica, and peripheral vascular disease may all provoke discomfort, which resembles hip pain.

Clinical examination

Carry out a general inspection to include general stature, height and weight. Examine the quality of the skin overlying the joint. Note any previous skin incisions.

"There is a well-healed right mid-lateral proximal thigh scar without any evidence of redness, heat or localized tissue swelling. The right leg appears shortened and externally rotated when the pelvis has been levelled. There is marked muscle atrophy present in the right thigh. There are gross bilateral prominent varicose veins with chronic venous ulceration of both lower legs."[5]

Gait should be carefully observed to look for antalgic gait, limb-length discrepancy or abductor deficiency. The onset of limb length inequality should be related to the time of the operation, as progressive shortening and muscle weakness may indicate subsidence of one of the components.

"When observing the right leg supine it was again noted to be in a position of slight external rotation in comparison to the left side. There was obvious right leg shortening present. Formal measurement of leg lengths revealed a true leg length discrepancy of 2 cm on the right side. Galeazzi's sign indicated that this shortening was in the

---

[5] It is important to notice these peripheral clinical findings and even more important to mention them to the examiners.

femur. Bryant's triangle test suggested that the discrepancy was proximal to the greater trochanter."

"The temperature of the joint and surrounding tissues appeared normal. There was no localized tenderness to palpation. There were well-preserved movements of the hip joint but they were painful at the extremes of movement."

Specific restrictions in ranges of movement may be related to impingement, contracture or heterotopic bone formation. Pain at the extremes of movement may indicate impingement or loosening of prosthetic components. Pain with jerking the leg into internal or external rotation is suggestive of femoral component loosening. Pain in the groin with resisted straight-leg raising is suggestive of acetabular loosening.

"Examination of motor power of the lower limbs revealed MRC grade 5 power on the left side but grade 4 MRC powers of the right gluteal and flexor muscles of the pelvis. The right abductor muscles were MRC power weak grade 4. Right quadriceps power was also reduced to grade 4 MRC but hamstring power was well preserved as was that of the foot dorsiflexors and plantar flexors."

"Sensation was normal in both lower limbs and straight-leg raising was full in both legs and did not produce any pain referred to either the legs or the lumbar spine. Femoral, popliteal, dorsalis pedis and posterior tibial pulses were all palpable and full in both legs with good capillary refill in the toes."

Radiographs

"This is an AP radiograph of the pelvis. It shows an obviously loose femoral component with luciencies present in all seven Gruen zones. There is cement outside the femur. The femoral component is a Charnley prosthesis. The long stem femoral component suggests that the hip is probably a revision-type prosthesis or custom prosthesis.[6] I would be interested in viewing previous radiographs to determine the amount of migration of both the femoral and acetabular components. I would also be interested in seeing a lateral radiograph."

---

[6] Use of a Charnley long stem prosthesis in a primary hip procedure is suggestive of the occurrence of significant complications during this index operation.

Discussion

- Indications and contraindications for revision hip surgery
- Differentiation between aseptic loosening and infection
- Preoperative planning
- Surgical approaches used and equipment necessary
- How are you going to get the acetabular component out and deal with the bony defect?
- How are you going to get the femoral component out and deal with the defect?

Long case 1

A 79-year-old man with right THA

Postoperatively the wound was oozy for a few days. This hip was thought to be loose at 18 months. Coagulase-negative *Staphylococcus* was obtained on aspiration of the hip. First-stage revision was performed using a Prostolac® spacer and intravenous vancomycin treatment. Second-stage revision was performed 3 months later. Dislocation of the right hip occurred 1 month following surgery. We are now 2 years on from successful revision for infection.

Long case 2

A 32-year-old African woman with revised right THA

The first THA was performed at the age of 20, which required revision surgery 2 years ago after 10 years of good results. She now presents with progressively worsening right hip pain, which had started 6 months after the revision surgery. The leg itself was shortened by 2 cm. The patient had a normal childhood. Her sister died young as a result of sickle cell disease.

Points to note:
- Discussion on the possible causes of initial hip pain leading to a THA being performed at the age of 20
- Was it a missed DDH, avascular necrosis of the hip secondary to sickle cell disease or infection?

- The examiners asked the patient themselves to confirm some of the history, mainly on possible childhood problems
- Management options now

Paget's disease

Memorandum

History

"Mr. McDonald is an 80-year-old retired farmer married with two grown-up children who presents with a 4-year history of increasing pain in his left hip."

"He was diagnosed as having Paget's disease 6 years ago and was started on regular bisphosphonates for the condition 2 years ago. His left hip pain was initially a dull ache but has become progressively more severe in recent months and now keeps him awake most nights. His walking distance is reduced to 200 metres and he finds he can no longer go to the shops with his wife because of his hip pain. Although his son runs the farm up until 18 months ago he was able to help out with some of the work but now finds this impossible because of his pain. He has used a stick in his left hand for the last year to increase his mobility."

"On enquiry about general health he denies any hearing difficulties, headaches or vertigo. He did complain of chronic intermittent low backache, which sounded like mechanical back pain rather than anything more sinister."

Pain in the hip associated with Paget's disease of the femur may cause diagnostic problems. It can be very difficult to distinguish whether the pain is due to Paget's disease or to degenerate arthritis of the hip. A therapeutic trial of calcitonin may be helpful to differentiate between the two causes. If the character of the pain changes and becomes much worse and continuous it is important to consider the possibility of sarcomatous change.

Examination

"On general inspection there is enlargement of the skull. There is also bowing of both the femur and tibia in both legs in both the AP and lateral directions. The sharp anterior edges of both tibiae are thickened and curved making them very prominent and giving an almost sabre tibia appearance to them."

"On palpation of both lower legs there was no suggestion of the presence of increased warmth (due to increased vascularity)."

"The spine has a uniform, even kyphosis present (vertebral involvement leads to loss of height and kyphosis from disc degeneration and vertebral collapse)."

"The shoulders are rounded and the head and neck protrude anteriorly. The skull enlargement occurs in the vault and the enlarged frontal bones make the forehead bulge forwards. His arms appear to be disproportionately long (because of the kyphosis)."

"Examination of his left hip revealed gluteal and thigh muscle wastage. He had a marked stoop present, attenuated by bowing of both his femurs. Examination of gait revealed that it was antalgic in nature. The Trendelenburg test was markedly positive on the right side and delayed positive on the left side. Examination supine revealed equal leg lengths. On palpation of the hip there were no obvious areas of tenderness. A Thomas test revealed a fixed flexion deformity of 30°. Flexion of the hip was painful and reduced to 70° actively, which could not be increased appreciably passively. Internal rotation in flexion was zero whilst external rotation in flexion was grossly reduced to a jog of movement only. Similarly adduction was limited to 20° and abduction to 30° passively and it was also painful. Distal pulses were palpable with good capillary refill and neurological examination of the lower legs was normal. There was marked restriction of all spinal movements, in particular forward flexion – he was only able to touch his knees. Straight-leg raising reproduced low back pain but no true sciatic nerve root irritation."

Discussion

Paget's disease is a chronic deforming metabolic bone disease characterized by increased osteoclastic bone resorption and compensatory increases in bone formation. In the later stages of the disease the involved bone becomes enlarged, dense, sclerotic with an irregular trabecular pattern, an obliterated medullary canal and thickened cortices. The poor structural integrity of the bone renders it prone to either pathological fracture or repetitive stress fractures. Progressive deformity and secondary osteoarthritis of the hip affects between 30% and 50% of patients. For Paget's disease that involves the hip with secondary degenerative changes, surgery is indicated to manage significant pain, joint stiffness, deformity or a pathological fracture.

Preoperative treatment with bisphosphonates or calcitonin has been used to reduce the incidence of intra-operative bleeding, HO and loosening. There is a potential for significant intra-operative bleeding from hypervascular and osteoporotic bone. Excessive bleeding may prove troublesome and may require additional cross-matching of blood.

Proper preoperative templating and planning are necessary to size an enlarged medullary canal and to determine the correct component size and amount of cement to be used.

A broad spectrum of deformities of the proximal femur or acetabulum may hamper dislocation of the hip, exposure of bone or component alignment. Trochanteric osteotomy may be required for adequate exposure and beware of the sciatic nerve, which is nearer the joint than normal. In the presence of protrusio acetabulum combined with coxa vara, dislocation of the hip can be extremely difficult and the neck may need to be cut in situ.

A marked deformity of the proximal femur with coxa vara or anterolateral bowing of the femoral shaft may require a corrective osteotomy prior to THA. This will allow for alignment of the femoral component properly at the time of THA. The presence of dense sclerotic bone may make reaming and bone preparation difficult. Sharp reamers will be necessary to shape the femoral canal.

If protrusio acetabulum exists ream to expand the periphery without deepening the socket to avoid causing added protrusio. Consider what method of cup fixation to use: either uncemented acetabular fixation with supplementary screws or a cemented cup. Reconstruct the acetabulum with the hip centre in the anatomical location and reconstruct cavitatory and segmental defects in the medial wall with supplementary bone grafting.

A widened femoral canal can be dealt with either by using extra cement or by primary impaction grafting with cancellous allograft chips. Obliteration of the femoral canal with bone as opposed to cement is thought to provide a much more durable anchorage of the stem but is technically more difficult to do and increases surgical time. A large cement restrictor or bone plug may be required. There is an increased incidence of HO in this condition, therefore prophylaxis should be considered.

Radiographs

Sclerotic appearance of the bone with cortical thickening; trabeculae are coarse and widely separated.

Differential diagnosis

Osteitis fibrosa cystica, fibrous dysplasia, osteoblastic secondaries, osteopetrosis and lymphoma.

Long case 1

Examiner: What are the indications for therapy in Paget's disease?
Candidate:
- Bone pain
- Deformity
- Fracture
- Osteolytic lesions in weight-bearing bones
- Immobilization hypercalcaemia
- Markedly increased alkaline phosphatase
- Nerve compression
- Young age especially if disease is very active
- Before orthopaedic surgery

Ineffective for:
- Deafness
- Fissure fracture
- Sarcoma

Examiner: What are the causes of a bowed tibia?
Candidate: True bowing due to softening of bone occurs in Paget's disease and rickets. Apparent bowing due to thickening of the anterior surface of the tibia secondary to periostitis occurs in congenital syphilis and yaws.

Examiner: What are the complications of Paget's disease?
Candidate: Progressive closure of skull foramina may lead to:
- Headaches
- Deafness
- Blindness (optic atrophy)
- Tinnitus
- Vertigo

Other complication include:
- High output cardiac failure
- Pathological fractures
- Sarcoma change in bone
- Urolithiasis

- Spinal stenosis
- Hypercalcaemia

The pattern of presentation is variable. Only a minority of patients become symptomatic.

Examiner: How common is sarcomatous change in bone?

Candidate: It is very rare, probably less than 1%, but it carries a very poor prognosis. The patient presents with increased pain and swelling.

Examiner: What biochemical abnormalities occur in Paget's disease?

Candidate: Serum alkaline phosphatase and urinary hydroxyproline are elevated except sometimes in very early disease. Serum calcium and phosphate are usually normal in mobilized patients but can occasionally be increased or decreased. Urinary calcium rises in immobilized patients.

Adult elective orthopaedics oral 1

- Discussion on Paget's hip
- Radiographic features
- Management options
- Bisphosphonates and their mechanism of action
- Precautions prior to THA
- Technical difficulties of THA

Short case 1

Paget's tibia

Examiner: Examine this man's leg. What is the diagnosis?

Candidate: Bowed, enlarged leg, no other deformities, only other clue was hearing aid.

Candidate: The examiner wanted me to mention sabre tibia. In the tibia the forward bowing confirmed in lateral radiographs may be referred to as a sabre tibia (since the front of the tibia is blunt not sharp this is hardly appropriate). Also this is not strictly correct, as sabre tibia is usually associated with syphilis disease of bone. Syphilitic osteoperiostitis occurs late in the disease, on average 6 years after untreated syphilis. Usually one bone becomes painful and tender. Often the bone gives an illusion of being bent, because new bone is deposited beneath the periosteum on one aspect.

Adult elective orthopaedics oral 2

- Pathogenesis of Paget's disease
- Complications

- Radiographic features
- Cause of bone bowing
- Management of pathological fractures
- Problems encountered in joint replacement: how do you control bleeding?

Post-traumatic osteoarthritis of the hip

Accidents involving high-energy trauma may cause fractures of the acetabulum and fractures/dislocation of the hip joint. The treatment of choice for post-traumatic osteoarthritis in patients over 50 is THA but a younger patient is more likely to place higher demands on any implant.

Memorandum

History

- Age
- Occupation
- A full history should be obtained starting with the presenting complaint and any symptoms or disability experienced by the patient
- Full details of the original accident should be taken, including the mechanism, all injuries sustained and the time course of subsequent treatment
- The timing and nature of all operative procedures and the development of any complications should be documented with specific enquiry about any systemic or wound infections or thromboembolism
- Progress since the injury
- The onset, nature, progression and aggravating and relieving factors or symptoms should be established
- Social (smoking, alcohol) and general history
- Systemic enquiry about general health
- Expectation and ambitions of the patient

Examination

- Comment on the patient's posture, stance and gait patterns. Scars inspected for site as this may interfere with subsequent surgery, look for any evidence of ongoing infection. Carry out Trendelenburg test for abductor function

- Measure true and apparent leg lengths for adduction contracture. The mechanical axis of the legs and true leg lengths should be compared for the effects of the hip pathology or any associated injury to either lower leg
- The Thomas test is used to detect a fixed flexion deformity. Examine the range of movement of the hip and the presence of pain or fixed deformity
- Muscle power, tone and distal neurovascular status should be checked for evidence of impairment due to nerve palsy or vascular injury
- Knees, the contralateral hip and the lumbar spine should be thoroughly examined especially if arthrodesis is being considered

---

Long case 1

A 16-year-old girl who had been involved in a road traffic accident 1 year previously and had developed AVN with secondary osteoarthritis of her left hip

She had sustained a closed fracture of the right femoral shaft, which was treated with skeletal traction, and a traumatic posterior dislocation of her left hip. The left hip had been reduced under GA fairly promptly after admission. She, however, continued to complain of left hip pain following relocation and 4 days later a further radiograph was taken, which showed a displaced fracture of the femoral head. This was fixed with a cannulated hip screw the following day.

Essentially her presenting complaint was of severe constant pain in her left hip interfering with every aspect of her life. Her walking distance was reduced to a few hundred yards, sleep was severely affected and she was taking regular analgesia with minimal benefit.

Extracting the history from the patient was taxing and clinical examination was difficult; she was in a fair amount of pain when the left hip was moved.

The whole thing collapsed on the examination side of the long case. The examiners seemed to lose patience very quickly. Forgetting to perform the Trendelenburg test was fatal. Despite recovering during the discussion afterwards the candidate couldn't drag the long case back to a pass.

Examiner: Can you take us through your examination of this patient?

Candidate: On general inspection we have a young girl of average height and build. There is an old longitudinal lateral scar present over the right proximal thigh. There are other numerous scars both surgical and non-surgical present over the left and right lower legs. Her pelvis is not level when standing: the ASIS is lower on the left side. She appears to have a leg length discrepancy: the left leg appears to be shorter than the right.

Examiner: Hold on! Hold on a minute! You are jumping too quick with things. You can't say this till later.

Candidate: She walks with an antalgic gait. Can you lie down for us now so that we can continue with the examination? On inspection supine …

Examiner: You did perform the Trendelenburg test, did you?

Candidate: I'm sorry I completely forgot.

The patient had a severe adduction contracture of her left leg, which gave the erroneous impression of severe shortening on the left side. However, most of this was apparent shortening. True shortening of the left leg was minimal and probably not significant.

There is real shortening of 1 cm in the left leg, which I think is occurring in the femur presumably above the trochanter. I do not think this is too significant as in a normal individual this leg length discrepancy can be present without any clinical concern.[1]

Examiner: What do you mean a leg length discrepancy of 1 cm is not significant? Are you sure this is true?

Candidate: A 1-cm difference is not clinically significant and could easily be caused by inaccuracies in measurements.

Examiner: I do not agree with you but let's move on. Why don't you demonstrate to us how you measure leg lengths?

Candidate: Measuring real leg lengths confirms my previous clinical finding of 1 cm shortening on the left side.

Examiner: How do you know the left leg is short? There was a femoral fracture on the right side. Could the left leg not be a normal length and the problem is a longer right leg secondary to the right femoral fracture? In fact the right leg could be shorter than normal but the left leg be even shorter because of the hip condition.[2]

Examiner: Could you demonstrate the Thomas test for me?

Candidate: She has a very painful hip and found it uncomfortable when the Thomas test was performed previously.

Examiner: Just go ahead and be gentle.

Examiner: You have not put your hand properly behind the lumbar spine. Let me show you: this is where your hand should be. It should go all the way behind the small of the patient's back. The patient has a fixed flexion deformity of 20°.

Examiner: Can you show us how you measured movements of the hip?

Candidate: I began by measuring flexion. She flexes the hip from 20° to 100°.

Examiner: You have not stabilized the pelvis when testing for flexion of the hip and the pelvis moves a lot sooner than you demonstrated. Here let me verify this to you. See the pelvis moves a lot sooner than you think. You are out 100% in your measurement: active flexion of the left hip is only 40°. You must stabilize the pelvis when measuring flexion of the hip.[3]

Discussion

Discussion centred on the management of this patient. She was too young for a THA and unlikely to be happy with a fusion. Secondary OA was too far advanced for an osteotomy and the condition was too painful to do nothing. No definite management plan was agreed upon.

Radiographs of the initial dislocation were shown. The day-4 radiographs showed a transepiphyseal fracture of the femoral head through the proximal femoral physis. The examiner described it as a type of SUFE. Delbert's classification of hip fractures in children was briefly mentioned. Discussion then followed of the postoperative radiograph, which showed the fracture adequately fixed with a single cannulated hip screw. I was asked about the entry point for cannulated screw fixation for SUFE (it is not the DHS entry point for a proximal femoral fracture, it is much more anterior).

Transepiphyseal fractures represent about 8% of all hip fractures in children. They may occur with or without dislocation of the femoral head and results are generally poor due to a combination of AVN and premature closure of the physis. The diagnosis is often delayed because of concomitant injuries. The patient had developed AVN of the left hip but we didn't discuss this.

I recovered in the discussion and gave a reasonably good account of myself but the examination part of the long case had not gone particularly well and a reasonable history and discussion are not able to compensate for a very poor clinical examination.

---

[1] With the retrospectoscope this was a dangerous thing to say; far better to have just stuck with the clinical findings.

[2] The candidate is definitely in serious trouble with the examiner.

[3] Definitely failed by this stage.

Arthrodesed hip

This is classic material for the hip long case, in which there are good clinical signs to demonstrate and enough to talk about in the discussion afterwards. At least one arthrodesed hip will be present in the short case examination hall.

Memorandum [7]

"On general inspection the patient has a walking stick visible in the corner. He also has a shoe raise in the right foot. Looking at his right leg he has gross muscle wasting of the thigh and gluteal muscles. There is a well-healed extended longitudinal scar over the right proximal thigh. He has an obviously shortened, flexed right leg. His pelvis is not level with stance. The ASIS is hitched up on the left side and he has a compensatory scoliotic curve of his spine apex to the right. He demonstrates a short-leg antalgic gait. He is Trendelenburg false-positive on the right side."

"Sitting down on the bed the pelvic obliquity does not fully correct and he still demonstrates a scoliotic curve of his spine, suggesting an element of fixed deformity to the spine."

"On inspection supine we can again see the quite obvious leg length inequality on the right side. On measuring leg lengths there is a 5-cm true difference. Thomas test reveals a fixed flexion deformity of his right leg of 30°. On attempting to flex the hip the pelvis moves immediately, which is very suggestive of a fused hip. In addition there is no adduction/abduction possible at the hip joint."

Salient clinical features

- Scar
- Fixed flexion deformity
- Shortening
- No movement
- Check nerve function

Pitfalls

Whatever method you use to measure hip movement you must stabilize the pelvis to detect its movement. It is absolutely vital to keep one hand over the ASIS

---

[7] Clinical findings will vary depending on whether the arthrodesis was surgical or occurred spontaneously.

when measuring flexion so as to detect tilting of the pelvis. It is possible to "flex" a completely fused hip by 30°–40° – the movement actually occurring at the spine. One will not pick up the diagnosis of a fused hip in this situation.[8]

The unsound arthrodesis (spasm of muscles)

The patient can sometimes have a pseudoarthrosis of the hip, which allows some movement to occur at the hip, and this may create confusion. If the good leg is flexed up and the patient holds their knee, use one hand to palpate the lesser trochanter and iliopsoas and then with the other hand smartly abduct the arthrodesed leg. If there is protective contraction of the muscle group then the arthrodesis is not sound.

I have most often seen this case with tuberculosis and a fixed contracture of the ipsilateral knee. Extreme caution is required when measuring leg lengths to place the opposite leg in the same position. This may require the use of pillows to flex up the opposite leg. It may even require you to measure the component parts of the legs separately: anterior superior iliac spine to medial joint line, medial joint line to ankle, etc. With fixed knee flexion when checking hip extension move the patient to the end of the couch. Often the ipsilateral knee is limited in motion and is painful on weight bearing in a strained valgus position.

Discussion

- Position of fusion
- Methods of arthrodesis
- Revision to THA (take down the hip)

It is important to make sure that the back or knee pain is not caused by another pathology such as HNP, which would not be improved by THA. Ensure that the patient has a good indication for conversion. Good-quality radiographs are needed to identify

bone stock, hardware and the status of the greater trochanter. A CT scan can sometimes be helpful for identifying bone stock, the proximity of heterotopic bone to neurovascular structures and abductor muscle mass. The abductors may be inadequate. The sciatic nerve is closer than normal during surgery and one may need to release the psoas with or without adductor tenotomy if abduction is less than 15°.

Complications following conversion

- Deep infection: 1.9%–15.3% (higher in conversion of surgical fusion)
- Dislocation: 1.7%–6.25%
- Sciatic nerve palsy: 1.8%–13.4%
- Femoral nerve palsy: 3.6%

The gluteal muscles are atrophied and usually require the use of crutches for three to six months until the abductor function is strengthened. It may take 2–3 years to gain the full benefit of surgery. The knee has a tendency for a valgus deformity if the hip is fused. If the hip is fused in a poor position consider corrective osteotomy first before arthrodesis. Patients whose hips were fused before puberty have less improvement in hip muscle function following THA because of underdevelopment of the greater trochanter.

Short case 1

Fused hip

- Scar over a stiff hip (surgical arthrodesis)
- Examine this hip
  - Stiff leg gait
  - Trendelenburg: false positive; able to maintain abduction with no abductor function
- Leg length discrepancy

Short case 2

- Hip arthrodesis
- Examine this man's left hip
  - Surgical scar: posterior approach hip
  - Supine: shortened left leg with no hip movement

---

[8] This is regarded as an absolutely classic examination error. If one mentions there is 30°–40° of flexion in the hip when it is fused one will definitely fail a short case, whilst in the long case you will be on the back foot and have your work cut out to recover.

Long case 1

Arthritic knee below a fused hip

The discussion centred around the pros and cons of whether to take down the fused hip first, perform a THA and then afterwards perform a TKA versus going straight ahead and performing a TKA above a fused hip.

TKA in patients with an ipsilateral hip fusion leads to a reduced range of motion and the frequent need for MUA because of stiffness. Moreover these artificial joints function under abnormal overstress, leading to early failure.

Studies on the results of TKA in the presence of a fused hip have reported high complication rates with an unpredictable outcome. Thus, the only exception to performing a TKA before converting the fused hip would be a patient with a satisfactorily positioned hip in whom abductor muscle function was questionable. In these patients, the results of THA are known to be inferior, with poor gait patterns and a decreased likelihood of adequate knee pain relief. If the hip is fused in a poor position and the patient has significant knee pain, the conversion THA is preferable because of the notably inferior results of a TKA in that setting.

Long case 2

Arthrodesis of the hip in an elderly male patient

Past history of tuberculosis. Fixed flexion contracture of the knee. Minor complaints of low back pain and knee pain.

Long case 3

Arthrodesis left hip (post SUFE fixation with LLD). Left THA and then periprosthetic fracture

Discussion

- Position of arthrodesis
- Work-up of the infected hip
- Classification of periprosthetic fractures
- Management of periprosthetic fractures
- Taking down the arthrodesis
- TKA with hip arthrodesis
- Risk of back pain
- Other joint arthrosis

Long case 4

A 71-year-old housewife in good general health

History

- Low back and ipsilateral knee pain
- Hip arthrodesis after tuberculosis aged 15 years
- Intra-articular arthrodesis
- Position: 35° flexion, 5° adduction and neutral rotation

Examination

- Measurement of leg lengths
- Demonstration of gait (short limbed gait)
- Demonstration of Trendelenburg test
- Perform Thomas test

Discussion

- Why convert the arthrodesis to arthroplasty?
- Is hyperlordosis the cause of her low back pain?
- Should antituberculosis treatment be used preoperatively? If so for how long?
- What are the side-effects of antituberculosis drug treatment?
- What consent issues are there preoperatively?
- Neurovascular problems; in particular, the need to expose the sciatic nerve or not
- Hip instability
- Infection
- Results of conversion
- Preoperative planning of the arthroplasty
- Plain films, CT scan
- Implant considerations relevant to a stable hip

Long case 5

A 68-year-old man with fibrous ankylosis of the hip following SUFE and proximal femoral osteotomy approximately 50 years previously

Discussion on:
- SUFE
- Osteotomies

- Surgical approaches to the hip
- Demonstration of flexor contracture of the hip
- THA
- Surgical approaches
- Management of difficulties in the case

Long case 6

A 24-year-old female presented with DDH aged 4 years

The patient had an open reduction, Salter's osteotomy and a femoral osteotomy. She developed AVN and growth arrest of capital femoral epiphysis. She had an arthrodesis aged 14 years, complicated by sciatic nerve palsy.

Take a history and perform an examination in front of the examiners, followed by an oral exam.

Discussion points

- Diagnosis?
- What operations has she had?
- Measurement of the centre-edge angle?
- How would you perform an arthrodesis of the hip?
- What do you think of the position of this patient's arthrodesis?
- Why did she develop a sciatic nerve palsy?
- Outline the options for further management
- Outcome following revision to THA (taking down the hip)

Primary osteoarthritis of the hip

The case of the poisoned chalice.

Introduction

Most likely a long case but equally a candidate could be asked to demonstrate the Trendelenburg test, the Thomas test or range of movement in a short case. Examiners view a straightforward long case of primary OA of the hip as an easy case, a gift.[9] Be professional and thorough in your pres-

entation. I agree it is an easy case – an easy case to fail.

Unfortunately the FRCS Orth exam does not always work like this. Primary OA of the hip is a condition that candidates will see on a day-to-day basis in clinic and they will be expected to know it inside out for an exit exam. The examiners will have a very low threshold for any mistakes or errors made. You are not a medical student, this is an exit exam and if you miss subtle details out of the history, do not demonstrate the Trendelenburg test particularly well, or botch-up the Thomas test you may well end up failing the long case. In comparison a very difficult esoteric long case may mean that the examiners are more likely to be forgiving if you should make the odd mistake during the history and examination.

History

Pain

The predominant and most important symptom.

"*How long have you had pain? Where is the pain felt?*" Pain from an OA hip is classically felt in the groin, around the greater trochanter and occasionally in the buttock (suspect either the lumbar spine or sacroiliac joints). "*Is the pain getting worse or staying the same? Does the pain radiate anywhere?*" Radiation to the front of the thigh and knee commonly occurs and at times pain may present solely in the knee. "*Was the pain of insidious or sudden onset?*" Differentiates between OA and AVN. Any aggravating and relieving factors, etc.

Decreased walking distance

"*How far can you walk before you have to stop?*" Sometimes patients do not have a restricted walking distance but get pain after 10 minutes or so. "*Does the pain stop you from walking any further or is it shortness of breath or chest pain?*" This relates to concerns about fitness for surgery.

---

[9] *Examiner:* If you get a straightforward long case of OA of the hip you should be rubbing your hands with joy. I can't understand how any candidate could possibly fail it. In fact you should be aiming for a good to excellent pass.

Sleep disturbance

"*Does the pain stop you from sleeping at night? How many times do you have to get up in the night because of the pain?*" Night pain can be particularly distressing to patients and is an important and strong indication for surgery.

Analgesia

"*What painkillers are you taking and how often are you taking them? When was the last time you took a painkiller?*"

Limp

Limp may be noticed early, but more often than not comes on later than pain or stiffness. It can be due to a variety of causes including pain, muscle weakness and capsular contractions. The limp is due to pain, or stiffness, or apparent shortening due to adductor spasm.

Stiffness

The patient may be unable to put on their shoes, socks or stockings, be unable to cut their toe nails, get in and out of a bath, or in and out of a car. Difficulty bending down to pick up objects off the floor or getting on/off the toilet. Stiffness and limp are relative indications for surgery and should not be regarded as the sole indication for surgery in the absence of pain.

Drug history and past medical history

These are carried out to assess a patient's fitness for surgery and the need for an anaesthetic assessment.

Miscellaneous and social history

"*Do you use a walking stick? For how long? In which hand do you hold it?*" Note the previous treatments tried and their success. Take a smoking and alcohol history. Do not forget to take the social history. Ask the patient whether they have stairs in their house, home help, meals on wheels, etc.

Memorandum [10]

History

As for OA hip above.

Examination

Make sure the pain is arising from the hip joint and is neither back pain nor knee pain. Move the knee in the plane of the knee joint (if there is pain, it is attributable to the knee). Move the knee as a pendulum (if there is pain, it is attributable to the hip). Be suspicious if back movements reproduce the pain. Occasionally patients are referred for THA with arthritis of the hip but examination and observation of gait will show that the patient is more limited by peripheral vascular disease, peripheral neuropathy or Parkinson's disease than by the arthritic hip. Under these circumstances THA is relatively contraindicated.

Discussion

Discussion would usually start with a description of the patient's radiographs:

Examiner: Why do osteophytes form?
Candidate: As the articular cartilage begins to degenerate the ability of the cartilage to distribute stress begins to fail and the stress on bone increases. The bone responds to increased stress by laying down increased bone (Wolff's law). Thus more surface area is produced to cover the increased stress.
Examiner: Why do subchondral cysts form?
Candidate: In areas of very high stress, stress fractures occur. Because of continued pressure the fractures cannot heal and cysts form.

---

[10] Basic standard history for OA of the hip. You've only got 10 minutes so practise beforehand. The FRCS Orth exam has changed now with the requirement to perform the history and examination in front of the examiners. Luck certainly played a part in the exam in the past. If one got a patient who had seen three or four previous candidates, you could extract the relevant history much faster and more efficiently compared to the first candidate.

From here there may be a discussion of the merits of conservative versus operative management for OA of the hip.

Examiner: How would you consent the patient? What would you tell them about the risks of the procedure?

This may lead on to what approach to use for a primary THA, followed by a general discussion about the advantages and disadvantages of each of the various surgical approaches to the hip.

Examiner: What type of THA you would use and why?[11]

The examiners may ask you about the rationale behind the use of cement versus uncemented hips versus metal-on-metal hip resurfacing. The oral may then move on to long-term published results of THA in the literature and end with survival analysis curves or how to set up a study to assess the long-term outcome of a particular THA.

Long case 1

An 80-year-old lady with a painful right hip and knee

History

Co-morbidity factors included a history of significant exertional angina and previous myocardial infarction.

Clinical examination

No pelvic tilt, ASIS level with no leg length discrepancy and a symmetrical stance.

Right hip

Antalgic gait, positive Trendelenburg test
No fixed flexion deformity of the hip but marked restriction of internal and external rotation in flexion with only a jog of

movement present. Abduction restricted to 20°, adduction similarly restricted to 20°; both were painful.

Right knee

Effusion, fixed flexion deformity of 5°, flexion reduced by 40° compared to the opposite side.

Spine

No evidence of spinal pathology.

Discussion

I was asked by the examiners to demonstrate all of the above clinical signs. The discussion focused on her cardiac condition and fitness for surgery. The management of the arthritic hip and the need for cardiology input before any hip surgery, as this was elective lifestyle surgery and not an urgent, life-threatening condition. This was then followed on with a discussion of the pros and cons of total hip arthroplasty and how the risks of surgery could be reduced.

Long case 2

Primary OA of the hip

The history and examination were relatively straightforward. Ten minutes was fine for the history. I was asked to demonstrate the Thomas test and was questioned about what I was doing as I performed it. Demonstration of abduction, adduction and internal/external rotation of the hip. In the discussion section I was asked virtually everything possible there was to know about THA in great detail, including what type of hip arthroplasty I would use and why.

SUFE

History

"Mr. Wade is a 60-year-old retired local government officer married with three grown-up children. He had a severe left SUFE, which was pinned as a 14-year-old boy."

"His main complaint now is of left-hip stiffness. He has difficulty putting his shoes and socks on and getting in and out of the bath. His walking distance is not restricted but he needs to take his time getting from place to place. Pain

---

[11] *Candidate:* I use the Exeter prosthesis because I am most familiar with this design from my training. The instrumentation is relatively straightforward; the neck cut is not critical. Most importantly it has successful long-term peer-reviewed published results. The straight stem allows controlled insertion and the highly polished taper... , etc.

is not a significant feature, there is no sleep disturbance and he is on no regular medication. He is otherwise fit and healthy."

Clinical examination

"On general examination the patient is of average height and build. He looks well for his years."

Standing

"On examination standing there is a well-healed left lateral hip scar present from his previous hip surgery. He stands up straight with a flexion attitude of his right leg, which on straightening up the pelvis revealed a left leg length discrepancy. A mild external rotation deformity of the affected leg was present. There is marked left thigh muscle wastage. He walked with an antalgic short-left-leg gait. He was Trendelenburg positive on the left side."

Supine

"Measurement of leg lengths using a tape measure confirmed 2 cm of real shortening. Galeazzi's test revealed this to be in the femur. Digital Bryant's test suggested the shortening was above the trochanter. The Thomas test demonstrated a fixed flexion deformity of 10°."

"Flexion was to 90° with the leg tending to go into fixed external rotation as it was flexed up. There was virtually no internal rotation or external rotation at 90° flexion. Abduction was limited to 30° and similarly adduction was limited to 20°. Pain was present at the extremes of movement. The leg was neurovascularly intact and examinations of the spine and both knees were unremarkable."

Discussion

- AP radiographs
- Aetiological factors of SUFE
- Dunn and Loder classification of SUFE
- Radiological findings in SUFE
- Management options of severe slips
- Various osteotomies

Management of this particular case

In the absence of significant pain this patient is not a candidate for total hip arthroplasty as this rarely improves range of movement significantly. Advanced changes of OA are too severe for osteotomy. Therefore, we propose to continue with conservative management at present.

Technical difficulties of performing a THA in SUFE

An anteverted femoral neck may mislead the surgeon during stem insertion and lead to component mal-positioning. There could be problems with metalwork removal so it is important to have special instruments available. Consider carrying out a two-stage procedure: metalwork removal first followed by THA 3 months later.

Consider the feasibility of incorporating the previous scar into the new scar. Soft tissue scarring and fibrosis mean that a longer surgical incision may be needed for hardware removal; assess LLD preoperatively and cement extruding from the breached lateral cortex of the femur. Extra theatre time should be scheduled as it is not a simple primary hip arthroplasty and will take a bit longer to perform (brownie points for thinking like a consultant surgeon and planning your lists!).

Rheumatoid patient with hip disease

Background

Despite numerous medical advances in the treatment of RA severe involvement of the hips is common. Fortunately THA provides excellent reliable relief of pain and functional improvement. Between 6% and 15% of THA are carried out for RA. The average age of onset of rheumatoid disease is 55 years and the average patient has had hip symptoms for 4 years.

In general forefoot deformity should be the first deformity to be corrected to ensure that patients are capable of comfortable weight bearing and to reduce sources of infection at a later date.

Thereafter the hip should take priority over the knee and hind foot. Knee pain referred from the hip is abolished and the restoration of knee anatomy and ligament balance at subsequent TKA is easier and more reliable when the hip above is mobile. Rehabilitation of TKA is difficult with a stiff, painful or deformed hip. The hind foot should be corrected last, as correction of hip and knee deformities may alter the dynamic position of the hind foot.

There are concerns regarding:
- The polysystemic/multiple joint nature of the disease
- Polypharmacy – patients often take a variety of medications that can affect surgery
- Immunosuppression from either the disease or its treatment
- Difficulties with rehabilitation

Memorandum

History

Insidious onset of groin, buttock or thigh pain. Subject to acute flare-ups.

Examination

Shake hands with the patient and at the same time observe their skin condition, i.e. is it dry, eczematous, psoriatic, scarred, etc.?

"On general inspection the patient has features of extensive rheumatoid disease affecting many joints. The buttock and thigh are markedly wasted with the limb held in external rotation and fixed flexion. The skin overlying the joint appears shiny, thin and atrophic with evidence of spontaneous bruising. All movements of the hip joint are restricted and painful."

Hip flexion and adduction contractures of various degrees may be present. It is important to examine the upper extremities to evaluate the patient's ability to use walking aids. The knees, ankles and feet should be examined for arthritic involvement.

Beware of the patient in a wheelchair
Some patients with severe multiple lower extremity involvement may be confined to a wheelchair.
- Can they walk?
- How?
- Do they use a stick?
- When did they last walk?

- Make the patient walk if possible

Radiographs

Radiographic findings in the rheumatoid hip can often be subtle. Osteopenia is seen in most cases. Typically there is concentric joint space narrowing due to generalized loss of articular cartilage without evidence of osteophytes or cyst formation. As the disease progresses, medial and/or superior migration of the femoral head with protrusio deformity occurs especially if steroids are used.

Management[12]

Often rheumatoid patients are generally disabled having various degrees of osteopenia, skin fragility, vasculitis and poor musculature. It is important to ensure that the patient is in as fit a state as possible for surgery. Synovitis should be controlled as well as possible and no chest, urinary, dental or skin sepsis should be present.

Management options include:
- Intra-articular injection of steroid/local anaesthetic
- Open synovectomy: not popular, risk of AVN of the femoral head
- Arthroscopic partial synovectomy: becoming more widely practised and may have a role in the young rheumatoid patient
- Osteotomy: contraindicated as the disease is generalized throughout the joint
- Arthrodesis: contraindicated, as it requires good joint functioning and no disease in neighbouring joints
- THA

Operative issues

Careful position on the operating table is vital due to the poor skin quality and other painful joints; pad all the pressure areas. Care must be taken with the neck during patient transfer and positioning.

---

[12] It is quite possible that you may be asked about management options for the rheumatoid hip other than arthroplasty.

Temporomandibular disease may make intubation difficult. Bone stock is often poor, being soft and osteoporotic, so great care is required during dislocation and relocation of the hip to avoid fracture of the femur. Dislocation may be difficult if protrusio is present. Care is needed not to bruise the skin and soft tissues of the leg. The femoral head and neck may be partially absent. Due to the reported high rates of non-union in RA the transtrochanteric approach should generally be avoided. Reaming can compromise the edges of the acetabulum and the acetabular bone is soft and easily penetrated. If protrusio acetabuli is present (2%–40%) bone grafting of the medial wall (with a bulk autograft or packed reamings from the femoral head) and in severe cases mesh and/or shell reinforcement may be required.

The rate of deep infection is approximately double (2.6) that of OA. Late infection is more common in rheumatoid disease, a fact possibly related to immune suppression or other sources of infection.

There is some debate as to whether the incidence of thromboembolism is reduced in rheumatoid disease due to a mild coagulopathy. Evidence in the literature is sparse. HO is less common in rheumatoid arthritis than in OA. The dislocation rate has been reported as more common compared to OA but there is little evidence for this.

Implants should in general be cemented as poor bone stock may not support cementless fixation. Uncemented components have not been widely used in the treatment of RA. Orthopaedic surgeons have been concerned that the osteopenia, contractures and bony deformity often seen in RA would make it difficult to safely and reliably obtain the initial stability necessary for bony ingrowth. In addition there have been concerns relating to how much bony ingrowth will occur in the presence of systemic inflammatory disease and the effects of anti-rheumatic medications. Cemented implants may be a wiser move but there is little evidence in the literature to support this opinion.

Mixed results have been reported for the survival of primary THA in RA compared to OA. In the Swedish hip registry an increased rate of revision of acetabular cups in rheumatoid patients, both young

and old, was noted.[13] Other studies have found no difference in survival between RA and OA.[14]

Long case discussion

Examiner:
   How do you assess the rheumatoid patient in general for THA surgery?
   What about the cervical spine? When do you order new X-rays?
   What about methotrexate? Would you stop it before surgery in order to decrease the risk of infection?[1]
Candidate: I would continue methotrexate.
Examiner: Yes that is correct.

Thereafter followed a 5-minute chitchat by the examiner on methotrexate, the essence of which was that continuation of methotrexate treatment did not increase the risk of THA infection occurring in patients with RA.

Examiner: In fact there is evidence to suggest that stopping treatment does in fact increase the risk of infection and also the general complications with disease control. Therefore methotrexate treatment should not be stopped under any circumstances before elective orthopaedic surgery.

The examiner mentioned the word "papers" on several occasions but didn't specifically quote any. There are several papers published on the subject and they report mixed results but the sample sizes were poor. The most comprehensive paper is the Wrightington paper in 2001 from Grennan *et al.*,[2] which would be the one to quote in the exam.

So the irony of the long case examination is that one can spend most of the oral discussing the medical treatment of RA and not cover any surgical principles at all.

[1] Difficult to appreciate out of context of the exam but the way the examiner phrased the question seemed to imply/suggest the correct answer to the candidate.
[2] Grennan DM, Gray J, Loudon J, Fear S (2001) Methotrexate and early postoperative complications in patients with rheumatoid arthritis undergoing elective orthopaedic surgery. *Ann Rheum Dis* **60**(3): 214–17.

---

[13] See www.jru.orthop.gu.se/
[14] Johnsen SP, Sørensen HT, Lucht U, Søballe K, Overgaard S, Pedersen AB (2006) Patient-related predictors of implant failure after primary total hip replacement in the initial, short- and long-terms: a nationwide Danish follow-up study including 36 984 patients. *J Bone Joint Surg Br* **88-B**: 1303–8.

AVN of the hip

Comes up fairly regularly as a long case. The patient typically would be young or middle aged and present with early AVN and worsening hip pain. Another possible case scenario would be progression of AVN with worsening hip pain following unsuccessful core decompression.

In a short case you may be asked to demonstrate fairly specific hard clinical signs such as measurement of leg lengths, the Thomas test or a restricted painful range of hip movement rather than go through a complete hip examination.

History

As with any diagnosis, the history is critical. A high index of suspicion is essential especially if the patient has one of the atraumatic conditions associated with AVN.

The standard hip questions should be asked. In addition the history should include a search for possible aetiological factors. Inquire about steroid use, alcohol intake and history of previous hip trauma.

The clinical presentation is of pain in the thigh, which is out of proportion to any radiographic changes, which may be minimal. The pain is typically deep seated; throbbing is felt at night, is unremitting and is similar to bone tumour pain. Pain is usually worse with ambulation.

Examination

The clinical findings on examination can be unremarkable or can include pain on internal rotation of the hip, a decreased range of motion, an antalgic gait and clicking of the hip when the necrotic fragment has collapsed. Pain with internal rotation of the hip and a limited range of hip motion are often signs that the femoral head has already collapsed.

Memorandum

Candidate: On general inspection the patient looks well for his years. He is of tall stature and muscular build. He is standing up straight with his pelvis level and taking weight equally through both legs. As we can see here there is a suggestion of possible left gluteal and thigh muscle wasting.

Examiner: Yes it is mild but clearly present.

Candidate: Examination of gait revealed that he walked with an antalgic gait. Trendelenburg testing of his lower limbs revealed a delayed positive response on the left side and negative Trendelenburg test on the right side.

Formal measurement of leg lengths supine revealed 2 cm of true shortening of the left leg. Galeazzi's test confirmed that the shortening was arising from the femur. Bryant's triangle testing suggested that the shortening was above the trochanter. Movements of the left hip were painful and grossly restricted, particularly abduction and internal rotation in flexion. The left hip demonstrated almost full internal rotation in extension but with the hip flexed it was grossly restricted.[15] The left hip had a tendency to twist into fixed external rotation during passive hip flexion.

Discussion

Following history and examination a candidate will usually be led into a separate room to discuss management of the case. The result of the long case has most likely already been decided in the majority of instances. However, in a borderline case a good discussion may pull you through.

Discussion will probably begin by reviewing hip radiographs. A candidate would be expected to describe the typical radiographic findings of AVN and then stage the disease. The examiners may also have an MRI scan of both hips and there are several possible lines of questions that can emanate from this.

The aetiology of AVN will probably be asked and possibly current theories of the pathogenesis of AVN brought up. It is almost certain that the candidate will be asked about the classification of AVN, possibly which classification system he/she uses and why.

Management options will definitely be discussed. Candidates will have to decide whether to simply go

---

[15] If internal rotation is full with the hip extended but restricted in flexion this suggests pathology in the anterosuperior portion of the femoral head, probably AVN, the so-called Sectorial sign.

through a list of possible management options or be more specific in their management plan for their particular case.

The oral can then go anywhere:

- The advantages and disadvantages of performing either a cemented or uncemented THA in a young patient
- Can you perform a hip resurfacing procedure in the presence of AVN? If so how much AVN is acceptable and how do you deal with the defect?
- How you would perform a THA? What approach would you use and why? What implant would you use and why? What are the long-term results of this implant? Do you know of any published results for this implant?
- Describe the advantages obtained by setting up the Swedish registry. Discussion of the potential benefits of the UK National Joint Registry
- What are the results like for THA in AVN compared to a normal standard group with OA?
- Describe the mechanisms involved in performing a study for your consultant who wants to find out how well the particular implant that they've been using for the last 10 years has been doing. This will lead on to the various different types of studies that exist and then probably on to statistics covering areas such as type I and II errors, the power of a study, numbers for statistical significance, etc.

Short case 1

Psoriatic arthropathy with AVN secondary to steroid use

Examiner: Examine this lady's hip.

Candidate:

- Bilateral AVN of the hips with scars on each side of the proximal thigh for core decompression

Shown AP pelvis radiograph of patient and asked to pass comment

Candidate:

- Radiographic features of AVN
- Discussion on Steinberg's classification system

Short case 2

Examiner: This man was involved in an RTA; just examine the range of movements of the right hip.

Candidate: I examined his hip movements and found a restricted and painful range of movement in his right hip particularly abduction (15°) and internal rotation in flexion (virtually nil). I mentioned the large proximal thigh scar present. For some reason and I have no idea why I asked the patient two or three questions about his hip pain: How severe was his hip pain? How far was his walking distance? Did it keep him awake at night? The examiner then led me through his radiographs.

Examiner: These are his radiographs. He had a severe posterior pelvic fracture, which has been fixed with pelvic reconstruction plates. The diagnosis is obvious looking at the femoral head. He has developed AVN.

(It wasn't that obvious and I may have struggled to get to it.)

Examiner: What would you do for the patient?

Candidate: His pain is not too severe at present and he seems to be coping reasonably well with things. He can walk up to 2 miles without too much difficulty. He isn't kept awake at night with this pain. I wouldn't do anything with him at the moment. I would review him regularly in the clinic and if his symptoms deteriorated significantly I would offer him a total hip replacement.

Examiner: Yes you are quite right. There is no need for any surgery at present as his symptoms are minimal.

Candidate: If your luck is with you it is with you in incredibly large amounts. I do not know why I started to ask the patient questions. The examiners certainly didn't ask me to but it gave me the information I needed to answer correctly the question about his current management plan. The examiner assumed that I had picked up on the fact he had developed AVN, which, in the stress of the examination, I hadn't quite managed to do!

Long case 1

Male aged about 60 years with history of Caisson's disease

- Painful right hip – moderate OA secondary to AVN
- Left THA
- Moderate bilateral varus OA knees

Most of above clinical finding were demonstrated to the examiners. In particular they were interested in the difference between true and apparent shortening of the right leg.

Discussion

The discussion focused mainly on the differential diagnosis, radiographic features, pathology, aetiology, classification, grading and management of AVN (detailed discussion on core decompression). Results of THA for AVN were also discussed, as were metal on metal resurfacing, concerns with femoral neck fracture, etc.

Long case 2

A 14-year-old boy with AVN and collapse with ankylosis of the hip following pinning for severe SUFE

The infected THA

Probably the most important complication following arthroplasty surgery with significant cost to the individual and to the health service.

Introduction

I think it is highly unlikely you will get a frankly acutely infected hip draining pus in the long case oral. More probably the hip will be painful due to a chronic low-grade infection or it will have been revised because of previous infection and the patient then had complications postoperatively such as a dislocation or periprosthetic fracture. The best way to deal with this type of long case is to go back to basics and try to keep things simple. Think in terms of how you would normally approach this type of case if you had seen it in the clinic.

History

How long has the hip been painful? Was the hip always painful after surgery or was there a pain-free interval? Is the pain getting worse? There is an increased risk of deep prosthetic infection as a result of delayed wound healing or large haematoma formation. Therefore, specific inquiry should be made about wound drainage, persistent fever, prolonged antibiotic administration, or delayed hospital discharge. Has the patient had a recent urine or chest infection? Has there been a reduction in walking distance and/or are walking aids now necessary? Pain at night or at rest suggests infection (or tumour).

Examination

"On examination we have an elderly male patient who has difficulty standing upright unaided. There is an old, well-healed left lateral hip scar. The surrounding skin and soft tissues appear normal. There is no evidence of a discharging sinus in the wound. There is marked left thigh and gluteal muscle wastage."

"Examining his gait revealed that it was antalgic and he was markedly Trendelenburg positive on the left side but negative on the right side. Formal measurement of leg lengths with a measuring tape revealed that both real and apparent leg lengths were equal. The Thomas test failed to reveal any fixed flexion deformity of the left hip. Examination of the left hip movement demonstrated a globally decreased range of movement, which was painful but not stiff."

Investigations

Radiographs

Suggest taking AP and lateral radiographs and look for radiographic features highly suggestive of infection, such as endosteal scalloping and the new formation of multi-lamellar, periosteal bone in the femur.

Bloods

WCC, ESR/CRP.

Bone scan

In practical terms a bone scan isn't particularly helpful in differentiating between aseptic and septic loosening. A radioactively labelled white blood cell scan (leukocyte scan) is more sensitive and specific but its value is still somewhat limited.

Aspiration of the hip

This is carried out in theatre, under sterile conditions; blood culture bottles are required ±arthrogram.

Management

The FRCS Orth exam is much more than just presenting facts to the examiners. Just as important are the linking of words and sentences, to connect these facts together, and an attempt to establish a rapport with the examiners.

"My management would be directed towards trying to identify a cause for this painful hip. There are numerous possibilities; the most common causes would be infection, aseptic loosening or referred pain from elsewhere. Other causes could include impingement, instability or fracture. Features suggestive of infection would include . . . . It is potentially a very difficult problem to manage especially if deep infection is present in the medullary canal. The condition should not be underestimated. There are several ways to treat deep prosthetic infection, which may include . . . . I would perform a two-stage procedure. I think it is safer for the patient with a better chance of eradicating infection than a one-stage procedure."

Discussion

A large topic with plenty to discuss. Keep the discussion simple, straightforward and uncontroversial and avoid getting yourself into a corner. Examiners can sometimes focus in on fairly minor details. Five minutes discussing the value of ESR/CRP measurements in the diagnosis of hip infection can become very uncomfortable. Most candidates would dry up within a couple of minutes.

The painful THA

Unfortunately a number of patients following THA have persistent or new pain and some have disability. These problems remain a challenge.

History

- The hip is painful
- The patient's walking distance has become less and/or walking aids are necessary
- The hip is stiff or does not move at all
- Duration: how long has the hip been painful?
- Progression: is the pain getting worse?
- Site of pain. Pain localized to the trochanter region suggests bursitis, irritation secondary to underlying wires or sutures, osteolysis or fracture. Pain felt in the buttock or groin suggests vascular or neurogenic claudication, acetabular loosening or osteolysis. Less frequently it may indicate iliopsoas impingement or tendonitis secondary to acetabular retroversion, hernia or gynaecological or genitourinary cause. Thigh pain may be secondary to a loose femoral implant
- Pain felt at rest or during the night raises the possibility of infection or malignancy
- Were there any problems with the wound postoperatively? A history of persistent wound drainage, haematoma or a prolonged course of antibiotics following the operation should increase the index of suspicion for infection as a cause of the pain
- Ask whether there has been any recent bacterial infection or possible bacteraemia: urine or chest infection, dental procedure, etc.
- Has pain been present since the original index operation? This may indicate subclinical infection
- If there was a pain-free interval following the initial successful THA, there may now be aseptic loosening or late-onset infection
- With aseptic loosening a triphasic pattern is classic. Pain is sharp with the first few steps of ambulation, is reduced after the patient has walked a moderate distance and then gradually increases after the patient has walked a still greater distance
- With pain that is the same after surgery, the initial diagnosis may have been incorrect and other local disorders or referred pain may have been the cause of symptoms

The possible causes for pain are:

- Referred pain from elsewhere, e.g. the lumbar spine
- Aseptic loosening: one or both components
- Infection is present: subclinical, acute, delayed, etc.
- Broken trochanteric wires, non-union of the greater trochanter
- Some problem is present but it may be difficult to pin down, e.g. trochanteric bursitis, irritation of the psoas tendon or abductor muscle weakness

Examination

Look at the state of the wound, skin and soft tissues, noting inflammation and healed sinus tracks. Note if there is marked thigh atrophy from disuse.

Gait: Is there any asymmetry or abnormality of gait? Trendelenburg positive test?

Palpation: are there any hernias or defects in the deep fascia?

Is there tenderness on palpation? This may suggest a neuroma or an area of osteolysis. Tenderness over the pubic rami may suggest a stress fracture. Pain at the extremes of hip motion suggests aseptic loosening. Extreme pain with any hip range of motion suggests active synovitis and raises the concern of infection. Pain over the greater trochanter may indicate a bursitis or tendonitis. The spine may be a source of referred pain. Carry out a neurovascular examination of both lower limbs. Peripheral vascular disease may occasionally present as discomfort in the hip or thigh area.

Investigations

"My investigations would be directed towards trying to identify a cause for this painful hip."

Radiographs

"I would start by reviewing up-to-date, good-quality AP pelvis and true lateral radiographs of the relevant hip and, if possible, compare these to previous radiographs as this may document migration of either the acetabular or the femoral component, which is pathognomonic for loosening."

Look for radiographic signs of aseptic loosening.[16] Look again for any radiographic features suggestive of infection.[17]

Bloods

"I would then want to perform some routine bloods: ESR/CRP, WCC."[18]

Bone scan

A bone scan is a reasonable option to suggest but be careful to follow through and mention that a bone scan may not always be particularly helpful in differentiating between aseptic and septic loosening.[19] Consider a leukocyte scan, or a radioactively labelled white cell scan.

Hip arthrography and aspiration

This is carried out in theatre, under sterile conditions, and requires blood culture bottles ±hip arthrogram.[20] Arthrography of the hip can demonstrate pocketing of the radio-opaque medium in the area of the pseudo-capsule, which suggests infection. Unfortunately this finding is uncommon.

---

[16] If you want to spin out the discussion talk about the Harris classification of loosening (definite, probable or possible) but do not make it too obvious, as it will irritate the examiners. Better still is to bait/tempt the examiners with a tit bit of information and see if they respond.

[17] Make a general comment to the examiners that radiographs are not particularly helpful in diagnosing infection and that features suggestive of infection would include endosteal scalloping, generalized osteolysis and periosteal new bone formation, but that in this particular case none of these features were present.

[18] It is not unreasonable to explain why you are performing these tests and what you are looking for. Be prepared to discuss sensitivity, specificity, etc. Throw a couple of recent references in if you can but be sensible – it may not be particularly appropriate to do so.

[19] It is easy for the examiners to back you into a corner with this one especially if you don't get your phrasing just right. Again be prepared to talk about sensitivities, specificities, etc. What is the sensitivity of a test? What is specificity? What do we mean by accuracy? What are the typical values quoted in the literature for the various scans, etc.?

[20] All cases or just selectively – have an opinion – you will have to decide yourself in 2 years or so when you become a consultant.

Table 10.1 Pain following THA

Differential diagnosis of pain following THA	
Intrinsic causes	Extrinsic causes
Aseptic loosening	Lumbar spine disease: stenosis, spondylolysis/spondylolisthesis, HNP
Infection	Peripheral vascular disease
Trochanteric bursitis	Stress/insufficiency fracture
Non-union of the greater trochanter	Iliopsoas tendinitis
Wear/debris synovitis	Hernia: femoral, inguinal, obturator
Instability	Malignant tumour: primary or secondary
	Metabolic disease
	CRPS

Differential diagnosis

Divided into intrinsic and extrinsic causes (Table 10.1).

Extrinsic causes

Spinal stenosis and nerve root irritation can cause pain in the buttock, thigh and sometimes the groin. Vascular disease commonly causes buttock or thigh pain. Neurological complications occur following <1% of primary THA. They can be caused by a direct injury from a surgical instrument, haematoma, cement or scar entrapment or can occur secondary to lengthening. Metabolic disorders such as Paget's disease can occasionally cause symptoms on their own, which may persist after THA.

Intrinsic causes

Soft tissues can occasionally become irritated by the prosthesis. The psoas tendon may become irritated by a prominent anterior flange of an insufficiently anteverted acetabular component. Instability can result in pain from capsular stretch and from soft-tissue impingement. Stress fractures can develop at the sites of cortical perforation and the pubic ramus secondary to disuse osteopenia and increased patient activity after THA.

Nothing wrong with the hip

The salient feature was that the pain was never relieved by the THA. Examination may show features suggestive of a problem with the THA, such as a limp and some limitation of motion, but nevertheless none of these signs is likely to be gross. Review of the case notes and plain radiographs of the original hip may reveal that the hip before replacement was minimally, if at all, arthritic, so that with the retrospectoscope it is clear that the original symptoms did not come from the hip.

Management

Obviously this depends on the cause. If no obvious cause is found then suggest a second opinion. The examiners can now choose a number of paths to go down:
- Preoperative planning for revision hip surgery
- A review of the surgical approaches that can be used
- A review of the choice of implant
- Complications of revision surgery

Protrusio acetabuli

Present the case to the examiners as if you are speaking to an equal about a straightforward case.

Memorandum

Candidate: I would like to present my long case.

This is Mrs. Brown, who is a 32-year-old married housewife with two young children who presents with progressively worsening bilateral hip pain, right worse than left. The pain is felt in both the groins and the anterior aspect of both thighs. It has been present for the last 5 years but has become much more severe in the last 18 months. The pain is present every day as a dull intermittent pain worse with activity.

Walking distance is reduced to one mile and there is sleep disturbance most nights. Putting shoes and socks on can be difficult and the patient is unable to go for long rides in a car. Getting in and out of a shower is not a particular problem. She takes paracetamol and ibuprofen when required for pain control. A walking stick is not used.

She was seen 3 years ago by an orthopaedic surgeon regarding her hip condition and it was decided at that time to soldier on with things, persevering with conservative management and not to go ahead with hip surgery. In the last year there has been a marked deterioration in her pain such that she now wishes to be considered for surgery.

Relevant past medical history is unremarkable. She has had no previous operations or medical conditions. In particular there is no history of diabetes, asthma, epilepsy, tuberculosis or hypertension; there is no family history of note.

She smokes 10 cigarettes a day and drinks 20 units of alcohol a week. She is a housewife who looks after two children aged seven and four. Her husband is an electrician and in good health. She has worked in a sweet shop in the past but had to give this up because the hip pain was exacerbated by standing on her feet for long periods of time. There are stairs in the house, which she is able to manage by going up one step at a time.

Examiner: Is there a family history of hip disease?

Candidate: I did ask the patient this question and she says that she thinks her cousin might have had Perthes disease as a child but there is nothing else that comes to mind.

On general examination we have a fit looking woman who is of average height and thin build. She walks with a limp but the gait itself is neither antalgic nor Trendelenburg.

Examiner: What do you mean exactly by a limp?

Candidate: During normal midstance the hip is displaced laterally by approximately 2 cm to the weight-bearing side. With a hip limp this lateral displacement is accentuated and results in an exaggerated limp.

Trendelenburg test was strongly positive bilaterally. I then examined the patient lying supine on the couch. After squaring up the pelvis with the bed and making sure the legs were square with the pelvis, there was a difference in heel height. Measurement of leg length revealed a true right leg shortening of 2 cm and an apparent leg length discrepancy of 1 cm. Galeazzi's sign suggested that the shortening was in the femur; the femora were parallel so the discrepancy was not below the knee. Digital Bryant's triangle palpation suggested that the shortening was above the trochanter. There was a reduced distance between my thumb and the tip of my index finger on the right side compared to the left.[21]

Examiner: Could you demonstrate these tests for me to confirm your clinical findings?

Candidate: Thomas test revealed a fixed flexion deformity on the right of 20° and 15° on the left. Right hip movements were grossly restricted and painful, in particular abduction. Active flexion was limited to 60° with only 70° obtained passively.

There was no internal or external rotation in flexion. Passive abduction was markedly limited to only 10°, whilst adduction was greater at 20°. On the left side movements were again restricted and painful but to a lesser degree. Active flexion was only possible to 90°. No internal or external rotation in flexion was possible. Passive abduction was again markedly limited to 10° with adduction restricted to 20°.

Discussion

- Aetiology of the condition
- Classification of protrusio
- Principles of THA reconstruction
- Bone graft
- Results of THA
- Technical issues specific to THA in protrusio

Tuberculosis of the hip

A case of old tuberculosis of the hip enrolled for the examination.

---

[21] One needs to talk to the examiners during one's clinical examination. Do not examine in silence! In this case the candidate is letting the examiners know in an indirect way that they understand Bryant's triangle.

Memorandum

"On examination we have an elderly man of average height and build. There are several well-healed scars over the lateral aspect of the left hip. There is a discharging sinus present in the groin/greater trochanter. There are puckered scars suggestive of healed sinuses. The left leg is shortened with gross generalized wasting, particularly of the thigh and buttock. There is a pelvic obliquity with the ASIS lower on the left side and a compensatory scoliosis which does not fully correct when sitting down on the couch, suggestive of a fixed element to the scoliosis."

"Inspection of gait revealed a short leg gait. There was also a suggestion of lack of movement of the left hip, with the trunk being thrown forwards to aid walking."

"On examination supine, again as mentioned previously, there is a gross left leg length shortening. The left leg has a flexed attitude and in order to measure leg lengths correctly both limbs need to be placed in equivalent positions. I am therefore using a pillow to fix the right leg in the same position of flexion as the left. There is a combination of real and apparent shortening of the left leg. Galeazzi's test demonstrated that most of the shortening is in the femur but there is however a suggestion of a small amount of tibial shortening. Bryant's triangle suggests most of the femoral shortening is above the trochanter. There is a definite decreased difference between my thumb over the ASIS and my fingers over the trochanter on the left side compared to the right. The hip is flexed, adducted and medially rotated. All movements are grossly restricted by pain and spasm."

Muscle spasm in the early stages can be elicited by rotating the extended hip when the muscles around the joint as well as the abdominal muscles exhibit spasmodic contraction (Gauvain's sign [22]). If no hip movement occurs at all consider bony ankylosis. Usually a combination of real and apparent shortening exists. In the initial stages of the disease there is slight flexion, abduction and

[22] Described by Sir Henry Gauvain in 1910. This test is of value in early doubtful cases of tuberculosis of the hip. In active tuberculosis of the hip, on initiating rotatory movements the muscles around the hip and lower abdomen go into spasm. The lower end of the thigh is rotated internally and externally. The movement is then checked and any further slight sharp rotation is followed by spasmodic contraction of the joint muscles as well as those of the lower abdomen.

lateral rotation. The earliest clinical sign is a limp, which comes on after walking. Flexion is concealed by an exaggerated lumbar lordosis. Adduction is corrected by tilting the pelvis upwards, which results in a scoliosis of the lumbar spine with convexity towards the normal side. If the hip has been fused the patient may develop back or hip pain several years later. In a young patient if there is mal-position of the fusion consider corrective osteotomy rather than arthroplasty. If a painful pseudoarthrosis exists consider fusion rather than arthroplasty.

Radiographs

The earliest sign is a general haziness of the bones as seen in a bad film but with a normal joint space and line with or without an area of rarefaction in Babcock's triangle (inferior aspect of the femoral neck). There is increased joint space due to an effusion.

Later on there is gross enlargement of the acetabulum roof with the femoral head migrating into the dorso-ilium (*travelling or wandering acetabulum*). The combination of partially destroyed femoral head, destroyed acetabulum and muscle spasm can lead to a posterior dislocation of the hip. In some situations the femoral head is destroyed and becomes small and contained in an enlarged acetabulum, giving rise to a *mortar and pestle* appearance. Softening and destruction of the medial wall of the acetabulum can lead to *protrusio*. With healing, bony ankylosis may occur.

Clinical features

Presenting complaint

Disease is insidious in onset and runs a chronic course. One of the first symptoms is stiffness of the hip. A child may be pale and apathetic, with loss of appetite before definite symptoms pertaining to the hip appear. Pain may initially be absent or be referred to the knee. Pain occurs around the hip particularly with weight bearing.

Gait

There is a stiff hip gait. While walking the hip is kept stiff and a forwards-backwards movement at the lumbar spine is used for propulsion of the lower limb. Because of the flexion deformity of the hip the patient stands with a compensatory exaggerated lumbar lordosis. Later on an antalgic gait may develop to quickly take the weight off the affected side.

Muscle wasting

The thigh and gluteal muscles are wasted.

Swelling

There may be swelling around the hip because of a cold abscess.

Discharging sinus

There may be discharging sinuses in the groin or around the greater trochanter. More likely there may be puckered scars from healed sinuses.

Shortening

There is a true shortening of the hip in tuberculosis except in stage I. There may be a combination of true and apparent shortening of the limb. Be able to measure true and apparent lengths of a limb and be quite clear on the difference between the two.

Stage 1. Synovitis: the stage of apparent lengthening

Initially the clinical features are common to all diseases producing synovitis. There is a joint effusion, which demands the hip to be in a position of maximum capacity and comfort. This is obtained by a position of *flexion, abduction and external rotation of the hip.*

Since the flexion and abduction deformities are only slight and are compensated for by the tilting of the pelvis, these do not become obvious. Flexion is concealed by a lumbar lordosis and by tilting the pelvis forwards. Abduction is corrected by tilting the pelvis downwards and scoliosis of the lumbar spine with convexity towards the affected side.

As the pelvis tilts downwards to compensate for the abduction deformity, the affected limb looks longer (apparent lengthening) than the normal opposite hip, though on measuring true limb lengths the two limbs are found to be equal. This stage lasts only for a short length of time and it is rare to see a patient in such an early stage of the disease.

Stage 2. Arthritis: the stage of apparent shortening

The effusion subsides. There is involvement of the articular cartilage. This leads to spasm of the powerful muscles around the hip to protect its movement. Since the flexors and adductors are stronger muscle groups than the extensors and abductors the attitude of the hip is one of *flexion, adduction and internal rotation.* The flexion and adduction may be concealed by the compensatory tilt of the pelvis but the internal rotation of the leg is obvious.

Adduction is corrected by tilting the pelvis upwards, resulting in scoliosis of the lumbar spine with convexity towards the sound side.

As the pelvis tilts upwards to compensate for the adduction the affected limb appears shorter (apparent shortening) than the normal opposite hip, although on comparing the limb lengths in similar positions, true shortening is usually absent or not more than 1 cm.

Stage 3. Erosion: the stage of real shortening

In this stage, the cartilage is destroyed and there is erosion of the upper part of the acetabulum and the femoral head becomes dislocated by the spasm of the adductors (wandering acetabulum or pathological dislocation). The attitude is similar to that seen in stage 2 but exaggerated. There is true shortening of the limb because of the actual destruction of bone. In addition, the apparent length of the limb is further reduced because of the adduction deformity.

Management

THA

Consider:

- The possibility of reactivation of infection following THA
- Shortening of the limb
- Deformed greater trochanter
- Distorted anatomy placing the sciatic nerve and femoral artery at risk of injury
- Acetabular defect
- Antituberculosis treatment 3 months pre-surgery and for 9–12 months post surgery
- A disease-free interval of 10 years before THA is recommended

Excision arthroplasty

This is an option for patients who will not accept stiff joints. Culturally it will allow them to sit cross-legged and also squat. It provides a mobile and painless hip joint but produces shortening and instability leading to tiredness and the need for a walking aid.

Arthrodesis

This is a possible option in a young patient with a deformed painful hip. The rate of pseudoarthrosis is high because of poor bone stock.

Long case 1

Tuberculosis in the left hip as a child

- Underwent arthrodesis of the left hip aged 20
- Deformity of spine
- Leg length discrepancy
- Valgus deformity of the left knee
- Osteoarthritis of the right knee

Long case 2

Arthrodesis of the left hip with ipsilateral knee OA

Young patient with rheumatoid hip disease

This is classic long case material with a lot to talk about and discuss with the examiners. In juvenile RA the problem relates to the onset of the disease. The younger the onset the more severe the growth retardation and deformity. These patients are often severely affected with multiple joint disease and severe osteoporosis. In the FRCS Orth examination a patient seen as a long case may be under consideration for surgery, therefore a specific general physical examination should be undertaken.[23]

Specific attention should be paid to the following:

Anaesthetic concerns

- Cervical spine instability. It is important to assess stability of the cervical spine preoperatively and exclude the presence of a cervical myelopathy.[24] Evaluate for neck pain, neurological signs and symptoms and radiographic changes
- Hypoplasia of the mandible and stiffness of the TMJ may make intubation difficult
- Pulmonary involvement
- Restriction in movement of the upper limb so as to avoid injury whilst establishing IV access

Orthopaedic concerns

- Medication (steroids, etc.)
- Rheumatoid disease distorting hip anatomy
- Implanting THA in a young patient

Steroid use

- General debility
- Fragility of the skin
- Osteoporosis
- Poor musculature

---

[23] Make sure you leave yourself enough time to do this at the end of your clinical examination.

[24] Long case of rheumatoid disease mainly affecting the shoulder and elbow. A large part of the clinical examination was directed towards a cervical myelopathy present.

- Increased risk of wound infection
- Wound healing prolonged

Distorted anatomy

- Hypoplasia of the pelvis and femur
- Gross anteversion and valgus angulation of the femoral neck may lead to difficulty controlling the alignment of a femoral component
- Generalized severe osteoporosis and marked soft-tissue contractures
- Marked anterior bowing of the upper femoral shaft
- Acetabular dysplasia: small size but possible protrusio
- Coxa magna and/or subluxed femoral head
- Premature closure of the growth plate
- Fibrous ankylosis of the hip necessitating in situ osteotomy of the neck

Implanting THA in a young patient

Patients are polyarthritic, often underweight, and often put less stress on their components, so that wear is less than expected.

Indications

Pain is the major indication for surgery. Loss of function and reduced range of movement are secondary indications. Mobility may not be greatly improved post THA because of limitations due to disease in other joints and an improvement in mobility may depend on the replacement of other joints in the lower limb.

Technical concerns when performing THA

Great care is needed when dislocating the hip to prevent a femoral shaft fracture or damage to the ipsilateral knee. Reaming the femur is easy because the femoral canal is usually wide but the cortex is soft and easily penetrated or fractured. The femur is often underdeveloped and a smaller implant may be required. Intra-operative pelvic fracture can occur. If acetabular protrusio

is present avoid penetration of the medial wall and be prepared to do a bone graft if necessary. Some authors suggest it is preferable to avoid trochanteric osteotomy since during the re-wiring of an osteoporotic trochanter there is a risk that the bone may become fragmented. Others would suggest that trochanteric osteotomy decreases the risk of femoral shaft fracture or perforation from malposition of the femoral reamers. There is an increased risk of trochanteric displacement (15%) and non-union (10%).[25]

When the acetabular floor is extremely thin bone grafting with multiple morselized segments cut from the excised femoral head may help to preserve bone stock. If there is a large medial wall deficiency a single solid bone graft fashioned from the femoral head may be used for reconstruction.

If the roof of the acetabulum is deficient then it can be reconstructed by screwing on segments of the patient's femoral head or similar allograft bone to reconstruct the roof. Where the acetabular floor has become completely fragmented or destroyed but the rim of the acetabulum remains intact use of an acetabular ring may prove useful.

Results

The survival of the prosthesis is less than that seen in elderly rheumatoid patients, just under 50% are loose at 5 years, and the 10-year survival as measured by revision is ~75%.

Recurrent dislocation THA

History and examination

The history should begin with details of the last episode of dislocation and any previous episodes of instability. When was the index hip procedure performed and what was the original diagnosis?

[25] Sochart DH, Porter ML (1997) The long-term results of Charnley low-friction arthroplasty in young patients who have congenital dislocation, degenerative osteoarthrosis, or rheumatoid arthritis. *J Bone Joint Surg Am* 79(11): 1599–617.

What approach was most likely used (check scar) and which components were used (check operation notes)? What was the direction of the dislocation (anterior, posterior, other)? What was the prior treatment for the dislocation? Clinical examination should include a full bilateral lower extremity examination with particular attention paid to scar, leg length, gait, range of movement, strength of muscles (particularly abductors) and neurovascular exam. Look for clinical evidence of infection.

Imaging

AP view of the pelvis, AP view of the hip and a cross table lateral view of the hip. Check for component mal-alignment, evidence of eccentric wear, osteophytes, bone quality and integrity, femoral offset and leg length, component geometry, trochanteric non-union, osteolysis and component loosening. Identify the components (must confirm).

Time to dislocation

Time to dislocation is important. Early dislocation (weeks or months) suggests problems with soft-tissue tension such as muscle weakness and inadequate capsular healing and scarring, component mal-position, infection or patient noncompliance. Late dislocation (beyond 1 year) suggests stretching of the soft tissues or polyethylene wear.

Discussion

Discussion would start with a review of the radiographs. This will lead on to the causes of recurrent dislocation. There may be an obvious cause but often the reason is complex and multifactorial. Next up would be the management of recurrent dislocation in general and in this particular patient.

There is a lot to talk about:
- Component alignment
- Early versus late dislocation
- Treatment options
- Posterior approach versus anterolateral approach
- How do you perform a posterior approach to the hip?
- Constrained acetabular cup liner
- Revision surgery
- Jumbo heads

11

Knee clinical cases

Deiary F. Kader and Leo Pinczewski

Anterior cruciate deficiency

Usually there will be one or two patients with an ACL-deficient knee in the short cases.

Memorandum

"This patient is a young, typically male, sporty type of person in shorts. They usually have obvious quadriceps wasting with possible medial and lateral arthroscopic portal scars."

"The patient has a normal gait and knee motion, a minor effusion and no specific areas of tenderness in the knee. The anterior drawer test and Lachman's test revealed an increase in translation of the tibia on the femur compared to the opposite side and no firm end point was felt. The pivot shift test was positive for anterior cruciate deficiency (describe what you are doing as you are doing it). A pivot shift demonstrates a non-functioning ACL. With the leg extended there is an anterior subluxation of the tibia on the femur. Flexion with a valgus stress and axial load to the knee causes the anteriorly subluxed knee to spontaneously reduce into its normal position with respect to the femur with a sudden visible jump or shift at 20°–30° flexion."

Discussion

- Indications for ACL reconstruction
- Technique
- Pivot shift

Short case 1

Examiner: This is a 20-year-old male who sustained an injury to his right knee 1 year ago. Examine his knee for instability.

Candidate: I would normally start my examination by walking the patient.

Examiner: Don't bother, just examine on the couch.

Candidate: I mentioned quadriceps wasting. Patellar apprehension was test negative. Knee flexed to 90°, negative sag, normal step off.

The anterior drawer test was positive and there was a soft end point on Lachman's test.

I continued examining the knee testing the collateral ligaments (which were normal).

I asked the patient to lie prone to test for posterolateral corner injury.

I performed the dial test at 30° and 90° (which was normal).

Management of the case was discussed:

- It was agreed that the role of an MRI scan should not be routine but only used to confirm findings following an equivocal pivot shift test or to identify associated injury for surgical planning
- Noyes' "rule of thirds"
- Physiotherapy initially and, if this is unsuccessful, then consider ACL reconstruction

---

Osteoarthritis of the knee

This can be a short or long case. There is little room for any error. The candidate would be

Postgraduate Orthopaedics: The Candidate's Guide to the FRCS (Tr & Orth) Examination, Ed. Paul A. Banaszkiewicz,
Deiary F. Kader, Nicola Maffulli. Published by Cambridge University Press. © Cambridge University Press 2009.

expected to be very familiar with this type of case from clinic.

Memorandum

"On examination from the front, with the patient adopting a weight-bearing stance, I see that this is an elderly gentleman of average height and build. There is a bilateral varus deformity of both knees. There are no scars, no skin discoloration or varicose veins. He walks in a slow plodding manner suggestive of loading his knees on the lateral compartment."

"There is no effusion present in either knee but generalized synovial thickening. He has a fixed flexion deformity in both knees of 10° and demonstrates a range of movement from 10° to 70° flexion."

"The knees are tender globally with osteophytes over the joint lines. There is a grating sound with crepitus when the knees are moved. Both knees are stable when the anterior drawer, posterior drawer and Lachman's test are performed with a firm end point noted. The varus deformity is not fully correctable."

"The distal circulation is good with dorsalis pedis and tibialis posterior pulses strongly palpable, good capillary refill, no dystrophic changes in the nails and no distal hair loss. Likewise sensation to fine touch is normal."

Discussion

Candidate: These are AP and lateral radiographs of the weight-bearing left/right knee, which demonstrate severe changes of osteoarthritis. There is marked loss of joint space, subchondral sclerosis, gross osteophytosis and bone cysts are present. The leg is in overall varus alignment with preferential loss of the medial joint line space. The patella also shows loss of joint space and osteophytes.

Examiner: How are you going to treat this patient?

Candidate: With such severe changes of osteoarthritis, the only realistic option, assuming failure of conservative management, would be a total knee arthroplasty, but you would need to go back to the patient and take a detailed history and examine him as you cannot base management decisions purely on radiographic findings.

We also need to assess the patient better. Questions I would like to ask include whether he is getting any pain at all in this knee and if so how much. I would ask

what painkillers he is taking; how much and when he last took any. I would ask whether he is sleeping well at night or whether he is woken up by the knee pain. I would ascertain how his activities of daily living are affected and whether he has difficulty going up and down stairs, rising from a chair, and getting in and out of a car. I'd also ask how far he can walk, and if he can get to the shops.

We need to get more information from the patient before we commit ourselves to surgery. We need to take a full history from the patient. Salient features would include ... , etc. The most important symptoms would be pain, stiffness ... , etc. Other symptoms the patient may complain about to a lesser degree include ... , etc.

Features on examination to which I would pay particular attention are the state of the skin and surrounding soft tissues and any foci of infection such as an infected ingrowing toenail or skin lesion. From the surgical point of view, I would assess how large the knee was and if there was a severe varus or fixed flexion deformity that would make the operation more difficult.

Examination corner

Long case 1

An 81-year-old male with bilateral varus osteoarthritis of the knees

Gross deformity present with associated fixed flexion deformity of approximately 20° in each knee. Thorough history including recreation, social, stairs in house, etc.

Demonstration of:
- Varus/valgus instability
- Anterior drawer test
- Lachman's test

The usual questions were asked on possible spinal/vascular/hip aetiology for knee pain.

Asked to take informed consent for TKA in front of the examiners.

Discussion

- Shown radiographs of both knees
- What type of TKA would you do?
- What problems do you anticipate (patella eversion, rectus snip, etc.)?
- How do you sequentially release the medial structures?

- How do you correct for a fixed flexion deformity intra-operatively?
- How do you re-create the joint line in TKA?

Long case 2

A 63-year-old male with severe bilateral varus osteoarthritis knees with fixed flexion deformity

- Demonstration of full hip and knee examination
- Discussion of radiographs
- Discussion of all management options
- Discussion of recently published literature on the subject
- Discussion about thromboprophylaxis including relevant literature on the subject

Short case 1

A 41-year-old lady with posttraumatic osteoarthritic left knee

- Varus mal-alignment
- Antalgic gait
- No fixed flexion deformity, effusion or patellofemoral joint tenderness
- Normal range of movement
- Tenderness limited to medial joint line
- Varus was correctable
- Cruciates and collaterals were stable

Management

I suggested conservative management and then, if there was significant severe symptomatic deterioration, either osteotomy or UKA.

Long case 3

This was a gift. The patient was an otherwise fit and healthy 79-year-old female with predominantly right-sided osteoarthritis of the knee. I took a full history. I examined her back and hips thoroughly and noted that she has bilateral varus knees with a mild fixed flexion deformity on the right.

I was asked to demonstrate the Thomas test and correctable varus. The second examiner discussed investigation, long leg films, non-operative options, evidence for the benefit of arthroscopic washout and UKA. I was asked what type of knee prosthesis I would offer her, which led to a discussion of PCL retaining versus posterior stabilized total knee replacement.

Short case 2

Varus knee with osteoarthritis

- Examine this patient's knee
- What investigations would you order and why?

PCL injury

Memorandum

"On examination there is a young athletic gentleman of average height and build. What we can see from the front is fairly marked quadriceps muscle wasting of his right knee. There appear to be well-healed arthroscopic portal scars over the medial and lateral joint lines."

"On inspection of his gait he demonstrates a varus thrust of the right knee during walking."

"Examination supine reveals a small effusion present in this knee. There is no fixed flexion deformity. A range of movement 0°–110° flexion compared to 0°–130° flexion on the opposite, normal side. Palpation reveals no specific areas of tenderness. On flexing his knees to 90° there appears to be a posterior sag sign. The tibial tubercle appears less prominent than usual whilst the patella appears more prominent than normal. Placing a flat card over the front of the right knee reveals a subtle concavity present with a gap between the card and the front of the knee. Also the step off sign is negative (the tibial plateau is flush with the medial femoral condyle) suggesting PCL disruption."

"Anteriorly directed force applied to the proximal tibia moved it anteriorly from an abnormal sagged back position to a normal alignment. As soon as the force was released gravity caused the tibia to sublux posteriorly with respect to the femur (dropback phenomenon)."

"The quadriceps active drawer sign was positive for PCL disruption. The tibia moved anteriorly when the quadriceps contracted actively extending the knee from a flexed position."

Discussion

- Surgical reconstruction for symptomatic chronic PCL injuries
- Acute bony avulsions
- Acute combined injuries
- Debate about the long-term history of the PCL-deficient knee: some studies suggest that there is significant activity-related pain and possibly degenerative changes especially in the anterior and medial compartments

Previous high tibial osteotomy

Memorandum

"A lateral scar or an L-shaped lateral scar suggests that the patient has had an HTO."

"Controversy remains as to whether the outcome after TKA following HTO is less successful than conventional TKA."

"Conversion to TKA may be technically demanding due to difficulty with patella eversion, soft-tissue balancing and infection."

Discussion

Technical problems include:
- Patella baja
- The need to respect a longitudinal scar: at least 6 cm should be allowed between a new midline scar and an old lateral scar
- Subperiosteal exposure is difficult
- Consider PCL sacrificing/substitution
- There may be a large uncontained bone defect on the tibia requiring augmentation
- Indications for HTO
- Results of HTO

Pigmented villonodular synovitis

Memorandum

"The knee is the most commonly involved large joint. Two types of pigmented villonodular synovitis exist: a localized form characterized by a solitary lesion and a diffuse form aggressive in nature usually involving the entire synovial membrane. Local disease presents with mechanical symptoms such as locking and catching, whilst the diffuse type is characterized by pain, swelling, stiffness and deformity."

Examination corner

Short case 1

Pigmented villonodular synovitis (PVNS) of the knee
- Examine the knee for effusion and history of recurrent bleed
- Clinical differentiation of effusion from synovial thickening
- Differential diagnosis of PVNS
- PVNS: clinical presentation, joints affected, management

Valgus knee

Memorandum

Look for walking aids. Typically this would be a rheumatoid patient or a young patient post-trauma.

Rheumatoid arthritis

The patient presents with polyarthropathy. Look for hand and wrist signs. Weight bearing leads to marked valgus deformity of the knee. Fullness of the knee suggests soft-tissue swelling due to a synovitis.

Discussion

- Radiographs of the knee
- Cervical spine evaluation
- Medical evaluation of the rheumatoid patient
- Methotrexate, steroid usage
- Sequential release of the valgus knee
- Type of knee replacement to use, i.e. PCL sacrificing with patella replacement
- A stemmed implant is necessary in severe valgus deformity

Examination corner

Adult elective orthopaedics oral

- Radiograph of the medial compartment and patello-femoral OA
- Management options
- Indications for osteotomy versus unicompartment knee replacement
- Results of Coventry osteotomy
- Criteria for osteotomy

Clinical short case 1

- Examine this man's knee
- Look at the patient (middle-aged, body-builder)
- Ask the usual questions about knee pain

Assess

- Gait: look for varus thrust
- The degree of varus deformity. Is it correctable?
- The range of movement in the knee
- Ligament laxity
- Leg length discrepancy
- Examine the hip and foot for fixed deformity

Radiographs

- Medial compartment OA
- What are you going to do?
- Why not carry out a unicompartmental knee arthroplasty? (Age and ACL are probably the main factors to consider here)

If the patient is <60 years old and has some articular surface preserved, in addition to the previous prerequisites one can offer HTO. However, if the patient is older and the degenerative arthritis is severe (bone on bone), unicompartmental knee arthroplasty would be a better choice.

12

Foot and ankle clinical cases

Paul A. Banaszkiewicz

Deformities of the foot

Equinus

The entire weight is borne by the forefoot, the hindfoot remaining off the ground. The equinus deformity may be compensatory for either quadriceps or gluteus maximus weakness, or due to shortening of the limb. The equinus deformity may also be caused by contracture of gastrocnemius and/or soleus.

Calcaneus

Here the weight is borne mainly by the hindfoot. The forefoot may have varying degrees of weight bearing, but definitely below normal.

Varus

The weight is borne mainly on the outer side of the foot. This deformity is mainly at the hindfoot.

Valgus

Weight bearing is borne mainly on the inner side of the foot. This deformity is of the hindfoot or of both the forefoot and hindfoot.

Inverted foot

When the hindfoot and forefoot are both in a varus position, the deformity is termed an inverted foot.

The accentuation of this position will gradually turn the sole towards the sky – supination of the foot. In these positions, i.e. in inverted and supinated foot, adduction of the forefoot and plantar flexion of the ankle will coexist.

Everted foot

The hindfoot and forefoot are both in a valgus position. The outer part of the sole bears increasingly less weight. In the exaggerated situation, the outer part of the sole acquires a tendency to face towards the sky. In this position, adduction of the forefoot and dorsiflexion at the ankle will coexist.

Pes cavus

A normal foot has a medial longitudinal arch that is higher than the lateral one. When this normal proportion is exaggerated, the medial side of the foot tends to assume the shape of a high arch and looks like a cave. It rarely occurs as a single deformity. It is a common accompaniment of equinovarus, equinus and clawing of the toes.

Pes planus

Collapse of the medial longitudinal arch. The normal concavity due to the medial longitudinal arch is absent and instead the medial side of the foot bulges as a medial convexity, particularly on weight bearing.

Postgraduate Orthopaedics: The Candidate's Guide to the FRCS (Tr & Orth) Examination, Ed. Paul A. Banaszkiewicz,
Deiary F. Kader, Nicola Maffulli. Published by Cambridge University Press. © Cambridge University Press 2009.

Arthrodesed ankle

Short case 1

- Examination of ankle and subtalar movements
- Complications of arthrodesis
- Position of fusion

Short case 2

I was asked to examine a 50-year-old man and to describe what I saw, which was Charnley clamps with a type of external fixator arrangement applied across the left ankle.

The examiners asked what I thought it was for, I replied, "ankle arthrodesis".

The examiners then asked what I would look for on the postoperative ward rounds, I said, "Pin site care/infection, neurovascular deficit, consider retightening the construct."

I was then asked if there was anything else to add. I noticed that the big toe was slightly plantiflexed and suggested checking the "range of movement" whilst commenting on the big toe's posture. Asked what could be causing this, I said that I would want to check neurology in the sural, saphenous, deep peroneal nerves and plantar nerve territory. Comparing both sides the patient could only achieve a jog of dorsiflexion/plantar flexion at the MTP joint with a little more possible passively. The IP joint was a little more flexible when passively tested. I mentioned pin tethering was a possible cause and that I would like to have known the range of movement preoperatively. I was asked if I thought the big toe was stiff anyway. I said it was, at the MTP joint.

Short case 3

A middle-aged man with an anterolateral surgical scar over his right ankle

I was asked to examine his ankle and hindfoot.
- No ankle movement and limited painful subtalar movement
- The patient had developed secondary osteoarthritis of the subtalar joint following a previous ankle arthrodesis
- I was asked about the incidence of subtalar arthritis after ankle arthrodesis and how long it usually takes before it presents (20 years)
- I was asked about the management of subtalar arthritis

Charcot foot

Memorandum

Make a quick scan of the surroundings for possible clues to the diagnosis. There may be a foot orthosis present.

"The ankle joint is grossly deformed and swollen. There is loss of the normal medial longitudinal arch of the foot, a valgus deformity of the forefoot and a rocker bottom deformity of the foot. There is a chronic painless ulcer present on the plantar surface of the collapsed midfoot caused by excessive pressure in this area (malperforans). It does not appear infected. No ulcers or blisters/skin breakdown are seen over the first, third or fifth metatarsal head. Movement is abnormally increased and associated with loud audible crepitus, but it is painless. There is loss of light touch, pinprick and vibration sense in the foot, markedly decreased joint position sense in the toes, but it is normal in the fingers, and absent ankle jerks. There is wasting of the intrinsic muscles of the foot and clawing of the lesser toes."

"This is a Charcot joint."

A Charcot joint (neuropathic arthropathy) is gross osteoarthritis with new bone formation. It is caused by repeated minor trauma without the normal protective responses that accompany pain sensation. The joint is painlessly destroyed. The foot may resemble osteomyelitis in that it appears swollen with overlying erythema and warmth.

Three stages

- Development stage
- Coalescent stage
- Reconstructive stage

Causes

Any loss of protective sensations of pain and proprioception in a joint may render it susceptible to the development of a neuropathic arthropathy.

Radiographs

Radiographs reveal bone fragmentation, joint subluxation or dislocation, resorption and coalescence of the bony fragments. The bone surrounding the joint becomes sclerotic.

Management

- Bisphosphonates
- Immobilization in total contact cast
- Mid foot or ankle arthrodesis

Charcot–Marie–Tooth disease

History 1

Patients complain of having tired feet and having difficulty buying shoes that accommodate their high arch and the clawing of their toes; they have metatarsalgia and callosities secondary to lateral weight bearing.

Examination 1

"On inspection, there is distal wasting of the lower limb muscles that stop abruptly (state where). The legs are stock or spindle shaped, and the calves have a fat bottle or inverted champagne bottle appearance. The feet show a pes-cavus-type deformity with associated clawing of the lesser toes. The patient has a bilateral drop foot gait (steppage gait). There is weakness of the extensors of the toes and feet. Ankle jerks are absent. The ankle is in equinus; there is midfoot and hindfoot varus and cavus. The forefoot is in valgus and there is a plantarflexed first ray."

"Weakness of the foot intrinsics and contracture of the plantar fascia add to the fixation of the cavus deformity and secondary clawing of the toes. There are no neuropathic ulcers present."

"The patient also demonstrates wasting of the small muscles of the hands. There is a tendency for the fingers to curl and the patient has difficulty in straightening and abducting them."

History 2

- The presenting complaint is of walking on the outer borders of the feet, difficulty in wearing shoes and painful callosities
- Walking distance is reduced to 100 yards
- Previous surgery of Jones procedures and PIP joint fusions

- No regular medication
- Otherwise fit and healthy

Examination 2

"On inspection, this gentleman stands with some difficulty. He has obvious wasting of both calves. On the left foot, he has a varus heel. Both feet are in equinus. Looking from behind, one can again see the obvious varus left heel."

"*Just tell me if you have any discomfort on palpation.*"

"There are thick callosities over the lateral border of both feet. The hindfoot will not come to neutral. The subtalar joints will not correct to a neutral position; they are fixed in 10° of inversion. There is a jog of movement of the hindfoot. He has grade 4+ power of tibialis posterior. There is almost no power of eversion."

"*Push your big toe down.*"

"He does appear to have good peroneus longus power. Coleman block test does not improve the hindfoot varus, suggesting that it is fixed."

Initially the hindfoot is in varus. The Coleman block test is performed by placing a block under the lateral column of the foot and allowing the first metatarsal to drop to the floor. Heel varus correction indicates that the hindfoot deformity is flexible and that the varus position is secondary to the plantarflexed first ray, or valgus position of the forefoot. A fixed hindfoot deformity will not correct.

Background

Hereditary neurological disorder characterized by weakness and wasting of intrinsic muscles of the foot, particularly the peroneal muscles, the dorsiflexors and plantar flexors of the foot and toes.

The end result is a progressive equinocavovarus foot with:

- Clawing toes
- Forefoot valgus
- Plantarflexed first ray
- Midfoot and hindfoot cavus
- Ankle equinus

Presentation

- Autosomal-recessive disease presents early
- Sex-linked recessive disease presents at 20 years of age

- Autosomal-dominant disease presents at 30 years of age

Management

Conservative

Insoles, orthotics, physiotherapy, etc.

Soft-tissue procedures

- Achilles tendon lengthening
- Split anterior tibial tendon transfer
- Plantar fascia release
- Claw toe procedures

Bony procedures

- Dwyer's calcaneal osteotomy
- Jones procedure: interphalangeal arthrodesis of the hallux and transfer of the EHL tendon into the distal first metatarsal (to decrease clawing of the big toe)

Short case 1

A candidate was asked to examine a patient's gait and to examine his lower legs. They could see bilateral foot drop and wasted anterior muscle compartments but they did not make the diagnosis of Charcot–Marie–Tooth disease. The examiners were critical of the candidate's neurological examination of the lower legs – they required prompting and appeared hesitant. The candidate failed to appreciate that the small muscles in the hand can be affected in this condition.

Short case 2

Cavus feet, young man with hereditary sensory-motor neuropathy

- Differential diagnosis and management
- Types of hereditary sensory-motor neuropathy
- Surgical management: Jones procedure

Short case 3

Examine this lady's feet

Very obvious pes cavus deformity bilaterally. I was just about to mention the possible causes of a pes cavus deformity when I noticed she had mild clawing of both hands. The examiners asked me why I was looking at her hands and what the likely diagnosis was. I mentioned HSMN.

Clawing of the lesser toes

A claw toe refers to a toe with flexion at the DIP and PIP joints and extension at the MTP joint.

A flexible deformity indicates an imbalance between extrinsic and intrinsic muscle forces, whilst a fixed deformity may result from joint damage, capsular and/or ligamentous shortening or tendon shortening.

Claw toe deformities are often associated with conditions that produce a muscle imbalance. Causes include neuromuscular disorders such as Charcot–Marie–Tooth disease, cerebral palsy and diabetic neuropathy. Other causes include compartment syndrome, poliomyelitis, cerebrovascular accidents and multiple sclerosis.

Memorandum

"On examination there is hyperextension at the MTP joints, plantar displacement of the metatarsal heads and distal migration of the fat pad. There are also plantar keratotic lesions and callosities present over the dorsal surface of the PIP joints of the 2nd/3rd/4th toes of the right/left foot. There are no ulcers under the metatarsal heads. There is plantar flexion of the PIP joints and the DIP joints are flexed/extended/neutral. The deformity is fixed/flexible."

Management

Try to identify an underlying cause if possible.

Conservative

Padding and protection of specific callosities, metatarsal pads, etc.

Surgery

The goal is to bring the MTP joints and PIP joints into a neutral position.

If there is a flexible deformity, consider FDL tenotomy or Girdlestone flexor-extensor transfer. To correct the MTP joint deformity extensor tenotomy and dorsal capsulotomy are required (MTP joint soft-tissue release).

If there is a fixed deformity, carry out a fusion or excision arthroplasty of the PIP joint; if the MTP joint is dislocated carry out Stainsby's procedure.

Short case 1

- Claw toes and mild claw foot
- Discuss the differential diagnosis of this condition
- Principles of management

Curly toe

Background

This is a common condition affecting one or more toes. It is often bilateral, symmetrical and familial. It involves malrotation of the toe with a digit flexion deformity at the PIP and DIP joints. Deformity may resolve as the child grows. It is usually asymptomatic but may occasionally cause discomfort if rotation of the toe is such that the nail becomes weight bearing. It can cause difficulty with shoe wear or may catch when putting socks on.

Memorandum

On examination the third to fifth toes are curled medially and plantar flexed with lateral rotation at the DIP joint. The third toe is flexed and deviated medially to under-ride the second toe, pushing it dorsally.

Management

Manage conservatively if possible. Surgery is indicated if there are significant symptoms and deformity such as toes under-riding adjacent medial toes. Delay surgery until after 4 years of age as at that stage the toes are bigger, and the condition may have improved in a number of patients.

Open flexor tenotomy of both FDL and FDB via incision over the proximal phalanx

- Be careful with skin closure

Transfer of flexors to extensors (Girdlestone transfer)

- No longer recommended; this has fallen out of favour as it is technically difficult and produces a toe stiff in extension

Diabetic foot

Despite being a common condition, this does not appear to be a particularly common short or long case.

Memorandum

"There is a well-circumscribed punched out ulcer approximately 4 cm in diameter on the sole/plantar surface of the right foot (most commonly at the site of maximal pressure under the head of the first metatarsal). The ulcer does not appear to be infected; there is no surrounding cellulitis or discharge from the ulcer base. There is thick callous formation over the pressure points of the feet. Two toes have previously been amputated and the remaining toes are clawed. There is loss of the normal medial longitudinal arch of the foot. Both the metatarsal and heel pads are atrophied. There appears to be reduced sweating of the foot. There is loss of sensation to light touch, vibration and pinprick in a stocking distribution.[1] The feet are cold, the pulses are not palpable and there is loss of hair on the lower legs, which are shiny."

"The toenails have no chronic changes present such as onychomycosis, ingrowing or incurvated changes. The patient has a peripheral neuropathy, a neuropathic ulcer

---

[1] In the neuropathic foot the pulses may be palpable or even bounding. The foot is warm, dry and insensate with pulses and distended veins.

on the sole of his foot and evidence of peripheral vascular disease. It is likely he has diabetes."

The neuropathic ulcer

- Thick hyperkeratosis
- Pink punched-out base, which readily bleeds
- Painless

The ischaemic ulcer

- Not surrounded by hyperkeratosis
- Dull fibrotic base, does not bleed easily
- Painful to touch
- Ulcers present over the curve on the first and fifth metatarsal heads

Factors that may contribute to the development of the diabetic foot lesion include:

- Injury
- Neuropathy
- Small vessel disease
- Large vessel disease
- Increased susceptibility to infection
- Foot deformity leading to increased possibility of mechanical stress and trauma

Causes of a peripheral neuropathy

- Diabetes (foot)
- Tabes dorsalis (lower extremity)
- Syringomyelia (upper extremity)
- Hansen's disease (leprosy)
- Myelomeningocele (ankle and foot)
- Congenital insensitivity to pain
- Other neurological problems
- Peripheral neuropathies (alcohol, amyloidosis, pernicious anaemia)
- Infection (yaws, tuberculosis)

Hallux rigidus

Memorandum

"On inspection of the weight-bearing foot and ankle from the front the left/right hallux is straight and the MTP joint bumpy. There is mild erythema and oedema seen at the MTP joint, but no ulceration present. There is a prominent dorsal/lateral osteophyte and an increased bulk of the joint. Dorsiflexion of the first MTP joint is restricted and painful. Likewise plantar flexion of the first MTP joint is limited. Sensation was normal, there was good capillary refill and there were strong palpable dorsalis pedis and posterior tibial pulses."

"The patient walks with an antalgic gait and is tending to walk on the outside border of the left/right foot to avoid loading the first MTP joint. In addition the big toe is not being used in the toe-off part of the gait cycle."

Other physical signs

- Prominent marginal osteophytes
- Affected feet are often long, narrow and pronated
- The first metatarsal is often long

Management options

Conservative management

- Adequate toe box, rigid and/or rocker bottom insoles, etc.

Surgery

Mild disease

- **Cheilectomy.** Especially for dorsal osteophytes and dorsal impingement. Excision of the proliferative bone about the metatarsal head, removing approximately 30% of the metatarsal head and lateral osteophytes flush with the metatarsal shaft. The bone is resected to obtain 70°–80° of dorsiflexion and to eliminate dorsal impingement. If severe arthrosis is present, a cheilectomy may lead to unsatisfactory results
- **Closing wedge osteotomy of the proximal phalanx.** Carried out if there is loss of dorsiflexion but no dorsal impingement
- **MUA and steroid injection.** Only for mild disease

Severe disease

- **Arthrodesis.** The gold standard: it resolves pain and provides stability of the joint. However, it is also accompanied by loss of motion, loss of pivoting sports and loss of ability to wear high heels. Position of fusion: 15° valgus, 25° dorsiflexion and the IP joint should be mobile.

- **Silastic® implant.** Not recommended because of the possibilities of transfer metatarsalgia, implant breakage, silicone synovitis, cock-up toe and stress fracture
- **Keller's excision arthroplasty.** For the elderly patient

---

Short case 1

Hallux rigidus

Demonstration of the range of motion in joints of the foot and ankle.

Short case 2

A middle-aged lady who had a spot diagnosis of hallux rigidus. I went through the look, feel and move scenario so I had asked her to stand up and then I described what I saw. The examiner then pushed me and asked, "Okay what is the diagnosis?", which I gave and the examiner then asked me how I would confirm it. I explained that first of all I would get her walking and this confirmed that there was no dorsiflexion in her big toe and that she actually supinated the foot to avoid any pressure on the first metatarsal head.

The examiner sat down next to the patient and asked me for a definition of hallux rigidus and again asked, "Show me how you would confirm that this is hallux rigidus". I continued with palpation but the examiner really wanted me to demonstrate that there was no passive extension of the MTP joint. I got there in the end. I was then asked what the sole of her foot would look like. I mentioned that there would be a plantar callosity over the metatarsal head.

My impression of this case was that although I went through the look, feel and move scenario the examiner really just wanted me to say, "Look this is a hallux rigidus deformity" and confirm it by bending up a painful toe within 30 seconds of actually introducing myself to the patient.

Short case 3

Arthrodesed left hallux in a middle-aged lady with continuing difficulties

Short history: instructed to ask three to four questions.

- What was the original problem with the big toe that required you to have surgery?
- What is wrong with your big toe now?
- Is it painful?
- Do you have trouble walking?

Examination

- What has gone wrong?
- What is the optimum position for arthrodesis of the great toe MTP joint?
- What are the complications from surgery?

Short case 4

Hallux rigidus

- Big cyst on great toe MTP joint
- History and examination
- Management options

Hallux valgus

Memorandum

"On inspection of the foot and ankle from the front, there is an obvious severe/moderate/mild hallux valgus deformity of the right/left big toe. There is lateral deviation of the big toe at the MTP joint and prominence of the metatarsal head and a varus deformity of the first metatarsal. The skin over the medial border of the metatarsal head is thickened and hyperkeratotic but not ulcerated. There is also over-riding of the second toe onto the hallux. There is pronation of the hallux. There are no lesser toe deformities or visible callosities. The longitudinal arch and hindfoot posture appear normal."

"On observing the patient's gait, the hallux is used in the normal push-off function. There are no other obvious features of note; in particular the gait is not antalgic or Trendelenburg."

"The deformity is fully correctable/not fully correctable at the MTP joint and is painful when moved. The patient demonstrates a positive grind test at the MTP joint suggesting arthrosis of this joint."

"The medial eminence, sesamoid complex and lesser MTP joints were non-tender to palpation. Inspecting the plantar surface of the foot, there were no callosities present. There was no metatarsalgia of the lesser toes."

"There is normal sensation of the foot particularly over the first metatarsal. There are palpable dorsalis pedis and posterior tibial pulses and the capillary refill at the toes is normal. The appearance of the skin and distribution of hairs suggest a good circulation distally. There are no obvious plantar callosities or other lesions on the plantar aspect of her foot. There is no Achilles tendon tightness, and there are otherwise normal ankle and subtalar movements. There is a normal metatarsocuneiform joint motion. There is no hindfoot valgus or collapse of the medial longitudinal arch of the foot."

Short case 1

Young female sitting on a chair in a corner. The examiner is looking around the hall for further patients and spots the young female.

Examiner: You will do. Examine this lady's foot.
Candidate: On inspection of this lady's feet she has an obvious mild hallux valgus deformity of her left big toe. The right hallux is normal. There is lateral deviation of the big toe at the MTP joint, prominence of the metatarsal head and a varus deformity of the first metatarsal. The skin over the medial border of the metatarsal head is thickened and hyperkeratotic but not ulcerated. There are hammertoe deformities of her second and third left toes with pressure lesions over the PIP joints.

The candidate lifts up the foot to inspect the sole. There are prominent plantar callosities over the metatarsal heads.

The candidate now checks for correctability deformity.

Candidate: The deformity is fully correctable and it is not painful when I correct it.
Candidate: Is it sore when I push on your joint? (grind test).
Patient: No.
Candidate: She has a negative grind test for the MTP joint.
Candidate: Is your big toe painful?
Patient: No.
Examiner: Come and have a look at her X-rays.

Candidate: The radiographs demonstrate a mild hallux deformity of her left big toe. There is no arthrosis at the MTP joint.
Examiner: So how are you going to manage her?
Candidate: She has a mild deformity and is not complaining of any pain so I would manage her conservatively.
Examiner: What do you mean by conservative management?
Candidate: I would not operate on her. I would give her some advice about appropriate shoe wear (wide fitting shoes) and bring her back to the clinic in 6 months if she had any concerns.
Examiner: Yes, she has minimal symptoms and minimal deformity in the big toe and she does not require surgery.

In this particular diet of examinations there was a shortage of good clinical material for both the long and short cases. This patient had only a mild hallux valgus deformity and it's debatable if she would have been included if better cases had been available.

You cannot always examine in as comprehensive a manner as you would like. There were quite a lot of things missed out in the above example. Sometimes it is just not practical to test for things like a tight Achilles tendon or the metatarsocuneiform joint. Sometimes you just forget to do so in the heat of the exam.

Keep talking and keep the examination running along smoothly. The candidate realized it was a mild deformity and was thinking ahead about management options. The candidate spontaneously asked the patient if she was getting pain in the big toe.

Short case 2

Severe bilateral hallux valgus deformities

- Examination and plan of management
- The patient had severe deformities and the examiner wanted to hear basal osteotomy

Hammertoe

A short case spot diagnosis.

Memorandum

A hammertoe refers to a toe with flexion at the PIP joint and extension at the MTP joint. The DIP joint is usually flexed although occasionally it is held in extension. The deformity can be flexible or fixed. Usually there are painful corns over the dorsum of the flexed PIP joint and callosities under the plantarly prominent metatarsal head.

Management

Flexible

- Conservative if possible. Flexor tendon transfer, e.g. Girdlestone-Taylor transfer of FDL to the extensor hood; variable results reported

Fixed

- PIP joint arthrodesis
- Partial proximal phalangectomy. It relieves symptoms but has poor cosmesis
- Excision arthroplasty of the PIP joint ±extensor tenotomy plus MTP joint capsular release
- DuVries metatarsal head arthroplasty

Complications of lesser toe surgery include swelling, reoccurrence of deformity, infection and neurovascular compromise.

Ankle osteoarthritis

History

- Pain is usually felt anteriorly and is made worse with activity and long periods of standing
- There is impingement due to osteophytes developing anteriorly on the joint line, first on the tibia, and then later kissing lesions develop on the talus, with impingement occurring in full dorsiflexion. It is worse in situations of increased dorsiflexion such as ascending slopes and stairs
- Deformity
- Restriction of movement (stiffness)
- Occasionally there is instability or weakness of the ankle

Examination

Both feet should be examined and ranges of movement compared. Any restriction of dorsiflexion is significant. Passive movement will often reveal crepitus. Active and passive movements are usually both restricted in ankle arthritis, and dorsiflexion is typically more affected than plantar flexion. An effusion may be present, which can be felt either anteromedially in the notch of Harty or anterolaterally. Osteophytes along with synovial thickening and swelling may be palpated. Pain is usually present on palpation of the anterior joint line. There is no significant valgus or varus deformity of the ankle. Test for ankle stability using the anterior drawer and tilt tests.[2]

Having assessed the ankle joint, assess both the subtalar and mid tarsal joints for signs of degenerative change as this will influence management options. Finally assess the neurovascular status of the foot.

Memorandum

A typical case would possibly be a middle-aged or elderly patient or a young patient post trauma.

The deformity would be either a valgus or varus deformity of the ankle best seen from behind. There may be scars from previous surgery in a trauma case. There may be swelling of the medial or lateral malleoli, or of both. Assess the patient with them standing on tiptoe, and then ask them whether they can roll back onto their heels.

"On inspecting this patient's gait, he does not demonstrate any asymmetry or abnormal contact with the ground. The patient walks with an externally rotated gait in order to avoid tibio-talar movements. The patient demonstrates a restricted painful range of dorsiflexion/plantarflexion of the ankle. The subtalar movements are well preserved. Tibialis posterior function is normal."

Management

Conservative

Conservative management consists initially of rest, physiotherapy, shoe modification, steroid injections, splints and orthosis, etc.

---

[2] Go to www.youtube.com (You Tube Broadcast Yourself™) and search for anterior drawer test to find some useful videos of this.

Surgery

- Open or arthroscopic ankle debridement
- Joint distraction using Ilizarov fixator
- Ankle fusion
- Ankle arthroplasty

Position of ankle fusion
- Neutral dorsiflexion: 10° plantarflexion (CP)
- 5° valgus – any more results in a stiff gait due to poor push-off
- 5°–7° external rotation
- Slight shift of the talus posteriorly on the tibia is recommended to preserve the heel prominence and improve gait (controversial)

There are many methods of ankle fusion but the key point is that if you are considering ankle fusion get the patient to wear AFO for a few weeks. If it relieves pain then one is much happier to go ahead and perform an arthrodesis. Postoperatively keep the patient in a plaster, non-weight-bearing for 6–8 weeks and then allow partial weight bearing for a further 6–8 weeks in plaster until there are radiographic signs of bony union. Try to delay arthrodesis in post-traumatic osteoarthritis for at least 2 years.

Complications

- Wound breakdown
- Non-union
- Delayed union
- Mal-alignment
- Infection
- Peripheral neurovascular complications

Short case 1

Post-traumatic osteoarthritis of the ankle

Examine this gentleman's feet. I was asked to demonstrate ankle and subtalar movements. The examiner was not entirely happy and made a point of demonstrating how they held the talar neck with their thumb and index finger rather than the tibia to isolate subtalar from ankle movement.

Short case 2

Osteoarthritis of the ankle

- Diagnosis
- Discussion of management
- I was then asked to take a consent for ankle arthrodesis

Short case 3

Ankle pain in an elderly woman

- Why are you making her stand on her toes?
- Assessment of tibialis posterior function
- Demonstration of active and passive range of movement of the ankle
- Demonstration of subtalar range of movement
- Discussion of the complications of ankle arthrodesis
- Take a consent for ankle arthroplasty
- What procedure (ankle arthrodesis or arthroplasty) would you do in this patient and why?
- Are there any recent papers that you know that compare the clinical outcomes of the two?

Pes cavus

Aetiology

- Idiopathic
- Congenital; arthrogryposis, residue congenital talipes equinovarus (CTEV)
- Traumatic: compartment syndrome, crush, burns
- Neuromuscular: disorder of muscles, peripheral nerves, spinal cord, central nervous system

History

- Congenital or acquired? When did you notice this deformity? Were you born with it? When did it develop?
- Progression: is it getting worse?
- Full family history: this often runs in families, so check the family history for neurological disease/neuromuscular disease

- Any problems with your back?
- Any problems with the bladder or bowel? (Bladder or bowel dysfunction)
- Have you any pins or needles or loss of power in your legs? (Sensation and motor power)
- Any difficulty with walking, weakness or tremor?
- Patient may complain of difficulty with footwear, of tired aching feet, of metatarsalgia and lateral foot pain due to area of contact with the floor, pressure over the dorsum of the PIP joints, or recurrent giving-way of the ankle

Memorandum

Look for orthosis, splints, and special shoes.

"On inspection of the feet there is a unilateral/bilateral accentuation (exaggeration) of the medial longitudinal arch of the foot. There is clawing of the lesser toes with callosities over the dorsal PIP joints and heads of the metatarsals (examine the soles of the feet). There is clawing of both halluces and prominence of the EHL, which is overactive as a dorsiflexor to compensate for a weak tibialis anterior. There is a varus of the hindfoot, as well as a high arch, clawing of the toes and callosities. There are no visible ulcers or surgical scars present. There is a generalized wasting of the calf muscles. On the double heel raise test, the hindfoot remains fixed in varus."

"I would like to examine this gentleman's spine please. On inspecting this man's spine, there are no obvious hairy patches, skin discoloration or swelling suggestive of either occult spina bifida or diastematomyelia."

Carry out a full neurological examination of the lower legs testing for sensation, muscle power and reflexes.

"On examination of gait, the patient demonstrates a drop foot gait. Examining his hands, he demonstrates intrinsic muscle wastage."

Coleman block test

The Coleman block test is used to check whether the subtalar joint is mobile or rigid. It is performed by placing the patient's foot on a wooden block with the heel and the lateral border of the foot on the block full weight bearing whilst the first, second and third metatarsals are allowed to hang freely into plantar flexion and pronation. If the heel varus corrects while the patient is standing on the block the hindfoot is considered flexible.

Two main patterns of deformity tend to occur: calcaneocavus and cavovarus.

Calcaneocavus

This mainly involves hindfoot abnormalities. Dorsiflexion of the calcaneum occurs due to a weak Achilles tendon with normal tibialis anterior. There is no pronation of the forefoot and therefore no varus deformity of the hindfoot. It is more common in polio.

Cavovarus

Mainly forefoot abnormalities. The forefoot is pronated and the heel is in varus. This is more common in HMSN.

Investigations

- Weight-bearing lateral radiograph
- X-ray of the spine for spina bifida
- MRI scan of the spine
- Neurological referral

Management

Conservative

- Moulded insoles, heel pads, etc.

Surgery

- Plantar fascia release (Steindler release) if mobile
- Jones procedure: fusion of the IP joint and proximal transfer of EHL to the neck of the first metatarsal
- IP joint fusions as part of claw toe correction
- Calcaneum osteotomy – closing wedge lateral osteotomy
- Triple arthrodesis as a salvage procedure for a severe deformity

Short case 1

Multiply operated bilateral cavovarus feet

- Examination features
- Differential diagnosis
- Suggest further surgery options

Short case 2

Bilateral pes cavovarus due to diastematomyelia

- Candidate asked to take a short history
- Assessment of gait
- Examination of motor and sensory function of the lower legs to locate the level of the lesion
- Demonstration of knee reflexes and ankle clonus
- Surgical scar from a previous Jones procedure: "What is this scar suggestive of, why is the operation performed?"

Short case 3

Young female in her early 20s, sitting down on a chair; unilateral pes cavus deformity

Candidate asked to examine left foot.

Candidate: On inspection of the left foot there is an obvious severe pes cavus deformity present with clawing of the lesser toes. There are callosities present over the dorsal surfaces of her PIP joints. There is a well-healed longitudinal surgical scar present over the dorsal surface of her big toe.

Candidate: I would like to examine her spine now.

Examiner: The spine is normal, don't bother. What operation has she had on her big toe and why?

Candidate: She has had a Jones procedure; this is where the IP joint is fused and the EHL tendon is transferred to the metatarsal neck to prevent hyperextension of the hallux.

The candidate was not asked to demonstrate anything else clinically, particularly the Coleman block test, gait or neurological examination.

Short case 4

- Postoperative resection of a spinal tumour
- Bilateral wasted calves with resolving neurology
- Stiff cavovarus foot – differential diagnosis and management

Short case 5

This is a young man with a foot problem. Would you like to examine his feet and just describe what you are doing as you go along?

Small foot with pes cavus deformity. Clawing of the lesser toes, high arch and varus hindfoot. Calf wasting and LLD. Normal neurology.

Candidate: I would like to examine this man's spine.
Examiner: Why? What are you looking for?
Candidate: Any features suggestive of spina bifida such as a hairy patch or dimple or a diastematomyelia with associated scoliosis.
Examiner: Are there any other causes of a pes cavus deformity?
Candidate: Cerebral palsy but he has no features of this. HMSN, but it is unilateral. Becker muscular dystrophy, but he has no features such as significant progressive muscle weakness or difficulty walking.

Rheumatoid foot

A classic short case. It is unlikely that you would go much further than a general inspection of the feet. You may then be asked about the management principles of the rheumatoid foot. Remember to mention the need to assess the hip and knee first before considering foot surgery.

Memorandum

Examination tip is to start from the ankle and work distally.

"On general inspection there is a bilateral symmetrical deforming arthropathy. There is a hindfoot valgus and localized swelling over both the medial and lateral malleoli. This could be due to tenosynovitis of the tibialis posterior and peroneal tendons. There is also collapse of the medial longitudinal arch of the foot suggestive of possible tibialis posterior tendon rupture."

"There is pronation of the forefoot (forefoot abduction). There are severe bilateral hallux valgus deformities and clawing of several lesser toes and a hammertoe deformity of the third left toe. There are pressure lesions over the dorsal surfaces of the PIP joints of the lesser toes. The lesser toes are dislocated/inflamed/ulcerated. There is swelling over the MTP joints with the appearance of possible subluxation of these joints."

"The skin appears papery thin and fragile with a possible vasculitis. There are no obvious rheumatoid nodules or ulcers present. There is normal sensation of the foot and ankle. Similarly the dorsalis pedis and posterior tibia pulses are present and capillary refill is less than 2 seconds."

"The patient was not able to perform a double heel raise test because of pain. On double heel raise test, the heel failed to invert and the medial longitudinal arch remained collapsed. This suggests tibialis posterior insufficiency. The patient demonstrates an antalgic gait with an externally rotated attitude of both feet. A roll over gait is present."

"On inspection of the plantar surfaces of both feet, there are callosities present over the metatarsal heads. There are no ulcers, scars or sinuses. There is crepitus, tenderness and swelling present over both malleoli. Movement, both actively and passively, of the ankle and subtalar joint is reduced. Specifically, dorsiflexion is painful and limited both actively and passively to neutral. Similarly, plantar flexion is limited to 20° bilaterally both actively and passively."

"The left/right subtalar joint is irritable with only a jog of movement present. There is reduced power of dorsiflexion, plantar flexion, inversion and eversion probably MRC grade 4 minus."

Check the vascular status foot. Perform a careful neurological assessment as there may be a neuropathic component.

Management

Surgical options include:
- Ankle arthrodesis
- Ankle arthroplasty
- Triple arthrodesis or subtalar arthrodesis
- Forefoot excision arthroplasty
- Arthrodesis of the first MTP joint

Ankle arthrodesis

Options include:
- Intramedullary nail through the heel
- Dowel arthrodesis. (Milling cutter passed across the ankle joint with the bone removed, rotated and reversed back across the joint)
- External fixation. Traditional technique of Charnley now superseded by internal fixation as this has lower rates of infection and a higher incidence of fusion
- Arthroscopic ankle arthrodesis
- Plate fixation

Short case 1

Examine the feet
- Hallux valgus with pronated great toe
- Clawed toes
- Callosities under metatarsal heads
- Varicose eczema

Tarsal coalition

Not an uncommon lower limb short case with usually at least one patient in the examination hall with the condition.

Examination corner

Short case 1

Young boy (approximately 11 years old) sitting on a chair

Examiner looks around and spots the young boy.

Examiner: Why don't you start by examining this young man's left foot and tell me what you find. He has been complaining of some vague pain in this foot for several months.

Candidate: (After a brief introduction and handshake with patient.) May I examine your foot? Would you stand up for us so that we can have at look at your feet?

Examination started with inspection from behind (the rules were immediately broken!).

Candidate: On inspection there is a marked pes planus deformity of the left foot with a valgus heel compared to a normal-looking right foot.

A spot clinical diagnosis – even at this early stage I picked up that it was a probable tarsal coalition. However, one cannot assume anything and has to carry on examining, but the rest of the examination should be directed towards confirming this clinical diagnosis.

Candidate: The medial longitudinal arch of the left foot is not visible.

Examiner: What do you think the diagnosis is?

Candidate: I think the diagnosis may be tarsal coalition.

Examiner: You have one test only to confirm this, which one will you use?

Candidate: Can you stand on your tiptoes for me? On double heel raise stance the left heel fails to invert and go into varus. The medial longitudinal arch of the foot remains flat. Jack's test fails to correct the pes planus deformity.

Examiner: Good.

I carried on examining the patient.

Candidate: The patient walks with an antalgic gait. Palpation revealed tenderness at the anterolateral aspect foot – the sinus tarsi (location of the coalition). There is no peroneal spasm/protective spasm of the peroneal muscles. There are normal ankle movements of both feet but no passive movement present in the left subtalar joint compared to the opposite side.

Examiner: Why don't you go on to test motor function of the feet?

Plantar flexion, dorsiflexion, inversion and eversion were tested whilst the patient was sitting in the chair. There was grade 4 MRC power compared to the opposite side. This was done very slickly as I had practised it before with somebody sitting in a chair.

Examiner: What are you going to do for this patient?

Candidate: Resection of the coalition.

Examiner: What about conservative management?

Candidate: The patient is markedly symptomatic and I do not think conservative management will work although it may have a role in less severe cases.

Discussion

The subtalar joint may be rigid and any attempt to bring the foot into inversion aggravates pain and causes peroneal muscles to go into spasm.

- Talocalcaneal coalition – accounts for two-thirds of cases; presents with pain under the medial malleolus and reduced subtalar movement
- Calcaneal navicular – pain in the anterolateral aspect of the foot in the region of the sinus tarsi
- Talonavicular – very rare

The natural history is unclear; it is not uncommon to find relatives with the condition who are entirely symptom free. Management depends on the severity of symptoms. Mild cases may initially be managed conservatively; observe with shoe modification and change in activity. Established symptomatic cases with pain would be an indication for surgery, usually excision of the bar. If symptomatic degeneration is present one could consider a triple arthrodesis, however this should not be done until late adolescence/adulthood. A talocalcaneal coalition is more likely to require arthrodesis due to disturbance of the weight-bearing relationship of the foot.

Tibialis posterior tendon dysfunction/rupture

Memorandum 1

"In the standing position from the front, we notice that the patient's feet are externally rotated, that her hind feet are pronated and that her forefeet are abducted. When seen from behind, these deformities are even more obvious. She demonstrates the sign of too many toes and requires assistance to rise up onto tiptoe. The hindfoot fails to supinate and the medial longitudinal arch remains flattened. She has even more difficulty in the single foot stance."

"As she walks in bare feet one notices the heel strikes briefly in supination before the foot goes into marked pronation during the stance phase. Toe-off is markedly reduced and the feet are in an attitude of external rotation with the forefeet abducted, which produces a roll over gait."

"I would like now to examine the patient's shoes, first of all from the plantar aspect; we see that there is outer heel wear confirming heel strike in slight supination. There is increased wear on the medial aspect of the sole with roll-over onto the medial side of the toe. The uppers are not broken but there are orthoses in the shoes, which show some evidence of wear on the medial side."

"We are now going to examine the patient in the seated position."

"The lesser toes are held in a somewhat flexed position and there are small pressure lesions on the dorsal surfaces of the proximal interphalangeal joints. The great toe is slightly extended at the interphalangeal joint and there is dystrophy of the toenail."

"There is some swelling around the tarsometatarsal region of the first ray. There is also some swelling around the outside of the left ankle. On examining the plantar aspect of her feet, there is obvious swelling on the medial aspect of the midfoot with overlying callosity formation. With the thumb on the neck of the talus, the hindfoot is put into the neutral position and when it is held there it is quite obvious that the forefoot is supinated."

"When we examine her for tenderness, we find marked localized tenderness just below the tip of the left lateral malleolus."

"Once more palpating the neck of the talus we can assess tibiotalar dorsiflexion and plantar flexion followed by talo-calcaneal supination and pronation. My hand now slides down to stabilize the hindfoot so that we can assess mid-foot inversion and eversion. I am moving my hand down to stabilize the hindfoot so that we can invert and evert the midtarsal joint. In this case, midtarsal eversion is pain-ful. The midfoot can be stabilized and the tarsometatarsal joint moved in a combined fashion and then individually. The metatarsophalangeal joint movements and the inter-phalangeal joint movements are full and pain-free. We will now look at the active movements of the foot and ankle. With the hindfoot held in neutral, active dorsiflexion is lim-ited to neutral. If the hindfoot is allowed to go into pronat-ion, dorsiflexion is markedly increased. There is a good range of plantar flexion and this can quite clearly be seen to be a combined movement of all the joints of the foot and ankle. There is a good range of inversion and eversion, but there is weakness of resisted inversion and the activity of tibialis posterior is substantially reduced."

Memorandum 2

"On inspection there is a plano-valgus deformity of the right/left foot. There is hindfoot valgus, forefoot varus, external rotation of the foot and forefoot supination. In addition, there is splaying of the forefoot. Medially, there is a swelling over the posterior tibial tendon, posterior and distal to the medial malleolus. From behind, the patient demonstrates the sign of too many toes."

"There is a rigid/flexible flatfoot and heel inversion is not/is occurring. The patient is unable to perform a single limb heel raise test (supported on wall)."

"On palpation with the foot in full plantar flexion and inversion, the tendon stands out. I am feeling for any areas of tenderness or crepitus; there is anterolateral ankle and sinus tarsus pain. There is loss of power and weakness of inver-sion from an everted position. Passive range of motion of the hindfoot and midfoot is reduced to about half normal."

Classification (Johnson and Strom 1989[3])

Johnson and Strom devised three classification stages, with Myerson[4] adding a fourth:

Stage 1 (tendinopathy)

- Tenosynovitis, mild symptoms
- Medial ankle and foot pain
- Swelling without deformity
- Still able to perform a single limb heel raise test
- Normal tendon excursion
- Radiographs normal, MRI shows oedema around the tendon ± intrasubstance degeneration of the tendon

Stage 2 (flexible deformity)

- Deformity still remains flexible
- Pain and tenderness over the tendon; palpable enlargement/defect
- Too many toes sign; single heel raise test abnormal
- Radiographs show increase lateral talocalca-neal angle; MRI shows tendon degeneration ± discontinuity

Stage 3 (fixed deformity)

- Rigid flatfoot deformity associated with hindfoot valgus and loss of subtalar joint motion
- Forefoot varus, absent single heel raise test, sec-ondary degeneration

[3] Johnson KA, Strom DE (1989) Tibialis posterior tendon dysfunction. *Clin Orthop* **239**: 196–206.
[4] Myerson MS (1996) Adult acquired flat foot deformity. *J Bone Joint Surg* **78A**: 780–92.

- Predominantly anterolateral ankle pain secondary to impingement of the calcaneus on the fibula and not anteromedial ankle or foot pain as seen in the earlier stages of the disease

Stage 4 (fixed deformity with generalized arthritic changes foot)

- Significant soft-tissue attenuation and loss of the deltoid ligament
- Valgus angulation of the talus
- Subtalar joint degeneration
- Fixed forefoot supination

Management

Stage 1

NSAIDs, physiotherapy, insoles, immobilization in a short leg walking cast, tendon decompression and debridement.

Stage 2

Non-operative, orthotic arch supports, etc.

FDL tendon transfer with medial-displacement calcaneal osteotomy, which re-directs the strong pull of gastrocnemius muscle; lateral column lengthening. Cobb's repair involves a split anterior tibial tendon transfer often combined with a calcaneal osteotomy.

Stage 3

Subtalar or triple arthrodesis depending on the degree of joint arthrosis and age of the patient.

Stage 4

Pan-talar fusion. Tibiotalocalcaneal arthrodesis may be required if the tibiotalocalcaneal joint is incongruent and arthritic.

13

Paediatric clinical cases

Paul A. Banaszkiewicz

Cerebral palsy

May come up as a long case; it is unlikely as a short case. If unlucky, you will be shown a video of the gait of a cerebral palsy patient near the end of the paediatric oral and asked to describe it.

Try to minimize moving backwards and forwards from the couch to reduce distress to the patient and look as though you have a system:
- General
- Standing
- Walking
- Supine on couch
- Lateral position on couch
- Prone on couch

General

Comment on the presence of wheelchairs, walking aids, gastrostomies, nappies, braces and orthotics, e.g. KAFOs, AFOs, spinal braces.

Look at pattern of involvement

- Monoplegic
- Hemiplegic
- Diplegic (lower limbs affected more than upper)
- Paraplegic (arms not affected)
- Quadriplegic
- Total body

Cerebral palsy can also be classified according to type:
- Spastic (60%)

- Athetoid (20%)
- Ataxic
- Hemiballismic
- Hypotonic
- Combination

Standing

- Ask whether the patient is able to stand first
- Look from behind, from the side and from the front for obvious deformities, e.g. obvious joint contractures, adduction of the hip, shortened leg, equinus and varus or valgus feet
- Note stability when the child is gently pushed forwards, backwards and from side to side (predicts the need for support when walking)
- Spine: is there a fixed scoliosis? Adams' test (bending over)
- Pelvic obliquity: if there seems to be a limb length discrepancy, use blocks to even up the pelvis and look from behind

Walking

- Look and describe walking in three planes

Sagittal: from the side
Transverse: from the front
Coronal: imagine looking from above

Supine on the couch

- Examine the passive range of motion of the hips, knees, ankles and feet

Postgraduate Orthopaedics: The Candidate's Guide to the FRCS (Tr & Orth) Examination, Ed. Paul A. Banaszkiewicz, Deiary F. Kader, Nicola Maffulli. Published by Cambridge University Press. © Cambridge University Press 2009.

- Hips: perform the Thomas test for fixed flexion of the hip
- Knees: perform the popliteal angle test to assess hamstring tightness
- Ankle: perform the Silverskold test for Achilles tendon tightness
- Feet: assess for deformities, e.g. planovalgus, collapsed midfoot

Lateral position on couch

- Perform Ober's test for TFL tightness
- The patient is in the lateral decubitus position with the side to be tested facing upwards. The patient's knee is flexed 90° and then the hip abducted to 40° and extended to its limit. The limb is then gently adducted towards the examination table. Normally the hip should adduct past the midline but inability to do so indicates contracture of the iliotibial band

Prone on couch

- Stahelis rotational profile
- Duncan Ely test. Tests for rectus femoris spasticity. The child is placed prone and then their knee is flexed. The pelvis will rise (hip flex) if the rectus is spastic or contracted

Congenital pseudoarthrosis of the clavicle

Note the heel-strike, foot-flat, toe-off sequence. The patient will be a child and it will almost always be the right clavicle. If it occurs on the left side it is associated with dextrocardia. There will be a non-tender swelling/lump over the middle third of the clavicle and possibly a gap across the clavicle. The shoulder may hang lower than on the opposite normal side. The clavicle is also effectively shortened.

The pseudoarthrosis is caused by failure of fusion of the medial and lateral ossification centres. Possible aetiology is an abnormally high subclavian artery. Differential diagnosis includes post-traumatic pseudoarthrosis, neurofibromatosis and cleidocranial dysostosis of the clavicle (skull abnormality).

This is a painless condition and produces little functional abnormality. There are parental concerns about the unsightly lump. The opposite ends of the clavicle fragments are enlarged just lateral to the midpoint of the clavicle. The larger sternal fragment is pulled upwards by the sternocleidomastoid and lies slightly superior to and in front of the shorter acromial fragment. The shoulder droops and is rotated forwards.

Management

Conservative

Observe; leave it alone, especially if the patient is asymptomatic, because of the risk of possible complications from surgery.

Surgery

Excision of the pseudoarthrosis, curettage of the bone ends and intra-fixation with plate and screws. A bone graft (tri-cortical iliac crest graft) is sometimes required to reconstruct the length and shape of the clavicle. A recon plate is then contoured and fixed with screws. Surgery can be carried out by the age of about 4 years although opinion varies as to the appropriate age for surgery. Brachial plexus neurapraxia has been reported following resection and fixation of the pseudoarthrosis. With skeletal growth the lump and instability at the pseudoarthrosis site increase. The overlying skin becomes atrophic and the deformity can become cosmetically unsightly. The affected shoulder droops. The patient may complain of mild pain and weakness in the shoulder. Surgery is generally advised, "*My preferred option would be to fix it*".

Examination corner

Short case 1

Classic short case. Spot diagnosis. The candidate should recognize the diagnosis immediately on inspection.

Examiner: Would you like to examine this young girl's shoulder and describe what you are doing as you go along?

She is a young girl about 5 years old and therefore it is vital to smile at the child to put her at ease no matter how stressed you may feel. Introduce yourself to both mother and child. Crouch down so you are at her eye level.

Candidate: On inspection from the front there is an obvious swelling over the middle of the right clavicle. *Is it painful? Can I touch it?* On palpation the swelling is bony, hard, non-tender, not attached to skin, its surface is uneven, its edge is distinct and it is non-pulsatile. There is a suggestion of a small amount of painless mobility between the two ends. The swelling is probably bony in origin and very suggestive of pseudoarthrosis of the clavicle. *Can you swing your arm outwards* (demonstrated whilst talking)? She has a good range of shoulder abduction which is non-painful.

Examiner: Good, let us look at her X-rays.

Candidate: This confirms a pseudoarthrosis of the right clavicle with smooth sclerotic enlarged deformed bone margins characteristic of the condition.

Examiner: How are you going to manage it?

Candidate: My preferred option would be to fix it. It's an unsightly deformity that tends to worsen when the child grows. It can also be painful and the shoulder tends to droop down.

Examiner: Is there any place for conservative treatment?

Candidate: That's certainly an option if it's painless and causing no undue problems and the parents are not concerned about its appearance.

Examiner: Why are they always right sided?

Candidate: That is because it is thought that the subclavian artery interferes with fusion of the medial and lateral ossification centres. They can occur on the left side with dextrocardia.

Short case 2

Pseudoarthrosis of the clavicle in a 6-year-old girl

- Discuss the case
- Discuss management, if at all
- Complications of surgical treatment

Klippel–Feil syndrome

Adult or child. Short web neck or no neck appearance with low hairline. Decreased neck mobility, neck stiffness with restricted range of movement.

Associated features include Sprengel's shoulder, congenital scoliosis/kyphosis of the cervical spine, congenital heart disease and renal anomalies.

Congenital failure of segmentation of the cervical vertebrae. Multiple fused cervical segments. Renal ultrasound and echocardiogram are recommended to rule out associated renal or cardiac anomalies which can be more serious.

Spot diagnosis: head on top of the shoulders. Full spinal and neurological examination required. High risk of instability especially if the malformation limits mobility at one level; these include atlanto-occipital fusion with C2-C3 block vertebrae, abnormal atlanto-occipital junction with several distal block vertebrae, and a single open interspace between two block segments. Subluxation of the cervical spine can occur with minor injury. Warn patients against contact sport (diving, gymnastics and rugby) and review annually with flexion/extension plain radiographs. Arthrodesis of unstable segments may be required if excessive instability and neurological abnormalities are present.

This is also a classic spot photograph diagnosis in the children's orthopaedics oral examination but does not seem to get asked as presumably there is more important material to cover in a limited amount of time available.

Congenital radial head dislocation

A classic short case. Possibly a radiographic spot diagnosis in the paediatric oral with discussion about its differentiation from a traumatic dislocation or acquired dislocation that gradually develops during infancy and childhood. Be familiar with the various management options available and their indications.

Memorandum

On examination of the left/right elbow there is a suggestion of a mass present posteriorly around the lateral epicondyle. The attitude of the left/right elbow suggests there is a loss of full supination.

I would like to confirm this clinically. There is both a restriction of full supination and loss of full extension of the elbow. Flexion and pronation appear full. The swelling itself is non-tender and bony hard. The ulna appears more prominent at the wrist.

Background

The radial head may be dislocated anteriorly, laterally or posteriorly. Posterior dislocations are nearly always congenital. Congenital anterior dislocations are usually associated with other congenital conditions. The primary defect in the condition is thought to be capitellum dysplasia. The anteriorly dislocated radial head is rounded, often with a deficient capitellum and a long radius. The posterior border of the ulna is concave instead of convex. The posteriorly dislocated radial head is thin and elongated, and the posterior border of the ulna is markedly convex.

Relocation is usually not successful. The condition predisposes to osteoarthritis of the ulnohumoral joint in later life. Can be bilateral.

Clinical features

The elbow is usually pain free with little loss of function. An anterior dislocation will usually have restricted flexion and supination due to a mechanical block. Posterior dislocation usually causes limitation of extension and rotation of the forearm. The radial head can usually be easily palpated. Associated conditions include arthrogryposis, Ehler–Danlos syndrome, diaphyseal aclasis and nail patella syndrome.

Management

Conservative

- In childhood, leave it alone, surgery should not be carried out because it may cause longitudinal growth disturbances
- In adulthood again preferably manage conservatively

Surgery

- Open reduction is difficult and recurrent dislocation is common. The flat or convex radial head and flat capitellum make relocation very difficult
- If necessary, excision of the radial head in the adult can be done to relieve pain and improve appearance, however the range of motion is not significantly altered

Radio-ulnar synostosis

An extremely common short case. Can be **congenital** or **acquired**, partial or complete, fibrous or bony, unilateral or bilateral and is usually an isolated defect. Congenital bilateral in 60% cases with males and females equally affected.

Classification

Traumatic radio-ulnar synostosis (Vince and Miller[1])

Type 1: Distal intra-articular part of the radius and ulna

Type 2: Middle third or non-articular part of the distal third of the radius and ulna most common

Type 3: Proximal third of the radius and ulna

Congenital radio-ulnar synostosis (Cleary and Omer[2])

Type 1: Fused clinically but not radiologically, small but normally developed radial head

Type 2: Similar but with clear bony synostosis

Type 3: Hypoplastic, posteriorly dislocated radial head

Type 4: Hyperplastic anteriorly dislocated radial head

---

[1] Vince KJ, Miller JE (1987) Cross-union complicating fracture of the forearm. Part I: Adults. *J Bone Joint Surg Am* **69**(5): 640–53.

[2] Cleary JE, Omer GE (1985) Congenital proximal radio-ulnar synostosis: natural history and functional assessment. *J Bone Joint Surg Am* **67-A**: 539–45.

Symptoms

The position of the forearm rotation is variable and determines the degree of disability.

- Difficulty turning doorknobs
- Difficulty buttoning shirts
- Difficulty using eating utensils

Predisposing factors for traumatic radial ulnar synostosis

- Badly displaced and comminuted fractures
- Both fractures at the same level
- Crushing injuries of the forearm
- Open fractures
- Single-incision exposure of both bones
- Fractures with concomitant head injury
- Delayed surgical fixation

Management

Results from surgery are poor and unpredictable even in the best of hands, especially for the congenital variety. Leave the synostosis alone if at all possible and manage conservatively.

With the congenital variety there is usually little functional deficit. The forearm is in fixed pronation (30°), neutral or in slight supination. This is generally less disabling than fixed supination. Patients with unilateral synostosis usually do not require surgery unless there is excessive pronation, which can be functionally and cosmetically disabling. Patients with bilateral synostosis may request surgical correction with the dominant limb fixed in 30°–45° of pronation whilst the other side is fixed in 10°–30° of supination.

Surgery

Rotational osteotomy

Realignment of the forearm by distal osteotomy; in adults both bones are realigned, with compression plating, whilst in children realignment of the radius is the preferred option. This can be complicated by vascular compromise if the correction is greater

than 45°. In children osteotomy through the fusion mass with K-wire fixation has been described but is generally not recommended.

Resection synosthosis

Resection of the bony bridge, interposition of fascia lata, plus resection of the radial head and division of the interosseous membrane. This is described in the textbooks but is not recommended; do not take down the synostosis.

Examination corner

Short case 1

A candidate in her first short case was asked to examine the left forearm of a middle-aged male patient. She commented on several well-healed surgical scars present over both the volar and dorsal surfaces of the wrist, which she was told to ignore and to just concentrate on the forearm. There was muscle wasting present over the flexor muscles of the forearm.

The candidate was a little confused as to what to do next and was told to examine forearm rotation. The patient demonstrated restricted forearm pronation. Asked what the diagnosis was she mentioned radio-ulnar synostosis. She was then asked the likely cause, to which she replied, "trauma". The candidate was then asked to check the patient's forearm rotation on the right side, which was similarly restricted.

The examiner then asked whether she still felt trauma was the cause and would it not be more likely to be congenital.

In retrospect the candidate felt that being asked to examine the forearm had unnerved her and she would have made a better account of herself if she had been asked to examine the patient's elbow.

Would you care to examine this gentleman's forearm?

Short case 2

A candidate was asked to examine the elbow of a young girl aged about 5. The lack of forearm rotation was immediately spotted when the patient was asked to "show me your arms". A slight loss of full extension was also noted after which the candidate was asked what the probable diagnosis was. The candidate was then shown radiographs, which confirmed a proximal radio-ulnar synostosis. There followed a brief discussion about treatment options. [Pass]

Over-riding fifth toe

This may be present at birth or develop during childhood. It is usually bilateral and familial.

Over-riding fifth toe may present as a cosmetic deformity; occasionally there are pressure problems over the toe or the toe is caught when putting socks on.

Memorandum

The fifth toe is hyperextended at the MTP joint with flexion of the IP joints. It is deviated medially to lie on top of the fourth toe. Often the toe is hypoplastic and there may be a rotational component so that the nail faces laterally. Usually the skin on the dorsal surface of the toe is contracted. The MTP joint is subluxed dorsomedially due to capsular contracture along with shortening of the common EDL tendon. In some cases there is an associated bunionette.

Management

- Will not correct without surgery
- Manage conservatively if at all possible; strapping, stretching, etc.

Butler procedure

Creates a dorsal racket-handle incision over the little digit, centred over the EDL tendon, which allows the toe to be de-rotated. The contracted extensor tendon and dorsal capsule are released and then skin repair with the toe can now be moved to a more plantar and lateral position.

SECTION 4

Adult elective orthopaedics oral

14. **General oral guidance**   135
    Paul A. Banaszkiewicz

15. **Shoulder and elbow
    oral core topics**   138
    Niall Munro

16. **Hip oral core topics**   155
    Paul A. Banaszkiewicz

17. **Knee oral core topics**   194
    Deiary F. Kader and Leo Pinczewski

18. **Foot and ankle
    oral core topics**   215
    Paul A. Banaszkiewicz

19. **Spine oral core topics**   237
    Niall Craig

14

General oral guidance

Paul A. Banaszkiewicz

General advice

Preparation

- The best preparation for the oral is practise, practise and practise as much as possible
- Know the basics well
- Use smaller textbooks, it's a mistake to discount them. In larger textbooks subjects should be covered sparsely
- If you leave your reading to the last 3 months there is far too much to read and learn in too little time

- Orals can be hit and miss affairs and the onus is on the examiners to enable you to show your knowledge
- Adopt the right mental approach and go in with a positive attitude
- I failed the oral and I am sure it was because I was not sure of myself and my answers were hesitant and indecisive
- Many candidates answer a question with one or two sentences and then wait for another question. You should take charge and outline your approach in full
- You should aim to home in on a subject you know well and keep talking
- Always keep talking
- If you feel that examiners want you to speed up then go for it
- nb Clear head
- You have 5 minutes between orals, you must put the last oral out of your head. They are not all going to go well but just forget about it

Mock orals

- Are important in improving one's ability to cope under pressure
- May reveal areas of weakness or unpreparedness
- Highlight mannerisms, which may distract or annoy the examiner
- Improve your spontaneity in responding to questions
- Allow you to sharpen up
- Invite criticism

Avoid

- Giving monosyllabic answers such as "yes" or "no"
- "Ums" and "errs"
- Becoming aphasic because of the shocking stress of the examination, since examiners expect you to function properly under the stress of orthopaedic emergencies and major operations, which is a similar if not greater stress than the examination

- Be smooth, comfortable and to the point
- The examiners want to cover as many oral topics as possible in the time available. Be prepared for them to cut you off in mid-sentence and move on to another topic. This will happen whether you are doing well or not!
- If you go down, go down fighting; get your bit in first
- It's important to put mistakes behind you and to take each question fresh

Postgraduate Orthopaedics: The Candidate's Guide to the FRCS (Tr & Orth) Examination, Ed. Paul A. Banaszkiewicz, Deiary F. Kader, Nicola Maffulli. Published by Cambridge University Press. © Cambridge University Press 2009.

Do not

- Produce bizarre facial expressions when asked a question and do not smile too much when answering a question. This is an irritating habit. Do not make unnecessary hand or body movements and do not lean on the examiner's table
- Touch the screen of the examiner's computer when describing a radiograph
- Be too friendly or casual with the examiner or be tempted to crack a joke; it may backfire. Be reserved, smile a little, be confident, relaxed and keep the discussion going
- Guess and avoid waffle. Cut your loses and admit if you do not know something
- Try to bullshit the examiners; they will spot it a mile away
- Let the examiners do too much talking

- If you are stuck try to go back to the basics and show that you are trying to work out the problem logically
- I felt the orals went well because I managed to steer the conversation on to home topics
- Be aware that the stress of the oral can cause you to "blurt out" things you do not really mean. Keep calm and think before you speak

The examiners

- Were very pleasant and friendly. They gave me a lot of feedback
- Were aggressive and determined to unsettle me
- The main problem was that the examiner always had one particular answer in mind and it became an exercise in mind reading
- I'm sure the examiners decide in 30 seconds whether they are going to pass you or not
- Most of the examiners know less than you and wouldn't be able to pass the exam themselves

---

- System overload with knowledge is a difficult problem and there are no easy solutions for this
- All oral questions were with props except some basic sciences. Most examiners set you scenarios to discuss. They quite often stop you in mid-sentence
- The orals were a very stressful experience, as they are relentless and after 2 hours solid your head is throbbing

Old chestnuts

There are some general questions, which have been recurring for many years. Even the answers are well known. The examiner may throw one in at the beginning of the oral while they are making their mind up about you.

Biblical stories

These are questions on well-established and everyday clinical practice. You cannot afford to make many mistakes in responding to straightforward biblical stories. Assess quickly what the examiner is getting at and therefore what to say.

Detective stories

When presenting this story the examiner usually has a specific diagnosis (what dunnit?) in mind and gives what he or she thinks is enough information for you to find your way to the diagnosis.

Historical stories

As the name suggests questions under this heading are related to historical events or personalities. You may invite these questions by name-dropping and using eponyms instead of descriptive titles.

Ghost stories

Two or more immediately obvious diagnoses that could fit the clinical picture and the actual one lurks in the shadows linked by some unusual but specific event in the story (the ghost link).

Wild stories

The questions mainly refer to uncommon orthopaedic conditions and the examiners usually have either personal or second-hand knowledge of the condition. The examiner almost invariably knows the correct answer.

Bedtime stories

The hallmark of these stories is the relaxed manner in which the examiner starts the question.

Tell me something about …

How would you deal with?

What do you think about?

These questions allow you some freedom.

Controversial subjects

These questions are asked to probe the depth of your knowledge of a subject, your ability to critically evaluate the available evidence and abstract it, and your competence to justify your opinions. Taking a clear dogmatic stance may annoy the examiners.

Specialist questions

As to be expected, the specialist always feels at home with their own special subject and are likely to ask questions in the field they know best. Be certain of your ground. If you do not know something, say so. You should only proceed to answer the question if you have a reasonable grasp of the subject.

The boundaries between each section are not rigid. The adult and pathology oral on total hip replacement may well merge imperceptibly into setting up a trial to assess results and then on to survival analysis. I was asked repeatedly about AVN whilst my colleague was asked about Enneking's classification for malignant tumours. This is not meant to occur as candidates carry a written sheet around with them, which the examiners are supposed to read in order to avoid repeating questions already asked.

Some candidates will end up with four continuous back-to-back orals whilst others may have

a lunch break or coffee break between the various orals. In some ways it is better to get on with it and sit them all together rather than hang around in the examination corridor ruminating on your performance.

General orthopaedics and pathology oral

This oral has a mixed reputation amongst candidates. Some view it as fairly straightforward whilst others regard it as a difficult and tricky oral to pass.

It covers a huge breadth of elective orthopaedics with a large volume of material from which examiners can choose. Also it would seem important that candidates are able to structure an answer/discussion as well as possible without jumping about. In addition many candidates felt they were never quite sure what exactly the examiners were "looking for" in any particular answer.

Feedback from candidates suggests several styles of oral. One style consisted of a series of rapid-fire clinical photographs and radiographs with hardly a second to catch your breath between topics.

Another oral style consisted of a series of impossibly complex clinical cases. Candidates were expected to provide almost instantaneous answers to difficult clinical problems with no time for a reflective thought process. In real-life clinical practice one would spend a considerable amount of time deliberating the correct course of action and probably discuss the case with senior colleagues.

Other candidates felt the importance of the oral (from the examiner's prospective) was based on obtaining a structured, logically ordered answer to a question rather than any specific detail. In other words if you jumped about all over the place with an answer, eventually covering everything, you would still fail that particular question.

In the end one can analyse things too much and maybe the best plan of action is to completely ignore all of this and just get on with answering the questions!

15

Shoulder and elbow oral core topics

Niall Munro

Acromioclavicular joint arthritis

The acromioclavicular joint (ACJ) contains a fibro-cartilaginous disc, which may be involved in the degenerative process. Stability of the joint depends partly on the superior (stronger) and inferior (weaker) AC ligaments, and partly on the conoid and trapezoid ligaments that connect the coracoid and the clavicle.

Causes

- Primary osteoarthritis
- Post-traumatic arthritis (e.g. after Grade I and II ACJ disruptions)
- Distal clavicular osteolysis, due to repetitive microtrauma or fatigue failure associated particularly with weight training
- Rheumatoid arthritis, in which ACJ pathology may be an under-diagnosed cause of pain

Assessment

The main symptom is pain. This is usually well localized to the joint, in contrast to the distally radiating pain of subacromial impingement. The two diagnoses frequently coexist, however, and inferior osteophytes associated with ACJ osteoarthritis may contribute to impingement. Patients have pain on working with their arms raised, and examination reveals a high painful arc above 120° on both active and passive movements. The cross body adduction test also produces localized pain, and local anaesthetic ACJ injection is useful both diagnostically and in terms of predicting likely response to surgery.

The ACJ is seen on standard AP and axillary shoulder radiographs. The Zanca view may be useful for specifically imaging the AC joint. This uses an X-ray beam angled 10°–15° superiorly and a decreased kilovoltage to avoid the overexposure typically found on standard radiographs.

Management

- Conservative, with activity modification, NSAIDs, steroid injections, etc. Physiotherapy may be used, although there is little evidence for its effectiveness in ACJ arthritis
- Open resection, carried out through a coronally or (better) sagittally oriented incision. The precise amount to remove is controversial, but around 2 cm is reasonable. Greater excision may damage the conoid and trapezoid ligaments and lead to instability. It is necessary to exclude coexisting subacromial impingement before embarking on isolated distal clavicular resection
- Arthroscopic resection (1.5 cm). This may be carried out using a subacromial (indirect) arthroscopic approach, or a superior (direct) approach. The former has the advantage of addressing coexisting subacromial impingement. Arthroscopic management may allow a quicker return to normal function than open surgery, but otherwise there does not appear to be a significant difference in outcome
- Complications of surgical treatment include instability (due to excessive resection) and

Postgraduate Orthopaedics: The Candidate's Guide to the FRCS (Tr & Orth) Examination, Ed. Paul A. Banaszkiewicz, Deiary F. Kader, Nicola Maffulli. Published by Cambridge University Press. © Cambridge University Press 2009.

continued pain (due to inadequate resection or coexisting pathology). The outcome may be poorer in post-traumatic than primary osteoarthritis. Distal clavicular excision alone is not suitable for treating symptoms due to ACJ injuries of Grade III or above: in this scenario a reconstructive procedure (e.g. Weaver and Dunn) is preferred.

Subacromial impingement

Subacromial impingement is probably the commonest cause of shoulder problems in middle and later life, and implies entrapment and inflammation of the rotator cuff (in particular supraspinatus) as it passes between the underside of the acromion, and the humeral head and greater tuberosity.

The aetiology is to some extent controversial. Intrinsic factors such as hypovascularity of supraspinatus (particularly at the so-called watershed area approximately 1 cm from its insertion) and extrinsic factors (compression by an abnormally shaped acromion and to a lesser extent ACJ osteophytes) are described. Bigliani described acromial morphology as follows:
- Type I: Normal-shaped acromion
- Type II: Curved acromion
- Type III: Hooked acromion

The type III acromion, however, may represent secondary pathological changes (due to stress on the coracoacromial ligament with subsequent calcification) rather than a primary occurrence.

The differential diagnosis of impingement syndrome includes ACJ arthritis (which may coexist), and other shoulder and cervical spine pathology. Apparent impingement may occur secondary to abnormal humeral head movement in other shoulder pathology such as adhesive capsulitis or shoulder instability. Primary rotator cuff impingement is rare in patients under 40 years.

Subcoracoid impingement is a separate condition, and occurs when the subscapularis tendon is trapped between the coracoid and the lesser tuberosity with the shoulder flexed and internally rotated.

It usually occurs in young patients engaged in competitive throwing sports.

Assessment

Symptoms include diffuse pain radiating distally to the mid-arm level, made worse on working with the arms raised. Examination reveals a painful abduction arc, lower than that for AC arthritis and classically from 60° to 120°, although in practice it is rarely so well defined. Neer's sign consists of pain on elevation of the arm. Hawkins' sign is pain on internal rotation of the arm in 90° of forward elevation: this brings the greater tuberosity under the acromion, and further exacerbates any compression of the supraspinatus tendon. Neer's impingement test involves abolition of pain from his aforementioned impingement sign on instillation of local anaesthetic to the subacromial space.

Impingement syndrome may lead to capsular tightness and a decreased range of movement. Rotator cuff tears (described later) may be a consequence of impingement, and careful assessment of the cuff is required.

Although isolated biceps tendinopathy is rare it is frequently found in association with rotator cuff disease. Clinical tests for biceps tendinopathy include those of Speed (pain localized to the bicipital groove on resisted forward elevation at the shoulder) and Yergason (pain on resisted supination with a flexed elbow), although they are somewhat non-specific. It is important to exclude other pathologies such as adhesive capsulitis or (particularly in young patients) instability.

Standard shoulder radiographs will help to exclude coexisting pathology such as ACJ arthritis. An anteroposterior film with 30° caudal tilt will visualize pathology on the undersurface of the ACJ, e.g. osteophytes. Acromial morphology is best shown by a lateral outlet view (taken as for a scapular lateral, with 10° inferior angulation of the tube). An axillary view will exclude the presence of an os acromiale, which may be an occasional cause of pain and which should be recognized prior to undertaking acromioplasty to prevent weakening of the acromion, causing a fracture.

Management

- Most patients will settle with conservative management. NSAIDs, physiotherapy and corticosteroid injections to the subacromial space have all been shown to be beneficial. Physiotherapy involves two phases, with initial emphasis on stretching exercises to regain movement and overcome capsular tightness. Only then are specific strengthening exercises performed, with an emphasis on the external rotators. Current physiotherapy programmes are somewhat controversial with a focus on rotator cuff and shoulder girdle strength prior to improving range of movement
- Open acromioplasty is an effective management for the majority of patients who do not respond to physiotherapy. Acromioplasty has historically been performed in different ways, but current techniques are all now based on the anterior acromioplasty and coracoacromial ligament resection popularized by Neer. The operation is performed through an anterior or anterolateral deltoid splitting approach, and involves detachment of a small amount of the deltoid from the acromion: it is important to reattach this carefully at the end of the operation. Complications include deltoid atrophy, acromial fracture and axillary nerve injury. It is important not to extend the deltoid split more than 5 cm from the acromion to avoid the last complication. Satisfactory pain relief is obtained in around 85% of patients, although rehabilitation may take 6 months or more
- Arthroscopic acromioplasty. The main advantage is a more rapid rehabilitation due to the absence of any deltoid detachment. Technically it is more demanding, particularly if a rotator cuff tear is present and requires repair

Rotator cuff tears

Rotator cuff tears occasionally occur following an acute traumatic injury, but are more commonly a chronic response to various insults. These factors can be intrinsic (hypovascularity of the tendon leading to poor tissue healing and tendinopathy), extrinsic (attrition from the anteroinferior acromion), and traumatic (traction leading to repetitive microtrauma to the tendon). Rotator cuff tears are associated with increasing age, frequent overhead use of the arms (work or sports related) and inflammatory arthritis.

Pathophysiology

Neer classified rotator cuff pathology into three progressive stages:
- Stage I with haemorrhage and cuff oedema
- Stage II with fibrosis of the cuff
- Stage III with tearing of the cuff

Tears are also classified according to size into small (<1 cm), moderate (1–3 cm), large (3–5 cm) and massive (>5 cm). Cuff tears may be either full or partial thickness and there has been recent appreciation of the importance of the latter.

Ellman's staging of partial-thickness tears may be helpful descriptively and as a guide to management:
- Grade I: Tear up to a quarter of the tendon thickness
- Grade II: Tear between a quarter and half the thickness
- Grade III: Tear more than half the thickness of the cuff

Tears most commonly occur in the supraspinatus tendon, close to its insertion in the greater tuberosity (corresponding to an area of relative hypovascularity) and to the bicipital groove. Partial-thickness tears may occur on the bursal side, the articular side or as intrasubstance tears. Articular-sided tears are 2–3 times more common than bursal tears. Bursal tears may be primarily due to the mechanical effects of acromial impingement, while articular tears may represent traction microtrauma or be an indirect effect of impingement.

The natural history of partial-thickness tears is of a gradual progression to full-thickness tears. Whether spontaneous healing occurs has proved controversial: bursal tears probably sometimes heal, but articular-sided tears rarely do so (possibly because of inhibitory factors in the synovial fluid). Cuff tears are much commoner in cadaveric studies than symptoms would suggest.

Assessment

There is considerable overlap in symptoms and signs with patients who have impingement without a cuff tear. The differential diagnosis also includes the much rarer suprascapular nerve palsy. Signs of weakness may be detected on testing the various cuff muscles if there are large tears. Suggested tests include the following:

- **Supraspinatus:** Jobe's test ("empty can" test) is performed with 90° abduction in the plane of the scapula and maximal internal rotation. The "full can" test is a variation where the shoulder is placed in 45° external rotation instead of full internal rotation: it is said to be better tolerated by the patient
- **Subscapularis:** Gerber's "lift off" test involves the patient placing the dorsum of their hand on the small of their back, and being asked to push the hand off against resistance. An alternative for patients who cannot reach behind their back is the "belly press" or "Napoleon" test where the patient places their hands on their abdomen and their elbows are brought anteriorly, resulting in internal rotation of the shoulder. The patient is asked to press into their abdomen. Subscapularis weakness is suggested by the arm falling posterior to the mid-coronal plane
- **Infraspinatus:** The elbow is flexed, keeping the arm at the patient's side, and the patient is asked to externally rotate against resistance

Radiographs may occasionally show superior migration of the humeral head and a narrowed sub-acromial space (best seen on an anteroposterior radiograph with 30° caudal tilt). This sign is somewhat unreliable, and only present in severe cases. Arthrography will detect many full-thickness tears but is poor for partial-thickness tears and is now rarely used.

Ultrasound has become the method of choice in most centres for the radiological diagnosis of cuff tears. It is capable of detecting both full- and partial-thickness tears, although the former are naturally easier to diagnose. It is highly operator dependent, but in good series has both sensitivity and specificity of over 90% when compared to arthroscopy. Dynamic ultrasound has a better diagnostic accuracy compared to static ultrasound.

MRI diagnosis of cuff tears has improved in recent years, but is more expensive and possibly less accurate than ultrasound. Techniques to improve results include the use of fat suppression sequences and MRI arthrography.

Management

Conservative

Although healing probably occurs only infrequently, authors report between 30% and 80% symptomatic success with conservative management and a 6-month trial of conservative management is appropriate for most patients with small or moderate tears. Management is similar to that for impingement syndrome, with physiotherapy (see earlier), NSAIDs and judicious corticosteroid injections.

Operative

This may be performed using an open deltoid splitting approach, or (increasingly, as techniques and expertise develop) arthroscopically. An ability to inspect the glenohumeral joint and detect articular-sided partial tears is an advantage of arthroscopy. Full-thickness tears are (if possible) repaired and reattached to bone using tissue anchors or drill holes. Mobilization of the relevant tendon is required, and relaxing incisions made within the rotator interval may be helpful. The management of partial-thickness tears is controversial. A reasonable approach is simply to debride tears of less than half the tendon thickness (Grades I and II), and to repair more severe injuries (Grade III). There is little evidence that healing occurs after simple debridement. Some authors have advocated converting them to complete tears and repairing them. Acromioplasty is performed in most patients in conjunction with cuff repair. It is particularly important after repairing full-thickness or bursal-sided partial tears, but may also be of benefit in articular-sided partial tears. Postoperative regimes vary, but it is reasonable to allow supine, active-assisted exercises immediately after full-thickness tear repairs, and to progress to active range-of-movement and strengthening exercises after 6 weeks. This is not necessarily more rapid after arthroscopic surgery because mobilization is limited by cuff healing rather than healing of the deltoid. Satisfaction rates of 85%–95% are typically reported with both arthroscopic and open surgery.

Salvage

If the cuff tear is too extensive for suture, a combination of debridement and acromioplasty may bring some relief. Acromioplasty should be modified to maintain the coracoacromial ligament and acromial curvature in patients with very severe tears to reduce the risk of further superior migration of the humeral head. Various tendon transfers have been described, including transfer of the upper two-thirds of the subscapularis for the reconstruction of large supraspinatus tears.

Cuff tear arthropathy

Approximately 4% of patients with massive cuff tears develop aggressive destruction of the glenohumeral joint. Originally described by Neer in 1977, although uncommon, it is without a direct counterpart elsewhere in the body.

Pathophysiology

Cuff tear arthropathy is found in conjunction with a massive tear of the supraspinatus, infraspinatus and long head of biceps tendons, with or without subscapularis and teres minor ruptures. Typically, the patient is an elderly female, and the dominant arm is affected more frequently. The humeral head is misshapen and has migrated superiorly. Wear of the greater tuberosity, acromion and superior glenoid may be seen. In very severe cases the distal clavicle, coracoid and humerus distal to the humeral head may also be involved. The bone may be osteopenic, and dislocation of the humeral head may occur, either anteriorly or posteriorly.

Various factors have been proposed as contributing to the development of cuff tear arthropathy:
- **Mechanical:** Rotator cuff loss leads to superior migration of the head and direct wear of the head on the underside of the acromion
- **Nutritional:** Leak of synovial fluid due to the deficient cuff may impair cartilage nutrition
- **Inflammatory:** Possibly a crystal arthropathy (young patients, e.g. Milwaukee shoulder)

Management

It is rarely possible to repair a severely damaged cuff in advanced cuff tear arthropathy, even if techniques such as transfer of the subscapularis are employed. Surgical management therefore is frequently aimed at "salvage" rather than reconstruction. Complications are higher than for other conditions with an intact cuff. Useful pain relief may be obtained, but there is frequently little improvement in range of movement or strength.

Management options include:
- **Total shoulder replacement.** This has been performed with standard unconstrained devices, fully constrained devices and partly constrained implants (with superior glenoid augments). All have a high rate of loosening due to the abnormal joint mechanics and the poor glenoid bone stock. As a result inability to reconstruct the rotator cuff is now considered a contraindication to glenoid replacement by most shoulder surgeons
- **Hemiarthroplasty.** This may be performed using standard or large-headed prostheses, or occasionally bipolar devices. Attempts have been made to augment either the superior glenoid or the coracoacromial arch using bone graft in small series
- **Arthrodesis** is occasionally performed, although it is technically difficult. Arthrodesis of the shoulder is performed with 20° abduction, 30° forward elevation and 40° internal rotation

- **Resection arthroplasty** is not recommended: it defunctions the deltoid, and traction brachial neuritis is a troublesome complication

Shoulder arthritis and osteonecrosis

Rheumatoid arthritis

Shoulder symptoms are common in patients with rheumatoid arthritis and are usually due to glenohumeral inflammation or destruction, although pathology relating to the cervical spine and ACJ also needs to be excluded. Neer described three clinical patterns of shoulder involvement in rheumatoid disease:

- "Dry": Stiffness, decreased joint space and presence of cysts on radiographs are typical
- "Wet": Characterized by extensive synovial involvement and glenoid erosion
- "Resorptive": This form shows extreme resorption of the humeral head and glenoid

Management follows similar lines to that for other joints. Conservative management involves controlling the inflammatory response to the disease (disease-modifying drugs, steroids) and local symptomatic measures (analgesics, NSAIDs, local heat, etc.). Steroid injections may be used to help patients through acute exacerbations or to delay surgery. Surgery usually takes the form of hemiarthroplasty since glenoid replacement is frequently difficult to undertake due to the degree of glenoid erosion. Improvement in pain is the major goal of treatment, and improved movement cannot be guaranteed. Other operations such as synovectomy (open or arthroscopic) and combined glenoid/humeral osteotomies have been described, but are now rarely used.

Osteoarthritis

OA of the shoulder can be primary or secondary (usually to fracture or dislocation). Maximal wear in the primary group tends to occur in the region of the head, which articulates with the glenoid between 60° and 100° of abduction (at which point maximal joint reaction force occurs) suggesting that excess pressure or wear is an aetiological factor. It is relatively uncommon in comparison to OA of the hip or knee, but management follows a similar course with symptomatic measures in the early stages and arthroplasty (as described separately) for end-stage disease.

Unlike patients with rotator cuff arthropathy, OA patients usually have an intact rotator cuff. Radiographically, they differ from rheumatoid patients in having osteophytes (especially posteriorly and inferiorly) and being generally sclerotic rather than osteopenic.

Osteonecrosis

The shoulder is second only to the hip in frequency as a site of atraumatic osteonecrosis. Unlike the hip, idiopathic osteonecrosis is rare and up to 70% have been associated with corticosteroid use. Other associations, however, are similar to those occurring with the hip, including alcohol, hyperlipidaemia, radiotherapy, decompression sickness, lymphoma, systemic lupus erythematosus and sickle cell disease.

Calcific tendinopathy

A condition leading to the deposition and subsequent resorption of hydroxyapatite crystals within the rotator cuff tendons.

Pathophysiology

Despite Codman's original suggestion that calcific tendinopathy occurred on a background of tendon degeneration, modern evidence suggests rather that it is a reactive condition that occurs within viable tendon. The precipitating factors are not fully understood, but it is thought that hypoxia or pressure may play a part.

Calcification may be preceded by metaplasia of tenocytes to chondrocytes and fibrocartilage. Histologically, calcific deposits consist of collections of hydroxyapatite crystals interspersed with areas of fibrocartilage. The surrounding tendon shows an inflammatory reaction, with multinucleated giant cells attempting to phagocytose the deposits. Resorption of the deposit results in granulation tissue, which is subsequently remodelled to new tendon.

The process of deposition and resorption can be divided into stages as follows:

- Formative phase. The calcium deposit is hard and chalk-like. Radiographically it appears well defined and homogenous
- Resting phase
- Resorptive phase. The deposit becomes soft and "toothpaste-like". Resorption at the edges of the deposit leads to a less defined, more "fluffy" appearance on X-ray

Clinical features

The peak incidence is in patients in their 40s, and up to a quarter of patients may have the condition bilaterally. Pain is the predominant symptom and is much more severe in the resorptive phase.

The diagnosis is made radiographically. Supraspinatus is the most commonly affected tendon (51%–82% of cases), and is most likely to be symptomatic due to compression by the acromion. Subscapularis calcification is very rare. Supraspinatus calcification is clearly seen on standard AP radiographs, while internal and external rotation views may show infraspinatus/teres minor and subscapularis calcification respectively. Occasionally a supraspinatus deposit may decompress into the subacromial bursa, giving a typical crescentic appearance.

The white cell count, ESR and CRP are normal in calcific tendinopathy.

Management

The majority of patients will settle with conservative management; indeed, the presence of severe acute pain usually indicates the beginning of the resorptive process.

- Analgesia. Pain may be exceedingly severe, and adequate analgesia is essential

- Subacromial injections. Although corticosteroids are frequently used, there is little firm evidence that they are effective, and they may slow resorption. Long-acting local anaesthetics may be just as effective
- Extracorporeal shock wave therapy. Evidence as to its effectiveness is mixed
- Aspiration of the calcific deposit may occasionally be possible during the resorptive phase when the deposit is soft and semi-liquid
- Removal, both arthroscopically or by open surgery, is possible and may bring relief, although it is infrequently necessary. Acromioplasty is not carried out routinely, but only if there is evidence of impingement in the chronic phase

Frozen shoulder

Codman first used the term "frozen shoulder" in his description of the condition in 1934. It is a condition characterized by gradually resolving pain and stiffness within the joint. Primary frozen shoulder or adhesive capsulitis is to be differentiated from secondary frozen shoulder (capsulitis), which follows surgery, trauma, arthritis or rotator cuff pathology.

Pathophysiology

The cause of frozen shoulder is unknown. One current theory is that hyperlipidaemia may be the main trigger, as increased lipid levels are found in many of the conditions associated with frozen shoulder.

Histologically, frozen shoulder is a disease of the joint capsule, which is thickened and shows increased vascularity. The picture is strikingly similar to Dupuytren's disease, with proliferation of fibroblasts, transformation to myofibroblasts and increased collagen deposition. The anterior capsule (particularly the rotator interval) is most affected. The synovium is normal, and there is no evidence of inflammation.

Other conditions associated with primary frozen shoulder include:

- Endocrine conditions: most commonly diabetes mellitus (which is associated with a poorer prognosis and greater resistance to treatment), hyperthyroidism and hypothyroidism
- Metabolic conditions such as hyperlipidaemia
- Dupuytren's disease
- Trauma (frequently affecting the limb more distally)
- Cardiac disease, subarachnoid haemorrhage and other conditions

Clinical features

Frozen shoulder is commonest in middle to old age (40–70 years), with a slight female preponderance. The diagnosis is largely clinical, and limitation, particularly of external rotation (both active and passive), is the critical diagnostic feature, although movements in all directions are affected. Capsular contraction may cause the humeral head to ride high leading to secondary impingement symptoms. Plain radiographs may help exclude other conditions. Arthrography, although rarely performed, reveals a decreased capsular volume.

Three clinical phases in the disease are described:

- Painful phase, characterized particularly by pain. Night pain is a prominent feature
- Stiffening phase, characterized by an improvement in pain, but increasing stiffness
- Thawing phase, with gradual resolution of symptoms. Symptoms classically resolve over 48 months, although recent studies have demonstrated that most patients are left with some background stiffness and discomfort

Management

Various management modalities have been used including:

- **Physiotherapy.** The goal of this is to maintain and improve movement. There is little objective evidence of its value, although the physiotherapist probably plays a useful role in supporting the patient through the natural course of the condition

- **Steroid injections.** Again, there is little evidence of long-term benefit, but they may be effective in providing pain relief
- **Manipulation under anaesthetic.** This may be beneficial in patients with persistent symptoms. It is probably best performed in association with a supraclavicular nerve block for pain relief and intensive postoperative mobilization, in an attempt to maintain gains in movement. Manipulation aims to re-establish external rotation before abduction: as it is difficult to abduct the arm if the greater tuberosity cannot be rotated from under the acromion, possibly resulting in dislocation. Humeral fracture is the major complication
- **Arthroscopic release.** This may be performed where closed manipulation fails, or in patient groups who tend to be recalcitrant to closed manipulation, notably diabetics. Release of the anterior capsule, and particularly the rotator interval, is usually sufficient, although the posterior capsule can also be released if required. Care is needed to avoid injuring the subscapularis and the axillary nerve. Simple arthroscopic distension may be of some value
- **Open release.** This is rarely performed, but release of the rotator interval may again result in significant improvement in movement. Open surgery may, of course, be required in cases of secondary frozen shoulder where a specific mechanical obstruction needs to be overcome

Recurrent shoulder instability

Recurrent shoulder instability usually falls into one of two main categories, each described by an acronym as follows:

- TUBS. This is usually due to a discrete **T**raumatic episode, and is **U**nidirectional (and Unilateral). It is associated with the presence of a **B**ankart lesion, and frequently requires **S**urgery. Ninety-eight percent of acute traumatic shoulder dislocations are anterior, and recurrent anterior instability is much more common than posterior

- AMBRI. This is **A**traumatic in origin, and is **M**ultidirectional. Symptoms are frequently **B**ilateral. The mainstay of treatment is conservative (**R**ehabilitation), although an **I**nferior capsular shift procedure may on occasion be performed

Recurrent unidirectional instability

The risk of subsequent dislocation is strongly dependent on the patient's age at the initial presentation. Typically quoted figures for recurrence are:
- <20 years at first dislocation: up to 80% (even higher in some studies)
- >30 years at first dislocation: up to 20%

Pathological features that may predispose to further instability include the presence of a Bankart lesion, a SLAP lesion, a Hill–Sachs lesion and a glenoid rim fracture. There is some evidence also that redislocation may be commoner after reduction with Kocher's method than with less traumatic methods due to further soft-tissue injury. There has been recent interest in immobilizing patients in external rotation (rather than the traditional internal rotation) after a first anterior dislocation, and some limited evidence from Japan suggests that this may decrease the risk of recurrence. Redislocation is less common if the original dislocation is associated with a greater tuberosity avulsion fracture.

Assessment

Symptoms may vary from recurrent frank dislocation to episodes of subluxation or even just a feeling of instability and lack of confidence in the shoulder. Subluxations may be felt simply as pain. Symptoms are very variable in frequency, but are most likely to occur with the shoulder abducted and externally rotated.

Clinical examination involves anterior and posterior drawer tests, as described by Gerber and Ganz. With the patient supine, the examiner stabilizes the shoulder girdle with one hand and draws the proximal humerus anteriorly and posteriorly with the other.

The anterior apprehension test is best performed with the patient supine. The shoulder is passively abducted to 90° by the examiner, and then brought slowly into progressive external rotation. Instability is indicated by a feeling of impending subluxation. This is abolished by pushing posteriorly on the proximal humerus while holding the shoulder in the same position (Jobe's relocation test) with symptoms recurring dramatically if the posterior relocating force is suddenly removed.

To perform a posterior apprehension test, the patient's arm is flexed to 90° and fully internally rotated while the patient is supine. A feeling of apprehension when a posteriorly directed force is directed to the humerus with the arm in this position indicates a positive test.

Radiographic examination is aimed at excluding any bony injury, which might either contribute to or result from recurrent dislocation. The apical oblique and axillary views may show a glenoid fracture, while the Stryker notch view may help in identifying a Hill–Sachs lesion (impaction of the posterior part of the humeral head upon the anterior glenoid).

Management

Conservative management consists of activity modification and physiotherapy in the form of rotator-cuff-strengthening exercises. The current gold standard operation for anterior instability is the Bankart procedure, which involves reattaching the stripped Bankart lesion (capsule and ligaments) to the glenoid rim, using either tissue anchors or sutures through drill holes. The classical open technique involves a deltopectoral approach, repair of the Bankart lesion and a moderate capsular shift. Recurrence rates vary from 1% to 11%. Exercises are gradually reintroduced over the subsequent 3 months.

The Bankart repair may also be performed arthroscopically, and this approach has gained popularity in recent years. The initial arthroscopic series suggested a higher redislocation rate than for open repair, although more recent studies have suggested improved results as experience, techniques and equipment for arthroscopic repair have improved.

Alternatives to the Bankart repair include:

- **Putti–Platt procedure.** This involves shortening both the anterior capsule and the subscapularis
- **Magnuson–Stack procedure.** The subscapularis and anterior capsular insertions are moved laterally to the lateral border of the bicipital groove, tightening the anterior structures
- **Bristow–Latarjet procedure.** The coracoid and attached conjoint tendon are transferred to the anterior glenoid rim. The conjoint tendon then reinforces the anteroinferior capsule, particularly as the shoulder is externally rotated and acts as a dynamic sling
- **Glenoid or humeral osteotomies.** Particularly if there is excessive anteversion of the glenohumeral joint

Recurrent posterior instability is rare, but can be treated with a posterior approach and either a "reverse Bankart" procedure and capsular shift, or a "reverse Putti–Platt" procedure. The Boyd–Sisk procedure involves transfer of the long head biceps to the posterior glenoid rim and is technically difficult.

If a large Hill–Sachs lesion is present, transfer of infraspinatus to fill the defect may help prevent redislocation. A reverse Hill–Sachs defect (due to posterior dislocation) may similarly be managed by transfer of subscapularis or the lesser tuberosity. Alternatively a bone block may be inserted to increase the anteversion of the glenoid.

Multidirectional instability

The pathogenesis of multidirectional instability is probably multifactorial, and involves:

- Hyperlaxity. This may be congenital (frequently generalized) or acquired, as may occur in athletes with repetitive stretching
- Precipitating events such as trauma
- Proprioceptive loss

Exploration of shoulders in patients with multidirectional instability reveals a voluminous, lax capsule, particularly inferiorly and in the rotator interval.

Assessment

Patients with multidirectional instability exhibit symptoms including:

- Recurrent subluxation and dislocation, often with spontaneous or easy relocation
- Pain, which is not confined to end-of-range movements. Symptoms on carrying objects such as shopping bags may suggest inferior laxity and subluxation
- Neurological symptoms of weakness and dysaesthesia

Although the patient's shoulder is lax multidirectionally, symptomatic instability may be predominantly in one direction.

The pathognomonic clinical sign on examination is the sulcus sign, where inferior traction on the patient's arm produces a sulcus inferior and lateral to the acromion. This is due to laxity of the capsule in the rotator interval. Inferior translational force on the proximal humerus with the arm abducted to 90° may also produce subluxation, this time due to redundancy of the inferior capsule. Between half and three-quarters of patients requiring surgery show signs of generalized hyperlaxity.

Management

- Conservative. Physiotherapy is the mainstay of management, with exercises to strengthen the rotator cuff and deltoid (phase I) being followed by proprioceptive rehabilitation (phase II) over a period of at least 6 months. An 88% success rate with conservative treatment has been reported by Rockwood
- Open inferior capsular shift procedure. This may be done through a deltopectoral approach with medial reflection of the subscapularis. A T-shaped incision is made in the capsule and the two leaflets are overlapped to reduce the capsular volume
- Arthroscopic capsular shift
- A small percentage of patients with multidirectional instability may exhibit habitual (or voluntary) dislocation. Such patients may or may

not exhibit signs of psychological disease; if so, treatment is directed at the underlying psychological state. Physiotherapy may be beneficial, but surgery is generally considered to be contraindicated

SLAP lesions

The **s**uperior **l**abrum **a**nterior to **p**osterior lesion has been recognized only since the development of shoulder arthroscopy, and arthroscopy remains the primary means of diagnosis, classification and management. Various forms of SLAP lesions exist, and have been classified by Snyder:

- Type I: Fraying and degeneration of the edge of the superior labrum, with the labral edge and biceps anchor still firmly attached
- Type II: Detachment of labrum and biceps anchor from the glenoid
- Type III: Bucket-handle tear of the superior labrum, with the remaining labrum and biceps anchor still attached
- Type IV: Bucket-handle tear of the superior labrum involving the biceps tendon
- Complex: Combination injuries, such as type II–III, or II–IV

Pathophysiology

There is a history of precipitant trauma in approximately two-thirds of patients. The supposed mechanisms are highly variable, including:

- Traction. This may occur from a fall, which is checked by the patient holding on to something, from the deceleration phase of throwing, or from a dislocation of the glenohumeral joint
- Compression. SLAP lesions are described after falls onto the outstretched hand with flexion and abduction of the shoulder, and direct blows onto the side of the shoulder
- The condition may be seen in athletes involved in throwing sports. It is frequently found in association with other pathologies around the shoulder

Assessment

Symptoms include:
- Pain, especially if patients are working with their arm above their head, or if lying on the arm
- Mechanical symptoms such as a feeling of the shoulder catching or locking
- Transient episodes of weakness and numbness ("dead arm")

There is no pathognomonic clinical test for a SLAP lesion, although tests for other shoulder lesions are frequently positive, including tests for impingement, biceps tendon pathology, instability and acromioclavicular arthritis. A compression-rotation test has been described. The patient is placed in the lateral position with the shoulder abducted to 90° and internal and external rotation is applied while compressing the glenohumeral joint. Pain occurs if the test is positive (O'Brien's test).

MRI, or better still MRI arthrography, may detect a proportion of lesions, but the majority of SLAP lesions are diagnosed arthroscopically.

Management

As the diagnosis is almost invariably made arthroscopically, the management for a recognized SLAP lesion is also generally operative and arthroscopic. The approach depends on the type of lesion:
- Type I: Debridement
- Type II: Repair, typically using suture anchors or staples
- Type III: Debridement
- Type IV: If a large part of the biceps is torn, it may be possible to repair it; failing this, management is again debridement

Arthritis of the elbow

Osteoarthritis

Aetiology

- Primary osteoarthritis. Uncommon, but more commonly affects the radio-capitate than the

ulno-humeral joints. It predominantly affects the dominant limb of men undertaking manual work
- Post-traumatic OA. This is more common than primary osteoarthritis
- Secondary to septic arthritis or haematological disorders (haemophilia or sickle disease)
- Neuropathic joint. Causes include diabetes, syringomyelia, syphilis and surgical denervation

Assessment

The two main symptoms are pain at extremes of movement, and decreased range of movement (loss of extension tends to be more marked than loss of flexion). Mid-range pain occurs only in advanced disease.

Standard AP and lateral radiographs confirm the diagnosis.

Management

- **Conservative management.** This consists largely of symptomatic measures such as analgesics
- **Capsulotomy.** To improve range of movement. This may be performed arthroscopically (with some risk to the neurovascular structures) or open (through an anterior, medial or lateral incision)
- **Joint debridement.** Three main options are available:
  1. **Outerbridge–Kashiwagi (OK) procedure.** The elbow is approached through a posterior triceps splitting approach and the tip of the olecranon is removed. The plate of bone between the coronoid and olecranon fossae is removed with burrs or drills, giving access to the anterior aspect of the joint and the coronoid and allowing debridement of osteophytes. An approximately 20° mean increase in range of movement has been obtained at the Mayo Clinic with this procedure
  2. **Lateral column procedure.** Although uncommonly performed in the UK, the trend in the USA is towards performing debridement through an extensile lateral approach. This is a more major undertaking, although larger improvements in

movement may be obtained. A lateral incision is made and triceps and anconeus are elevated. Brachioradialis and the carpal extensors are reflected distally. The lateral collateral ligaments are divided in Z-fashion, and an extensive joint debridement is performed
  3. **Arthroscopic debridement.** This has been described recently, but is challenging and there is some risk to the adjacent neurovascular structures
- **Interposition arthroplasty.** Interposition grafts include dermal graft, tibial periosteum and fascia lata. Interposition may be combined with application of a hinged distraction device. The technique is now used infrequently because it usually achieves only a moderate improvement in pain
- **Lateral resurfacing procedure**. Experimental procedure for isolated lateral joint arthritis
- **Total elbow replacement.** Survival, however, is poorer than in the rheumatoid patient due to increased demands
- **Arthrodesis** is difficult to achieve and is rarely used. The classical position for fusion of the elbow is 110°. If both elbows are fused, the second elbow is fused in a greater degree of extension

Rheumatoid arthritis

Twenty percent of patients with rheumatoid arthritis have severe elbow symptoms. Assessment and pathology are analogous to those for other joints.

Management

- **Conservative**, utilizing analgesics, NSAIDs, local and systemic corticosteroids and disease-modifying drugs
- **Synovectomy and radial head excision.** Usually performed through a lateral approach. Initial pain relief is obtained in 70% patients. This procedure may delay or avoid the need for elbow replacement in many patients
- **Interposition arthroplasty**, as described above, is rarely performed
- **Total elbow replacement,** as described separately

Elbow instability

The elbow is second only to the shoulder in terms of major joints that undergo acute dislocation. Although chronic instability is much less common than in the shoulder, it has been increasingly recognized as a clinical entity in recent years.

Stability of the elbow depends on the bony congruency of the elbow as well as the medial ligament complex (anterior, posterior and transverse parts) and the lateral ligament complex (the radial collateral, lateral ulnar collateral, annular and accessory lateral collateral ligaments).

Pathogenesis

Chronic instability of the elbow can arise from:
- Acute dislocation of the elbow. Associated fractures of the radial head or coronoid may also contribute to instability
- Chronic attrition of particularly the medial collateral ligament complex, as may occur in athletes involved in throwing sports
- Iatrogenic causes, such as removal of the radial head
- Arthritis

The typical instability pattern following acute dislocation is one of posterolateral instability due to tearing of the lateral ulnar collateral ligament in particular. O'Driscoll has classified the severity of the instability as follows:
- Stage 1: Posterolateral subluxation of the radius and ulna
- Stage 2: Impending dislocation, with the coronoid poised balanced on the trochlea
- Stage 3: Frank dislocation, which implies associated injury to the medial collateral ligament (divided into 3A and 3B, depending on the integrity of the anterior band of the ligament)

Assessment

The patient may complain of pain, "clunking" or catching of the elbow on certain activities.

Posterolateral instability is assessed with the patient supine, the arm above the patient's head, and the elbow at 20°–30° of flexion. Axial compression, valgus force and supination lead to subluxation which can be felt to reduce on further flexion of the joint. If the test is also positive in pronation, an associated injury to the medial collateral ligament is suggested. General anaesthesia is often required to permit full assessment of the elbow.

Management

Most acute elbow dislocations respond well to a brief (up to 2 week) period of immobilization. There is no evidence that longer periods of immobilization or routine surgical repair in the acute setting are of benefit. Those patients who do progress to chronic instability may have ligamentous repairs carried out. It may be necessary to reconstruct the torn ligaments using tendon grafts such as palmaris longus. Fractures should be fixed if contributing significantly to instability.

Miscellaneous pathologies around the elbow

Lateral epicondylitis (tennis elbow)

Pathophysiology

Tennis elbow produces lateral-sided elbow discomfort on activity. It is common, and has a peak incidence in patients in their 40s. Historically, many theories as to the cause of the pain have been advanced, but current feeling is that it usually represents degeneration within the tendon of ECRB, and occasionally EDC.

Histologically the finding is of angioblastic hyperplasia with tendon fibres invaded by fibroblasts and vascular granulation tissue. Of note is the absence of inflammatory cells.

Assessment

There is frequently a history of heavy occupational or sporting use of the arm. Men are affected twice as commonly as women. The complaint is of pain in the lateral aspect of the elbow, particularly on activities such as lifting. Maximal tenderness is anterior to the lateral epicondyle, and resisted extension or extreme passive flexion of the wrist may reproduce symptoms.

The differential diagnosis includes radiocapitellar pathology (arthritis or osteochondritis dissecans) and radial tunnel syndrome, which may occasionally coexist with lateral epicondylitis. Pain with the middle finger extension test (resisted extension of the finger) helps to identify radial tunnel syndrome. Radiographs may occasionally show abnormal calcification in the ECRB tendon, but are useful mainly for excluding other conditions.

A "mesenchymal syndrome" is described, whereby patients appear to develop multiple, related conditions including lateral and medial epicondylitis, Achilles tendinopathy, rotator cuff pathology and carpal tunnel syndrome.

Management

Conservative management includes rest and NSAIDs, physiotherapy and braces. The last of these may function either by altering the direction of extensor muscle pull or by providing a rigid constraint preventing over-contraction of muscles. The reported response to these methods is extremely variable. Steroid injections appear to bring short-term relief, although there is little convincing evidence of long-term benefit.

Standard surgical release is performed through a small lateral incision, although percutaneous release has also been described. The common extensor origin is reflected from the lateral epicondyle. Improvement is presumed to be due to lengthening and consequent de-tensioning of the ECRB tendon. Alternative explanations for the effectiveness of the operation include the initiation of an inflammatory response (conspicuously absent from the primary pathology) leading to healing; or simple denervation. Between 60% and 80% of patients have good results following the procedure.

Alternative procedures that have been carried out for tennis elbow include radiocapitellar synovectomy, partial division of the annular ligament, decompression of the posterior interosseous nerve, and distal lengthening of ECRB.

Medial epicondylitis (golfer's elbow)

Medial epicondylitis can be regarded as analogous to lateral epicondylitis in terms of pathophysiology, assessment and management, but it is less common.

Pain is felt on the medial side of the elbow. There may be symptoms (and signs) of ulnar nerve entrapment, which frequently coexists (10%). Pain can be reproduced on resisted flexion or passive extension of the wrist. The differential diagnosis again includes intra-articular pathology, and injuries to the medial collateral ligament of the elbow. Management follows the usual course of conservative management, steroid injection and surgical release. Care should be taken not to injure the ulnar nerve while injecting steroid.

Olecranon bursitis

Although there are multiple bursae around the elbow, the olecranon bursa is the one that most commonly gives rise to pathology. The bursa is a discrete structure, which does not usually communicate with the elbow joint, although in rheumatoid arthritis it may do so.

Aetiology

The primary causes of olecranon bursitis include:
- Infection. This accounts for approximately one-quarter of cases. *Staphylococcus aureus* is responsible for some 90% of these, although streptococci, anaerobes and other organisms may also be responsible
- Inflammatory. Due to an underlying inflammatory condition such as rheumatoid arthritis or gout
- Traumatic. This may be acute or due to repetitive trauma ("student's elbow")
- Haemodialysis
- Idiopathic

Assessment and management

The primary requirement is to distinguish between infected and non-infected cases. Symptoms and signs of systemic upset, haematological and biochemical markers of inflammation and aspiration may be beneficial. Organisms may not always be seen on Gram stain of infected cases, although a high white cell count in the aspirate (>1000/mm³) may be indicative.

Management options for septic olecranon bursitis include:

- Antibiotics, splintage and elevation
- Aspiration, which may need to be repeated
- Drainage. If possible this is avoided due to problems with prolonged fistulas, although it may be necessary
- Excision. This is used in cases of prolonged discharge after incision and drainage, or in cases of recurrent infection

Management of non-infected cases includes:

- NSAIDs and compressive bandages
- Steroid injections have been used, but may lead to dermal atrophy
- Excision

Arthroscopy of the shoulder and elbow

Shoulder arthroscopy

Improvements in technology and surgical techniques have led to the rapid expansion of arthroscopic shoulder surgery in recent years.

Indications

- Diagnostic in cases of instability or pain coming from suspected intra-articular or subacromial pathology
- Washout for septic arthritis
- Subacromial decompression and/or ACJ excision
- Rotator cuff repair
- Bankart repair for recurrent anterior instability, and on occasions capsular shift procedures for multidirectional instability

- Debridement or repair of SLAP lesions
- Removal of loose bodies

Technique

Shoulder arthroscopy may be performed either with the patient in the lateral decubitus position with their arm distracted by traction, or with the patient in the "beach-chair" position.

Most commonly used portals include:

- Posterior portal (2 cm inferior and 1 cm medial to the posterolateral corner of the acromion). This is the main port used for the arthroscope, and it gives good access to most of the shoulder joint
- Anterior portal (just lateral to the midpoint of a line between the antero-inferior border of the acromion and the coracoid but superior to subscapularis). This is usually used for surgical instruments
- Lateral portal (3 cm lateral to the lateral border of the acromion). This allows good access to the subacromial space
- Superior portal (1 cm medial to the medial border of the acromion, posterior to the clavicle and anterior to the spine of the scapula)

Complications include articular cartilage damage, brachial plexus palsy (from incorrect portal placement or excessive traction on the arm) and infection.

Elbow arthroscopy

Indications

- Diagnostic, looking for intra-articular pathology or in the assessment of instability
- Washout, e.g. septic arthritis
- Removal of loose bodies due to trauma, osteochondritis dissecans or arthritis
- Synovectomy
- Capsulotomy or joint debridement for primary or post-traumatic arthritis

Arthroscopy of the elbow is technically demanding due to the enclosed space of the elbow joint and the close proximity of numerous major neurovascular structures. This and the easy accessibility of the joint using open techniques mean that arthroscopy is less commonly performed than in the shoulder. A 10% complication risk has been quoted, including damage to major or cutaneous nerves, vascular damage, synovial fistula formation and compartment syndrome.

Technique

Elbow arthroscopy may be performed with the patient in the mid-lateral or prone positions, or with the patient supine and their arm suspended from above. A tourniquet is usually used to decrease bleeding, although it does not have to be used. The risk of neurovascular injury can be decreased by opening ports using blunt dissection, and by keeping the elbow flexed on entry to the anterior ports to ensure that the neurovascular structures are relaxed.

Multiple portals have been described:
- Direct lateral portal (at the centre of a triangle defined by the lateral epicondyle, the radial head and the olecranon). This is frequently used as the initial entry portal to inflate the joint with saline
- Anterolateral portal (1 cm distal and 1 cm anterior to the lateral epicondyle, between the radial head and the capitellum). This gives good access to the anterior aspect of the joint
- Anteromedial portal (2 cm distal and 2 cm anterior to the medial epicondyle). This is often created using an "inside out" technique by cutting down onto the tip of the arthroscope inserted using the anterolateral portal
- Proximal medial portal (2 cm proximal to the medial epicondyle along the anterior surface of the humerus towards the radial head)
- Direct posterior portal (1.5 cm proximal to the tip of the olecranon)
- Posterolateral portal

Arthroplasty of the shoulder and elbow

Shoulder arthroplasty

Design

Various options for replacement are available

- **Shoulder hemiarthroplasty**. This consists of a stemmed head, which may achieve fixation either with cement or by press-fit/porous coating. Many modern designs are modular, allowing stems of varying thickness to be matched to heads of different diameter and thickness. Bipolar prostheses are occasionally used
- **Total shoulder replacement**. Humeral components are generally capable of being used as a hemiarthroplasty or in conjunction with glenoid replacement as part of a total shoulder replacement. Metal-backed glenoid replacements have fallen out of favour, and cemented all-polyethylene components are now generally used. Glenoid loosening remains a real problem due to the small area of bone for fixation (often compounded by glenoid erosion) and the high forces generated due to the large range of movement in the shoulder joint. Total shoulder replacement is therefore less commonly used for most shoulder pathologies than is hemiarthroplasty, although it may provide superior pain relief in the early stages postoperatively
- **Resurfacing**. Humeral head resurfacing has become popular recently due to the reported success of the Copeland prosthesis. This is a hemispherical cup, which is implanted onto the reamed humeral head. Fixation is by means of hydroxyapatite coating and a central press-fit cruciform peg. As well as conserving bone stock, it may be easier to maintain correct retroversion/anteversion than with a standard hemiarthroplasty

Approach

Hemiarthroplasty or total shoulder replacement is generally performed using a standard delto-pectoral approach. The prosthesis is inserted in approximately 30° of retroversion to reproduce the normal anatomy and minimize the chances of dislocation.

Complications

Complications are similar to those for other joint replacements including infection, aseptic loosening (particularly of the glenoid) and dislocation. Care needs to be taken to ensure adequate room for the prosthesis if a stemmed elbow replacement is in place. The results (particularly in terms of regaining movement) are strongly related to the integrity of the rotator cuff.

Elbow arthroplasty

Design

The deficient bone stock frequently encountered during elbow arthroplasty is not attractive for cementless fixation, and most implants are designed to be inserted with cement. Entirely unstemmed components are prone to early loosening, and most modern designs include stems of variable lengths.

There are three broad philosophies of design:

- **Constrained**. Original designs were rigidly linked metal hinges, somewhat akin to early knee replacement designs. They also had the same problems of early loosening, and fully constrained devices are no longer used
- **Unconstrained** (more correctly minimally constrained). Examples of such unlinked prostheses include the Kudo and Souter–Strathclyde prostheses. Early minimally constrained designs often included replacement of the radial head, but this is usually now avoided due to problems with loosening and subluxation
- **Semi-constrained** ("sloppy hinge"). These are linked by a coupling that allows a certain amount of varus/valgus and rotational laxity. Forces are therefore absorbed by the soft tissues rather than by being transferred in their entirety to the implant–bone interface. The Coonrad–Morrey prosthesis is perhaps the best-known example

Semi-constrained devices are perhaps easier to insert, and typically result in a greater range of movement due to a greater soft-tissue release being possible. They can be used where there is deficiency of the collateral ligaments or bony integrity of the condyles (as in severe arthritis or after fracture), and largely avoid the risks of prosthetic dislocation. Greater forces are still theoretically transferred to the implant–bone interface than with minimally constrained devices, but relatively low rates of loosening have been observed in practice.

Approaches

- **Campbell's posterior approach**. This classical approach involves leaving a tongue of triceps aponeurosis attached to the olecranon and splitting the triceps underneath
- **Mayo approach**. The triceps is mobilized and reflected laterally after identifying and protecting the ulnar nerve. This involves partial release of the triceps tendon from the olecranon
- **Lateral approach**

Complications

Complications are higher than for other joints and include:

- Poor wound healing and infection, particularly in rheumatoid patients (rates of over 10% have been reported)
- Neurovascular injury. Some degree of ulnar neurapraxia is very common
- Dissociation of unconstrained devices
- Aseptic loosening, which is more common in osteoarthritis than in rheumatoid arthritis. Salvage may involve revision with linked semi-constrained devices, or in severe cases resection arthroplasty, leaving the patient with a flail elbow
- Periprosthetic fractures have been reported in up to 5% of cases

16

Hip oral core topics

Paul A. Banaszkiewicz

Anatomy of the hip

Blood supply of femoral head

This is a favourite question in either the basic science or the adult/pathology oral. This may lead into a discussion about avascular necrosis (AVN) of the femoral head. The blood supply has three sources:

1. Medial circumflex femoral artery is the most important supply; it is a branch of the profunda femoris artery
2. Lateral circumflex artery supplies the inferior portion; it is a branch of the profunda femoris artery
3. Artery of the ligamentum teres is a minor blood supply in the adult; it is a posterior branch of the obturator artery

The extracapsular arterial ring gives off ascending cervical arteries known as retinacular arteries. Injury to the retinacular arteries may lead to AVN.

Examination corner

Basic science oral 1

Second question after an initial discussion on the position that a leg assumes after a traumatic posterior and anterior dislocation of the hip.

Examiner: What is the blood supply to the femoral head?

Candidate: The blood supply to the femoral head is derived from the medial and lateral femoral circumflex arteries; these are branches of the profunda femoris artery. They form an extracapsular arterial ring around the base of the trochanter.

Ascending cervical arteries are given off this ring and then branch into retinacular arteries, which form a subsynovial intracapsular arterial ring …

The candidate was stopped in mid-sentence by the examiner, who was satisfied with the answer and wanted to move on to another question. This led on to a discussion of AVN of the hip, types of THA to use in a young patient, survival analysis curves, etc.

Basic science oral 2

Anatomy of the posterior thigh. The examiner had a colour, laminated photocopy of the whole of the posterior thigh from an atlas.

- Popliteal fossa: anatomy, approaches and the neurovascular structure arrangement
- Posterior approach of the hip: structures going above and below the piriformis muscle, and anatomy of the superior and inferior gluteal nerves and arteries. Identification of pudendal nerve and nerve to obturatus internus beneath the piriformis muscle
- Safe zones for acetabular screws
- Femoral head blood supply

Basic science oral 3

- Anatomy of posterior hip and thigh
- Surface markings for the sciatic nerve
- Causes of superior gluteal artery injury
- Hamstring origin
- Approaches to the hip

Postgraduate Orthopaedics: The Candidate's Guide to the FRCS (Tr & Orth) Examination, Ed. Paul A. Banaszkiewicz, Deiary F. Kader, Nicola Maffulli. Published by Cambridge University Press. © Cambridge University Press 2009.

Basic science oral 4

Picture of a hemipelvis with the outline of muscle origins – candidate was asked to identify approximately six muscles.

Basic science oral 5

Name the structures on the posterior aspect of the hip. A colour figure was provided with bare labels.

Basic science oral 6

• Anatomy of the gluteal muscles and pelvis
• Surgical approaches to the hip joint and complications of the direct lateral approach

Adult elective orthopaedics oral

Various surgical approaches to the hip joint

Basic science oral 7

• Blood supply to the femoral head
• Anterior approach to the hip

Avascular necrosis of the femoral head

Introduction

This is a controversial topic because the aetiology of AVN remains unclear and management is still somewhat unpredictable and uncertain.

Definition

AVN is the death or necrosis of bone secondary to the loss of its vascular supply or more simply "death of bone from ischaemia".

Causative factors

A variety of aetiological associations with AVN have been demonstrated.

Pathogenesis

1. **Idiopathic:** most common cause (up to 40% in total)
2. **Arterial insufficiency**. Due to fracture, dislocation or infection
3. **Intraosseous arteriolar occlusion**. Sickle cell disease or other haemoglobinopathies, Caisson's disease, vasculitis
4. **Capillary occlusion**. Due to fatty infiltration from excessive alcohol, steroids and hyperlipidaemia
5. **Venous occlusion**.

Bilateral in 50% of idiopathic AVN and as high as 80% if steroid induced.

Aetiology

The cause is still uncertain. Several theories have been put forward:

1. Intraosseous hypertension theory, the so-called compartment syndrome of bone
2. Abnormality of extraosseous blood flow
3. Fat emboli in subchondral arterioles
4. Fat cell hypertrophy
5. Direct cytotoxic effect on osteocytes (alcohol)
6. Clotting abnormalities such as deficiencies in protein S, protein C and antithrombin III

Clinical features

Usually non-specific with insidious onset of hip pain worse with weight bearing, often present at rest and eventually at night. Associated with a decreased or painful range of hip movement, limp, muscle weakness and antalgic gait.

Radiology

• **Plain radiographs.** Normal in the early stages of disease
• **Bone scan.** Cold area (initial loss of blood perfusion)
• **MRI scan features.** Ischaemic marrow changes evident before bone changes become apparent

Classification

Ficat

The original classification in 1968 did not include stage zero:

0 Preclinical: positive functional exploration of bone

I Pre-radiological: radiographs normal, MRI/bone scan positive

II Pre-collapse: osteopenia/sclerosis, head spherical

III Collapse: flattened head, crescent sign

IV Secondary degenerative changes of osteoarthritis

Management

Steinberg classification 0–6 (7 stage system)

0. Normal X-ray, bone scan and MRI, diagnosed on histology

1. Normal X-ray diagnosed on bone scan or MRI scan (minimal pain)

2. Sclerosis and/or cyst formation

3. Subchondral collapse (crescent sign) without flattening

4. Flattening head without joint narrowing or acetabular involvement

5. Flattening head with joint narrowing and/or acetabular involvement

6. Advanced degenerative change

Plus:

Area involved: A, minimal <15%; B, moderate 15°–30°; C, extensive >30°

Surface collapse 2 mm, 2–4 mm, >4 mm

Location

Observation (protective weight bearing)

Non-operative management. This is not a particularly good option as most patients do poorly with only approximately 20% obtaining a satisfactory clinical outcome (success rates for Ficat stage I, 35%; stage II, 31%; and stage III, 13%). The remaining 80% progress to collapse within 2 years. Observation may be indicated in those with very limited disease or if the patient is not fit enough for surgery.

Electrical stimulation

Despite being around for several years electrical stimulation has failed to gain widespread acceptance. Very few additional studies have been published in recent years and therefore it remains experimental and requires further evaluation as part of a randomized controlled clinical trial.

Hyperbaric oxygen therapy

This may be an effective management for stage I AVN. It is experimental and needs further evaluation.

Core decompression

This is simple, safe and a relatively successful way of managing early-stage AVN. It effectively relieves intraosseous venous hypertension, which reduces hip pain. In core decompression, an intraosseous wound is created that stimulates vascular neogenesis and may allow healing of the infarcted area. There is some controversy over the effectiveness of the procedure, but there is a reasonable body of evidence to support its use. Mont *et al.*[1] published a meta-analysis of patients treated with core decompression covering 1206 hips. Survival rates reported for Ficat stage I were 84%; for stage II, 65%; for stage III, 47%. Approximately two-thirds do well, half if you exclude centres of excellence with the most experience dealing with the condition.

Cortical strut grafts

Cortical strut grafts (non-vascularized) are carried out using either the fibula or tibia to provide mechanical support.

Free vascularized fibular grafts

These may be superior to non-vascularized grafts. The procedure is technically difficult, time con-

[1] Mont MA, Carbone JJ, Fairbank AC (1996) Core decompression versus nonoperative management for osteonecrosis of the hip. *Clin Orthop Relat Res* **324**:169–78.

suming and requires special equipment and micro-vascular surgical techniques.

Trapdoor procedure

This is indicated for pre-collapse (Ficat stage II). The break in the articular cartilage is exposed following hip dislocation and opened like a trapdoor. Necrotic bone under the flap is excavated and then removed with a power burr to expose bleeding bone. The defect is then filled with cancellous bone graft.

Proximal femoral osteotomy

A proximal femoral osteotomy attempts to shift most of the involved portion of the head medially. It is performed using a combination of varus, valgus, flexion, extension and rotation. It is usually indicated for patients with Ficat stage II or III AVN. Results are best with patients aged 45 years or younger, with unilateral disease, with idiopathic or traumatic aetiology and with a small to medium area of infarction. The reported success rate is 70%–80%. However, the procedure is only applicable to a small number of patients. The Sugioka transtrochanteric rotational osteotomy[2] shifts the diseased portion of the head medially, inferiorly and posteriorly.

Bipolar hemiarthroplasty

This is possibly best indicated in elderly unfit patients whose AVN has resulted from chronic alcohol abuse.

Hemiresurfacing arthroplasty

This is a bone-preserving procedure reserved for young active patients with femoral head collapse and minimal acetabular cartilage damage. It is potentially indicated for Ficat stage III disease or early stage IV disease. Controversial option, pain

[2] Sugioka Y, Hotokebuchi T, Tsutsui H (1992) Transtrochanteric anterior rotational osteotomy for idiopathic and steroid-induced necrosis of the femoral head. Indications and long-term results. *Clin Orthop Relat Res* **277**: 111–20.

relief is not as predictable as after THA but the procedure preserves bone stock and any subsequent revision is relatively straightforward.

Total hip resurfacing

When the acetabular cartilage grading is poor, total resurfacing arthroplasty using metal-on-metal designs is a possible option. It will address the pathology on both sides of the joint whilst preserving bone stock on the femoral side.

Cemented THA

This is relatively less successful in patients with AVN. Likewise results of uncemented THA have been mixed with no clear advantage over a cemented design for AVN.

Arthrodesis

Arthrodesis may be indicated in young patients with unilateral disease, e.g. trauma. Many cases are bilateral. This is more of a theoretical option for advanced disease than a practical one.

Examination corner

Adult elective orthopaedics oral 1

There had been previous discussion on how an MRI scanner works, with the usual questions about T_1- and T_2-weighted images. Coronal MRI scans of the pelvis were shown and the candidate was asked to point out various anatomical features of the spine: disc space, vertebral bodies, spinal cord and psoas muscle.

Examiner: This is in fact the scan of a 40-year-old gentleman who was complaining of a history of groin pain for several weeks. Are there any features of note that could account for his pain?

Candidate: These are T_2-weighted coronal images of the pelvis. The most obvious abnormality is decreased signal intensity from both femoral heads.

Examiner: What do you think the diagnosis is?

Candidate: The MRI features are suggestive of AVN of the femoral head.

Examiner: What is the Ficat classification system of AVN?

Candidate: The Ficat system is a 5-stage classification system for AVN. Stage 0 was not in the original classification of Ficat but was added later. The diagnosis is based on functional exploration of bone with core biopsy, an intramedullary venogram and bone marrow pressures. Stage I is called pre-radiological: the radiographs are normal, but the MRI/bone scan is positive. Stage II is a pre-collapse stage with osteopenia/sclerosis of the head but the head is still spherical. Stage III is collapse and a flattened femoral head with a crescent sign and finally in stage IV secondary degenerative changes of osteoarthritis are present.

Examiner (who had got bored after the first sentence): what nationality was Ficat?

Candidate: He was French.

Examiner: Yes, and the French have a very high incidence of AVN, much higher than in this country. So what do you think is probably the most likely reason for this?

Candidate: They drink a lot of wine.

Examiner: Yes alcohol, they drink a lot of wine, usually a nice, fine full-bodied red wine. So quickly tell me how do you treat Ficat stage I and Ficat stage IV? (I think the examiner had decided to pass the candidate at this stage and was making life easy for them or maybe was thinking about quaffing a few glasses of red wine at lunch!)

Candidate: I would treat Ficat stage I by core decompression and Ficat stage IV with a total hip arthroplasty.

Examiner: What are the published results of hip arthroplasty in patients with AVN?

Candidate: They do not do as well when compared to a standard hip replacement for osteoarthritis.[1] This is because there are histological bone changes of AVN further down the proximal femur, not just confined to the femoral head.

Calder *et al.* from Imperial College London first published these findings in the *Journal of Bone and Joint Surgery* British edition in 2001.[2] Cancellous bone biopsies were taken from four regions of the proximal femur in patients undergoing THA with a diagnosis of AVN and compared to a control group. Histological examination showed extensive AVN in the proximal femur extending up to 4 cm below the lesser trochanter compared to the control group. He postulated that the presence of AVN in the proximal femoral canal may reduce the remodelling capacity of bone at the bone–cement interface and impair the establishment of osseointegration and therefore adequate long-term fixation of the prosthesis.

Mont and Hungerford have extensively studied AVN. In his systematic review of 27 published series, all except two studies reported a higher rate of failure in patients with AVN than in age-matched patients with other disorders.[3] He reported

wide differences in failure rates of THA of between 10% and 50% at 5 years. Recently better short-term results have been reported with new cementing techniques and cementless component designs.[4]

Examiner: Yes you are forcing cement into dead bone. This gentleman is young at 40 years of age; how will you manage him?

Candidate: I would manage him with either a cemented THA telling him it would last between 10 and 15 years before requiring revision, or a metal-on-metal resurfacing hip procedure.

Examiner: If you get 15 years out of a cemented hip replacement you will be doing very well. Are there any published results of the second-generation metal-on-metal hip replacements?

Candidate: I have not come across any published articles as such. I know it was debated earlier this year at the BOA conference and there was some concern about aneuploidy and the subsequent risk of developing neoplasm.[5]

Examiner: That is not the only concern about this type of hip arthroplasty. Several surgeons have serious concerns about the amount of metal particles released into the local soft tissues from this prosthesis and the possibility of ALVAR and pseudotumours/massive granuloma disease developing. Do you know of any guidelines in place that will give you advice about what type of hip replacements to use in clinical practice?

Candidate: No I'm sorry.

Examiner: You're from Scotland so you may not have heard of the NICE guidelines from England and Wales but you must have heard about the Scottish Executive Home Office Guidelines.

Candidate: Yes, of course sir.[6]

Examiner: These are very important documents that give you valuable information about issues in clinical practice. It is important to read them before you start practising as a consultant. Anyway let's move on to another topic.

This examiner was essentially very benign and guided me through this topic but by this stage of the oral all the hard work had been done previously and I think he had already decided to pass me provided I did not say anything suicidal.

Basic science oral 1

The first question in the basic science oral was presumably a warm-up one.

The candidate was shown a gross histology picture of AVN of the femoral head.

Examiner: Just describe the picture to me; what do you see?

Candidate: (After a fairly longish pause.) This is a photograph of a gross histology picture of the femoral head. (Pause) It shows a space between the articulating surface of the femoral head and the subchondral bone. It is very suggestive of AVN.

Examiner: Yes of course it is. What is the aetiology of AVN?

Candidate: The aetiology is still uncertain but it's thought that it is due to arterial insufficiency, to intraosseous arteriolar occlusion or capillary occlusion.

Examiner: Go on, what other aetiologies are there?

Candidate: Certainly trauma can cause AVN.

Examiner: Yes, that is the commonest cause of AVN particularly around the hip. However, what is the current thinking for the aetiology of AVN?

Candidate: (After a long pause.) Most recently work has concentrated on clotting abnormalities as a cause of AVN such as deficiencies in protein S and protein C.

Examiner: Yes of course, you knew the answer all along! Now do you know a classification system for AVN?

Candidate: I am most familiar with the Ficat classification system. It is the classification system that I have most widely come across when reading articles on the subject.

Examiner: Any others?

Candidate: (Pause) The Steinberg classification system.

Examiner: Yes this is much more useful, detailed and comprehensive. How do you treat early AVN?

Candidate: I would treat Ficat stage I, II and some early cases of III with core decompression.

Examiner: What are the results like for core decompression?

Candidate: For Ficat grade I the success rate is 84%; for grade II, 65%; and for grade III, 47%.

[Fail]

Candidate debriefing

The candidate gave a slightly substandard answer albeit by no means a disastrous one. The content was reasonable, the candidate may just not have been confident enough in his/her answers or else the delivery may have been poor.

The candidate got off to a bad start as he/she was too slow and cautious in describing the initial clinical photograph as it was very obvious what the diagnosis was. He/she was too slow coming up with the latest thinking about clotting factors as an aetiological factor; the examiner was looking for a snappy quick answer.

In addition this examiner does not appear to be particularly candidate friendly. A different examiner may have coaxed out a better answer and the candidate may have gone on to do him/herself more justice and passed the oral. Unfortunately candidates have no control over who will

viva them. Candidates will almost certainly come across one or two examiners with whom they do not connect and who are on a different wavelength. One has to hope in this situation that a good rapport is developed with the other examiner so that at least you can scrape through your oral.

Adult elective orthopaedics oral 2

Same examiner we think! Different candidate, different examination, different year, different outcome (a pass this time).

The same slide and same questions were asked as outlined in Basic science oral 1, but presumably the candidate gave better answers! In addition:

- A cut section of femoral head showing subchondral collapse was presented
- The following were discussed:
    Radiographic findings in AVN
    The grading of AVN
    Management for this grade
    The role of fibula grafts, decompression

There was a very superficial discussion throughout.

Adult elective orthopaedics oral 3

Avascular necrosis:
- Classification
- Causes
- Management

Basic science oral 2

- Causes of AVN
- Classification
- Pathophysiology of AVN, specifically steroid-induced AVN
- Management of AVN

Adult elective orthopaedics oral 4

AVN of the femoral head:
- Classification
- Your management of a 48-year-old man with AVN

Adult elective orthopaedics oral 5

AVN hips – everything!

Basic science oral 3

AVN following fractured neck of femur: histological changes

Adult elective orthopaedics oral 6

AVN (Ficat classification and management)
Principles of classification systems

Adult elective orthopaedics oral 7

Clinical and MRI differences between AVN and bone marrow oedema syndrome

Trauma oral 1

Posttraumatic AVN (fractured neck of femur, managed with AO cannulated screws)
Stage [ARCO (Association Research Circulation Osseous), Ficat]
Management options

[1] Keep on talking, you know what the next question is going to be – "why?"
[2] Calder JD, Pearse MF, Revell PA (2001) The extent of osteocyte death in the proximal femur of patients with osteonecrosis of the femoral head. *J Bone Joint Surg Br* **83**(3): 419–22.
[3] Mont MA, Hungerford DS (1995) Non-traumatic avascular necrosis of the femoral head. *J Bone Joint Surg Am* **77**(3): 459–74.
[4] Kantor SG, Huo MH, Huk OL, Salvati EA (1996) Cemented total hip arthroplasty in patients with osteonecrosis: a 6-year minimum follow-up study of second-generation cement techniques. *J Arthroplasty* **11**: 267–271.
[5] The British Orthopaedic Association conference is a meeting that may be useful to attend prior to the exam, but it is not vital. However it is important to talk to someone who has attended the conference to find out the latest hot topics discussed; it may just get you out of a tricky situation!
[6] No I had not!

Protrusio acetabuli

Definition

Normally on an AP radiograph the medial wall of the acetabulum lies *2 mm lateral* to the *ilioischial line* in a male and *1 mm medial* to this line in a female. Protrusio is present if the medial wall of the acetabulum is 3 mm or more medial to the ilioischial line in a male or >6 mm medial to it in a female.

Classification: Hirst grade I–III[3]

Radiological classification based on plain radiographs of the pelvis:

Grade I: mild

- 3–8 mm medial ♂, 6–11 mm ♀
- 5–10 mm protrusion

Grade II: moderate

- 9–13 mm ♂, 12–17 mm ♀
- 10–15 mm protrusion

Grade III: severe

- >13 mm ♂, >17 mm ♀ (with fragmentation)
- >15 mm protrusion

Aetiology

The primary idiopathic form of protrusio is termed Otto's pelvis. The female-to-male ratio is 10:1, with the majority of cases being idiopathic. It has been reported as being present in approximately 22% of rheumatoid patients requiring arthroplasty.

[3] Hirst P, Esser M, Murphy JC, Hardinge K (1987). Bone grafting for protrusion acetabuli during total hip replacement. A review of the Wrightington method in 61 hips. *J Bone Joint Surg Br* **69**(2):229–33.

Associations

Decreased bone density

- Osteoporosis
- Osteogenesis imperfecta
- Osteomalacia
- Rickets
- Rheumatoid disease (19%)
- Marfan's disease
- Ankylosing spondylitis

Normal density

- Osteoarthritis
- Otto's disease (idiopathic, 75%)

Increased density

- Hypophosphatasia
- Paget's (4%)

Investigations

Standard AP and lateral radiographs of the pelvis will confirm the diagnosis and will permit staging.

Principles of THA reconstruction

Hip dislocation can be difficult: the neck may need to be cut in situ. Placing the hip centre back into the correct anatomical position is essential for restoration of joint biomechanics. The general principle is to bone graft the floor and lateralize the cup.

Examination corner

Adult elective orthopaedics oral

Idiopathic protrusio (Otto's pelvis)

- Surgery
- Approach
- Use of bone graft
- Cementing technique

Dysplastic hip

The hallmark of the dysplastic hip is lack of coverage of the femoral head, whether it is subluxed or dislocated.

Anatomical considerations

Acetabulum

Shallow, anteverted, deficient, small and poor bone quality.

Femur

Small deformed head; short anteverted valgus neck; small and posteriorly displaced greater trochanter; and narrow, straight, tapered femoral canal.

Soft tissues

Muscles are usually shortened and contracted and the hip capsule is elongated and redundant.

Classification

Crowe 1–4

This is useful in assessing the degree of subluxation in the end-stage arthritic hip and to predict perioperative complications (Table 16.1).

Management

Conservative

In the absence of pain, subluxation or dislocation (in the adult) is not itself an indication for surgery.

Osteotomy

This is possibly indicated for a young adult in their early 20s. Osteotomy is usually performed on the acetabular side.

Arthroplasty

End-stage arthritis is generally treated with THA.

Table 16.1 Crowe classification of acetabular dysplasia

Crowe classification	
Grade 1	<50% subluxation
Grade 2	Between 50% and 75% subluxation
	Usually patients do not have leg length inequality or loss of bone stock
Grade 3	Between 75% and 100% subluxation
	Complete loss of superior acetabular roof
	Possibly a thin medial wall
	Anterior and posterior columns are intact
Grade 4	Dislocated
	True acetabulum is deficient but remains recognizable

Arthrodesis

If unilateral disease is present, arthrodesis for end-stage arthritis is certainly an option worth considering in a young patient with high activity levels.

Total hip arthroplasty

Anatomic position (low hip centre)
Advantages: facilitates lengthening, better hip function, best available bone stock, diminished joint reaction forces.
Disadvantages: difficult surgery, osteotomy of the greater trochanter and resection of the proximal femoral metaphysis may be necessary.

Non-anatomic position (high hip centre)
A hip centre located at least 35 mm proximal to the inter-teardrop line.
Advantages: technically easier than the anatomic position; allows the component to be more completely covered by native bone and so may avoid the need for bone grafting and also decreases the need for a concomitant shortening femoral osteotomy.
Disadvantages: increased shearing forces may lead to early loosening; a higher rate of dislocation than the anatomic location; further revision surgery is difficult as bone stock not restored; affords a limited amount of leg lengthening, can only use a very small acetabular component with therefore thin polyethylene or the ceramic bearing surface option often not possible as a bigger acetabular shell is needed.

Oral questions

What are the advantages and disadvantages of placing the acetabular cup in either the anatomic position (low hip centre) or non-anatomic position (high hip centre)?
Is the cup going to be cemented or uncemented?
How much are you going to lengthen the patient?
Does the femur need subtrochanteric shortening?

Examination corner

This can be either a long case or an oral topic. Once the preliminaries of the radiographic description of the condition and Crowe's classification are out of the way, discussion will turn to management. A large part of the discussion will probably centre on the technical issues of performing a THA in this type of hip.

Adult elective orthopaedics oral 1

Radiograph of a 23-year-old female complaining of severe arthritic left hip pain secondary to DDH

- Discuss management options including the role of pelvic osteotomy

Adult elective orthopaedics oral 2

Patient who had a right THA at 30 years of age for DDH. THA has now failed

- Discuss the management

Adult elective orthopaedics oral 3

Radiograph shown of a 60-year-old female with a deformed arthritic left hip secondary to DDH

- Outline your management of this hip

Primary THA

Indications

Disabling pain refractory to conservative treatment, severely affecting the patient's quality of life.

Contraindications

Absolute

- Active infection

Relative

- Neuropathic joint
- Progressive neurological disease
- Significant co-morbidity factors
- Non ambulators
- Abductor muscle loss

Informed consent

Local risks

- Dislocation 3%
- Infection 0.5%
- Eventual failure due to wear (aseptic loosening)
- Leg length inequality
- Nerve or vascular injury

Systemic risks

- Death (<0.5%)
- Deep vein thrombosis
- Non-fatal pulmonary embolism
- Fatal pulmonary embolism
- Cerebrovascular accident
- Myocardial infarction
- Urinary tract and chest infection

Surgical approach

Trochanteric osteotomy (Charnley approach)

Advantages
- Hip is easy to dislocate
- Excellent acetabular exposure

- Cement is easy to insert
- Good femoral component alignment
- Trochanteric advancement permitted
- Useful in complex primary and revision hip surgery

Disadvantages
- Increased blood loss
- Increased operating time
- Technically difficult to reattach the trochanter particularly with scarred tissue and osteoporotic bone
- Possibility of trochanteric non-union causing Trendelenburg gait
- Wire breakage
- Trochanteric bursitis

Transgluteal Hardinge approach

Advantages
- Lower rates of dislocation and sciatic nerve injury compared with the posterior approach
- Preservation of the posterior soft tissue hip envelope
- Avoids the technical difficulties of trochanteric reattachment

Disadvantages
- Potential damage to the superior gluteal nerve if the gluteus medius division is extended >5 cm above the greater trochanter
- Damage to abductor musculature leading to a Trendelenburg limp post surgery
- Increased risk of heterotopic ossification
- Limited proximal acetabular exposure
- Unsuitable if a large amount of femoral lengthening is necessary
- Inability to adjust trochanteric tension
- Some concern regarding the security of reattachment of the abductor muscles

Posterior approach

The gluteus maximus is split bluntly in line with its fibres; the short external rotators are released at their insertion site and then a posterior capsulotomy is performed. The sciatic nerve should be identified and protected.

Advantages

- Avoids cutting the abductor muscles
- Avoids the complications of trochanteric osteotomy
- Relatively low incidence of heterotopic ossification
- Wide exposure of the acetabulum and femur
- Easier exposure, faster rehabilitation and diminished operating time compared to the Hardinge approach for primary THA

Disadvantages

- Increased risk of infection
- Increased risk of posterior dislocation

Anterolateral (Watson Jones) approach

Originally described for ORIF of femoral neck fractures, biopsy and arthrotomy. In this approach, the interval between gluteus medius and tensor fascia lata (both supplied by superior gluteal nerve) is exposed. Gluteus medius and minimus are retracted superiorly and laterally to expose the fat pad overlying the anterior joint capsule of the hip joint.

Advantages

- Possibly minimizes the amount of dissection between muscle groups
- Its use offers no real advantage to patient or surgeon over the Hardinge transgluteal approach

Disadvantages

- Exposure of the acetabulum depends on heavy retraction of the soft tissues and can be associated with damage to the femoral vein, artery and nerve
- Difficult exposure in obese or very muscular patients

- Access to the femur is restricted and possible only with strong lateral rotation, adduction and flexion so that orientation of the femoral component may be difficult
- Role in revision THA is extremely limited

Technical tips primary THA

Acetabular preparation

Failure to ream up to the true acetabular floor will have three negative effects:

- Lateralization of the acetabular cup (increasing joint reaction forces)
- Uncoverage of the superior acetabular cup or inappropriate abduction of the cup to achieve coverage
- Positioning of the cup in an area of suboptimal vascularity

Too small an offset will reduce the movement arm of the hip abductors and cause a limp. Too large an offset will result in an increased bending movement arm during weight bearing, which produces increased stresses within the stem that may lead to stem fracture or femoral loosening. Avoid excessive cup medialization. Decreasing the offset by more than 1 cm will weaken the abductors, increase joint reaction forces and may lead to THA instability.

Cup orientation

Generally accepted values are acetabular abduction of between 30° and 50° and acetabular anteversion of between 5° and 20°.

Femoral preparation

Femoral offset

This is the perpendicular distance between the long axis of the femur and the centre of rotation of the femoral head.

Increased offset:

- Increases the range of motion
- Decreases the incidence of impingement
- Increases stability by improving soft-tissue tension

Examination corner

Basic science oral 1

Several femoral prostheses were set out on the table:
- Discussion of uncemented femoral stems
- Methods of porous coating of the stem

Basic science oral 2

Comparison of the biomechanics of the Charnley and Exeter THA

Basic science oral 3

Discussion of metal-backed cups
- Wear
- Creep
- Osteolysis
- Fatigue failure

Adult elective orthopaedics oral 1

- History of THA
- Judet hip – manufacture and mode of failure
- Bone cement

Basic science oral 4

Cementless femoral stems: bone ingrowth, surface patterning, coatings, etc.

Adult elective orthopaedics oral 2

Examiner: What type of THA would you use?

Candidate: I would use a ***** femoral stem because:
- Good long-term, peer-reviewed follow-up results have been published (probably the most important reason for using it and should be stated first)
- I am familiar with the instruments and find them easy to use

Most of my training has been with the ***** hip.

Then go on and talk about the design features of your first-choice hip.

Complications of THA

Infection

- Overall in UK ~1%

Dislocation

- Incidence ~3%

Limb length discrepancy

Possible effects:
- Patient dissatisfaction
- Short leg limp
- Vaulting-type gait pattern
- Low back pain
- Groin pain

Nerve injuries

Incidence of sciatic and femoral nerve palsies:
- 0.7%–3.5% in primary THA
- 2.9%–7.5% in revision THA
Risk factors include:
- Revision procedures
- Female gender
- THA for DDH
- More than 4 cm lengthening of the extremity

Aseptic loosening

- Most serious long-term problem with THA

Haemorrhage and haematomas

Common sources of venous and arterial bleeding are branches of obturator and femoral vessels, medial circumflex vessels, inferior and superior gluteal vessels.

Vascular injuries

Extremely rare (0.2%–0.3%). Most vascular injuries occur during revision surgery because of distorted anatomy and scarring. The femoral vessels are primarily at risk from retraction and dissection over the front of the acetabulum. Penetration of the medial wall of the acetabulum may injure the common iliac artery or superficial iliac vein.

Urinary tract complications

- Bladder infection most common complication ~7%–14% after THA
- Urinary obstruction should be treated before THA

Trochanteric non-union and migration

- This is a concern with the Charnley approach

Heterotopic ossification

- Incidence is variable (3%–50%)
- Only 2%–7% have significant symptoms
- Candidates need to know risk factors, classification, prevention and management of HO of the hip

Gastrointestinal

- Bleeding gastric ulcer, acute cholecystitis and postoperative ileus (usually neurogenic)

Myocardial infarction and/or congestive heart failure

- Preoperative cardiac opinion is advisable if the patient has a significant history of ischaemic heart disease

Fat embolism syndrome

- In fat embolism syndrome fat particles and bone marrow are forced into the circulation at the time of femoral preparation and stem insertion

---

Examination corner

Adult elective orthopaedics oral 1

- Describe your preferred approach to the hip for THA
- Can you quote a dislocation rate for your approach?
- What prostheses would you choose for the femur and acetabulum and why?
- Can you quote survival rates from the Swedish hip register for your implant?

Adult elective orthopaedics oral 2

Examiner: What are the complications following THA?
  The candidate went through the various complications that can occur and their incidence.
Examiner: What is the overall complication rate?
Candidate: Overall 10% of patients are not happy with their THA.
Examiner: Are you going to tell your patient that?
Candidate: I would warn the patient that 1 in 10 of patients who get a THA either have a significant complication or are not entirely happy with the outcome of surgery.

Adult elective orthopaedics oral 3

Radiograph of an arthritic right hip

- Describe the radiographic features
- What are the radiographic differences between an osteoarthritic and a rheumatoid hip?
- What are the indications for THA?
- Give a detailed preoperative assessment of the patient

Adult elective orthopaedics oral 4

- Go through obtaining informed consent for a THA
- General discussion about the Swedish hip register

Adult elective orthopaedics oral 5

- How would you plan if you were to start using a different type of THA?

- Survival analysis – details, methods, Kaplan–Meier curve, etc.
- Draw survival analysis curve and describe it
- Confidence intervals

Dislocation of THA

Introduction

Early dislocation occurs within the first year after THA, and is usually due to malpositioning of components before full muscular strength is attained or to a technical error during surgery.

A dislocation is considered late if it occurs >5 years after surgery, and is usually associated with increased soft-tissue compliance, trauma, neurological decline and polyethylene wear.

Incidence

The reported incidence varies widely from <1% to >9% with 3% a generally accepted figure for primary THA. This figure increases dramatically after each revision operation and can be as high as 25% after multiple operations.

Patient-related factors[4]

- History of previous hip surgery
- Revision hip arthroplasty
- Pre-existing neurological disease
- Muscular weakness
- Patients with an acute fractured neck of femur
- AVN
- Age >70 years (relative risk 1.3)
- Female gender (relative risk 2.1)
- Inflammatory arthritis
- Alcoholism

Surgeon factors

- Experience of the surgeon. Surgeons who have performed fewer than 30 procedures have approximately double the dislocation rate of their more experienced colleagues[5]
- Poor technique

Surgical factors

- Surgical approach
- Soft-tissue tension
- Component position
- Impingement
- Head size

Hip stability

Depends on four major factors:
1. Component design
2. Component alignment
3. Soft-tissue tensioning
4. Soft-tissue functioning

Management

Management depends on the reason for dislocation. As a general rule, if the hip dislocates more than twice, recurrent dislocation is likely, and the hip should be revised to enhance stability. Remember to rule out infection and look for an obvious cause such as component malposition, retained osteophytes or cement.

Do nothing: In elderly and medically unfit patients.

Closed reduction under GA/spinal: It is important to screen the hip under image intensification to access for stability.

Revision of the arthroplasty components to improve position: Applicable if there is component malpositioning.

Removal of sources of impingement: Cement, osteophytes, etc.

---

[4] *"Several patient risk factors for dislocation after THA have been identified and these include …"* Practise the talk. The FRCS Orth is not just about reading facts in a book.

[5] Hedlundh U, Ahnfelt L, Hybbinette CH, Weckstrom J, Fredin H (1996) Surgical experience related to dislocations after total hip arthroplasty. *J Bone Joint Surg Br* **78**: 206–9.

Augmentation of the acetabulum lining – posterior lip augmentation device (PLAD): Reasonable option for a medically unfit patient with recurrent posterior dislocations of a Charnley prosthesis. Unlikely to be successful in other situations.

Confined/constrained acetabular socket design: Not a good choice for a young patient as it has a high failure rate after 5 years due to significant forces transmitted to the bone–prosthesis interface. There is a restricted range of movement and residual hip pain can be very problematic. Consider as a last chance bail-out option when other procedures have failed. Can be technically difficult surgery, and is usually successful in preventing dislocation but patients do not tolerate them very well. Complications include displaced liner coming out of a cup or a cup coming out of the acetabulum. When dislocations occur with a constrained device they are difficult to manage.

Lengthening of the femoral neck (with modular heads)/increasing head size: To improve head-to-neck ratio and/or femoral offset and to lessen the risk of impingement.

Advancement of the greater trochanter: When soft-tissue tension is inadequate.

Bipolar hip arthroplasty: May have a role in the salvage treatment of complex recurrent instability of a hip in which other stabilization procedures have failed. This procedure does however have a high rate of failure in this situation, and offers only modest improvement in function. Uses an oversized femoral head to increase stability, ROM and jump distance.

Resection arthroplasty: Usually used in the multiply revised patient with significant soft-tissue and bone deficiency. Not a good option as it leaves the patient with a shortened leg and significant limp.

Infection complicating THA

Incidence

- Approximately 1% after primary and 3%–4% after revision hip surgery

Classification

Fitzgerald

- Acute postoperative period (up to 3 months)
- Delayed deep infection (3–24 months)
- Late haematogenous >24 months

Approximately one-third of the infections fall into each group.

Coventry

I: first 30 days

Immediate postoperative period – the infected haematoma and the superficial infection that have progressed to deep infection.

II: 6–24 months

Smaller inoculum or lower virulence at the time of surgery, chronic indolent infection.

III: >2 years

Least common, usually haematogenous spread, although bacteria implanted at the time of the original surgery may have remained dormant until a change in host immunity occurs (onset of diabetes, malignancy, etc.).

The glycocalyx

The polysaccharide biofilm that permits increased adherence to and survival of bacteria on biosynthetic surfaces, thereby conferring resistance to the host's humoral and cellular defences.

Oral questions

What factors are involved in reducing the infection rate in THR surgery?

This is an absolutely classic FRCS Orth oral question. Dividing your answer into preoperative, perioperative and postoperative factors greatly simplifies things and more importantly demonstrates to the examiners a more structured approach in your answering technique.[1]

[1] Most candidates, even if they mention factors in a random haphazard manner, should obtain a pass mark for this question.

Table 16.2 Prophylactic measures for hip arthroplasty infection

MRC trial[a]	Factor
Antibiotic-loaded cement	11
Systemic antibiotics	4.8
Ultra clean air	2.6
Plastic isolators	2.2
Body exhaust suit	2.2

[a] Lidwell OM, Lowbury EJ, Whyte W, Blowers R, Stanley SJ, Lowe D (1982) Effect of ultraclean air in operating rooms on deep sepsis in the joint after total hip or knee replacement: a randomised study. *Br Med J (Clin Res Ed)* **285**(6334):10–14.

Prevention of infection in THA

Prophylactic measures to reduce hip arthroplasty infection are given in Table 16.2.

Preoperative factors

- Same-day admission
- Separation of elective from trauma cases
- All septic lesions should be examined and treated (feet, urinary, dental)
- Shave in the anaesthetic room (not night before)

Perioperative factors

- Antibiotic prophylaxis: systemic antibiotics, antibiotic-loaded cement
- Surgical technique: gentle handling of tissues, careful haemostasis, limitation of haematoma formation, avoid cremation of tissues/necrosis, length of surgery, wound lavage, etc.
- Movement: avoid unnecessary theatre personnel movement during surgery
- Face masks: BOA guidelines
- Gowns: modern, weaved patterns
- Gloves and hands: two pairs of gloves, changing the outer ones frequently
- Head gear: no hair exposed
- Body exhaust systems
- Sterile drapes: disposable non-woven drapes

- Drainage wound: arguments for and against
- Ventilation system: laminar-flow, ultra-clean-air system
- Ultraviolet light: bactericidal[6]

Postoperative factors

- Antibiotic cover for urethral catheterization
- The risk of infection is increased in rheumatoid arthritis, diabetes, those with immunosuppression and those with a history of previous joint infection

Diagnosis

Can be difficult, especially if a subclinical infection is present. The surgeon's clinical diagnostic skills and judgement are more important than any specific test.

Investigations

History

Type 1
Continuous pain, usually fevers, erythema, swollen and tender fluctuant wound; either an infected haematoma or deep spread from a superficial wound.

Type 2
Gradual reduction in function of the hip with increasing pain. Hip never "feeling right" from the time of original operation. Prolonged period of wound discharge postoperatively.

Type 3
History of sepsis. Dental extraction, chest or urine infection.

---

[6] Be sensible (and practical) with your answers: one candidate mentioned that we should perform elective joint replacement under UV light to reduce the risk of infection (this would required eye protection in addition to being a danger to the staff), which did not go down well with the examiners and spoilt an otherwise reasonable answer.

Blood tests

White blood cell count
Usually normal and not helpful unless the infection is acute.

Erythrocyte sedimentation rate
An ESR >35 mm/h 1 year after THA in the absence of any other systemic illness suggests hip infection until proven otherwise. However, the ESR may not always rise in the presence of deep sepsis.

C-reactive protein
This acute-phase reactant peaks 48 h postoperatively and returns to normal in 2–3 weeks. Based on multiple studies, >10 mg/l is significant. Sensitivity is 96%; specificity, 92%.

Radiographs

These are of limited value with respect to the infected hip. Both infected and aseptic hips can have similar appearances. However, some radiographic signs suggestive of infection include:
- Localized or irregular, scalloped pattern of endosteal bone erosion
- Rapidly progressive radiolucent lines
- Periosteal new bone formation (considered by some to be pathognomonic of deep infection)
- Evidence of early loosening
- Lacy pattern of new bone formation
- Area of bone erosion >2 mm about entire cement mass of stem or cup

Radiographic signs of loosening are seen in two-thirds of late infections, but <50% of early infections.

Radionuclide imaging

Technetium-99m scan
Very sensitive but non-specific. Increased uptake can be found in stress fractures, tumours, loosening, heterotopic bone formation and other inflammatory and metabolic disorders. A technetium scan can remain positive for up to 2 years following an uncomplicated THA. The technetium scan is most

useful if negative, as infection is unlikely, and it allows elimination of many of the component-related causes of pain at the site of a THA.

Gallium-67 citrate
Gallium-67 citrate is preferentially taken up in areas of infection and inflammation. Again this is very non-specific.

Indium-111-labelled white cell scan (leukocyte scan)
In theory in a labelled leukocyte scan indium-111 should not accumulate at sites of increased bone turnover in the absence of infection. The usefulness of this scan remains controversial. It has a limited role because of its sensitivity of 44%, its specificity of 100% and accuracy of 82%.[7]

Radiolabelled immunoglobulin G indium
Its role remains uncertain and is still under development, but it may supersede leukocyte scans in the future.

Hip aspiration, arthrogram and needle biopsy

Aspiration should not be performed routinely for all patients with pain at the site of a THA because the false-positive rate is unacceptably high. Most useful where there is clinical or radiographic evidence of infection or elevation of either the CRP or ESR. If aspiration is to be performed, all antibiotics should be stopped for at least 2–3 weeks. Transport should be rapid to allow immediate incubation and to minimize the risk of a false-negative aspiration. A spectrum of sensitivity (67%–92%) and specificity (94%–97%) is reported in the literature.[8] Follow the standard protocol. The accumulation of dye in pockets with an arthrogram may suggest abscess formation (pseudobursa).

[7] Glithero PR, Grigoris P, Herding LK *et al.* (1993) White cell scans and infected joint replacements. Failure to detect chronic infection. *J Bone Joint Surg Br* **75**(3): 371–4.
[8] Robbins GM, Masri BA, Garbuz DS, Duncan CP (2002) Evaluation of pain in patients with apparently solidly fixed total hip arthroplasty components. *J Am Acad Ortho Surg* **10**: 86–94.

*Biopsy at operation, frozen section
and Gram stain*

Intraoperative cultures are not always positive and frozen section is not available in all centres but can be a valuable diagnostic adjunct in equivocal cases.

Mirra *et al.*[9] reported on the use of intraoperative frozen sections, defining infection as being present if more than five neutrophil polymorphs per high-powered field were seen.[10]

More recent studies[11] recommend increasing the number of neutrophil polymorphs to 10 per high-powered field to improve specificity.

Management

Suppression treatment

Long-term oral antibiotic suppressant treatment alone will not eradicate deep infection but may control the sepsis and may have its place in an elderly patient medically unfit for major surgery.

Debridement and antibiotics with retention of prosthesis

This is carried out for either early postoperative infection or acute haematogenous infection if the duration of clinical signs and symptoms is less than 3 weeks, the components are stable at the time of debridement, the organism sensitivity is known and the overlying soft tissues and skin are of good quality.

Debridement involves removal of fibrous membranes, sinus tracts, and devitalized bone and soft tissue, and exchange of the polyethylene liner and femoral head. If one or both components are loose, both components, all cement and all infected and necrotic tissue should be removed (essentially a

first-stage revision). The success rate is very variable from 16% to 89% depending how strictly treatment criteria are adhered to.[12] Following debridement antibiotics are continued for 6 weeks.

First stage revision

Advantages
- Only one major operation
- Quicker return to normal function
- Avoids disuse atrophy, limb shortening and soft-tissue scarring associated with a second procedure

Disadvantages
- Demanding, prolonged procedure
- Antibiotic sensitivities must be known pre-operatively
- Uncemented prosthesis cannot be used

Contraindicated
- If antibiotic sensitivities are not known pre-operatively
- Doubt about the adequacy of debridement
- Massive bone loss requiring grafting (due to increased risk of sepsis)

Results

One-stage exchange arthroplasty has been popularized by Buchholz,[13] whose group reported a 77% success rate in 583 patients. Wroblewski[14] reported a 91% success rate.

Second stage revision

First stage consists of excision of the sinuses, the drainage of all abscesses and the meticulous removal of all foreign material: membranes, cement, plugs and any potentially infected soft tissue. The timing

---

[9] Mirra JM, Amstutz HC, Matos M, Gold R (1976) The pathology of the joint tissues and its clinical relevance in prosthesis failure. *Clin Orthop Relat Res* **117**:221–40.
[10] Polymorphs are only a significant component of the inflammatory cell infiltrate in infection.
[11] Lonner JH, Desai P, Dicesare PE, Steiner G, Zuckerman JD (1996) The reliability of analysis of intraoperative frozen sections for identifying active infection during revision hip or knee arthroplasty. *J Bone Joint Surg Am* **78**(10): 1553–8.

[12] Zimmerli W, Trampuz A, Ochsner PE (2004) Prosthetic-joint infections. *N Engl J Med* **351**: 1645–54.
[13] Buchholz HW, Elson RA, Engelbrecht E, Lodenkämper H, Röttger J, Siegel A (1981) Management of deep infection of total hip replacement. *J Bone Joint Surg Br* **63**:342–53.
[14] Wroblewski BM (1986) One-stage revision of infected cemented total hip arthroplasty. *Clin Orthop Relat Res* **211**:103–7.

of the second stage depends on the response to antibiotics, the patient's general wellbeing, wound healing and blood results (ESR/CRP).

Advantages
- Adequacy of debridement – can be repeated at the time of re-implantation
- Infected organism is known and the appropriate antibiotic given
- Persisting foci of infection can be identified
- Allows clinical assessment of treatment prior to re-implantation
- Allows uncemented reconstruction
- Augmentation with allograft may be carried out with greater confidence

Disadvantages
- Prolonged period of bed rest between the two stages
- Prolonged hospital stay
- Increased cost

Most reported protocols advise a 6-week gap between operations but this can be increased if necessary. Recently it has been suggested that shortening the interval period to 3 weeks does not increase the rate of re-infection.

A delayed exchange (two-stage procedure) is indicated for:
- Resistant organisms
- Gram-negative organisms (*Pseudomonas, E. coli*)
- Draining sinus
- Unhealthy or oedematous soft tissue
- Well established osteomyelitis with loss of bone stock

Results
McDonald *et al.*[15] studied 81 patients with 82 infected THA and reported an 87% resolution of infection at an average follow-up of 5 years. Two-stage revision is probably safer and more successful than a single-stage revision and the majority of surgeons would perform a two-stage revision. A single-stage revision

---

[15] McDonald DJ, Fitzgerald RH Jr, Ilstrup DM (1989) Two-stage reconstruction of a total hip arthroplasty because of infection. *J Bone Joint Surg Am* **71** (6): 828–34.

is possibly indicated for elderly patients who are not able to withstand multiple operations or prolonged bed rest.

Both methods in experienced hands give similar results and both methods have advantages and disadvantages.

As yet no randomized clinical trial exists to compare the two methods of treatment. The complexity of the operative procedure and the many factors involved have discouraged investigators from evaluating the timing of surgery.

Antibiotic spacer
A cement spacer, the most common being PROSTALAC (*prosthesis of antibiotic loaded acrylic cement*) can be inserted between first and second stage revisions to maintain soft-tissue balance and leg lengths. Allows local delivery of a high concentration of antibiotics. A custom-made spacer in the operating room can be used, which consists of coating a small, inexpensive sterile femoral component with antibiotic-laden cement. Allow touch or partial weight bearing only postoperatively to reduce the risk of either dislocation or periprosthetic fracture.

Salvage

If definitive treatment fails the following salvage operations may be required.

Resection arthroplasty
This is an occasionally necessary salvage procedure. It often provides marked relief of pain but results in the use of ambulatory aids, patients fatigue easily and have a Trendelenburg gait. Patients may experience hip joint pain and have a large leg length discrepancy.

Arthrodesis
This is a technically demanding procedure and is rarely performed.

Amputation
Occasionally performed on patients with a life-threatening or limb-threatening infection or

who have massive soft tissue and bone loss or vascular injury. The presence of systemic co-morbidities is strongly associated with the rate of amputation.

Antibiotics in cement

This is a controversial issue. The use of antibiotic-impregnated cement in primary THA may lead to the emergence of resistant organisms.

The prophylactic use of antibiotics with dental treatment

In 1997 a panel of experts adopted by the American Academy of Orthopaedic Surgeons (AAOS) and the American Dental Association decided that antibiotic prophylaxis was not routinely indicated for dental patients with total joint arthroplasties, but should be considered in a small number of patients undergoing procedures with a high incidence of bacteraemia.

Examination corner

Adult elective orthopaedics oral 1

Infected THA

• Investigations
• Management

Adult elective orthopaedics oral 2

Infected THA

Most of this oral seemed to be spent in discussing the investigations and various management options of the infected THA.

Adult elective orthopaedics oral 3

Examiner: How would you manage the infected THA?

A major part of this oral answer is to be able to discuss the advantages and disadvantages of one-stage versus two-stage revision hip surgery for infection:

• Conservatively on long-term antibiotic suppression: low virulence organisms, patient unfit for surgery
• Incision and drainage and wash-out: only applicable in the early postoperative stage or within 4 weeks of an acute haematogenous infection
• One-stage or two-stage procedure
• Resection arthroplasty
• Arthrodesis

Candidate: Arthrodesis is described in the textbooks but I would have reservations about suggesting it as a possible management option in the oral examination. I have never seen it carried out, in practice it is very rarely performed and it is a difficult procedure to do with the potential for major complications. More applicable in the knee (ligament, tendon and muscle loss with scarring) where, if reconstruction is performed, it is likely to have a poor outcome.

You have to be critical at times with your general orthopaedic reading and just because a particular management option is mentioned in a book it does not necessarily mean that it is an appropriate thing to refer to in the exam. Ask yourself if you have ever seen a hip fused for sepsis. Try to avoid inviting the scorn of the examiners. Worse would be to mention fusion as a second or third management option whilst omitting the more conventional methods of management.

• Amputation: for uncontrollable life-threatening sepsis

Adult elective orthopaedics oral 4

Comment on a THA radiograph
• Painful
• Why?
• Infection
• Investigations and management

Adult elective orthopaedics oral 5

Infection control in theatres including MRC trial on the effects of laminar flow, antibiotics and exhaust suits.[1]

Adult elective orthopaedics oral 6

- Prevention of sepsis following THA: pre- and intra-operative measures
- Management of wound haematoma following THA

Basic science oral 1

- General discussion about the prevention of infection in THA
- Discussion of laminar flow

Basic science oral 2

Examiner: What will you do if five infections occur in close succession after THA?

Examiner: How do you know that this is not a random occurrence and is probably due to a system failure?

Candidate: The organism; I would want to know if all the five hips were infected by the same organism.

[1] Lidwell OM, Lowbury EJ, Whyte W, Blowers R, Stanley SJ, Lowe D (1982) Effect of ultraclean air in operating rooms on deep sepsis in the joint after total hip or knee replacement: a randomised study. *Br Med J (Clin Res Ed)* **285**(6334): 10–14.

Periprosthetic femoral fractures

Cemented implants tend to fracture late (5 years or so). They occur most commonly at the stem tip or distal to the prosthesis.

In revision cases fractures tend to occur at the site of cortical defects from previous operations. Fractures also occur if the new stem does not bypass a cortical defect by >2 cortical diameters.

Uncemented implants tend to fracture within the first 6 months after implantation.

Incidence

- 1% primary THA
- 4.2 % revision THA

Table 16.3 Vancouver classification

Type	Location	Subtype
A	Trochanteric	A_G: Greater trochanter
		A_L: Lesser trochanter
B	Around or just distal to stem	B_1: Stable prosthesis
		B_2: Unstable prosthesis
		B_3: B_2 + inadequate bone stock
C	Well below the stem	

Classification

Many classification systems are descriptive and give information about the site of the fracture but are of little value in formulating a strategy for management.

1. Johansson (Types 1–3)

Type 1 fractures: Occur proximal to the tip of the prosthesis with no distal extension

Type 2 fractures: Extend from the proximal portion of the shaft to a point beyond the distal tip of the prosthesis

Type 3 fractures: Occur entirely distal to the tip of the prosthesis

2. Duncan and Masri (Vancouver)

More complex but gives a better guide to management options (Table 16.3). It takes into account the fracture site, the status of the femoral component and the quality of proximal femoral bone.

Type A_G and A_L (trochanteric)

Usually stable and minimally displaced. Displaced fractures are commonly related to osteopenia, and can usually be fixed adequately by cerclage wires supplemented by screws or plates if required.

Type B (around the stem)

B_1 prosthesis well fixed: This occurs in the region of the tip of a well-fixed stem. Spiral and long oblique fractures can be fixed by cerclage wires or cables and crimp sleeves. Supplementary fixation can be obtained by using either an onlay cortical strut graft or by cable plate. Short, oblique or transverse fractures can be slow to heal, and are treated with biplanar fixation on the anterior and lateral aspects with any combination of plates and cortical onlay grafts. Bone graft may also be used to enhance fracture healing.

B$_2$ prosthesis loose and good bone stock: The best method of treatment is to use a revision stem, which bypasses the site of the fracture, by at least 5 cm or twice the outer diameter of the diaphysis.

In most cases a long uncemented stem, which achieves good diaphyseal fixation with or without locking screws, provides the most effective contemporary method for managing these fractures. Occasionally, a cemented long stem prosthesis is used.

B$_3$ prosthesis loose and poor bone stock: A challenging fracture to manage with a high rate of complications. Best managed surgically, if the patient is medically fit, with proximal femoral replacement or so-called mega-prosthesis. In a young patient, an allograft–prosthesis composite is an attractive option.

Type C (distal to stem): Fractures well distal to a solidly fixed stem. Type C fractures are best managed with internal fixation such as a LISS or locking plate with or without femoral strut allograft, *morselized* cancellous femoral head allograft and demineralized *bone* matrix.

Complications
- Mal-union 5%–30%
- Non-union 10%–30%
- Periprosthetic re-fracture
- Infection 10%
- Reduced function in one-third
- Plate failure 15%
- Instability/dislocation 10%
- Death

Examination corner

Trauma oral 1

Radiograph of a supra-condylar fracture in an 80-year-old female distal to a THA

For management of this case, ORIF was suggested in order to avoid problems with a stress riser above the supra-condylar nail and difficulty with proximal locking so close to the fracture.

I was then shown a radiograph of a retrograde nail with substandard fixation. I was asked how I would manage this if the patient was still on the operating table – would I remove the fixation? I answered that I would not but that I would consider supplementary fixation and/or a cast brace.

Adult elective orthopaedics oral 1

AP radiograph demonstrating complete fracture of the femoral prosthesis stem of a THA

Candidate: This is an AP radiograph of the pelvis, which demonstrates Gruen mode IV failure, bending cantilever fatigue with complete stem fracture of the femoral prosthesis. This mode of failure is the most common type. It is caused by proximal loss of support of the stem while distally the stem is securely fixed.

Radiolucent zones develop proximally, medial and lateral to the stem progressing to stem failure. Other modes of failure include mode IA subsidence of the stem in the cement mantle, and IB subsidence of cement mantle and stem.

Mode II failure is medial stem pivot and mode III failure is calcar pivot.

Looking at the acetabulum there appears to be loosening in DeLee and Charnley zones 1–3, suggesting that the acetabular component is also loose.

Examiner: You need to look a little bit more closely on the acetabular side especially superiorly.

Candidate: There is a large lytic defect superiorly.

Examiner: There is obviously a large amount of bone loss superiorly and one would also have to revise the acetabular component at the time of surgery using bone graft. Tell me what you know about types of bone graft.

Short answer question

Classify periprosthetic femoral fractures following THA and discuss their management

Aseptic loosening of THA

Wear debris

The generation of particulate debris after THA occurs as a result of two processes:
- Wear
- Corrosion

The fundamental mechanisms of wear include adhesion, abrasion and fatigue. Wear debris sources include polyethylene (PE), cement and metal particles. PE-bearing surfaces are thought to be the major factor responsible for periprosthetic osteolysis and aseptic loosening in TJA.

Studies have shown there is a critical size of particle. Small particles that can be phagocytosed, 0.5–10 μm in size, are more active than large (>10 μm) or very small particles (<0.5 μm). Particles greater than 10 μm stimulate a giant cell response with the formation of multinucleated giant cells but no osteolysis. Below 0.5 μm the particle size is too small to significantly activate a response. Irregularly shaped particles are more active than spherical particles.

Modes of wear

The mechanical conditions under which the prosthesis was functioning when the wear occurred have been termed the wear modes.

Mode 1

The generation of wear debris that occurs with motion between the two bearing surfaces as intended by the designers.

Mode 2

Refers to a primary bearing surface rubbing against a secondary surface in a manner not intended by the designers. Usually this mode occurs after excessive mode-1 wear. An example would be a femoral head articulating with a metal acetabular backing following the wearing through of the PE.

Mode 3

Refers to two primary surfaces with interposed third-body particles. This is known as third-body abrasion or third-body wear.

Mode 4

Refers to two non-bearing surfaces (non-primary) rubbing together. This includes the back-sided wear of an acetabulum liner, the fretting and corrosion of modular taper connections, and fretting between a metallic substance and a fixation screw. Particles produced by mode-4 wear can migrate to the primary bearing surfaces and induce third-body wear (mode 3).

Osteolysis

Osteolysis occurs following the stimulation and differentiation of osteoclasts and inhibition of osteoblasts by cytokines that are produced primarily by macrophages in response to phagocytosis of submicron wear particles of PE.

Modes of cemented femoral stem loosening

With cemented femoral implants Gruen *et al.* described four modes of failure.[16]

Mode 1 Pistoning behaviour

1a: A radiolucent line is seen between the stem and cement at the superolateral part of the stem. The stem is displaced distally, producing the radiolucent zone and a punched-out fracture of the cement near the tip of the cement mass.

[16] Gruen TA, McNeice GM, Amstutz HC (1979) "Modes of failure" of cemented stem-type femoral components: a radiographic analysis of loosening. *Clin Orthop Relat Res* **141**:17–27.

1b: A radiolucent zone can be seen about the entire cement mass, often with a halo or thin line of reactive sclerotic bone about the radiolucent zone.

Mode II Medial stem pivot

Caused by medial migration of the proximal portion of the stem. Lateral migration of the distal tip results from inadequate superomedial and inferolateral cement support. This may produce a fracture of the cement at the midstem and a fracture of the sclerotic bone lateral to the tip of the stem.

Mode III Calcar pivot

Caused by medial and lateral toggle of the distal end of the stem. The distal stem lacks support and a bone reaction develops. Adequate proximal support produces a windscreen-wiper type of reaction at the distal stem with sclerosis and thickening of the cortex medially and laterally at the level of the tip of the stem.

Mode IV Cantilever bending

Caused by proximal loss of support of the stem while distally the stem is securely fixed. Radiolucent zones may develop proximally, medially and laterally to the stem, and may progress to stem failure.

Examination tip

During your general discussion of revision hip surgery if radiographically the cup is seen to be loose it will impress the examiners if you can mention acetabular safe zones and also fit in somewhere the method by which these are calculated.[1]

[1] One line is drawn from the anterior superior iliac spine to the centre of the acetabular socket. A second line is drawn perpendicular to line 1, also passing through the centre of the socket.

Radiographic features of femoral stem loosening

Definite loosening

- Stem failure (fracture)
- Cement mantle fracture
- Radiolucency at the cement–component interface >1 mm
- If a new radiolucent line of any size appears at the cement–prosthesis interface which was not present on initial postoperative radiographs then suspect loosening
- Changes in stem position (usually into a more varus position)
- Pistoning, medial midstem pivot, calcar pivot

Probable loosening

- Continuous radiolucent line at the bone–cement interface. Typically these lines will be surrounded by lines of increased density
- Endosteal cavitation (linear osteolysis and focal osteolysis)

Possible loosening

- Radiolucent lines at the bone–cement interface: 50%–100%

Technical problems that contribute to stem loosening

- Failure to remove adequate cancellous bone medially so that the column of cement does not rest on dense cancellous or cortical bone
- Inadequate quantity of cement
- Cement laminations and voids
- Failure to prevent cement motion while the cement is hardening
- Failure to position the component in a neutral or mildly valgus position

Radiographic features of acetabulum loosening

- Bone/cement lucency >2 mm and/or progressive
- Medial migration (and protrusion) of cement and cup (into the pelvis)
- Change in inclination of the cup (indicating component migration) greater than 5°
- Eccentric polyethylene wear of the cup
- Fracture of the cup and/or cement (rare)

Zones of loosening

Gruen zones (femur)

The femur is divided into seven zones on the anteroposterior radiograph: zone 1 is the greater trochanter whilst zone 7 is the lesser trochanter.

DeLee and Charnley zones (acetabulum)

The acetabulum is divided into three zones: superior I, middle II and inferior III.

Examination corner

Adult elective orthopaedics oral 1

The candidate was shown a radiograph demonstrating gross aseptic loosening of a THA.

Candidate: This is a difficult and challenging situation. A postoperative film would be useful for comparison, to see whether these changes are progressive or were present immediately postoperatively. A lateral radiograph would also be useful. I would be very concerned about catastrophic failure occurring in the near future and regard the case as urgent. Looking at the acetabular side there are AAOS grade 3 bone loss changes present (brief pause). The cup has rotated and is obviously loose.

The candidate briefly mentioned the "AAOS classification of bony acetabular defects" to the examiners. The candidate was baiting the examiners to see if they would rise to the challenge and ask him about this classification system. The candidate thought this gamesmanship wasn't too obvious

but some examiners are much cleverer than they appear. They simply ignored it and let the candidate continue talking. After a while the examiners began to get mildly irritated by the candidate. He was discussing sensible issues but the examiners thought he was talking too much so as to waste time and prevent them probing him. They began to ask very specific focused questions and abruptly cut him short if he failed to precisely answer the question asked.[1]

Examiner: What surgical approach would you use?

Candidate: There are many surgical approaches that one can use with revision hip surgery.

Examiner: Answer the question! What approach would you use and why?

Adult elective orthopaedics oral 2

Small 5×7 inch postoperative photograph was shown of an AP radiograph of the pelvis.

Examiner: This patient had revision surgery to his right hip performed with impaction bone grafting of the femur 3 months previously. What do you think of the radiograph?

Candidate: My mind went blank. There was nothing very obvious to say about the radiograph. I mumbled something nonsensical and almost immediately the examiner jumped in to screw me.

Examiner: Well it is quite obvious that the femoral stem has subsided and sunk into the femur. Can't you see this here on the picture? (The examiner pointed out the subsidence with their pencil.) It is quite clearly seen. It is very obvious. This is one of the worries and concerns of impaction grafting along with the increased risk of infection. Anyway you evidently have not picked this up.[2]

What type and size of bone graft would you use for impaction grafting?

Candidate: Small particles.

Examiner: The term you are looking for is "crouton size" particles.[3] Let us move on and talk about types of bone graft. Can you name the various types of bone graft that exist?

Candidate: Autograft is from the same person; allograft is from another person; xenografts, from a different species; and isograft from an identical twin. Or you can describe this in terms of tissue composition, i.e. cortical, cancellous, corticocancellous and osteochondral, etc.

Examiner: Which graft is best in terms of incorporation?

Candidate: Cancellous autograft.

Examiner: Why?

Candidate: It is best in terms of osteoconductive, osteoinduction and osteogenesis potential.

Examiner: What do you mean by these terms that you have just used?

Candidate: I went on to describe fairly well osteoconductive, osteoinduction and osteogenesis. Unfortunately the examiner wasn't really listening and remained unimpressed.

In retrospect the massive subsidence of the femoral stem should have been spotted straight away and commented on. This was a spot diagnosis, which was the pass/fail bit of the topic straight away at the beginning. I failed!

Adult elective orthopaedics oral 3

X-ray of massive subsidence after impaction grafting

Examiner: What is impaction grafting?

Examiner: What are the complications, etc.? (The examiner was getting bored at this stage.)

Know your impaction grafting: one or two of the examiners like to ask you about it and it can be a tricky topic if you are unsure of it. This was probably the same examiner and same photograph as in Adult elective orthopaedics pathology oral 2 (see above). I presume the candidate picked up on the spot diagnosis as they passed the oral.

Long case oral discussion 1

Aseptic loosening of THA

At the beginning of the long case discussion, an AP radiograph of the relevant patient will usually be shown to the candidate and he/she will be invited to pass comment.

Candidate 1: This is an AP radiograph of the pelvis. It shows a THA in situ but I am not familiar with the type of prosthesis used. Turning towards the femoral component what we can see is a straight-stem prosthesis with a modular head. The head size would appear to be large, possibly 28 mm. The tip is blunt and there is no cement plug suggesting first-generation cementing techniques. There are trochanteric wires present, which would be in keeping with a trochanteric approach.

We can see lucencies in Gruen zones 1, 2, 4 and 7. There is bony sclerosis around the tip of the prosthesis and the tip is in contact with the lateral cortex of the bone. This is suggestive of Gruen mode-2 failure of the medial stem pivot.

A lateral radiograph of the hip would be helpful at this stage.

Turning towards the acetabular component there are lucencies present in all 3 DeLee and Charnley zones. A post-operative radiograph would be helpful in deciding whether these changes were present postoperatively or are progressive. There is obvious wear of the acetabular cup as shown by superior migration of the femoral head. There are also significant acetabular bony defects present probably AAOS type III, a combination of segmental and cavitatory defects.

Candidate 2: This radiograph demonstrates gross aseptic loosening of a THA of both the acetabular and femoral components.

Comment

The diagnosis is obvious but Candidate 1 has given an altogether much more complete and comprehensive answer. Answering this type of question is rather like passing your driving test, demonstrating to the examiner that you are looking in the mirror before you pull out. Rather than the examiners "assuming" that Candidate 2 knows their stuff, Candidate 1 has put them at ease by demonstrating that they do indeed know what they are talking about.

Adult elective orthopaedics oral 4

Radiograph of broken femoral prosthesis

Candidate: This is an AP radiograph of the pelvis. It shows a broken femoral prosthesis. This is Gruen mode-4 failure, a bending cantilever failure. It is the most common form of failure. The other modes of failure are pistoning, either the stem within cement or the stem within bone, a medial stem pivot and a calcar pivot.

Examiner: What do you think is happening at the neck of the prosthesis? *(It was obvious osteolysis.)*

Candidate: Bone resorption is taking place here and this has led to cantilever failure. Bone resorption is also present superolaterally. The acetabular component is loose also. There are lucencies in DeLee and Charnley zones 1, 2 and 3.

Examiner: What do you think of this area here? *(Large lucency in acetabular bone superiorly.)*

Candidate: There is probably a segmental and possibly also a rim defect in the acetabulum caused by osteolysis. A bone graft will be needed when revising the cup.

Examiner: Yes that defect will definitely need bone grafting. Now tell me what types of bone graft do you know?

Adult elective orthopaedics oral 5

How would you investigate and manage a patient with early loosening of a THA?

Basis science oral 1

Retrieval of THA – discussion on reason for failure
Osteolysis
Why would you not have a complete cement mantle? Canal too small, prosthesis too big, malalignment, and poor surgical technique.

Basis science oral 2

Candidate was given a worn plastic acetabular cup and asked to comment.
Discussion on aseptic loosening of THA, wear particles, sources, etc. then followed.

Long case oral discussion 2

I was asked how I would assess wear of a THA at follow-up clinic. My mind went blank and I waffled on about nothing in particular. I thought the examiners were looking for a complicated answer. Keep things simple: all they were looking for was a comparison of the degree of migration of the femoral head into the acetabular component on serial radiographs. We eventually got there but I didn't do too well with it. This is basic stuff that can catch you out if you are not careful.

Basic science oral 3

Wear in THA

Name the causes of wear in different types of hip arthroplasty

[1] I believe most examiners prefer candidates to take the initiative in any discussion. It can be quite tiring (and boring) to have to drag out answers all day long from candidates. Very occasionally the reverse is true and a candidate can talk too much and irritate the examiners.

[2] This was obviously still in the good old exam days of accepted un-political correctness. The examiner would probably not get away with this behaviour now and would probably remain silent. I am not sure what is worse for a candidate: to know they are performing badly or to receive no feedback at all.
[3] The examiner is looking for a very specific term and wants this term to be mentioned and nothing else. At least they did not spend 5 minutes trying to drag it out of the candidate. This in fact can be quite a common scenario and can cause extreme distress to candidates. *"We kept talking away for 5 minutes and I still did not get the term they wanted. They should have told me and we could have moved on from this instead of wasting valuable time labouring a point."* The examiner is looking for a key word or phrase to magically unlock the door.

Design features THA

Femoral component design

Cross-section of the stem: broad medial border and preferably a broader lateral border to load the proximal cement mantle in compression.

Surface finish: matt or polished. There are higher failure rates in stems with a rough surface finish. Changing the Exeter stem from a polished to a matt finish resulted in a much higher failure rate.

Modularity (non-modular, modular): modular heads allow for adjustment in neck lengths.

Shape stem: straight (curved only in the frontal and not sagittal plane) or curved.

Tip: tapered or blunt.

Cement centralizer: provides a more uniform cement mantle.

Neck shaft angle: typically about 135°.

Longitudinal slots/grooves: improve the rotational stability of the stem within the cement mantle.

Neck length: measured from the centre of the head to the base of the collar.

Medial (head stem) offset or femoral offset: perpendicular distance between the centre of the femoral head and the long axis of the distal part of the stem. Primarily a function of stem design.

Ratio of femoral head diameter to the femoral neck diameter: if this is increased there is a greater primary arc of motion.

Head size

Head size influences range of motion, wear and dislocation.

Small head (22.25 mm)
- Low frictional torque
- Higher rate of dislocation
- Greater linear wear and creep

Large head (32 mm)
- Greater stability and range of movement but increased volumetric wear
- Less space is left for the acetabular component resulting in a thinner layer of polyethylene

The 28-mm head
The 28-mm head is a reasonable compromise as it produces the least linear wear and volumetric wear rates similar to those for the 22-mm head.

Cementless femoral component

Initial mechanical stability is achieved by one of two ways:
1. Diaphyseal press fit
2. Metaphyseal press fit

Acetabular component

Metal-backed cemented acetabular sockets have higher failure rates compared to all PE cups. Elevated posterior lip designs are thought to reduce the risk of dislocation. Flanges on the acetabular components are designed to improve pressurization of cement.

Cementless design

The initial stability of an implant is achieved by mechanical interlock with the host bone. This is then converted to long-term secondary stability by the ingrowth/ongrowth of a stable biological interface.

Attempts to improve bone ingrowth into metal implants have centred on either porous coating or coating with hydroxyapatite (HA). The optimum thickness of HA for coating is approximately 50 μm.

A pore size of 50 μm is accepted as the minimum for bony ingrowth with an ideal pore size of between 50 μm and 400 μm to enhance bone ingrowth.

1. Threaded designs
Threaded cups can be either non-porous or porous coated.

Non-porous-coated, threaded cups rely on a mechanical interlock between the acetabular bone and the implant threads for both initial stability and long-term fixation. They have fallen out of favour in recent years, as a number of studies have shown unacceptable high early revision rates.

2. Hemispheric designs
The majority of acetabular components are hemispherical and available in incremental sizes.

Initial fixation of the acetabular component is usually accomplished by either a *press-fit technique* or *line-to-line fit*. The press-fit technique involves the bone prepared being sized slightly smaller in diameter than the actual component. A line-to-line fit involves preparing bone to the same size as the implant and securing with screws.

Hybrid THA

Hybrid THA, combining a cemented stem and a cementless socket, were introduced because of concern about the long-term fixation of the cemented all-PE cups. Although progress in cementing techniques has improved the fixation of implants, this improvement has been more significant for the stem than for the socket. A survival rate for a cemented stem of >90% at 10 years follow-up is common.

Exeter prosthesis

This is a highly polished collarless, double-tapered, straight stem. The straight stem allows for controlled insertion. A highly polished tapered stem allows implant subsidence, cement creep and stress relaxation. Once the stem is loaded, "hoop stresses" are set up within the cement mantle as the stem engages. This allows the uniformity of hoop stresses, a cone-like configuration of the stem and cement mass. Within the cement mantle, the stem migrates distally in response to creep without disruption of the cement–bone interface (and may in fact protect the bone–cement interface).

Metal-on-metal hip resurfacing articulations

Introduction

The main reason for the reintroduction of the metal-on-metal bearing surface is the aseptic loosening seen with PE-particulate-induced osteolysis. Metal-on-metal particle debris is much smaller in size (0.015–0.12 μm) and induces a much less intense osteolytic reaction. Mean total wear rate is 1–6 μm per year, compared to >0–200 μm for a PE cup.

Absolute and relative contraindications to resurfacing

- Inadequate bone stock
- Femoral head too deformed, e.g. SUFE
- Acetabular morphology unsuitable, e.g. severe DDH
- Chronic renal failure
- Female of child-bearing age
- History of metal hypersensitivity
- Large femoral head cysts
- Large BMI

Complications

AVN

Femoral neck fracture (1.5%)
Most common mode of failure. Most occur in the first 6 months. Technical issues (neck notching, varus component positioning, adequate pin centring technique, incomplete seating of the femoral component, cement over-penetration with thermal necrosis, uncovered reamed bone), head perfusion issues (posterior approach, cylindrical reaming), host issues (age, female, bone quality, anatomy) and surgeon issues (experience, learning curve).

ALVAR (aseptic lymphocyte-dominated vasculitis-associated lesions)
A delayed hypersensitivity-like reaction. Histological analysis of soft tissues retrieved at revision surgery demonstrates an immunological response, which leads to periprosthetic osteolysis. Presents with progressively increasing groin pain 2–3 years following metal-on-metal hip resurfacing. Affects a small number of patients and is a low-probability event, but the BHS in 2008 recommend that the surgeon writes on the consent form that the risks have been discussed with the patient.

Pseudotumour (massive granuloma, neocapsule tissue reaction)
Catastrophic complication of metal-on-metal hip resurfacing. It has been suggested that approximately 1% of patients who have a MOM hip resurfacing will develop a pseudotumour within five years. A locally highly destructive lesion. Aetiology is unknown but is thought to be related to severe metal hypersensitivity and/or to be a wear issue due to component mal-alignment or a severe toxic reaction to an excess of particulate metal wear debris. Presents with hip pain, a lump in the groin, dislocation, and sciatic or femoral nerve palsy or destruction. Findings at surgery are of a massive granuloma with extensive soft-tissue destruction. More common in females.

Risk of neoplasm
At present the concern of long-term induction of neoplasm is unfounded but it remains an unproven worrying issue. There is no documented increased risk of neoplasm. Chromosomal abnormalities in peripheral blood are more common with metal-on-metal bearing articulations.

Metal hypersensitivity
Must be discussed preoperatively. Approximate risk is 1 per 500; it can be a very severe reaction with intense lymphocyte infiltration. Presents early; not many metal ions are needed. Must be differentiated from a wear issue due to component malposition or edge loading, which presents later with high ion levels.

Examination corner

Adult elective orthopaedics oral 1

The examiner handed me a metal-on-metal prosthesis

Examiner: What is this prosthesis?
Examiner: What are its characteristics?
Examiner: What is the advantage of metal-on-metal articulation?
Candidate: Less wear debris.
Examiner: Do you know any literature evidence?
Examiner: What are its problems and those of metal debris?
Examiner: What do the NICE guidelines say about this?

(I had looked at the BOA website on all the various guidelines.)

Adult elective orthopaedics oral 2

Metal-on-metal hip prosthesis

- The candidate was asked to describe the prosthesis
- There then followed a discussion about metal-on-metal joint articulations
- The candidate was asked to describe HA coating principles
- The candidate was asked to describe the posterior approach to the hip

Revision of total hip arthroplasty

Surgical goals in revision hip surgery

1. Removal of loose components without significant destruction of host bone and tissue
2. Reconstruction of bone defects with bone graft ±metal augmentation
3. Stable revision implants
4. Restoration of normal centre of rotation of the hip

Indications

Indications for revision hip surgery include:
- Painful aseptic loosening of one or both components
- Fracture or mechanical failure of the implant
- Recurrent dislocation or instability
- Infection

Table16.4 AAOS classification system for acetabular deficiencies in total hip arthroplasty

Type	Lesion	
Type I	Segmental deficiency Peripheral (rim) Central (medial)	Allograft/support ring
Type II	Cavitary deficiency Superior Anterior Posterior Medial (protrusio)	Morsellized bone/support ring
Type III	Combined deficiencies	Structured allograft/reconstruction plates and support rings
Type IV	Pelvic discontinuity	Reconstruction plates/metal cage
Type V	Arthrodesis	

- Periprosthetic fracture
- Progressive loss of bone
- Excessive wear of components

Contraindications

Contraindications for revision surgery would include:
- Referred pain from elsewhere
- Medically unfit patient
- Caution with painless LLD
- Rarely indicated for painless loss of motion

Acetabular reconstruction

Table 16.4 gives the AAOS classification system for acetabular deficiencies in THA.

Femoral reconstruction

Table 16.5 gives the AAOS classification of femoral abnormalities in THA.

Type I: These defects are segmental in nature, typically involving the proximal part of the femur.

Type II: These defects typically involve ballooning of the cortex to create an ectasia femur. An intact

Table16.5 AAOS classification of femoral abnormalities in total hip arthroplasty

Type	Lesion
Type I	Segmental (any loss of bone in the supporting shell of the femur)
	Proximal
	Partial
	Complete
	Intercalary
	Greater trochanter
Type II	Cavitary (loss of cancellous or endosteal cortical bone stock without penetration of the cortex)
Type III	Combined segmental and cavitary
Type IV	Mal-alignment (loss of normal femoral geometry) due to prior surgery (osteotomy), trauma
	Rotational
	Angular
Type V	Stenosis (occlusion of canal following trauma, fixation devices or bony hypertrophy)
Type VI	Femoral discontinuity (loss of femoral integrity from fracture/non-union)

proximal femoral tube with endosteal loss and cavitation.

Type III: A proximal femur, which is both ballooned and deficient in its cortical integrity.

Type IV: These defects are characterized by mal-lignment involving either rotatory or angular deformity.

Type V: These features are often the sequel to previous periprosthetic fractures.

Type VI: Characterized by periprosthetic discontinuity between the upper and lower halves of the femoral shaft.

Postoperative complications

Failure rates of revision of THR are three times that of primary surgery.
- Infection (12%–17%)
- Dislocation (5%–10%)
- Vascular injury

- Nerve palsy
- Cortical perforation
- Fracture
- Heterotopic ossification
- LLD
- DVT/PE rate similar to those for the primary operation

Conversion of hip arthrodesis to THA

Indicated if a fused hip causes severe persistent low back pain, pain in the ipsilateral knee, or the arthrosis is painful (rule out infection).

Pain in the contralateral hip is rarely an isolated problem. The contralateral joints are especially vulnerable if the hip has been fused in a poor position (flexed more than 30°, adducted more than 10°, or abducted to any extent). In this situation osteotomy should be considered first to correct the position.

One needs to try to assess the function of the abductors preoperatively. Inadequate strength of the abductor muscles results in a Trendelenburg gait, a feeling of instability of the hip, the probable need for a walking aid and the inability to stand on one leg. The patient should be informed that if the abductors are inadequate the procedure will be abandoned.

Results

The complication rate for conversion can be high. One study reported a 33% failure at 10 years with a previous history of surgical fusion because of loosening, infection or recurrent dislocation. Nerve palsy has been reported as high as 7% in some series.

Hip arthrodesis

A hip arthrodesis when performed correctly provides pain relief, enables an active lifestyle and may permit later conversion, if indicated, to a THA.

Indications

Young patient with unilateral OA hip. Especially suited in the young male with OA secondary to trauma, who is involved in heavy manual work. The long-term results of THA in this patient population are disappointing.[17]

Prerequisites

Must have a normal contralateral hip, a normal ipsilateral knee and normal spine, as a fused hip increases the stresses on these joints and the clinical results of hip fusion can be compromised.

Contraindications

Active infection, obesity, poor bone stock.

Advantages

Painless and stable joint for many years.

Disadvantages

- Immobile joint
- LLH
- Pain in adjacent joints with long-term follow-up

Techniques[18]

Arthrodesis is a technically demanding procedure to undertake. Fusion of the hip may be obtained by extra-articular, intra-articular or combined intra-articular and extra-articular methods.

AO Cobra head plate technique

This is a fixation spanning the pelvis and the proximal femur. It is stable but disrupts the hip abductors and requires a bone graft.

---

[17] The management dilemma of the young arthritic hip. A difficult problem and very common clinical hip scenario. Go through your answer as a series of management options outlining the pros and cons of each procedure.
[18] *Examiner*: What are the various techniques that can be used for hip fusion? Don't just read this book passively always keep in the back of your mind what likely question the examiners will ask you and rehearse your answer.

Transarticular sliding hip screw

The lag screw is inserted just superior to the dome of the acetabulum. Poor fixation is achieved due to a large lever arm and increased torque, therefore hip spica casting may be required postoperatively.

Anterior plating technique

An extended Smith–Peterson approach is used and although the femoral head and acetabulum can be prepared for hip arthrodesis the abductor mechanism is not violated. The fusion plate is taken across the anterior column of the pelvis superiorly into the sacroiliac joint.

Combined intra-articular and extra-articular fusion

Combination of plating and lag screw fixation.

Position

- Avoid abduction and internal rotation
- 20°–30° flexion
- Neutral – 5° external rotation
- Neutral – 5° adduction

An arthrodesis in an abducted position produces pelvic obliquity and a limp. More flexion produces a greater LLD and lumbar lordosis, whilst less flexion creates sitting difficulties.

Complications

Most patients will have complications from this surgery, which may be either major or minor:
- Malposition (most common)
- Neurovascular injury
- Femoral fracture in the first year following surgery
- Failure of internal fixation
- Non-union (pseudoarthrosis rate of 15%–25%)
- OA of the hip, knee and/or spine
- Instability of the ipsilateral knee
- LLD (common)

Informed consent

Warn the patient about the variable amounts of LLD, and the possible need for a shoe lift postoperatively.

Examination corner

Adult elective orthopaedics oral 1

The candidate was shown a radiograph of pelvis demonstrating an ankylosed right hip, possibly due to old tuberculosis.

Examiner: What is the position of the hip for fusion?

Candidate: 30° flexion, neutral to 5° external rotation and neutral or slight adduction.

Examiner: What effect does arthrodesis have on a contralateral total hip arthroplasty?

Candidate: Mechanical loosening occurs at a slightly higher rate when the opposite hip has been arthrodesed.

Heterotopic ossification following THA

Definition

Heterotopic ossification is the formation of mature bone outside the skeleton.

Incidence

The radiographic incidence of HO following primary THA has been reported to vary between 8% and 90% (21% in Brooker's original paper[19]) but only ~2% have significant symptoms.

Predisposing risk factors

- Male (2×>F)
- Hypertrophic OA
- Ankylosing spondylitis
- Diffuse idiopathic skeletal hyperostosis (DISH)

- Post-traumatic OA
- Prior hip fusion
- Paget's disease
- History of previous HO
- Intra-operative muscle ischaemia
- Direct lateral approach (direct lateral approach[20])

Pathology

The process of bone formation is essentially the same as fracture healing. Haematoma after surgery is organized, converted to osteoid and ultimately bone.

Clinical features

Usually painless but can limit hip motion. Surgical excision is rarely indicated due to the high incidence of recurrence.

Surgery may be indicated in the rare cases of:
- A severe restriction of hip range of motion
- Severe pain from impingement

Allow the process to mature (sharp cortical and trabecular markings) before operative resection. Some authors recommend waiting 12 months before operative resection.

Radiology

Calcification of soft tissues can occur as early as 2 weeks postoperatively, maturing fully by 1 year.

Classification Brooker 1–4

Brooker *et al.*[19] described four stages based on an AP radiograph of the pelvis:
- Islands of bone within the soft tissues about the hip
- Bone spurs from the proximal femur or pelvis with at least 1 cm between opposing bone surfaces
- Bone spurs with a gap of less than 1 cm
- Apparent bony ankylosis of the hip

[19] Brooker AF, Bowerman JW, Robinson RA, Riley LH Jr. (1973) Ectopic ossification following total hip replacement. Incidence and a method of classification. *J Bone Joint Surg Am* **55(8)**: 1629–32.

[20] Horwitz BR, Rockowitz NL, Goll SR *et al.* (1993) A prospective randomized comparison of two surgical approaches to total hip arthroplasty. *Clin Orthop Relat Res* **291**: 154–63.

Prevention

- External beam radiation therapy 8 Gy (800 rad) in a single dose (treatment within 3 days)
- Indomethacin 75 mg for 6 weeks

Examination corner

Adult elective orthopaedics oral 1

The candidate was shown an AP radiograph of a primary THA performed several months previously. There were severe Brooker grade 4 heterotopic ossification changes on the radiograph.

The candidate was asked about predisposing causes, Brooker classification and what symptoms the patient was likely to complain of.

Candidate: Pain is an uncommon feature of the condition. Stiffness may be present but it would need to be of a significant disability before one would consider surgery. With Brooker grade 4 changes the patient may complain of difficulty with sitting, ascending stairs, or putting on shoes and socks.

Adult elective orthopaedics oral 2

I was shown an AP pelvic radiograph with a THA in situ that had evidence of severe heterotopic ossification. I was asked about predisposing causes and the Brooker classification.

Basic science oral 1

Discussion of the management and prophylaxis of heterotopic ossification after a pelvic fracture.

Osteotomy

Introduction

Osteotomy aims to improve congruency and reduce point loading by restoring proper biomechanics. This is achieved by increasing the surface area available to transfer loads, decreasing muscle forces across the joint and re-orienting the weight-bearing surfaces of the joint to allow normal areas to articulate, moving away the diseased areas from the weight-bearing axis. Proximal femoral osteotomy, pelvic osteotomy or both can achieve these goals. Proximal femoral osteotomy should be considered when the predominant deformity is in the proximal femur. Patients with inflammatory arthritis are not suitable candidates for osteotomy. Timely intervention is required as the prognosis is adversely affected by the presence of advanced arthrosis.

Indications for proximal femoral osteotomy

- Young patient with advanced OA of the hip to avoid THA
- Post Perthes hinged abduction disease (valgus extension osteotomy)
- SUFE (flexion osteotomy)
- Avascular necrosis
- Idiopathic protrusio (valgus extension osteotomy)
- Mal-union of trochanteric fractures
- Congenital coxa vara

Indications for pelvic osteotomy

Congenital dislocation of the hip rarely involves a primary femoral deformity; hence it is usually managed with a pelvic osteotomy rather than isolated femoral osteotomy. Acetabular osteotomies in the adult patient have been classified into two groups: reconstructive and salvage osteotomies. Peri-acetabular osteotomy has recently emerged as the method of choice for young adults with significant hip dysplasia and minimal arthritic changes.

Clinical

With osteotomy motion is neither lost nor gained but its range is altered. The patient must have sufficient preoperative motion so that correction leaves a functional range of movement. Mechanical hip pain commonly occurs with weight bearing and may be associated with a subjective feeling of instability or weakness and clicking or locking. Exclude painful hip conditions other than mechanically induced pain. Chondral defects and loose bodies may also mimic the symptoms of mechanical hip pain. In the assessment of the patient's active and passive range of motion, the presence of flexion, abduction and external rotation contractures should be noted along with any LLD.

Radiographs

AP and lateral radiographs should be taken of the pelvis and the proximal femur.

On the femoral side assess for:
- Poor bone quality
- An abnormal femoral neck shaft angle
- Incongruity of the femoral head
- Unusual trochanteric anatomy
  Whilst with the acetabulum evaluate for:
- Poor bone stock
- The presence of cysts and osteophytes
- Degree of dysplasia

Functional radiographs (maximum abduction and adduction) are helpful in establishing which position of the proximal femur will improve the congruency of the hip joint and coverage of the femoral head. Other studies include a three-dimensional CT scan, CT arthrogram or MRI scan.

Contraindications

- Stiffness
- Obesity
- Inflammatory joint disease
- Presence of significant arthrosis
- Stiff hip (minimum 90° flexion, 15° abduction/adduction)

Technical considerations

The aims of surgery are:
- Elimination of impingement
- Correction of deformity
- Restoration of a pain-free range of movement
- Maintenance of the mechanical axis of the femur in both coronal and sagittal planes
- Maintenance or restoration of equal leg lengths
- Restoration of proper rotational alignment

Types of osteotomies

The major types of femoral osteotomy are:
- Flexion
- Extension
- Varus
- Valgus
- Rotational
- Combinations of the above

Varus osteotomy

A prerequisite for surgery is congruency of the joint in the re-aligned position. This is confirmed with improved femoral head coverage seen on the functional abduction-view radiographs. The patient should have a minimum of 15° abduction preoperatively. The osteotomy works by shifting the greater and lesser trochanters upwards, reducing the tension of the adbuctors and iliopsoas and therefore vertical compression forces. This improves a Trendelenburg gait pattern. A disadvantage is that this osteotomy usually shortens the leg by at least 1 cm. The most common technique is to excise a medially based wedge of predetermined size, and fixation of the osteotomy with a blade plate device. Varus osteotomy displaces the centre of hip rotation medially and should be combined with medial displacement of the femoral shaft to maintain the mechanical axis of the lower extremity passing through the centre of the knee. This avoids overloading the medial compartment of the ipsilateral knee but results in a laterally prominent proximal femur, which may cause cosmetic concerns.

Valgus osteotomy

Usually indicated as a salvage procedure in a young patient for an OA hip or post Perthes disease deformity with coxa magna, hinged abduction and a large medial osteophyte. An acceptable passive range of motion is required with a minimum flexion of 90° and adduction of 15° preoperatively. An adduction functional film should show improved congruency of the joint. Valgus osteotomy generally lengthens the limb. If lengthening is undesirable a closing wedge can be used but this may shorten the leg by as much as 2 cm.

A valgus osteotomy displaces the centre of hip rotation laterally and should be combined with lateral displacement of the femoral shaft to align the mechanical axis of the limb through the centre of the knee to avoid overloading the lateral compartment.

Flexion osteotomy

Indications include hip extension contracture, AVN with anterior involvement in the sagittal plane and posterior sparing of the femoral head. The apex of the osteotomy is located posteriorly and so a wedge of bone is removed anteriorly. The shaft of the femur is flexed and the proximal femur is extended. A posterior closing wedge may be better, and less likely to compromise future stem insertions.

Extension osteotomy

Indications for extension osteotomy include hip flexion contracture and deficient anterior acetabular coverage (seen frequently with CDH). The apex of the osteotomy is located anteriorly so that the shaft of the femur is extended and the proximal femur is flexed.

THA after previous osteotomy

A previous femoral osteotomy may render subsequent conversion to THA technically difficult because of distortion of the proximal femoral anatomy. Varus and valgus osteotomies may alter the neck shaft angle and be rotationally mal-aligned. Rotational mal-alignment can affect the estimation of anteversion of the femoral component. A custom-made femoral prosthesis or intra-operative femoral osteotomy may be necessary for success.

Pigmented villonodular synovitis of the hip

Introduction

Pigmented villonodular synovitis (PVNS) is a proliferative disease of synovial tissue, which affects the knee, hip, ankle and elbow. A slow-growing benign, locally invasive tumour of the synovium, the disease usually presents as a monoarticular haemarthrosis, and may exist in a nodular or a diffuse form. The hip is involved in 15% of cases.

Clinical features

Acute episodic attacks of hip pain and swelling. Groin pain and restriction of movement. Always consider PVNS in a younger patient with unexplained hip pain.

There are two sub-types: the diffuse and nodular forms.

Diffuse form

- The disease may be active or inactive
- Look for periarticular erosions on radiographs
- A diffuse mass may be present on examination

Nodular form

- Less common than the diffuse form of PVNS
- Does not show the same destructive changes as the diffuse form
- May cause recurrent haemarthrosis and aspirate may be of normal colour (instead of the classic brown colour)

Radiology

Radiographs show cysts on both sides of the joint that are not confined to the weight-bearing areas. MRI will demonstrate hyperplastic synovium.

Management

Ultrasound-guided biopsy is recommended for histological diagnosis. Conservative management of symptomatic PVNS of the hip in the young patient has included external beam radiation and open synovectomy, with THA reserved for aggressive end-stage disease. Arthroscopic synovectomy or open synovectomy is viewed as the management of choice for the active form of diffuse disease. Radiation may control PVNS in extensive recurrent disease.

Examination corner

Long case 1

PVNS of the right hip

Adult elective orthopaedics oral 1

- The candidate was shown an AP radiograph of the hip of a young woman with rapid deterioration in hip function
- Radiographic features included joint space narrowing and lytic defects in the bone on both sides of the joint
- What findings at surgery would you expect?

Tuberculosis of the hip

Introduction

The hip is the most commonly affected joint and accounts for 15% of all cases of osteoarticular tuberculosis. The initial lesion usually starts as an osteomyelitis in one of the bones adjacent to the joint (osseous tuberculosis). In some cases, the disease may begin in the synovium (synovial tuberculosis) but spreads quickly to involve the articular cartilage and bone (articular tuberculosis). A progressive pattern of destruction of the hip occurs in patients who are not treated. Treatment must be instituted early with the aim of salvaging the hip.

Clinical features

Insidious onset with aching in the groin and thigh and limp. Later on the pain becomes more severe and causes sleep disturbance. A child may complain of "night cries", the so-called starting pain.

All movements of the hip are grossly limited by pain and spasm. The leg is scarred and thin and shortening is often severe because many factors can contribute (adduction deformity, bone destruction, damage to the upper femoral epiphysis).

Radiology

Often non-specific. Earliest change is *diffuse osteoporosis* but with a normal joint space. There may be a *lytic lesion* involving either the head of the femur or the acetabulum. The outline of the *articular ends* of the bone becomes *irregular* because of destruction by the disease process.

Management

Chemotherapy is the main basis of management.

Skin traction in a Thomas splint

- Provides rest of the affected part
- Relieves muscle spasm
- Prevents and corrects deformity
- Maintains joint space
- Minimizes the chances of developing a wandering acetabulum

Joint arthroplasty[21]

Joint arthroplasty is not performed in the active stage and should only be considered after a safe period of absolute disease quiescence. Ankylosis of the hip/knee may occur spontaneously; it may be unnecessary to perform arthrodesis. Conversion of ankylosis or arthrodesis should be covered by anti-tuberculosis treatment for 3 months presurgery and 9 months postoperatively.

---

[21] Kim YY, Ko CU, Ahn JY, Yoon YS, Kwak BM (1988) Charnley low friction arthroplasty in tuberculosis of the hip. An eight to 13-year follow-up. *J Bone Joint Surg Br* **70**(5): 756–60.

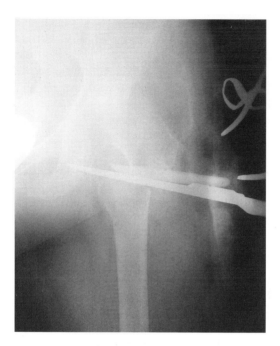

Figure 16.1 Brittain's arthrodesis of the hip

Hip arthroplasty has a 12% sepsis rate. There is a low probability of reactivation if:

- >10 years since infection
- Solid arthrodesis
- Previous medical treatment

Examination corner

Adult elective orthopaedics oral

Radiograph demonstrating a Brittain ischiofemoral arthrodesis

This is a classic and distinct spot diagnosis of the adult and pathology oral (Figure 16.1). It is an extra-articular arthrodesis hip used to treat tuberculosis infection. This concept was first popularized by Brittain of Norwich in 1941 and involved a sub-trochanteric osteotomy and medial displacement of the femoral shaft with a tibial graft bridging the femur and ischium. It is a clever concept based on the principle that compression provided by the adduction forces will induce hypertrophy of the tibial graft as opposed to iliofemoral grafts, which are under distraction. The graft was also extra-capsular, i.e. it could be performed away from the tuberculous infection. The structure that is particularly at risk when performing an ischiofemoral arthrodesis is the sciatic nerve. This is put at even more risk if there is a severe fixed flexion deformity of the hip, as this effectively drags the nerve forward into the plane of the strut graft between the femur and the ischium.

General orthopaedic and adult oral

This was actually a spot MRI diagnosis of spinal tuberculosis with a discussion of the differential diagnosis.

Examiner: What are the current recommendations for antituberculosis treatment?

Candidate: Either a triple or four-phase drug treatment. This is the initial intensive phase, which is for a period of 2 months. This is followed by a continuation phase with rifampicin and isoniazid, which is usually continued for a period of 6–9 months.

Examiner: What about long-term therapy of 12–18 months?

Candidate: Orthopaedic surgeons initially favoured long-term therapy but the short-course therapy of 6–9 months, as used successfully for pulmonary tuberculosis, has been shown to be equally successful with osteoarticular tuberculosis. It is now thought that extending chemotherapy beyond a year is required in only rare circumstances.

Examiner: What are the side-effects of treatment?

Candidate:

Rifampicin: rashes, hepatitis, orange discoloration of urine, sweat and saliva

Isoniazid: hepatitis, peripheral neuropathy

Pyrazinamide: anaemia, arthralgia, hepatitis, gout

Ethambutol: optic neuritis (red–green colour blindness)

There were much more interesting things to discuss about this topic. The characteristic MRI differences between secondary metastatic disease, infection and tuberculosis, the indications for surgery with tuberculosis spine, etc. The examiners were having none of this and more or less just concentrated on drug treatment of the disease. I must admit I did struggle a bit and the examiners would not let go of it and move on to something else.

Basic science oral

Management of tuberculosis (including drugs)

Outcome measurements

A number of questionnaires have been developed to evaluate the outcomes of interventions for OA hip. Six broad dimensions are important: pain, ability to walk, level of activity, walking capacity, patient satisfaction and clinical examination.

Types of patient-based measures outcome

Disease-specific questionnaires

Most traditional hip outcome measures (e.g. Harris, D'Aubigne, Mayo and Iowa hip scores) are disease specific. Most disease-specific outcome measures have not been validated. The WOMAC hip assessment is a newer, validated, disease-specific outcome measure. It consists of 24 items assessing three dimensions: pain, stiffness and physical function.

Patient-specific outcome measures

An example of a patient-specific outcome measure would be the MACTAR scale in which the patient is asked to list the primary reasons why he or she is undergoing THA.

Region-specific questionnaires

The Oxford hip score is a questionnaire designed to assess patients' perceptions in relation to outcomes of THA.

Functional capacity outcome

This measures functional capacity before and after a medical treatment. The 6-min walk utilizing the same course and prompts has proven useful in assessing THA patients.

Global outcome measures (generic health status questionnaires)

The SF-36 is a typical global outcome measure.

Examination corner

Basic science oral 1

Examiner: Do you know any outcome measurements that can be used to assess the success of primary THA?

Candidate: No.

Examiner: Have you heard of the SF-36 or Nottingham Health Profile or Oxford hip score?

Candidate: I have heard of the Oxford hip score.

Examiner: What type of outcome measurement is it?

Candidate: Sorry I am not sure of your question.

Examiner: Lets move on. How does heparin work?

[Fail]

17

Knee oral core topics

Deiary F. Kader and Leo Pinczewski

Knee arthroplasty

Aims of TKA

The primary aim of arthroplasty is to achieve:
- Weight-bearing line through knee centre
- Joint line perpendicular to the weight-bearing line
- Soft-tissue balance
- Restoring normal Q angle and joint alignment

Anatomic and mechanical axes

The valgus cut angle is the angle between the femoral anatomical and mechanical axes. The normal anatomical axis or tibiofemoral angle measures *5°–6° of valgus.*

The mechanical axis, or weight-bearing line, is the line from the centre of the hip to the centre of the tibiotalar joint; it typically measures *1.2° of varus.* Hence, 60% of weight goes through the medial compartment.

Femoral roll-back

Femoral roll-back is the posterior shift in the femoral–tibial contact point in the sagittal plane as the knee flexes.

Aetiology of arthritis

- Idiopathic
- Post-traumatic
- Avascular necrosis
- Inflammatory arthritis

Contraindications to TKA

- Infection
- Neurogenic genu recurvatum
- Deficient quadriceps mechanism (polio)

Constraint ladder within knee implant design

- PCL-retaining (cruciate-retaining, or CR)
- PCL-substituting (posterior-stabilized, or PS)
- Unlinked constrained condylar implant (varus-valgus constrained, or VVC) provides anteroposterior and varus-valgus stability (substitute for deficient collaterals), e.g. CCK, TC3
- Linked, constrained condylar implant (rotating-hinge knee, RHK). Rarely indicated. Used for global instability (total collateral disruption/recurvatum) and severe distal femoral bone loss, osteolysis/fracture

Posterior cruciate ligament (Leo Whiteside)

- A major stabilizing ligament in the normal and pathological knee
- It tightens the flexion space only
- It is a secondary mediolateral stabilizer in flexion
- The only mediolateral stabilizer after releasing collateral ligaments
- PCL function cannot be corrected by polyethylene post

Postgraduate Orthopaedics: The Candidate's Guide to the FRCS (Tr & Orth) Examination, Ed. Paul A. Banaszkiewicz, Deiary F. Kader, Nicola Maffulli. Published by Cambridge University Press. © Cambridge University Press 2009.

PCL retaining (CR)

Advantages (compared to PCL substituting design)
- Provides least constraint
- Lowered shear forces at the tibial component–host interface
- Preserves proprioceptive fibres (intact PCL)
- Greater stability during stair climbing (quadriceps strength)
- Fewer patellar complications
- Preserves bone stock on the femoral side
- Better kinematics but relatively less predictable
- Avoids the tibial post–cam impingement
- Ease of management of supracondylar fracture (plate/nail)

Disadvantages
- Less conforming surfaces to allow roll-back
- Slide increases contact stresses and polyethylene delamination
- Technically difficult to balance

PCL substitution (sacrificing)

Indications

- Previous patellectomy
- Rheumatoid arthritis
- Stiff knee in post-traumatic arthritis
- Previous high tibial osteotomy (HTO)
- Large deformity, over-released PCL

Advantages

- Conforming surfaces allowing roll-back
- No component slide
- Provides a degree of VVC
- The cam-post mechanism improves anterior-posterior stability
- Uses more congruent joint surfaces than CR, which reduces wear
- Facilitates any deformity correction
- Better range of motion
- Technically easier than CR and reproducible
- Higher degree of flexion

Disadvantages
- Increased constraint associated with high stresses at fixation interface leading to increased loosening
- Femoral bone loss
- Tibial peg increases wear
- Post dislocation
- Three times greater joint line alteration compared to CR
- Patella clunk syndrome

Mobile bearing tibial components

Advantages

- Maximum conformity without an increase in component loosening
- Increased contact area in both sagittal and coronal planes
- Minimal constraint
- Reduced component sliding during flexion
- Reduced shear stresses on the polyethylene insert
- Allows self-correction of tibial component in rotational malalignment
- Facilitates patella tracking
- Better kinematics in gait
- Low polyethylene wear

Disadvantages

- Bearing dislocation and spin-out if the soft tissues are imbalanced
- Underside bearing wear creating small debris, hence more osteolysis
- Technically difficult, less forgiving soft-tissue imbalance

Skin incision

- Anterior longitudinal midline skin incision
- Skin blood supply is in the subcutaneous fat so avoid undermining
- Medial vessels are relatively large so in cases where there are multiple scars use the most lateral

Table 17.1 Balancing the flexion and extension gaps

	Flexion gap loose	Flexion gap OK	Flexion gap tight
Extension gap loose	Thicker plastic	Augment femur/downsize femur	Convert to PS design of knee/downsize femur
Extension gap OK	Resect more distal femur Oversize femoral component	Perfect	Downsize femur/increase tibial slope
Extension gap tight	Resect distal femur Thicker plastic insert Release capsule posteriorly	Resect distal femur/release posterior capsule	Thinner plastic insert/cut more tibia

Deep dissection

- Medial parapatellar in most cases
- Subvastus, midvastus
- Lateral parapatellar (very valgus knee, laterally subluxed patella)
- Tibial tubercle osteotomy (Whiteside)
- Rectus snip
- Quadriceps turn-down

Soft-tissue balancing

- Collateral ligaments are no longer isometric but act as a sleeve
- Sleeve release affects both flexion and extension gaps
- Medially, posteromedial release affects extension only
- Laterally, iliotibial tract and posterolateral release affect extension only
- In FFD release the tight posterior corner first

Equal flexion/extension gap (Table 17.1)

- If the flexion and extension gap is symmetrical, adjust tibia
- If the gap is asymmetrical, adjust the femur (majority of cases)
- Downsize the femur, cut more off the posterior femoral condyle
- Resect the distal femur to increase the extension gap
- Increasing the tibial slope increases the flexion gap
- PCL excision increases the flexion gap by roughly 5 mm

Tibia cut

- Posterior slope 3°–5° generally, but depends on knee design
- PS knee performs better with no slope
- CR knee needs 5° slope

Distal femoral cut

- Valgus angle 5°–7° from anatomical axis
- Perpendicular to mechanical axis
- Intramedullary alignment jig
- Cut less femur in CR knee
- Cut 2 mm more femur in PS knee

To make flexion gap rectangular

- External rotation femoral cutting block 3° or parallel to femoral epicondyles
- Flexion/extension gaps should be rectangular and equal
- Never internally rotate the tibial component

Malalignment

- Coronal malalignment (varus valgus) causes a 24% failure rate at up to 8 years (Jeffrey *et al.*[1])
- The optimum AP position of the femoral component is in line with the anterior cortex of the femur
- A forward femoral implant leads to overstuffing of the patella and instability in flexion

[1] Jeffery RS, Morris RW, Denham RA (1991) Coronal alignment after total knee replacement. *J Bone Joint Surg Br* **73B**: 709–14.

- A medialized femoral component leads to patella maltracking
- A >10° posterior tibial slope leads to premature failure
- Tibial medial overhang causes impingement and pain (minor lateral overhang is acceptable)
- A slight posterior overhang is acceptable
- A posterolateral overhang may cause popliteus muscle impingement

Coronal plane ligament balancing

Medial release for varus knee

- Osteophytes excision
- Deep MCL to posteromedial corner
- Semimembranosus aponeurosis
- Superficial MCL
- Pes anserinus insertion
- PCL

Mostly 1 and 2 but if still tight proceed to 3–6. Check stability at each stage.

Lateral release for valgus knee

See "Valgus knee" below.

Fixed flexion deformity

- Less than 10° can be corrected by cutting bone
- May need to resect more bone from the femur
- Remove posterior osteophytes
- Severe FFD needs posterior capsular cutting (with great care) with the knee in extension and the capsule under tension (lamina spreader)
- For very severe FFD, use a Cobb to lift posterior capsule of femur

Patellofemoral maltracking

A potential major problem after TKA. To prevent maltracking:
- Externally rotate the femoral component
- Lateralize the femoral component
- Avoid anterior placement or oversizing of the femoral component

- Avoid internal rotation of the tibial component (increases the Q angle)
- Avoid an excessive valgus angle
- Avoid raising the joint line
- Medialize the patella button
- Avoid inferior placement of the patella component

The following cause increased anterior displacement of the patella:
- Oversized femoral component
- Overstuffing the patella

Patella resurfacing debate[2, 3, 4]

For:
- Reduces anterior knee pain
- Improves knee strength in flexion (stair descent)
- Less likely to revise the knee for anterior knee pain

Against:
- No difference in outcome
- Increases wear particles
- Long-term problems with patellar fracture

Historically extensor mechanism problems occurred in up to 10% of patients and accounted for up to 50% of the long-term problems of TKA:
- Patella avulsion
- Patella fracture and AVN
- Patellofemoral instability
- Component loosening

Indications for selective patella replacement:
- Advanced osteoarthritic patella
- Rheumatoid arthritis
- Preoperative patellofemoral pain
- Obese patients
- Overweight females
- Chondrocalcinosis

---

[2] Wood DJ, Smith AJ, Collopy D, White B, Brankov B, Bulsara MK (2002) Patellar resurfacing in total knee arthroplasty. A prospective, randomized trial. *J Bone Joint Surg Am* **84**: 187–93.

[3] Barrack RL, Betot AJ, Wolfe MW, Waldman, DA, Milicic M, Myers LJ (2001) Patella resurfacing in total knee arthroplasty. *Bone Joint Surg Am* **84**: 1376–81.

[4] Keblish PA, Varma AK, Greenwald AS (1994) Patellar resurfacing or retention in total knee arthroplasty. *J Bone Joint Surg Br* **76 B**: 930–7.

Patella baja

- Shortened patella tendon, which is hard to evert
- Knee flexion is limited by patella impingement on the tibia
- Seen most often following prior HTO, fracture of the proximal tibia, or tibial tubercle osteotomy
- Avoid cuts that raise the joint line
- Increases the difficulty of TKR

Managing patella baja

- Use a small patella dome superiorly
- Trim anterior tibial and patella polyethylene at the impingement points
- Lowering the joint line by cutting more off the proximal tibia and using distal femoral augmentation (rarely necessary)

Raising the joint line affects:

- PCL function
- Collateral ligaments tension
- Patellofemoral joint mechanics

Valgus knee

- Normal tibiofemoral angle is 5°–6°
- Normal knee mechanical axis is 1.2° varus
- Valgus knee can be defined as a tibiofemoral angle greater than 10°
- Is associated with bony and soft-tissue abnormality
- Acquired or pre-existing bony deficiencies
- Lateral subluxation of the patella
- Lateral capsule and ligament contracture
- Elongated PCL may become dysfunctional in severe valgus
- Distal femoral rotational deformity with externally rotated epicondylar axis up to 10°

Aetiology

- Primary arthritis mainly
- Inflammatory arthritis and osteonecrosis (small proportion)
- Post-traumatic arthritis (loss of lateral meniscus)
- Over-correction after HTO
- Childhood metabolic disorder (rickets)

Alignment

- No greater than 5° femoral cut
- Component rotation is best achieved using the AP axis (Whiteside)
- Do not use additional 3° of external rotation, as the distal femur is externally rotated already
- Be careful not to internally rotate the femoral component by posterior referencing off a deficient lateral condyle

Approach and soft-tissue release

- Medial parapatella gives good access to the whole knee and better soft-tissue cover (preferred approach)
- Lateral parapatella is a direct approach. Theoretically it preserves the neurovascular supply to the extensor mechanism and enhances postoperative rehabilitation
- Make pre- and intra-operative assessments of the deformity. If the deformity is passively correctable and the flexion–extension gaps are equal then a lateral release is unnecessary
- There is no consensus regarding the sequence of soft-tissue release

Soft-tissue release in valgus knee

- Osteophytes excision
- Lateral patellofemoral ligament release
- Sacrifice PCL in moderate–severe valgus

Flexion and extension tightness

- Release lateral collateral ligament (LCL) from the femur

Extension tightness

1. Release iliotibial band from Gerdy's tubercle
2. Release popliteus

Flexion tightness

- Release posterolateral capsule off the tibia
- Cut PCL
- If it remains tight, you rarely need to proceed to:

- Biceps femoris tendon – Z lengthening
- Detachment of lateral head of gastrocnemius

Complications

- Same as for varus knee
- There is a high risk of peroneal nerve stretching after severe valgus correction
- It is best to use a loose bandage postoperatively and to keep the knee in slight flexion

Unicompartmental knee arthroplasty (UKA)

It is important to understand that UKA is not "half a total knee" (Cartier *et al.*[5]). It is a ligament-balancing procedure more than a realignment procedure and cannot correct an extra-articular deformity.

Advantages

- Avoids patellofemoral overload
- Retains knee kinematics
- Restores function and range of movement
- Rapid recovery: 3 times faster than after TKA
- Less blood loss and hence transfusion
- Cheaper than TKA
- Quicker operation than TKA
- Quicker return to work than after TKA
- Lower infection rate (halved) compared with TKA
- Allows minimally invasive approach
- Easier to revise than HTO
- No patella fractures or dislocations
- Maximizes the longevity of total knee arthroplasty
- Reduced mortality from pulmonary embolism
- High flexion lifestyle

Prerequisites

- Intact ligaments (especially ACL and PCL)
- Correctable varus deformity

---

[5] Cartier P, Sanouiller JL, Khefacha A (2005) Long-term results with the first patellofemoral prosthesis. *Clin Orthop Relat Res* **436**: 47–54.

- Less than 10° FFD
- Flexion beyond 100°
- Preservation of the articular cartilage lateral compartment, as demonstrated on a valgus stress radiograph
- Clinically asymptomatic patellofemoral joint and contralateral compartment

Contraindications

- Inflammatory arthritis
- Sepsis
- Young age
- High level of activity

Relative contraindications

- ACL degeneration
- Chondrocalcinosis
- Lateral meniscectomy
- Osteonecrosis
- Combined obesity and small bone size in some females

Principles

- Appropriate for 25% of osteoarthritic knees needing replacement
- Never release the MCL
- Dislocation rate is 1/200 after medial compartment UKA (Oxford unicompartmental knee)
- Dislocation rate is 10% after lateral compartment UKA (Oxford unicompartmental knee)
- Dislocation rate can be reduced by using a fixed bearing for lateral UKA
- Intact ACL preserves articular cartilage at the posterior aspect of the tibia, which keeps the MCL stretched on roll-back at flexion

Management options for medial compartment OA

- HTO suitable for high-demand, young patients
- UKA (better functional results, much better 10-year survival – 98% versus 66%)
- TKA

Patellofemoral disorders

Patellofemoral joint (PFJ) dysfunction

PFJ dysfunction is loss of tissue homeostasis in the various innervated patellar and parapatellar tissues.

Anatomy and biomechanics

Patellar articular cartilage is the thickest in the body. It has two main facets separated by a ridge. The medial facet is convex and the lateral facet is concave. The femoral trochlea has a higher and longer lateral facet compared with the medial side. The patella increases the efficiency of the extensor mechanism by 1.5 times and the muscles around the knee are capable of absorbing more than three times the energy generated. Fifty percent of the quadriceps tendon inserts into the upper pole of the patella and the rest blends into its anterior surface.

Joint reaction forces

- 0.5 times body weight with level walking
- 3–4 times body weight when using the stairs
- 7–8 times body weight with squatting
- 20 times body weight with jumping

Common causes of PFJ dysfunction

- Overloaded subchondral bone due to articular lesions
- Patellar or quadriceps tendinopathy
- Retinacular pain from overload/neuroma
- Peripatellar pain related to instability analogous to multidirectional instability of the shoulder
- Synovitis or fat pad pain
- Referred pain from the hip/back

Examination

- Standing: valgus/varus alignment, gait, leg length inequality, Q angle
- Sitting: VMO/quads atrophy, lateral patella tilt, patella tracking, J sign
- Supine: patellar glide test, patellar tilt test, Clarke's test, apprehension test, compression test and trochlea depth

A patella deviates laterally in terminal extension (J sign), suggests significant malalignment that may benefit from a distal realignment. Patella tilt associated with lateral patella compression, if severe, can be treated with lateral retinacular release.

Patella instability

- Patellofemoral subluxation or dislocation

Risk factors

1. Bony factors (static)
   - Shallow trochlea groove
   - Hypoplastic femoral condyle
   - Patella shape
   - Patella alta
2. Malalignment
   - Patella malalignment is an abnormal rotational or translational deviation of the patella along any axis
   - External tibial torsion
   - Increased femoral anteversion
   - Increased genu varum
   - Increased Q angle
3. Soft tissue (dynamic)
   - Ligamentous laxity (medial patello-femoral ligament rupture)

Investigations

- A lateral radiograph is the most helpful view for assessment of patella tilt and trochlear depth
- Axial radiographs (Merchant's view) to assess patella tilt angle (normal <10°), congruence, sulcus angle (normal 138°) and trochlea dysplasia
- MRI for articular lesion
- CT scan to assess:
  - Rotational malalignment of femur and tibia (normal femoral anteversion is 5°–15°)
  - TT–TG distance (tibial tuberosity–trochlea groove (distance) more than 20 mm is significant
  - Knee rotation (normal value is 3°)

- Patella tilt more than 20° is pathologic
- Lateral trochlea tilt (less than 14° is pathologic) (David Dejour and Xavier Meyer CT protocol, personal communication)
- A bone scan measures bony activity and homeostasis within the knee and can sometimes be useful

Management

Conservative

Indicated for first-time dislocation. Possible aspiration, immobilize in extension for 3–4 weeks. In cases of recurrent dislocation, supervised rehabilitation for 6 months is recommended.

Proximal re-alignment procedure

- Lateral release (open/arthroscopic) rarely performed nowadays
- Best results when there is pain and lateral retinacular tightness. Medial imbrication (open/arthroscopic)
- For mild–moderate mal-tracking

Combined proximal and distal re-alignment procedures

Indicated for tubercle malalignment and traumatic incompetency of the medial restraints.

Distal re-alignment procedures

Direction of tibial tubercle (TT) transfer:
- Medial: for malalignment
- Anteromedial: for malalignment and arthrosis
- Anterior: for arthrosis

Elmslie Trillat: Medialization without posteriorization of TT

Fulkerson: Medialization with anteriorization of the TT in arthritic patella. To maximize anteriorization and minimize medialization in patients with arthrosis that is greater than malalignment, the obliquity of the cut should be a maximum of approximately 60°. However, when there is more problem with malalignment than with arthrosis the cut can be less oblique

Hauser: Transfer of the TT to medial, distal and posterior position. This has been abandoned. It increases the PFJ reaction force and causes patellofemoral degenerative joint disease

Goldthwait 1899 – Roux 1888: Medial transposition of the medial half of the patella tendon, lateral release/medial reefing. Now the lateral half is placed under the medial half and medially (historic procedure)

Maquet: Anterior transportation of TT, which decreases patellofemoral (PF) contact forces. Not performed nowadays (historical) as it has a high incidence of skin necrosis, compartment syndrome and no effect on the Q angle

Summary

Identify the cause of instability and take the following actions accordingly:
- Manage tight lateral structure with lateral release
- Manage Q angle >20° or TT–TG >20 mm by medialization of TT (Elmslie Trillat)
- Manage patella alta Caton/Deschamp or Insall/Salvati ratios >1.2 by distalization
- Manage patella OA with elevation of TT (Fulkerson)
- Manage immature knee using soft tissue re-alignment procedures
- Manage patella tilt and subluxation (CT scan proven) of more than 20⁰ by medial patellofemoral ligament reconstruction.
- Manage trochlea dysplasia (true lateral X-ray and CT scan proven) by trochleoplasty

PF arthroplasty

Effective in isolated PF arthritis, post-traumatic arthrosis and severe chondrosis after an extended period of supervised and non-operative measures.

Contraindications

- Inflammatory arthritis
- Chondrocalcinosis of menisci or tibiofemoral surface

- Patients with inappropriate expectation
- Considerable patella maltracking or malalignment
- Patella tendinitis, synovitis and patella instability

Outcome
- 90%–95% good and excellent results in isolated PF arthrosis at midterm follow-up
- Obesity and ACL deficiency do not seem to increase failure rate
- It is an excellent alternative to patellectomy and TKR in patients younger than 55

Patellectomy

Salvage, last-resort surgery – may not eliminate pain. Reduces extension power by 30%–50%. Tibiofemoral joint reaction force may increase by 250% causing OA. Satisfactory results in 77% (Blatter *et al.*[6])

Lateral patella compression syndrome

- Pain due to tight lateral retinaculum. Normal mobility. Normal Q angle and alignment
- Imaging : abnormal patella tilt without subluxation

Patellofemoral arthritis without malalignment

Difficult problem to treat in young patients. The treatment should be individualized.

Management

Non-surgical
- Patient education, physiotherapy, activity modification
- Optimize body weight

Surgical
- Arthroscopic debridement (careful), lateral release (tilt and arthritis), Fulkerson tibial tubercle elevation (focal distal lesion), patella resurfacing, TKR (older patients) and patellectomy (rarely)

[6] Blatter G, Jackson RW, Bayne O, Magerl F (1987) Patellectomy as a salvage operation. *Orthopade* **16**(4): 310–16.

ACL injury

Anatomy

- Intra-articular ligament. May heal to PCL after rupture
- Inserts just anterior to and between tibial intercondylar eminences
- Attaches to posteromedial aspect of lateral femoral condyle
- 33 mm long, 11 mm in diameter
- Two bundles anteromedial bundle – tighten in flexion
- Posterolateral bundle – tighten in extension
- Supplied by middle geniculate artery
- 90% type I and 10% type III collagen
- Isometric – constant length with flexion
- Prevents anterior translation and internal rotation of the tibia

Clinical features

- Mechanism of injury – low velocity, deceleration and pivotal injury, usually non-contact
- Valgus external rotation or hyperextension force in contact injury
- High-energy RTA
- Audible or feeling of "popping"
- Acute haemarthrosis in young within 1–2 h, less dramatic in older patient
- Inability to continue playing sport
- Females more susceptible
- 20% of ACL injury associated with MCL injury
- 80% incidence of lateral meniscal injury with combined ACL–MCL
- In chronic ACL deficiency medial meniscal injury is more common

Examination

Lachman

- Check PCL sag and medial tibial step-off before the test
- Maintain the knee in neutral rotation during the test

Pivot shift – non-functioning ACL

Place a valgus stress, axial load and internal rotation on the tibia as the knee is slowly flexed. In full extension, gravity pulls the femur posteriorly resulting in anterior subluxation of the tibia. With further flexion, posterior pull by the iliotibial tract reduces the tibia at about 20°–30° (shift).

Partial tear and lax MCL lead to positive Lachman and negative pivot.

Complete tear leads to positive Lachman and pivot. The knee cannot be pivoted if there is complete disruption of the iliotibial tract or MCL.

Differential diagnosis of acute haemarthrosis

- ACL rupture
- Intra-articular fracture
- Patella dislocation
- Capsular tear
- Peripheral meniscal tears

McDaniel and Dameron[7, 8] – rule of thirds

Patients with ACL-deficient knee
- One-third is able to compensate, and can pursue normal recreational sports
- One-third is able to compensate but will have to reduce their sporting activities
- One-third does poorly and develops instability with simple activities of daily living

However, in reality:
- Few are able to compensate and pursue normal recreational sports
- Most are able to pursue sporting activities within "envelope of stability"
- Some do poorly and develop instability with simple activities of daily living

[7] McDaniel WJ, Dameron TB (1980) Untreated ruptures of the anterior cruciate ligament. A follow up study. *J Bone Joint Surg Am* **62**: 696–705.
[8] McDaniel WJ, Dameron TB (1983) The untreated anterior cruciate rupture. *Clin Orthop Relat Res* **172**: 158–63.

Management

Management should be individualized based on age, activity level, laxity, instability, associated injuries, and other factors.

Conservative

- Almost always requires restriction of activity level
- Associated with high incidence of instability in younger patients
- Potentially may lead to meniscal tear, articular injury and subsequent degenerative changes
- Fallen out of favour as advances in surgical technique and physical therapy have reduced operative morbidity and improved outcome

Surgical

1. Primary repair of bony avulsion lesion
   - In young patients, manage with bent K-wires or fiberwire
2. Primary repair ± augmentation
   - Definitely out of favour
3. Extra-articular reconstruction (MacIntosh, Ellison)
   - Involves tenodesis of the iliotibial tract
   - Pass a mobilized strip of iliotibial band to the posterolateral corner of the knee through a tunnel deep to LCL
   - Reduces or eliminates pivot shift but there is concern regarding its effectiveness in addressing anterior translation
4. Intra-articular reconstruction
5. Arthroscopic/open ACL reconstruction
6. Graft types
   - **Autografts**: PTB (bone patella tendon-bone), hamstring, quadriceps
   - **Allograft**: PTB, Achilles tendon, hamstring, tibialis anterior
   - **Synthetic**: Gore-Tex®, Dacron® or polyester
   - **Xenograft**
7. Graft fixation
   - Interference screw (metal or bioabsorbable)
   - EndoButton®

- Cross-pin
- WasherLoc™ (tibia)
- None (Press-fit)

8. Bone patella tendon bone (PTB) autograft
   - Advantages:
     - Easy to harvest
     - Bone-to-bone healing
     - Direct rigid fixation
     - Faster biological integration in 6 weeks
   - Disadvantages:
     - Donor site morbidity from graft harvest
     - Anterior knee pain 30%–50%
     - Patellar tendonitis 3%–5%
     - Fracture patella, rare
     - Patella baja (shortening of patella tendon)
     - Development of late OA
9. PTB allograft
   - Slower incorporation
   - Less stability in 6 months
   - Risk of disease transmission
   - Role in revision surgery
   - Weaker after having been irradiated and not biologically active
10. Hamstring graft
    - Advantages:
      - Small incision
      - Large cross-sectional area of tendon
      - Relatively easy passage graft
      - Less donor site morbidity
    - Disadvantages:
      - Slow tendon-to-bone healing in the tunnel in 8–12 weeks
      - No bone graft in the tunnels
      - Hamstring weakness after operation
      - Possibility of injury to saphenous nerve (poor technique)
11. Synthetic grafts (Gore-Tex®/Dacron®)
    - High failure rate
    - Expensive
    - Osteolysis
    - Risk of infection
    - Atraumatic effusions
    - No disease transmission
    - No harvest site morbidity
12. Quadriceps graft

Thick tendon but short, with good biomechanical properties. The graft is associated with decreased anterior knee pain. However, graft harvest weakens the quadriceps and can be technically difficult. In most centres, it is used for revision.

Principles of ACL reconstruction

- Graft: biologically active graft
- Tunnels: anatomically and isometrically placed tunnels
- Fixation: the graft should be adequately tensioned and fixed in extension
- Rehabilitation should respect fixation choice

Surgical technique

- Graft placed in the footprint of the posterolateral bundle of ACL
- Keep posterior to the "Resident's ridge"
- Notchplasty is unnecessary if the graft is correctly placed. Remove osteophytes
- Tensioned in extension

Complications

- Anterior placement of the femoral tunnel limits flexion
- Anterior placement of the tibial tunnel limits extension
- Graft rupture from impingement
- Flexion contracture and arthrofibrosis
- Failure of fixation
- Cyclops lesion from residual tissue anterior to the ACL block extension
- Infection
- DVT and PE
- Osteoarthritis

KT 1000

- An instrument used to measure anterior knee translation objectively. Anterior displacement at 30 lb (133 Newtons) and manual maximum are recorded and compared to the unaffected knee
- Side-to-side difference of more than 5 mm is significant

Examination corner

Adult orthopaedics and pathology oral

Shown lateral radiograph of knee with interference screws
- Comment on tunnel positioning
- What are the indications and principles of ACL reconstruction?
- Methods of fixation of the graft and advantages and disadvantages of each
- Types of graft

PCL injury

Anatomy

- The strongest ligament in the knee
- It is regarded as "a central stabilizer"
- Originates from a broad crescent-shaped area in the posterolateral medial femoral condyle
- Inserts centrally posteriorly 1–1.5 cm below articular surface of the tibia
- Has an average length of 38 mm and diameter of 13 mm
- Vertical
- PCL and quadriceps are dynamic partners in stabilizing the knee in the sagittal plane

Three components:

- Antero-lateral: long and thick part, twice the size of the posteromedial bundle; tightens in flexion
- Posteromedial: tight in extension
- Meniscofemoral ligaments: mechanically very strong
  - Anterior: Humphrey's ligament
  - Posterior: Wrisberg's ligament

Mechanism of injury

- 3% of all knee injuries
- Direct injury against the dashboard when the knee is flexed 90° is the most common
- Falling on a flexed knee with foot in plantar flexion
- Forced hyperextension (>30°) is associated with multi-ligament injury

Examination

- Tibial step-off sign (medial tibial plateau is anterior to the femoral condyle at 90° flexion in a normal knee)
- Posterior drawer test at 90° and 30°
- Quadriceps active drawer test at 30°–60°. Tibia reduces when the foot is controlled
- Posterior sag sign (step-off)
- Posterolateral rotatory instability (Dial test prone)
- External rotation recurvatum test

Grading of PCL instability

- Normal tibia step-off is 10 mm at 90° flexion
- Instability could be mild, moderate or severe
- Grade I instability is when there is a 5-mm step-off
- Grade II instability is when there is no step-off (flush)
- Grade III instability is when there is –5-mm step-off

Management

In isolation, it often causes minimal long-term instability. However, it may lead to medial or PFJ pain at a later date. More troublesome in soccer players due to difficulty in deceleration.

Most surgeons treat an acute, isolated PCL injury conservatively (quadriceps rehabilitation). Knee is kept in extension until the pain subsides then early motion is reintroduced.

Outcome is poor after meniscectomy, with patella chondrosis, gross laxity and weak quadriceps. If associated with posterolateral or posteromedial injuries, knee stability is dramatically reduced.

Surgical reconstruction

PCL open/arthroscopic reconstruction is recommended for acute combined injuries, acute bony avulsion and symptomatic chronic PCL injuries that failed rehabilitation. Arthroscopic reconstruction is technically demanding. Most surgeons are unfamiliar with the procedure. Any of the grafts can be used in ACL reconstruction.

Complications

Immediate

- Neurovascular injury → popliteal vessels
- Infection
- Technical error → imprecise tunnel placement, graft tensioning, insecure fixation

Delayed

- Loss of motion
- Avascular necrosis (medial femoral condyle)
- Recurrent or persistent laxity (common) when a combined injury is not adequately addressed

Knee dislocation

ACL, PCL, MCL, LCL and posterolateral corner are the main stabilizers of the knee. Any triple-ligament knee injury constitutes a frank dislocation. This is relatively rare but a severe and potentially limb-threatening injury.

There is a 50% incidence of vascular compromise and a 20%–30% incidence of nerve injury. The incidence of any fracture may be as high as 60%. It usually happens as a result of a high-energy injury such as an RTA. It may occur following lesser injuries such as a sporting accident. May be missed on initial assessment.

Classification

Classified on the basis of the direction of tibial displacement (displacement of the tibia with respect to the femur):

- Anterior and posterior (most common), also medial, lateral and rotatory or combined
- Closed or open
- High or low energy

- Dislocation or subluxation
- Neurovascular involvement

Mechanism of injury

Hyperextension leads to anterior dislocation. Dashboard injury leads to posterior dislocation.

Examination

Must examine carefully looking for:
- Valgus and varus laxity
- Anteroposterior translation
- Recurvatum
- >10° hyperextension suggests ACL injury
- >30° hyperextension indicates PCL injury
- Rotation indicates MCL and LCL injury

Management

- Surgical emergency
- Deal with life-threatening injuries first
- Assess circulation using Doppler in A&E
- Radiography before manipulation (assess direction and associated fracture)
- Reduction as soon as possible in the Emergency Room
- Check for the dimple sign medially, indicating posterolateral dislocation and medial condyle buttonholing which preclude close manipulation
- Immobilization in an extension knee splint
- Check radiograph to confirm congruity
- Involve the vascular surgeon with a view to arteriography
- Conservative management is going out of favour as it leads to gross instability
- Timing of intervention is critical
- During the first week there is a likelihood of late vascular compromise
- Surgical dissection after 3 weeks becomes very difficult
- Ligament surgery is best performed as soon as the vascular surgeon allows
- Early motion is allowed to prevent arthrofibrosis if the integrity of the ligament and vascular reconstruction permit

- Most ACL/PCL/MCL can be treated with a brace for MCL followed by combined ACL/PCL reconstruction once range of movement is restarted, usually after 3 months
- Alternatively, repair the capsule and repair or augment the collateral ligament early and reconstruct the ACL later after 10–12 weeks
- ACL/PCL/posterolateral corner should be treated surgically as soon as possible
- Open dislocation may require staged procedures

External fixator

- If tibiofemoral joint is incongruent after reduction
- Vascular injury (plus fasciotomy)
- Massive soft-tissue injury

Proximal or high tibial osteotomy (HTO)

This is an excellent operation for relatively young or highly active individuals, with isolated medial compartment OA and varus alignment of the knee.

The principle is to realign the weight-bearing axis from varus to slight valgus.

Realignment can be achieved either by closed lateral HTO or an open medial HTO. Many surgeons prefer closed wedge osteotomy because of the disadvantages of an open wedge HTO (see below).

Open wedge osteotomy

Advantages

- Preserves bone stock (subsequent TKR is technically easier)
- Makes tightening of the MCL easier
- Preserve the lateral side for LCL or posterolateral reconstruction if insufficient
- Less risk to peroneal nerve

Disadvantages

- Requires a bone graft (substitute, autograft, allograft)
- Plate fixation makes TKR harder

- Increased incidence of delayed union
- Large correction may affect leg lengthening
- Recurrence of varus deformity
- Worsens patella infra
- Slow rehabilitation

Prerequisites for HTO

- Age <60 years
- Less than 15° FFD knee
- >90° flexion knee

Patients should be able to use crutches and have no major varicose veins or peripheral vascular disease.

Contraindications

- Severe OA changes in the lateral compartment or PFJ
- >1 cm medial bone loss
- Incompetent MCL
- Subluxation of tibiofemoral articulation (tibial subluxation >1 cm)
- Inflammatory arthritis
- Crystal arthropathy
- Osteochondral injuries involving more than one-third of the condylar surface
- Obesity. Valgus knee is poorly tolerated due to medial thigh contact
- Large varus thrust
- If more than 20° correction is needed

Radiology

- Standing, long leg views, patella facing forwards
- Mechanical axis (normal = 1.2° varus)
- Anatomical axis (6°–7° valgus)
- 64% across tibial plateau from medial side
- Laterally based closing wedge osteotomy above the level of the tibial tubercle
- Final alignment should create 10°–13° valgus. Overcorrection of 3°–5° above the 6°–7° normal valgus angle
- Medial tibial cortex represents the apex of the bony wedge and should be left intact

Methods of osteotomy fixation

- Cast immobilization
- Staples
- Plate and screw
- External fixator
- Distraction osteogenesis. Correction can be adjusted after surgery. But pin tracts create a potential problem for subsequent TKA

Surgical technique for closed wedge HTO

- Computer-aided measurement of the wedge size can be used
- A 10-mm wedge excision leads to 10° correction in 57-mm-wide tibia
- An angular jig is more accurate
- Tourniquet. Knee flexed to 90°
- Curved incision from the head of the fibula to 2 cm below the tibial tubercle
- Peroneal nerve protected
- Identify the bare area of the fibula head (safe landmark)
- The tibia is dissected subperiosteally anteriorly and posteriorly
- Proximal fibular head is excised at the superior tibiofibula joint or the proximal tibiofibula joint separated using a cob elevator
- A calibrated osteotomy guide must be used for the bone cut
- Leave 15–20 mm of tibial plateau to avoid fracture
- Fix with a plate or staples

Complications

- Inadequate valgus correction aim for tibiofemoral angle 11°–13° valgus
- Overcorrection – PFJ derangement
- Alteration in patella height
- Intra-articular fracture
- Osteonecrosis of the tibial plateau
- Vascular injuries – anterior tibial artery, popliteal artery
- Peroneal nerve palsy

- Delayed or non-union
- Compartment syndrome
- TKR more difficult
- Varus laxity (loose LCL)

Valgus deformity

Less than 12° can be dealt with by varus tibial osteotomy.

A deformity of 12° or more needs distal femoral varus osteotomy to address a lateral femoral condyle deficiency and to prevent joint-line obliquity and gradual lateral tibial subluxation.

Either lateral open wedge using a Puddu plate/Tomofix or medial closing wedge.

Coventry *et al.*[9] found a 5-year survival of 87% and a 10-year survival of 66%. However, 5-year survival was reduced down to 38% when valgus angulation at 1 year was less than 8° in a patient whose weight was more than 1.32 times the ideal weight.

Knee arthrodesis

Indications

- Failed knee replacement
- Uncontrollable sepsis
- Neuropathic joint
- Young patient with severe articular joint disease and ligamentous damage
- Disruption of extensor mechanism
- Poor soft-tissue envelope
- Systemically immunocompromised
- Resistant microorganisms
- Post-traumatic arthrosis in a heavy manual labourer

Contraindications

- Bilateral knee disease
- Ipsilateral ankle or hip disease

[9] Coventry MB, Ilstrup DM, Wallrichs SL (1993) Proximal tibial osteotomy. A critical long-term study of eight-seven cases. *J Bone Joint Surg Am* **75**: 196–201.

- Ipsilateral hip arthrodesis
- Severe segmental bone loss
- Contralateral limb amputation

Ideal position of fusion

- "Neutral range"
- 7° ± 5° of valgus
- 5° ± 5° of flexion

Techniques

1. Intramedullary arthrodesis
   - Long custom-made nail through piriform fossa
   - Intramedullary fixation with modular and non-modular nails
   - Linked nail through the knee is easier to apply
   - More reliable in achieving union than external fixation
   - Technically difficult
   - 40% complication rate (nail breakage and migration)
   - May cause wide spread osteomyelitis in the tibia and femoral shaft
   - The nail has to be inserted after removing implants and infection treatment
2. External fixation
   - Conventional or circular frames
   - Allows for arthrodesis in the presence of infection
   - Can be applied at the time of implant removal
   - 20%–60% complication rate (neurovascular injury, pin site infection and fracture through pin site)
3. Plate fixation
   - Main drawback is recurrent or new infection
   - Single anterior or dual plating

Complications

- Non-union
- Mal-union
- Delayed union
- Recurrent infection

Menisci

Anatomy

Crescent-shaped *fibrocartilaginous* structures that are triangular in cross-section. Peripheral border attached to the joint capsule. Lateral meniscus is more circular, and the medial meniscus is more C shaped.

The anterior horns are connected to each other by the short, transverse, anterior intermeniscal ligament. The anterior horn of the lateral meniscus and posterior horn of both menisci attach to the intercondylar eminence.

The popliteus is attached to the lateral meniscus. The semimembranosus is attached to the medial meniscus.

The lateral meniscus excursion is twice that of the medial meniscus. The medial meniscus is torn three times more frequently than the lateral meniscus.

Differentiate between traumatic tears (younger patient, sporting injury) and degenerative tears (older age group, 60% of the population over 65 years, majority asymptomatic and occur in degenerative joint disease).

Blood supply

- Branches of the lateral, middle and medial genicular arteries
- Peripheral portions of the meniscus are vascularized (20%–30% medial meniscus, 10%–25% lateral meniscus)
- Perimeniscal capillary plexus penetrates through the peripheral border

Classification of meniscal tears

Vascular zones

- Red zone (outer), red-white zone, white zone (inner)
- Red zone can heal via fibrovascular scar formation

Orientation

- Longitudinal, radial, horizontal or oblique

Appearance

- Complete longitudinal, bucket handle, displaced bucket handle
- Parrot beak, flap and displaced flap
- Radial, double flap and incomplete longitudinal

Composed of collagen type 1 fibres arranged radially and longitudinally (circumferential). Longitudinal fibres help to dissipate hoop stresses in the meniscus. A combination of fibres allows the menisci to expand under compressive forces and increases the contact area of the joint.

Proteoglycans trapped within collagen fibres absorb energy. The extracellular matrix consists of proteoglycans, glycoproteins and elastin.

Functions of menisci

- Joint stability and congruity
- Load transmission: 50% in extension and 85% in flexion
- Aid lubrication and nutrition
- Shock absorber during gait cycle
- Limit extremes of flexion/extension
- Reduce contact stresses
- Proprioception

The compression of the menisci by the tibia and femur generates outward forces that push the meniscus out from between the bones. The circumferential tension in the meniscus counteracts this radial force. The hoop tension is lost when a single radial cut or tear extends to the capsular margin.

Meniscal repair

Consider the following:
- Patient's age
- Occupation
- Chronicity. Better results if carried out <8 weeks (may be due to spontaneous healing)

- Type, location and length of tear
- Associated ligamentous injury

Relative contraindications to repair

- Stable tear (partial thickness tear)
- Peripheral tear <10 mm long that cannot be displaced more than a few millimetres
- Complex, degenerative and central/radial tears are best excised partially

Types of meniscal repair

- Open repair: vertical mattress sutures
- Inside out
- Outside in. Versatile access, less expensive instruments and safe
- All inside

To optimize healing could use

- Fibrin clot
- Rasps and shavers are used to freshen both sides of the tear prior to repair
- Vascularized synovial flaps
- Autologous blood clot
- Parameniscal synovial abrasion
- Endothelial cell growth factor
- Fibrin sealants
- Notch microfracture/bleeding

Complications

- Excluding failure to heal and re-tearing, neurovascular injury is the commonest
- Medially: saphenous nerve and its infrapatellar branch injury 1%–2.5%
- Laterally: popliteal artery and peroneal nerve

Meniscal allograft transplantation

This is still regarded as an experimental procedure. It is carried out to prevent joint deterioration following total meniscectomy and to help improve knee stability in patients with ligamentous instability.

Indications

Consider

- Patient's age (best results if <20 years old)
- Symptoms (in the future may be done prophylactically)
- Knee stability and alignment
- Compartment wear (Outerbridge I and II better outcome)

Graft

- Fresh-frozen
- Freeze-dried grafts
- Collagen or synthetic grafts

The meniscus is immunologically privileged due to dense matrix isolating the cells.

Technique

- Open
- Arthroscopically assisted

Examination corner

Basic science oral

Composition and structure of the menisci including arrangement of the collagen fibres. Biomechanics of the menisci in the knee and the role of load distribution. How meniscectomy affects the load distribution.

Plus questions about the repair of the meniscus.

Meniscal cyst

Aetiology

- Cause unknown
- Myxoid degeneration of stressed fibrocartilage
- Probably traumatic in origin
- Meniscal tear creates a one-way valve

Pathology

- Contain gelatinous fluid, surrounded by thick fibrous tissue
- Nearly always associated with a small, horizontal cleavage tear in the meniscus

- Isolated cysts without meniscal pathology have been reported
- Much more likely to occur laterally

Clinical features

- Insidious onset of discomfort
- Point tender cyst
- Symptoms are intermittent or related to activity
- Lump is situated at or slightly below the joint line
- Usually anterior to collateral ligament
- Seen most easily with the knee slightly flexed (<45°)
- Lateral cysts are firm, medial cysts are usually larger and softer
- Pisani's sign (cyst size decreases with knee flexion)

Differential diagnosis

- Ganglia: superficial, not as hard and unconnected to the joint
- Calcified deposits in the collateral ligament: show on radiographs
- Prolapsed torn meniscus (pseudocyst)
- Sebaceous cyst
- Bursitis
- Various tumours: sarcoma, lipoma, fibroma and histiocytoma
- PVNS

Management

- Depends on symptoms, size, location and relation to meniscal tear
- If contiguous with the meniscal tear the meniscus is debrided and the cyst is decompressed arthroscopically or with a needle aspiration
- If the cyst is distinct or very large, an open excision is more successful

Congenital discoid menisci

In children, most meniscal tears are due to a congenitally discoid menisci (5% Anglo-Americans, up to 20% Asians).

Aetiology

Possibly failure of resorption of the central portion of the meniscus during development; or secondary to instability of the meniscus during development, subsequent to failure of attachment of the meniscotibial (coronary) ligament to the posterior horn (type III).

Classification

Type I – complete

With the meniscus covering the whole lateral tibial plateau, causing inadequate visualization on arthroscopy.

Type II – incomplete

The central portion extends further across the tibial plateau than normal.

Type III – Wrisberg's variant

Involves deficiency of attachment to the posterior horn meniscotibial ligaments, so the posterior horn is only secured by the meniscofemoral ligaments.

Clinical features

Snapping knee syndrome (popping knee syndrome) in children <10 years old, whose knee snaps spontaneously causing momentary pain and apprehension. A characteristic clunk may be felt at 110° as the knee is bent, or at 10° as the knee is straightened.

A McMurray test may cause an obvious pop, with temporary subluxation of the posterior horn, and locking can occur.

In older children, the discoid meniscus usually presents with the symptoms of a meniscal tear. Types I and II commonly have longitudinal or horizontal tears. Type III usually have no tears, but may exhibit degenerative changes. All types may have radial, bucket-handle or complex tears.

Radiographs

- Widened joint space
- Squaring of the lateral condyle
- Ridging
- Cupping of the lateral tibial plateau
- Hypoplastic lateral intercondylar spine

MRI appearance

- A black image across the entire lateral compartment

Management

- If asymptomatic or there is only a clunk (not associated with a tear) leave it alone
- Symptomatic patients with a type I or II discoid meniscus may be treated with arthroscopic debridement and contouring of the central portion, leaving a rim of 6–8 mm (saucerization). Peripheral tears in the vascularized zone should be repaired. Often the remaining rim is degenerate and may necessitate total meniscectomy
- Type III menisci, traditionally treated with total meniscectomy, are now usually managed with meniscal repair and reattachment of the posterior horn to the tibial plateau
- Further surgery is often required for recurrent tears
- OA is common following meniscectomy
- No increase in the risk of OA in asymptomatic patients

Osteochondritis dissecans (OCD) and articular cartilage injury

Definition

- A lesion of subchondral bone that results in subchondral delamination and sequestration with or without articular mantle involvement (Stanitski)
- Subgroups: juvenile, adolescent and adult types
- Peaks in preteen years

- Male:female ratio is 5:3
- Bilateral 20%
- Medial:lateral condyle ratio is 80:20
- Patella lesion in 10%

Aetiology

- Aetiology is unknown
- Lesion is thought to be due to macrotrauma or repeated microtrauma
- Possibly AVN
- Or there may be abnormal epiphyseal ossification
- The condition tends to occur in children during increased physeal activity

Clinical presentation

- Non-specific, poorly localized pain
- Activity-related pain
- Stiffness
- Swelling
- Mechanical symptoms with locking
- Antalgic gait
- Effusion in unstable lesion
- Localized tenderness
- Wilson's sign (pain relieved by external rotation of tibia)

Pappas classification (according to age at detection)

- Category I: below age 12 (excellent prognosis)
- Category II: between 12 and 20 years
- Category III: above 20 years

Prognosis

- Healing potential is high in juveniles (75%)
- Adolescent prognosis is unpredictable (50% heal)
- Healing is markedly reduced in those with a mature skeleton with possible premature OA

Radiographs

- Preferred radiographic view is the tunnel view

Guhl arthroscopic classification

- Intact lesion 1–3 cm (in situ, soft area covered by intact cartilage
- Early separation (stable flap)
- Partially detached (flap attached by hinge)
- Complete detachment (full-thickness loss within bed or displaced)

Stage the lesion: radiographs, MRI and arthroscopy.

Management

- Young patient (open physis, category I, juvenile OCD) → activity modification
- OCD in young adults is usually symptomatic and almost invariably leads to early-onset OA unless treated:
  - In situ lesions → retrograde drilling
  - Early separation stage → secured K-wires, special screws
  - Incompletely detached → removal of underlying fibrous tissue, some form of chondroplasty and then reduction and fixation flap
  - Completely detached → removal of the loose body (often too damaged to replace), some form of abrasion chondroplasty ± osteochondral allograft, autologous chondrocytes culture implantation
  - Needs careful follow-up

Options

- Abrasion
- Abrasion and K-wire drilling
- Abrasion and microfracture
- Mosiacplasty
- Osteochondral graft
- Autologous chondrocyte graft from the periosteum of the tibia and fibrin glue

Cartilage injury

- This is a separate entity. Usually related to rotational force in direct trauma
- Located in weight-bearing area such as medial femoral condyle

- Classified as linear, satellite, flap, crater, fibrillation and degrading lesions
- Treatment is still evolving
- Debridement, microfracture and contouring of the sides of the lesion are recommended (only remove loose flaps)
- Chondroplasty has been tried with promising early results

Examination corner

Trauma oral

Clinical photograph fracture/subluxation knee

- Classification
- Management of knee dislocation
- When to perform arteriography
- Which ligament to repair

Clinical examination of the knee

You must have a system.

Ask the patient to stand

- Look for clues (brace, sticks, calliper, RA hands and shoe raise)
- Inspection (front, side and behind)
- Alignment (varus, valgus or windswept knees)
- Patella rotation
- Swelling (position in relation to patella)
- Skin changes (psoriasis)
- Scars are very helpful but sometimes they are not visible (get closer)
- Skin grafts or flaps and sinuses
- Quadriceps wasting, especially VMO
- Look at the knee position from the side: is it flexed or in recurvatum?
- Look at the popliteal fossa and calf muscles

Ask the patient to walk

- Look at the knee position in flexed posture
- Thrust (dynamic instability)

Ask young patients to squat

- Patients cannot do this if they have a meniscal tear or patella problems

Ask the patient to sit on the couch

- Check patella tracking during extension
- J sign
- Palpate for crepitation during extension

Ask the patient to lie supine with their knee flexed 50°–60°

- Look for sag. Double check with card test or palpate a step-off at the joint line
- Palpate the knee
- Drawer test flex to 70°–80°

Ask the patient to extend the knee

- Check extensor mechanism (leg raise)
- Feel and measure the quadriceps bulk
- Q angle
- Effusion, milk or bulge test/patella tap
- Patella grind test
- Patella mobility
- Iliotibial tract tightness
- Check active and passive range of movement
- Fixed flexion in OA
- Check collateral ligaments
- Lachman's test
- Provocative meniscus tests – McMurray test if meniscal injury is suspected
- Compartment loading

Ask the patient to lie prone

- Dial test in prone position
- Externally rotate the knee at 30° and 90° flexion
- More than 10°–15° difference in external rotation is abnormal
- If one side is rotated more at 30° this suggests posterolateral corner injury
- One side rotated more at 90° suggests both posterolateral corner and PCL injury
- Finally, examine the lumbar spine, hips and peripheral circulation

Examine the PFJ

- Follow your routine concentrating on patella abnormality
- Tenderness around the patella
- Hypermobility
- Tracking
- Apprehension (symptom)
- Patellar tilt

18

Foot and ankle oral core topics

Paul A. Banaszkiewicz

Introduction

There is a large recommended syllabus from the British Orthopaedic Foot Surgery Society for the FRCS Orth Examination. This syllabus is very detailed and comprehensive and if you learnt everything on it you would have no time to revise any other subject. Most candidates are not intending to become foot and ankle surgeons. It is difficult to know exactly how much detail needs to be learnt to pass the exam.

Whilst a candidate may not be expected to know all the details of every condition, he or she should at least be prepared to answer questions in general on most conditions and in particular on the more common foot and ankle disorders.

At least one foot/ankle condition is likely to be encountered in the short cases. As with all cases, asking appropriate questions and properly examining the affected part go a long way to securing a pass even if you only know a few of the managements available.

It is also a relatively common oral topic, usually the adult and pathology oral (hallux valgus, chronic ankle instability, etc.) or paediatric oral (juvenile hallux valgus, tarsal coalition, lesser toe deformities, pes planus, etc.).

It helps immensely if you have specifically worked for a foot and ankle surgeon, however it is not a disaster if you have not. Good overall examination technique, going through set answers for particular topics and being aware of where you can end up digging a hole for yourself can compensate for practical weakness in the subject.

Foot and ankle biomechanics

Windlass mechanism

Normally dorsiflexion of the big toe increases the tension of the plantar aponeurosis, which causes the longitudinal arch to rise. Failure to do so suggests a disrupted Windlass mechanism. A less effective Windlass mechanism can be caused by a variety of different conditions, e.g. abnormal stretching and elongation of the plantar aponeurosis, hallux deformity and Keller's excision arthroplasty. A less effective Windlass mechanism with a depressing metatarsal head and weight transfer to the hallux results in transfer metatarsalgia.

Ankle arthroscopy

Indications

Diagnostic

- Investigation of ankle pain of unknown aetiology
- Unexplained swelling, stiffness, instability, locking or popping
- Negative work-up in a patient with significant ankle symptoms unresponsive to conservative care

Therapeutic

- Evaluation, debridement, drilling or pinning of osteochondral defects of the talus
- Removal of loose bodies
- Excision of osteophytes

Postgraduate Orthopaedics: The Candidate's Guide to the FRCS (Tr & Orth) Examination, Ed. Paul A. Banaszkiewicz,
Deiary F. Kader, Nicola Maffulli. Published by Cambridge University Press. © Cambridge University Press 2009.

- Arthroscopic ankle arthrodesis
- Evaluation and debridement of soft-tissue impingement lesions
- Synovectomy

Portals

Five portals have been developed for use.

Anteromedial

- Least dangerous portal
- Just medial to the tibialis anterior tendon and lateral to the saphenous nerve and vein
- Dangers: damage to tibialis anterior tendon, saphenous nerve and vein

Anterolateral

- Lateral to peroneus tertius tendon and extensors
- Dangers (risks): damage to superficial peroneal nerve
- By flexing and inverting the foot it is possible to put stretch on the nerve and to visualize it subcutaneously so as to avoid injury

Anterocentral

- Rarely used
- Medial or lateral to EHL tendon
- Danger: damage to anterior tibial artery and deep peroneal nerve; to EHL and EDL; to terminal branches of the superficial peroneal nerve

Posterolateral portal

- Lateral to the Achilles tendon, 2 cm above the tip of the lateral malleolus
- Danger: damage to short saphenous vein and sural nerve

Posteromedial portal

- Medial to Achilles tendon
- Not commonly used due to its close proximity to the posterior tibial artery and nerve and risk of injury

Distraction

- Good distraction of the joint is necessary for adequate visualization
- Invasive methods use pins to distract the joint but there is a possibility of direct neurovascular injury
- Non-invasive methods use skin traction via commercially available straps with one loop over the heel and the other over the dorsum of the foot

Complications

Studies have reported variable complication rates ranging from 7.6% to 17% including:
- Infection
- Nerve injury
- Scarring of the peroneal tendon from use of a distraction device
- Painful scars
- Broken pins

Ankle arthritis

Symptoms

- Pain
- Stiffness
- Deformity
- Limitation of ADL

Severe disabling ankle pain interfering with ADL with or without deformity.

Causes

Primary osteoarthritis of the ankle is rare. It is usually secondary to another predisposing cause. Look for features of a secondary cause on any radiographs studied.[1]
- Post-traumatic arthritis: displaced ankle fractures, talar neck fractures with AVN, chronic ankle ligamentous instability

---

[1] Attempt to subtly mention this fact to the examiners when describing radiographs to them without being too obvious.

- Inflammatory arthritis: rheumatoid arthritis, etc.
- Joint sepsis
- Charcot joint
- Osteochondritis dissecans of the talus
- As a result of bleeding and bleeding diathesis, e.g. haemophilia
- Can occasionally be affected by generalized osteoarthritis and pyrophosphate arthropathy

Conservative management

- Modification of footwear, e.g. cushioned heel inserts with a stiff rocker bottom sole
- Splints and orthosis, e.g. moulded ankle–foot orthosis
- Intra-articular steroid injections or visco supplements
- Non-steroidal anti-inflammatory medication, painkillers
- Physiotherapy possibly in cases of instability or weakness to improve muscle strength, proprioception and range of movement[2]

Limited surgical approach

A limited surgical approach can be used to improve symptoms in the short term and buy time.

Arthroscopic ankle debridement

- Can be technically difficult to get into the ankle joint especially if it is a tight arthritic joint
- May be useful if there is an obvious cause that could be corrected, e.g. anterior osteophytes
- Resection of osteophytes, inflamed synovium, areas of impingement, loose osteochondral fragments
- Buys time, 90% good/excellent results reported at 2 years

Open ankle debridement

- More invasive. Occasionally still required if there are large loose bodies, especially posteriorly

Joint distraction using Ilizarov fixator

- Improves symptoms of post-traumatic OA. The fixator is applied for a period of 3 months. The articular surfaces do not come into contact with one another during this time. The patient is allowed to weight bear
- At 6 weeks hinges are applied to the construct to allow movement whilst maintaining distraction
- The increased hydrostatic pressure within the joint is thought to stimulate proteoglycan production. Improvements in range of movement and pain as well as increased radiological joint space are seen at 2 years

Definitive surgical procedures[3]

More definitive surgical procedures would be an ankle arthrodesis or arthroplasty.

Ankle arthroplasty

Total ankle arthroplasty (TAR) is useful in low-demand patients with rheumatoid arthritis, in non-obese less active patients over the age of 60 years with osteoarthritis, in patients with bilateral arthrosis and in patients with degenerative disease in other joints. Poor candidates include young active patients with post-traumatic arthrosis. Prerequisites for TAR include a stable subtalar joint and limited deformity. It is sensible to proceed with caution for high-risk cases.

Contraindications include active infection, peripheral vascular disease, inadequate soft-tissue envelope, Charcot neuropathy, severe lower limb malalignment, marked ankle instability, marked osteoporosis and AVN of the talus.

---

[2] Be careful mentioning physiotherapy in an oral; qualify your answer. "*Examiner*: Come on now – is physiotherapy really going to be of any use in a patient with significant severe ankle arthrosis? It could make matter worse – more ankle movement, more pain" Don't just mention physiotherapy blindly as a conservative treatment for everything without first thinking through its role.

[3] Talking the talk. The options for management of ankle arthrosis would include conservative management, a limited surgical approach such as arthroscopic ankle debridement or a more definitive surgical procedure such as ankle arthrodesis.

Early designs had a bad reputation for the following reasons:

- Reports of severe osteolysis, component loosening, impingement, infection and soft-tissue breakdown. Failures were believed to be a result of poor prosthesis design, inadequate fixation, poor soft-tissue management and lack of soft-tissue balancing
- Poor long-term survival of the prosthesis
- Poor functional results
- Difficulty in salvaging a failed TAR often led to below-knee amputation

Types of ankle arthroplasty

1. **STAR (Scandinavian total ankle replacement).** Uncemented, minimally axially constrained, fully conforming mobile bearing implant
2. **Agility.** Porous-coated, fixed bearing implant with a partially conforming articulation. The distal tibiofibular joint is fused to create a stronger supporting base but there are reports of delayed and non-union in up to one-third of patients. A lateral plate is used to further compress the fibula against the arthrodesis site and lateral component developed to reduce the risk of non-union
3. **Topez total ankle replacement**
4. **Eclipse total ankle implant**
5. **Buechel-Pappas™.** Uncemented titanium resurfacing prosthesis with a polyethylene meniscal bearing between the tibia and talus. Reasonably encouraging results have been reported. Ten-year results are available but reflect isolated small series

Complications of ankle arthroplasty

- Recurrent pain, component migration, loosening, malalignment, infection, neurovascular injury

Ankle arthrodesis

Historically the gold standard. A large number of surgical techniques have been described. A fusion rate between 80% and 90% has variously been reported. Relief of pain is usually excellent but most have limited hindfoot motion that makes walking on uneven ground difficult and few are able to run effectively. Gait analysis shows that walking speed is decreased, as are step length and single stance duration. The normal leg mirrors the arthrodesed side.

Types of ankle fusion

- Compression arthrodesis using rigid internal fixation, e.g. cross screw or parallel screw compression, anterior tension plate
- Arthroscopically assisted ankle fusion (only in the absence of gross deformity)
- Compression arthrodesis with external clamp (Charnley). High incidence of pin tract and superficial infections
- Ilizarov technique. Allows tibial lengthening at the same time
- Intramedullary nail. Best suited for patients with soft tissue compromise, failed prior arthrodesis or diabetic neuropathy. Difficulties include providing adequate compression across the arthrodesis site, risk of neurovascular injury during nail insertion and stress fracture of the tibia
- Blair technique. The talar body is discarded and a sliding bone graft from the anterior aspect of tibia is inserted into the talar neck. Most frequently used to salvage AVN due to talar neck fractures
- Baciu and Filibiu. Dowel technique in which a K-wire is passed under image intensifier control through the medial malleolus, across the ankle joint and out through the lateral malleolus. A milling cutter is then passed over the K-wire through the medial malleolus, distal tibia and proximal talus and into the lateral malleolus. The graft is extracted, reversed and rotated 90° and then re-inserted

Position of fusion

The foot position when fused is extremely important. Small tolerances of position are compatible with good function:

- Neutral position: dorsiflexion/plantar flexion (10° equinus if patient cannot stabilize the knee) (CP)
- 5° valgus
- 5° external rotation – similar to contralateral limb
- Traditional teaching recommends slight posterior translation of the tibia

Complications

- Non-union, mal-union, infection, poor wound healing, pin tract infection, tibial fractures, amputation, painful neuroma, posterior tibia nerve injury, vascular injury
- Wound infection and breakdown with a reported incidence of up to 40% in some series. Non-union occurs in one-third of cases in some series

Salvage of non-union

High-risk cases for repeat ankle fusion following initial failure include:

- Bony defect
- Deformity
- Infection
- Diabetic neuropathy (use a nail)
- Sensory deficit – Charcot–Marie–Tooth disease, lumbar disc disease

Repeat surgery increases the risks of neurovascular damage, infection and further non-union. Additional loss of bone may lead to peroneal, posterior tibial or flexor tendon incompetence. The worst-case scenario is amputation.

Chronic ankle instability

Introduction

This is a must-learn key B list topic for the oral part of the examination. It is a much loved favourite topic of examiners although I am not entirely sure why. I can think of many other more important topics that hardly ever crop up in the exam. Perhaps it is an important practical topic that we manage badly.

Ankle sprains are very common conditions, which we deal with on a daily basis in the fracture clinic and the vast majority can be managed conservatively without any functional instability developing. Perhaps the examiners feel that we should be able to recognize the few patients that present with features of instability who require additional investigation and management. Possibly it is a question that differentiates a good candidate who knows the subject well from a poor one who has briefly skimmed over the topic without fully understanding it.

Anatomy

The lateral aspect of the ankle capsule is reinforced by three ligaments:

- Anterior talofibular ligament (ATFL)
- Calcaneofibular ligament (CFL)
- Posterior talofibular ligament (PTFL)

A forced inversion injury leads first to damage to the ATFL. In more severe injuries this is followed by damage to the CFL. It is almost impossible to injure the CFL in isolation. Disruption of the PTFL is rare.

Acute inversion injuries can be graded as either unstable or stable.

Unstable injuries are further subdivided according to the degree of talar tilt and anterior drawer present under stress. A partial or complete tear of the ligament complex heals in a lengthened position causing lateral joint laxity. If only the ATFL is involved anterior subluxation of the talus in the ankle mortise will occur. When both the ATFL and CFL are injured talar tilt will also be present. An important component of the injury is proprioceptor damage.

Investigations

- Plain radiographs
- Stress views

Anterior talar shift stress test (anterior drawer test)

ATFL is the primary restraint to anterior shift. Forward displacement of the talus greater than 3 mm from the normal ankle or an absolute value of 9 mm is significant and indicates a torn ATFL. This is determined on a lateral stress radiograph by measuring the perpendicular distance from the talus to the posterior articular margin of the tibial plafond.

Talar tilt stress test

CFL is the primary restraint to tilt. Talar tilting >15° is significant and indicates a torn ATFL and CFL. If >30° then all three lateral ligaments have been ruptured. However, just because there is gross tibiotalar tilting on stress radiographs does not necessarily mean that the patient is symptomatic and requires an operation.

A high degree of variability in laxity in normal ankles makes it difficult to establish strict criteria for ligament reconstruction on the basis of stress measurements alone. Comparing laxity with the normal side if the other ankle is asymptomatic is useful.

Symptoms

- There are three common presentations of chronic ankle instability: pain, pain and instability or mechanical instability symptoms alone
- Pain can be felt on climbing stairs, when walking on uneven ground, during exercise, with swelling and recurrent giving way
- Ask specifically about the exact location of the ankle pain
- Ask whether a feeling of instability occurs first followed by pain or whether pain is felt first and then instability. Ask whether there is just a feeling of instability (giving way) or whether the patient actually falls to the ground
- Locking (loose body); ask the patient whether their ankle locks
- In the history try to differentiate between true mechanical instability and functional instability. Functional instability is a subjective sensation of the ankle giving way. It is thought to be due to poor motor coordination or disordered ankle proprioception. Mechanical instability is an excessive laxity of the lateral ligamentous complex. There is often a positive anterior drawer test

Indications for surgical reconstruction

- Disabling symptoms of chronic instability
- Positive clinical examination (anterior drawer sign, positive varus tilt test)
- Positive stress radiographs
- Failure of conservative management

Ankle pain alone is usually not an indication in itself to reconstruct an unstable ankle as most patients continue to have significant pain after reconstruction.

Some foot and ankle surgeons would proceed with EUA and ankle arthroscopy before reconstruction. A significant number of patients with instability symptoms may have a different pathology, e.g. osteochondral lesion, chronic synovial hypertrophy, scar tissue, etc.

Proceed with ankle arthroscopy and then reassess the patient in the outpatient clinic before proceeding with reconstruction or carry on after ankle arthroscopy depending on the amount of soft-tissue swelling and findings at arthroscopy. Another option would be to order an MRI scan which would demonstrate whether there was a normal or a torn ATFL and CFL.

Techniques

Reconstruction methods fall into two general types:
1. Anatomic repair (augmented or non-augmented)
2. Non-anatomic

Anatomic repair

Attempts to reconstruct normal anatomy (with or without augmentation) without sacrificing the peroneal musculature or other tendons.

Non-anatomic reconstruction

In which another structure or material is substituted for the injured ligament. This is accompanied by significant loss of eversion and inversion because of the non-anatomical placement of tissue across the joint.

Watson–Jones tenodesis

This procedure reconstructs both the ATFL and CFL ligaments. The peroneus brevis tendon is divided proximally and threaded through a drill hole in the fibula back to front and then through a vertical hole in the neck of the talus from above to below and then back to the fibula, where it is secured.

Evans procedure

The peroneus brevis tendon is divided proximally and re-routed into the fibula through a bony tunnel. The procedure requires less length of tendon and is a good operation for varus tilt without anterior subluxation at the loss of inversion. Reconstructs only the CFL. This is a good operation that is not too technically difficult, and can be used as a back-up procedure if required and indirectly limits anterior tibial translation.

Fitton's operation
Uses an isolated graft of peroneus brevis or plantaris. The ATFL is reconstructed by passing the graft through four drill holes made in the fibula and talus. A good operation for pure anterior translation only.

Chrisman–Snook repair
Both ligaments are reconstructed in a split tenodesis of peroneus brevis to reconstruct the ATFL and CFL. Peroneus brevis is passed posteriorly through a horizontal hole in the fibula. Another hole is drilled postero-anteriorly through the lateral ridge of the os calcis. This is a good procedure for anterior laxity and varus tilt although it restricts inversion. It is a challenging operation, which is technically difficult. There is little room for error, and it is sometimes difficult to get enough length of tendon for the operation and if the tendon graft ruptures the procedure is difficult to salvage. Freeze-dried fascia lata has been used as a substitute in certain situations.

Brostrom repair
A mid substance late repair with shortening of the free ends of the ligaments (anatomical repair).

Brostrom–Karlsson repair
Modification of the Brostrom repair. Shortening of the ligaments with re-attachment onto the roughened fibula through drill holes.

Brostrom–Gould repair
Modification of the Brostrom technique to include repair of the lateral talocalcaneal ligament and suturing of the lateral extensor retinaculum to the distal aspect of the fibula. This limits excessive subtalar motion whilst preserving normal anatomical relationships and subtalar joint function.

The Bostrom–Gould and Chrisman–Snook procedures remain the gold standards of lateral ligament reconstruction. Both restore excellent or good mechanical stability in 80% of patients. The Bostrom–Gould repair has however higher functional scores, less frequent complications and the best long-term results in terms of outcome.

Contraindications to reconstruction

- History of instability >10 years
- Generalized joint hypermobility

Complications of surgery

- Wound infection
- Ankle and subtalar stiffness
- Repair may stretch up in time and fail
- Scar tenderness
- Sural nerve injury

Differential diagnosis of persistent pain after ankle sprain

- Incomplete rehabilitation
- Osteochondral fracture talus
- Chronic instability
- Fracture of the fifth metatarsal bone
- Subtalar sprain
- Fracture of the lateral process of talus
- Syndesmotic sprain
- Peroneal tendinitis/tear
- Impingement problems
- Fracture of the anterior process of calcaneus
- Sinus tarsi syndrome
- Chronic tendon disorders
- Reflex sympathetic dystrophy
- Tumours
- Stress fractures

Examination corner

Oral question

Describe a surgical technique for chronic ankle instability
This topic always begins with a clinical radiograph of the ankle showing talar tilt (Figure 18.1). There may also be a lateral radiograph demonstrating anterior talar shift.

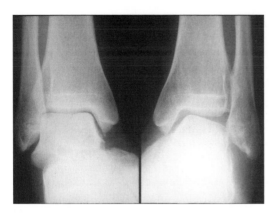

Figure 18.1 Radiograph of the ankle demonstrating talar tilt.

Adult elective orthopaedics oral 1

Examiner: This is a radiograph of an ankle, what does it demonstrate?

Candidate: This is a lateral stress radiograph of the ankle, which shows tibiotalar shift indicating injury to the lateral ankle ligament complex.

Examiner: How are you going to manage this patient?

Candidate: I would initially manage this patient with physiotherapy.

Examiner: Come on, is physiotherapy going to help in this situation with this amount of talar tilt?

Candidate: A patient may have significant talar tilt on stress views but not require surgery. The literature suggests that up to 80% of grade 3 injuries can be managed conservatively with good results.

Examiner: This patient is being seen in your fracture clinic 6 months following a lateral ligament injury which is not getting any better. She has severe symptoms of pain and instability and these are her stress views. Are you really going to manage her with physiotherapy, which she has had on two previous occasions?!

Candidate: In this case I would consider surgical reconstruction.

Examiner: Can you name any surgical procedures performed for chronic ankle instability?

Candidate: The Evans procedure.

Examiner: What is the concern about using the Evans procedure over a different procedure?

Candidate: I'm not sure.

Examiner: Different surgical procedures have different affects on subtalar movement. It is clear you do not fully understand the topic. Let's move on.

[Fail]

The first point would be to say that just mentioning physiotherapy as an initial management for the condition without qualifying your answer further is inviting trouble. A much better reply would have gone along the lines of *"The stress views show significant tibiotalar tilt and, if taken in conjunction with an appropriate history and clinical examination which are suggestive of chronic ankle instability, this may be an indication to consider surgical management."* Even better to continue on with *"Surgical options can be either an anatomical repair such as a modified Brostrom repair or a non-anatomical repair such as Chrisman–Snook repair."*

This examiner seemed to give the impression that a positive stress view equated with a surgical reconstruction. It is important to be quite clear that a positive stress view in itself is not an indication for surgery. Stress radiographs may show significant talar tilt and anterior subluxation but the patient may have minimal symptoms of ankle instability and may not require a reconstructive procedure. This point should have been mentioned in the general discussion in retort to the examiner's comments. The candidate obviously did not know the different techniques available to reconstruct the lateral ligament complex and the effect on subtalar movement.

Trauma oral

Clinical radiograph showing tibiotalar tilt

Candidate: This is a radiograph, which is a stress view demonstrating significant tibiotalar tilt suggestive of chronic ankle instability.

Examiner: You are seeing this patient in the fracture clinic 6 months following an ankle sprain with this X-ray. What are you going to do?

Candidate: If he has symptomatic, disabling ankle instability then I would offer him surgery.

Examiner: Is he likely to have anything else but symptomatic instability with this radiograph? (Not a question but a somewhat sarcastic comment.) What types of repair are you familiar with?

Candidate: A repair of the lateral ligament can be either augmented or non-augmented. (Slightly mixed-up answer, not entirely accurate.)

Examiner: (Not entirely happy with the answer.) What is the recommended type of repair to perform?

Candidate: It would probably be a modified Brostrom repair.

Examiner: An anatomical repair. What would you tell the patient the outcome is likely to be?

Candidate: In fact most ankle reconstructions do very well with a 90% success rate. It's one of those operations that tend to do well.

Examiner: Yes you are quite right about this. When would you allow a patient to return to playing football?

Candidate: Three months. (Complete guess.)

Examiner: Would you allow them to play unsupported or would you make them wear a support brace?

Candidate: I would allow them to play without any support.

Complete guess and wrong answer. Most athletes should continue to use a tape or brace indefinitely during sports activities, but a brace is not routine after 3 months for most work-related activities or activities of daily living. This oral took place in the old days when examiners were neither candidate friendly nor politically correct. How things have changed!

Adult elective orthopaedics oral 2

Clinical radiograph showing tibiotalar tilt

Candidate: This is a radiograph, which is a stress view demonstrating significant tibiotalar tilt suggestive of chronic ankle instability.

Examiner: How do you manage this patient? (Saved by bell.) We will leave it at that.

Adult elective orthopaedics oral 3

Clinical radiographs, AP stress view showing tibiotalar tilt and lateral stress view showing anterior subluxation talus on the tibia

Candidate: This is a radiograph, which is a stress view demonstrating significant tibiotalar tilt suggestive of chronic ankle instability.

Examiner: How much of a tilt is significant?

Candidate: A tibiotalar tilt of greater than 15°.

Examiner: You haven't commented on the lateral X-ray. What do you think about the talus?

Candidate: It's moved forwards.

Examiner: Yes, the radiograph demonstrates an anterior subluxation of the talus. What value of subluxation is significant?

Candidate: 3 mm.

Examiner: 3 mm compared to what?

Candidate: Compared to the normal contralateral side.

Examiner: What surgical operations do you know that can be used to manage this condition?

Candidate: You can either perform an anatomical repair or a non-anatomical repair. An anatomical repair is usually preferred and this can be either augmented or non-augmented. The classic operation was a Brostrom repair in which there was a mid-substance repair of the ligament but this tended to stretch out in time. Karlsson performed a modification of the Brostrom repair in which the ligaments were shortened and inserted into the fibula. Gould also modified the Brostrom repair in which the lateral talocalcaneal ligament was repaired and the repair reinforced with suturing of the lateral extensor retinaculum. This modification is important in patients who have excessive inversion and laxity of the subtalar joint. However there is very little to choose between the last two methods. There was a randomized controlled trial performed by Karlsson, which showed the Gould repair had more complications and slightly lower functional scores than the modified Brostrom repair.

Diabetic foot

Introduction

Approximately 10% of diabetic admissions to hospital are with foot problems. The severity of diabetic foot disease is not related to the severity of the diabetes but rather to the adequacy of blood sugar control.

Pathology

- One-third of diabetic foot ulcerations are neuropathic
- One-third are ischaemic
- One-third are mixed in nature

Neuropathy

Symmetrical distal polyneuropathy involving motor, sensory and autonomic nerves.

Autonomic dysfunction

Results in reduced sweating, leading to dry plantar skin, which can fissure. Autonomic neuropathy alters nail growth and inhibits the local vascular response to injury.

Sensory disturbance

Usually a painless sensory neuropathy causes a stocking-distribution sensory loss with reduced ability to sense pinprick, light touch and vibration. Those with a painful neuropathy do not tend to get ulcers. The neuropathic foot is a warm, dry, insensitive foot with clawed toes and increased pressure under the metatarsal heads. Superficial veins are often distended. The claw toes expose the metatarsal heads to further mechanical insult.

Motor involvement

Results in intrinsic muscles weakness and imbalance between the long flexors and extensors, which may lead to a cavus foot and claw toes. The metatarsal heads are pulled forwards, decreasing cushioning and increasing vertical and shear forces.

Peripheral vascular disease

Diffuse affecting both upper and lower extremities. Appears earlier in diabetes, bilateral involvement and progresses quicker.

Pathophysiology

Mechanical stress is the triggering factor for ulceration in both the neuropathic and ischaemic foot. In the ischaemic foot low pressures over a period of time may lead to necrosis. Most common sites are the curve of the first and fifth metatarsal heads. The sole of the foot has a relatively good blood supply and tends not to ulcerate early. In the neuropathic foot ulceration is triggered by direct high-pressure injury or slowly through repetitive stress. Callosities develop under the metatarsal heads and heel. Subcutaneous tissue trapped between bone and thick non-pliable skin produces high shear forces, leading to a sterile deep haematoma. This deep ulcer then tracks to the skin.

Clinical assessment

- Is the ulcer ischaemic, neuropathic or a combination?
- Is infection present?
- Assess pulses: if absent refer to vascular surgeon
- The size and depth of the ulcer along with the area of skin breakdown and any exposed structures should be documented

Neuropathic ulcers

These typically occur under metatarsal heads and are surrounded by thick hyperkeratosis; they have a pink punched-out base, are painless and readily bleed. The patient has a warm foot with palpable pulses and distended veins.

Ischaemic ulcer

This is not surrounded by hyperkeratosis, has a dull fibrotic base, doesn't bleed easily, is painful to touch, and there is hair loss in the affected area.

Infection

Surrounding cellulitis, discharge, erythema.

The most widely used classification system for diabetic ulceration is that of Wagner, which depends on ulcer depth:

- Grade 0: No ulcer, but patient at risk because of neuropathy. Educate the patient and advise them to modify their footwear
- Grade 1: Clean, uninfected ulcer. Antibiotics for cellulitis
- Grade 2: Some necrotic tissue. Treat by debridement
- Grade 3: Bone palpable through ulcer with immediate risk of osteomyelitis
- Grade 4: Forefoot gangrene
- Grade 5: Gangrene of the entire foot

Investigations

For nerve function
- Biothesiometer. Measures vibration perception threshold. The calculated standard deviation score evaluates the risk of ulceration
- Semmes–Weinstein hairs: nylon monofilaments of the same length but different diameters. If the 5.07 hair can be felt, the patient has protective sensation
- Nerve conduction studies. Can give spurious results if some fibres are conducting and others are not

For vascular status
- Doppler ultrasound
- Ankle/brachial index. Normal value is 1 and a value <1 indicates peripheral vascular disease. Treat with caution in diabetics as calcification of the arteries makes them relatively incompressible and gives spurious results
- Angiography

For infection
- Culture and stain. There is usually a polymicrobial colonization of foot ulcers. Most common organisms are *Staphylococcus aureus*, *Escherichia coli*, *Streptococci* and anaerobes. Give antibiotics only if there is clinical evidence of cellulitis, abscess or evidence of osteomyelitis
- White cell count, ESR
- Plain radiographs looking for osteomyelitis
- Bone scan or labelled white cell scan

Management

- Eliminate infection
- Remove infected bone
- Drain abscesses

Neuropathic ulcers
These are healed by limitation of causative mechanical forces. Strict bed rest is expensive and has a risk of complications. Advise non-weight-bearing on crutches and a total contact plaster cast. Apply a below-knee plaster cast with minimal padding, a rocker for walking, and a hole cut where the ulcer is.

Ischaemic ulcers
These are made worse by total contact plasters. Arteriography is helpful to determine whether angioplasty or bypass surgery is possible.

Ulcers of mixed aetiology
Usually there are more ulcers of one type than of the other. If it does not bleed, it is likely to be ischaemic; if it does, neuropathic. Aim for prevention of further ulceration through good diabetic control and well fitting shoes.

Surgery

- Debridement of infected ulcers, drainage of abscesses and excision of infected bone
- Revascularization of ischaemic foot
- Amputation for gangrene

Oral questions

- Discuss the role of amputation in the diabetic foot
- Describe how to salvage "the foot at risk"

Hallux rigidus

Hallux rigidus is a degenerative arthritis of the first metatarsophalangeal (MTP) joint of the big toe. There is painful limitation of first MTP joint movement particularly dorsiflexion. Later on osteophytes appear on the dorsal and/or lateral articular margin and block extension.

Aetiology

Precise aetiology unknown but may include:
- Single traumatic event
- Repeated minor trauma
- First ray hypermobility
- Metatarsus primus elevatus
- Osteochondritis dissecans
- Gout/pseudogout

History

- Activity- and shoe-related pain that is increased with dorsiflexion
- Stiffness
- Difficulty in wearing high heels
- Increased bulk of the joint, which makes shoe wearing difficult
- Difficulty in the push-off phase of running
- Patient's expectations of surgery

Examination

- Confirm painful limitation of movement at the MTP joint
- Assess the presence of marginal osteophytes, which are typically dorsally and laterally
- Is there increased bulk of the joint?
- Check motion at IP joint (it should be mobile)
- Assess the neurovascular status of the foot
- Dorsal medial cutaneous nerve is often sensitive
- Assess the presence of other foot pathology, e.g. lesser toe deformities, metatarsalgia, etc.

Investigations

Weight-bearing AP and lateral radiographs. Assess the degree of arthrosis at the MTP joint and any other foot pathology.

Management

Conservative treatment

Do nothing, reassurance. Advise the patient to use rigid, moulded and stiff insoles or rocker bottom insoles.

Limited surgical procedure

MUA and intra-articular steroid injection

May provide relief of symptoms in mild/moderate cases. Not proven to be effective if severe changes are present.

Cheilectomy

Removal of the dorsal osteophyte and part of the metatarsal head. A large portion of the motion achieved intra-operatively will be lost postoperatively. The principle is to change the arc of motion of the joint. Some patients, because the range of motion is increased in an arthritic joint, may complain of increased pain rather than relief of pain postoperatively. Need to warn patients about this preoperatively.

Closing wedge osteotomy of the proximal phalanx

Again this operation changes the arc of motion from flexion to extension.

More definitive surgical procedure

Keller's procedure

Particularly suited for the elderly patient with limited ambulatory capacity.

Arthrodesis

Gold standard for severe disease. Position of fusion: 15° valgus and 25° dorsiflexion with respect to the metatarsal. The IP joint should be mobile. An arthrodesis resolves pain, however at the expense of loss of motion. There is a loss of pivoting movement during sports and the loss of an ability to wear high heels.

Silastic® implant

This procedure has variable clinical success. It could possibly be used in a low-demand, elderly patient. Complications include silicone synovitis, implant wear and deformity, implant breakage, infection, recurrent deformity and loss of motion.

MTP joint replacement

This is a ceramic implant. It is an acceptable procedure in most centres. There is limited evidence on the durability of the newer implants. Complications include persistent pain, infection, implant loosening, implant fracture, osteolysis, bone over-production, cyst formation and transfer metatarsalgia.

Complications of surgery

- Transfer metatarsalgia
- Inability to wear high heels (fusion)
- Loss of pivoting sports (fusion)

- Non-union/delayed union (fusion)
- Stability variable (Silastic® implant)
- Cock-up toe (Silastic® implant)
- Stress fractures (Silastic® implant)
- Silicone synovitis (Silastic® implant)

Hallux valgus

Introduction

This is an important topic that tends to crop up in either the short cases or adult and pathology oral. It is an oral topic you can easily botch up if you say something silly or your answer jumps about back and forth. In the FRCS Orth oral there is a typical case scenario that the examiners usually present, with rules to follow and a specific set answer required in order to negotiate your way through this topic. If you break the rules there is only one winner and it will not be you. Familiarize yourself with the case scenario and practise your answer. Better still go through a dry run with your consultant so that you become more confident with your answer.

Hallux valgus is a lateral deviation of the big toe at the MTP joint. It is associated with other anatomical deformities, which occur concurrently. These include:
- Medial deviation of the first MTP joint
- Subluxation or dislocation of the first MTP joint
- The capsule becomes contracted laterally whilst attenuated medially
- Pronation of the big toe
- The sesamoid ridge on the plantar surface of the first metatarsal head (crista) flattens and the sesamoid complex shifts laterally
- Abductor hallucis tendon (plantar and medial) shifts further plantar-wards accentuating the pronation deformity
- Adductor hallucis tendon pulls the great toe into valgus
- ± Changes at the cuneiform metatarsal joint

Angle values

- Normal hallux valgus angle <15°
- Normal inter-metatarsal angle <9°

- Distal metatarsal articular angle <100°

These angle values are important to learn as the examiners have a very low tolerance threshold if you get them wrong or mixed up. To confuse matters further these values were put the wrong way around in a couple of older orthopaedic textbooks.

Aetiology

Can be either idiopathic or secondary.

Idiopathic

Aetiology is uncertain/poorly understood. Undoubtedly there is a familial tendency. It is still unclear whether metatarsus primus varus is a causative or contributing factor.

Secondary

Rheumatoid arthritis, poorly fitted shoe-wear, connective tissue disorders and cerebral palsy.

Classification

Based on the severity of clinical deformity. Try to be objective and mention angles if possible to quantify things (Table 18.1).

Management

History

- How old is the patient?
- Occupation
- Activity level
- What is the principal/chief complaint: is it pain, deformity (cosmesis) or difficulty wearing shoes?
- Where is the pain felt: bunion, metatarsal heads (metatarsalgia), MTP joint, over a callosity?
- Where is the area of maximum discomfort and what is the character of the pain?
- Onset and progression of the deformity
- Patient's expectations from surgery
- Night pain or other non-mechanical pain should prompt a search for other causes

Table 18.1 Angle values in hallux valgus

	Hallux valgus angle (°)	Intermetatarsal angle (°)
Normal	<15	<9
Mild	20–30	11–13
Moderate	30–40	13–20
Severe	>40	>20

Examination

- Is the deformity fully correctable?
- What is the range of movement of the MTP joint in both uncorrected and corrected positions and the range of movement of the IP joint?
- Is it painful when correcting the deformity?
- Grind test on the MTP joint (be careful, do not hurt the patient)
- What is the neurovascular status of the foot, and the condition of the skin and soft tissues?
- Are there lesser toe deformities (particularly the second toe)?
- Are there plantar callosities?
- Is there a tight tendon Achilles (dorsiflexion of the big toe)?
- Is there ulceration over the medial eminence?
- Pronation of the big toe
- Dystrophic changes nails, etc.
- Is there a bursitis around the metatarsal head?
- Splaying forefoot, metatarsalgia?
- With the patient standing: observe the hallux deformity, longitudinal arch foot and hindfoot posture
- Gait pattern

Radiographs

Standing (weight-bearing) anteroposterior and lateral radiographs foot. Comment on:
- Hallux valgus (HVA) angle, interphalangeal angle
- Intermetatarsal (IMT) angle
- Distal metatarsal articular angle

- Congruency of the MTP joint (radiograph looks like an ice cream scoop on top of a cone)
- Presence of arthrosis of the first MTP joint?
- Is the first MTP joint subluxed or dislocated?
- Are the sesamoids dislocated?
- Relative lengths of the first and second metatarsals (some osteotomies will shorten the first ray)
- Angulation of the first metatarsocuneiform joint
- Lesser toe deformities

Management

Based on:
- Patient's age
- Severity of the deformity
- The presence of first MTP joint arthrosis
- Whether the MTP joint is congruent or not

Conservative

Reassurance. Modification of shoe wear – soft, wide, toe box, stretching the shoe over the bunion region, sandal type of shoe, etc.

Progression

Progression tends to occur with a hallux valgus angle >25° or associated subluxation of the joint.

Surgery

This is indicated for a painful, progressive deformity that is unresponsive to conservative management in which a patient accepts the risks of surgery.

Types of procedures
- Medial eminence resection
- Distal soft-tissue realignment (STR) procedure: McBride, Mann
- Distal metatarsal osteotomy: Chevron, Wilson, Mitchell
- Proximal metatarsal osteotomy: crescentic osteotomy, opening wedge medial osteotomy, closing wedge lateral osteotomy, Z osteotomy
- Scarf osteotomy
- Keller's excision arthroplasty

- Silastic® implant
- Arthrodesis

At the end of the chosen procedure, the position of the hallux is observed visually and if it is still in slight valgus or slightly malrotated, a "fine tuning" phalangeal osteotomy can be added. For very severe fixed deformities it is usually necessary to perform an osteotomy on the phalanx.

An Akin procedure is a closing wedge proximal phalangeal osteotomy and medial eminence resection.

Complications of surgery

- Recurrence
- Under- and overcorrection of the deformity (poor cosmesis)
- Transfer metatarsalgia
- Hallux varus
- AVN of the metatarsal head
- Mal-union, non-union of osteotomy
- Flat, floppy short hallux (Keller's)
- Stiffness and arthritis
- Hallux extensus

Self assessment question

Discuss the conservative management and appropriate surgery indicated for a given clinical example of hallux valgus.

Examination corner

Adult elective orthopaedics oral 1

Clinical photograph of a female patient with a severe hallux valgus deformity.

Examiner: This 48-year-old lady presents to your clinic complaining about this foot deformity.

Candidate: This is a clinical photograph, which demonstrates a severe left hallux valgus deformity. There is no obvious ulceration of her bunion but the skin over it appears atrophic, shiny and red.

Examiner: How are you going to manage this patient?

Candidate: I would take a full history and perform a clinical examination of the patient. I would want to know if she has

any pain in the big toe … (at this point the candidate was cut short by the examiner).

Examiner: She has pain and she cannot wear normal shoes.

Candidate: Although she has a severe deformity I would still like to try conservative management.[1]

Examiner: Come on now, is conservative management likely to be successful in this lady?

Candidate: Not really, no.

Examiner: These are her radiographs.

Candidate: I would need to calculate the hallux valgus angle and intermetatarsal angle.

Examiner: What are the normal values for these angles?

Candidate: The normal hallux valgus angle is 9° and the normal intermetatarsal angle is 15°.

Examiner: I think you are a bit confused and have got them mixed up. Never mind let's move on to another topic you may know more about.

[Candidate failed oral]

Standard examination protocol dictates that when discussing management options we are always told to mention conservative treatment first. Generally speaking to jump in and start discussing surgery without first reference to it can be an invitation for trouble. Equally so you can dig a hole for yourself if you mention conservative management for a severe hallux valgus deformity and do not quantify your answer as with the above candidate.

A better reply would be, *"This lady has a severe hallux valgus deformity and I would offer her a basal metatarsal osteotomy for the condition if she is willing to accept the risks of surgery."*

Or covering all bases, *"This lady has a severe hallux valgus deformity, conservative management is unlikely to be successful in this case and I would offer her surgery. Conservative management certainly has a place in a less severe deformity and is a perfectly acceptable form of management for mild deformities."*

Adult elective orthopaedics oral 2

Clinical photograph of a middle-aged female with severe hallux valgus deformity

Candidate: This is a clinical photograph, which demonstrates a severe hallux valgus deformity of her left big toe.

Examiner: She is complaining of severe pain in her bunion. How are you going to manage her?

Candidate: Even though it is a severe hallux valgus deformity and conservative management is unlikely to be helpful I still think we should initially consider it.

Examiner: It is not likely to be successful though, surely.

Candidate: No it is not but before I would consider surgery I would like to find out a little bit more about her pain, whether the MTP joint has arthrosis, how old she was …[2] (candidate was interrupted).

Examiner: She is 52; she has pain only in the bunion.

Candidate: I would like to examine the foot paying particular attention to the neurovascular status because if it is compromised I will not be performing any surgery on her.

Examiner: Good.

Candidate: She is 52 so a Keller's procedure would not be a good choice for her as she is too young. If there is arthritis at the MTP joint then my preference would be to perform a distal osteotomy such as a Wilson's procedure or Mitchell's osteotomy. I realize that a basal osteotomy is used by some surgeons to treat a severe hallux valgus but I am not familiar with this procedure. I have read about it but never seen one performed.[3]

Examiner: How do you do a Mitchell's osteotomy? Why don't you draw it out for us? Here is a pen and paper.

Candidate: This is the metatarsal and I would perform a double osteotomy here.[4]

Examiner: Where?

Candidate: At the neck.

Examiner: That's fine; it is not quite clear on your diagram.

Candidate: I would then displace the metatarsal laterally and secure the displacement with a screw through the two fragments.[5]

[Candidate failed]

They wanted the candidate to discuss more fully the various surgical procedures available to manage a severe hallux valgus and how to perform them. They were not particularly interested in the history or examination findings and wanted to hurry the candidate along so that they could discuss the technical details of the operation. It is much safer to go through the history, examination and investigations regime if they allow you to do so if only to avoid getting caught out in the technical details of an operation.

Examiners: The candidate was not confident in the management of hallux valgus

Adult elective orthopaedics oral 3

Hallux valgus in a young patient

- Diagnosis including radiographs

- Various angles to consider
- Management

Adult elective orthopaedics oral 4

Hallux valgus

- Detailed questioning
- Things to look for in history and examination
- Angles
- Scenarios for treatment
- Metatarsal cuneiform fusion

Adult elective orthopaedics oral 5

Clinical picture of mild hallux valgus deformity

- Full discussion on hallux valgus
- Pathogenesis
- Angles

Examiner: What would you do for this patient?

Candidate: A distal osteotomy.

Discussion about consent for the procedure then took place and the candidate was asked to draw a diagram showing the distal osteotomy.

Adult elective orthopaedics oral 6

Surgical options for a severe hallux valgus deformity.

[1] The oral topic was lost at this stage because the candidate's reply was not particularly well thought out. The candidate first failed to mention the need for standing weight-bearing AP and lateral radiographs and what he/she would look for with them. The examiner alluded to this later on.

[2] This candidate has an unfortunate turn of phrase with this answer. Be careful when mentioning conservative management for a severe hallux valgus deformity. The candidate has not explained clearly enough the role of conservative management either generally or in this patient's specific case.

[3] The candidate's answer jumps about too much. The candidate mentioned conservative management and then backtracked and started to discuss history and examination findings. No mention at all about the role of radiographs in the management of the procedure although they were right there on the table.

[4] You should be aware of basal metatarsal osteotomies and be able to describe how to perform one if asked. I presume the examiners were wanting to discuss this for the management of a severe hallux valgus deformity. The candidate's answer was more of an excuse than anything else and certainly not good enough for the examiners. Most foot and ankle surgeons prefer to perform either a basal osteotomy or a scarf procedure for a severe deformity.

[5] The candidate was not detailed enough in their description of how to perform a Mitchell's osteotomy. A few extra details were needed to safely satisfy the examiners.

Interdigital neuroma

You may be given a clinical photograph showing an exposed interdigital neuroma in the foot or an excised digital neuroma.

Definition

A neuroma consists of degeneration and fibrotic changes in the common digital nerve near its bifurcation.

Aetiology

Unknown. There may be similar changes in unaffected nerves. Several causative factors have been suggested, although none is universally accepted.

- Tethering of the third space nerve by an anastomotic branch between the medial and lateral plantar nerves
- Traction on the nerve by hindfoot valgus, interdigital bursitis or forced toe dorsiflexion in high-heeled shoes
- The edge of the transverse intermetatarsal ligament causing compression of the nerve

Symptoms

Can be non-specific:
- Burning, tingling pain over the involved toes, exacerbated by shoe wear
- Neuralgic sharp pain in a toe and/or interdigital space
- Colour changes
- Numb or dead toe
- Pain worse on walking, sometimes at night
- Vague forefoot tingling

Diagnosis

History

Trauma to the foot, spinal problems (nerve root entrapment), peripheral neuropathy (diabetes), tarsal tunnel syndrome, etc.

Examination

Examine for local pain and tenderness of the involved nerve in the intermetatarsal space. Look for any other factors likely to produce metatarsalgia.

Special investigations

- Standing AP and lateral weight-bearing forefoot films to exclude other forefoot pathology
- MRI (preferred over ultrasound scan)
- Ultrasound scan

Some surgeons would operate without obtaining an MRI scan if the history and examination were very suggestive of a Morton's neuroma.

Other surgeons would reserve an MRI scan for doubtful cases. Still others would obtain a scan in all cases, the reasoning being that it is preferable to attempt to obtain a diagnosis before committing yourself to surgery. There may be no evidence of a neuroma on a scan; in this case are you still going to operate based on history/examination findings?

Diagnostic tests

- A local anaesthetic injection into the affected space that relieves symptoms supports the diagnosis
- Mulder's click on metatarsal compression. Reproduces the patient's pain in the involved web space

Differential diagnosis

- Synovitis
- Bursitis
- Metatarsalgia
- Trauma to the foot

- Tarsal tunnel syndrome suggested by discomfort around the ankle
- Spinal disorder: HNP, history of nerve root entrapment
- Peripheral neuropathy, diabetes
- Chronic inflammatory disorders

Management

Conservative

Advise the patient to wear sensible shoes, a metatarsal pad, and to avoid high heels. Corticosteroid injection can be successful especially if the history is short.

Surgery

Interdigital neurectomy. The nerve is divided 2–3 cm proximal to the bifurcation and excised. Plantar or dorsal approach ±partial release of the intermetatarsal ligament.

Symptoms are commonest in the third interdigital space; the second space is the next most common site; symptoms are rare in the fourth space and are virtually unknown in the first space.

Consent

Warn patients of the 80% success rate and that it may take several months to realize the full benefit of the procedure. Patients may develop a painful scar. The neuroma can re-form and cause symptoms that are worse than the original problem. Warn about the area of numbness in the web space.

Short case 1

A 40-year-old female with a history suggestive of Morton's right foot (intermittent stabbing/burning in the forefoot aggravated with wearing high heels)

   Well-healed dorsal scar left third interspace.
- Diagnosis
- Demonstration of Mulder's click-pain and click when the involved web space was compressed between thumb and index finger while the forefoot was squeezed
- Differential diagnosis (stress fracture, Freiberg's disease, bursitis, tarsal tunnel syndrome)

Nerve supply foot and ankle[4]

Anatomy

Posterior tibial nerve

The posterior tibial nerve (branch of the sciatic nerve) enters the deep posterior compartment of the leg between the two heads of the gastrocnemius. It travels deep to soleus, between it and tibialis posterior. It branches into medial and lateral plantar nerves, and calcaneal sensory branches.

Medial plantar nerve
Motor to:
- Abductor hallucis
- Flexor hallucis brevis
- Flexor digitorum brevis
- First lumbrical
Sensory to:
- 3½ digits, like the median nerve in the hand

Lateral plantar nerve
Motor to:
- Adductor hallucis
- Dorsal and palmar interossei
- Second to fifth lumbricals
- Abductor digiti minimi
Sensory to:
- 1½ digits
Calcaneal sensory branches provide sensation to the heel pad.

Saphenous nerve (branch of the femoral nerve)

Supplies the anteromedial side of the leg down to the dorsomedial ankle and midfoot.

Deep peroneal nerve

Supplies the web space between the first and second toes (first web space).

---

[4] On several occasions I have seen examiners throw in the nerve supply of the foot and ankle during a discussion of a foot/ankle topic as a quick aside to test your anatomy knowledge.

Superficial peroneal nerve

Exits the deep fascia anterolaterally about 8–12 cm above the tip of the fibula. Supplies the dorsum of the foot except the first web space. It descends in peroneus longus until it reaches the peroneus brevis, and passes over the anterior border of peroneus brevis and descends between it and EDL.

Sural (medial) nerve

The sural nerve (a branch of the tibial nerve) pierces the superficial aponeurosis half-way down the leg between the two bellies of the gastrocnemius and is joined by the peroneal communicating nerve. It supplies the lateral aspect of the heel, the fifth metatarsal and small toe. It is accompanied by the small saphenous vein.

Charcot foot/ neuropathic foot disease[5]

Most likely a radiographic spot diagnosis of a Charcot foot. This may lead on to discussion of the various stages of a Charcot foot and the management of the condition.

A Charcot foot is a chronic painless but accelerated degenerative process affecting the weight-bearing joints of the foot.

Aetiology

- Diabetes (foot)
- Tabes dorsalis (lower extremity)
- Syringomyelia (elbow and shoulder, Horner's, wasted hand muscles, etc.)
- Progressive sensory neuropathy
- Myelomeningocele (ankle and foot)
- Congenital insensitivity to pain
- Neurofibromatosis (pressure on sensory nerves)
- Hereditary motor sensory neuropathy (Charcot–Marie–Tooth)
- Peripheral neuropathies (alcohol, amyloidosis, etc.)

---

[5] On several occasions I have seen examiners throw in the nerve supply of the foot and ankle during a discussion of a foot/ankle topic as a quick aside to test your anatomy knowledge.

- Infection (yaws, TB)

Diabetes is the most common cause of a Charcot foot. Usually patients are insulin-dependent diabetics in their fifth or sixth decade who have generally had diabetes for more than 12 years. It is still a rare complication of diabetes seen in only approximately 1% of patients.

Pathology

Repeated minor trauma in the neuropathic foot with loss of protective sensation allows abnormal mechanical stresses that are normally prevented by pain. This leads to spontaneous fractures, subluxations and dislocations.

Autonomic neuropathy can increase blood flow leading to a weakening of the bone by osteoporosis.

Stages of the natural history of a Charcot joint

Development stage

Acute inflammation characterized by a swollen, hot, erythematous and painless foot. Radiographs may reveal healing fractures.

Coalescent stage

The foot collapses, the arch flattens, and the foot has a rocker-bottom appearance. There is progressive bone destruction, new bone formation and subluxation/dislocation. There is a risk of ulceration. Radiographs reveal evidence of periosteal new bone formation and osteopenia.

Reconstruction stage

There is a stable but deformed shape to the foot, which can create pressure points for ulceration. Radiographs reveal a totally disorganized joint, the resolution of osteopenia and bone healing. The whole process may span 2–3 years.

Early management

Exclude infection by WCC, ESR, joint aspiration, white cell scans, etc. Elevation of the joint for 10 min causes a significant reduction in erythema in the Charcot joint. Clinical acumen is just as important as laboratory and radiological investigations.

Avoid surgery if possible. Avoid weight bearing to prevent progressive destruction of the joints or apply a total-contact cast to keep the patient active and to prevent disuse osteoporosis. Patients may require a plaster for several months.

Late management

- If rocker-bottom deformity is already present wait until the patient has a negative bone scan and then offer reconstruction (e.g. midfoot wedge osteotomy)
- Advise the patient to modify their shoe wear
- Offer bony reconstruction by arthrodesis only to salvage a severe, non-braceable deformity
- Amputation for gangrene or uncontrolled infection

Rheumatoid foot

Introduction

The two predominant symptoms of the rheumatoid foot are pain and deformity. Approximately 15% of rheumatoid patients present initially with foot symptoms. Eventually 70%–90% of those with long-standing rheumatoid arthritis have foot involvement. The disease starts in the forefoot and with time advances to involve the hindfoot.

Clinical features

- Valgus ankle, which often presents late with pain and instability
- Valgus hindfoot with synovitis and arthritis in the subtalar joint
- Swelling of tendons both medially and laterally around the ankle
- Tenosynovitis of tibialis posterior tendon
- Impingement of the peroneal tendons
- Collapse of the medial longitudinal arch of the foot due to rupture or weakening of the tibialis posterior tendon. The head of the talus can sublux

medially and inferiorly from the navicular and may weight bear
- Pronation of the forefoot (collapse of the medial longitudinal arch and valgus heel swings the heel into pronation)
- Dorsally subluxed MTP joints (synovitis of the MTP joints, weakening and stretching the capsule and collateral ligaments, volar plate laxity)
- Hammertoe and claw toe deformities of the lesser toes (contracture of intrinsic muscle)
- Distal migration and atrophy of the forefoot pad; metatarsal heads are forced plantar-wards leading to plantar callosities
- Large painful bursae develop between the skin and metatarsal heads
- Burning and paresthesia in the tibial nerve distribution secondary to tarsal tunnel syndrome
- Morton's neuroma
- Retrocalcaneal bursitis

Examination

Several issues need clarifying before committing oneself to surgery.

Assess the hip and knee before foot surgery. Assess the skin condition for risk of infection and wound healing.
Also:
- Assess the vascular status of the foot
- Make a careful neurological assessment as there may be a neuropathic component
- Look for tendinopathy or ruptured tendons
- Assess whether the primary deformity is in the hindfoot or forefoot
- Determine which joint is causing pain: this is not always easy and may need a diagnostic injection
- Take a drug history, in particular steroid therapy and methotrexate

Management

Conservative

- Special shoes/footwear
- Accommodating orthoses
- Steroid injections

Surgery

If both the forefoot and hindfoot are involved, care is needed to decide which to operate on first. If the hindfoot is correctable go for forefoot surgery first. If the hindfoot is severely deformed and rigid it is often necessary to correct this first.

Forefoot

In the early stages of the disease a synovectomy may alleviate symptoms. Carry out a forefoot resection arthroplasty. Brattstrom found that resection of the metatarsal heads and basal phalanx does better than resection of just the metatarsal heads alone. Excision arthroplasty of the first MTP joint rather than fusion is recommended,[6] because of failure of fusion in one-third of cases. Some surgeons, however, prefer a stable medial post and will fuse the first MTP joint. Pobble amputation[7].

Hindfoot

Talonavicular fusion is a good operation for early disease, as this will prevent 90% or more of motion in the subtalar joint. With a severe valgus or varus deformity a triple arthrodesis is required.

Oral question

Describe how rheumatoid arthritis affects the foot

Rheumatoid foot. What are main problems? How do you manage the patient?

---

[6] Hughes J, Grace D, Clark P, Klenerman L (1991) Metatarsal head excision for rheumatoid arthritis. 4-year follow-up of 68 feet with and without hallux fusion. *Acta Orthop Scand* **62**: 63–6.

[7] This operation involves amputation of all the lesser toes at the MTP joints. It is used for severe pain and deformity. I have been shown an old radiograph of a rheumatoid foot with the lesser toes missing and asked to comment on what operation was performed.

Examination corner

Adult elective orthopaedics oral 1

Radiographs of a rheumatoid foot with dislocated MTP joints

Discussion about surgical management

Adult elective orthopaedics oral 2

A strange question.

Examiner: A 53-year-old lady attends your orthopaedic clinic complaining of a painful and swollen second left MTP joint. The GP has mentioned a possibility of rheumatoid arthritis. How will you confirm the diagnosis?

Candidate: I would take a history from the patient, find out how long she has had symptoms in the toe.

Examiner: Several months.

Candidate: I would measure ESR, CRP and rheumatoid factor.

Examiner: All normal.

Candidate: I am not sure I would do anything at this stage. Possibly I would send her for an X-ray of the foot.

Examiner: The point here is that you may want to refer her on to a rheumatology colleague for a second opinion. Reviewing her in 6 months is also a reasonable option – she won't come to any harm. The radiograph shows proximal resorption of the proximal phalanx of this second toe.

Candidate: This can occur in rheumatoid disease.

Examiner: Are you just going to accept this?

Candidate: There are other causes for this resorption such as gout and I would measure her serum urate level.

Examiner: Would you not want to biopsy the toe?

Candidate: I would not want to jump in at this stage and biopsy without further information (I was struggling a bit here and wasn't sure what he was getting at).

Examiner: The point here is that other rare conditions can cause this appearance such as PVNS. Let's move on to something else.

Adult elective orthopaedics oral 3

Clinical photograph of rheumatoid forefoot

Splayed foot

Hallux valgus with pronation and under-riding, lesser toe hammering. Vasculitic lesions on shin. We discussed orthotic shoes then Fowler's excision arthroplasty.

Tarsal tunnel syndrome

Compression of the posterior tibial nerve as it passes behind the medial malleolus. This is an entrapment neuropathy (Carpal tunnel syndrome of the foot). The flexor retinaculum constricts the nerve (attached to the medial malleolus and calcaneal tubercle).

The tarsal tunnel is formed by the:

- Contents of the tunnel (behind and distal to the medial malleolus)
- Flexor retinaculum
- Nerve abductor digiti quinti

Patients can have both proximal (whole nerve) and distal (terminal branches especially the lateral plantar nerve 1½ digits) syndromes.

Aetiology

- Accessory FDL muscle
- Proliferative synovitis
- Ganglion in the tendon sheaths
- Varicosities
- Lipomas
- Neurilemma tibial nerve
- Calcaneal fractures

A mass effect within the tunnel, hard or soft. Nerve pain is diffuse and poorly localized, and there is a burning, tingling, numbness and cramping sensation that radiates into the plantar aspect of the foot.

Examination

- Make a general inspection of the foot to assess alignment and bone deformities that could affect nerve function
- Palpate along the medial aspect of the ankle and hindfoot to identify extrinsic sources of compression from tenosynovitis, ganglia, etc.
- Is there paraesthesia and atrophy of foot intrinsics?
- Positive Tinel's sign behind the medial malleoli?
- Manual compression over the tarsal tunnel may reproduce symptoms
- Deep tendon reflexes, muscle testing and straight leg raising

Investigations

Take radiographs to identify exostosis and other bone changes. Nerve conduction studies are 90% accurate in identifying well-established tarsal tunnel entrapment. MRI shows an abnormality in 85% of cases and allows evaluation of the mass effect. Get an MRI so that the diagnosis can be confirmed.

Management

- Steroid injection
- Surgical decompression

Surgery

Make a curved incision that follows the nerve posterior to the medial malleolus. The flexor retinaculum is divided proximal to distal down to abductor hallucis fascia. The calcaneal branches are protected. The medial and lateral plantar nerves are followed and freed beneath the abductor hallucis. The deep fascia of the abductor hallucis should be divided if it is tight. When symptoms dictate, further dissection along the plantar aspect of the foot through the master knot of Henry or beneath the plantar fascia is needed. The master knot of Henry secures the flexor digitorum longus crossing superficially over the flexor hallucis longus.

Re-exploration of the tarsal tunnel is seldom beneficial unless there is clear evidence of inadequate initial decompression.

Anterior tarsal tunnel syndrome

This is entrapment of the distal part of the deep peroneal nerve beneath the dense superficial fascia at the front of the ankle. It is relatively rare, but suspect it in patients with neuritic pain on the dorsum of the foot. There are several potential sites of entrapment, which result in slightly different clinical presentations. With medial branch entrapment there is altered sensation in the first web space. If the lateral branch of the nerve is involved, the extensor brevis will show signs of atrophy.

19

Spine oral core topics

Niall Craig

Surgical approaches

Cervical spine: anterolateral approach (Smith–Robinson)

Background information

- One of the most common approaches to the neck
- Extensile – allows access to all levels
- Uses – anterior discectomy and fusion, anterior corpectomy and fusion or cage insertion for burst fracture, tumour or infection, kyphosis correction and vertebral artery exposure

Technique

- Patient placed in supine position with their head slightly extended and fixed, i.e. in Mayfield clamp
- Skin incision is made along the transverse skin crease or longitudinally
- Risk of recurrent laryngeal palsy is lower with approaches from left
- Platysma incised in line of incision
- Fascia incised anterior to sternocleidomastoid
- Blunt dissection between omohyoid/sternothyroid and midline structures
- Dissect between carotid sheath (laterally) and thyroid (medially) to expose deep fascia
- Can ligate thyroid artery for access
- The prevertebral plane is behind the fascia deep to the posterior pharynx
- Anterior longitudinal ligament divided in midline, retracted laterally with periosteum ±longus colli to improve exposure

Complications

- Injury to recurrent laryngeal nerve, hypoglossal nerve, vascular or visceral injury
- Neck swelling with airway compromise requiring urgent decompression; early dysphagia due to swelling

Cervical spine: posterior approach

Background information

- Access to occiput and posterior elements of cervical spine
- Can access the lateral masses
- Carried out for posterior cervical fusion, decompression of the canal, reduction and fixation for trauma and removal of lateral discs by foraminotomy

Technique

- Skull traction recommended
- Patient prone, head supported (no pressure on eyes)
- The shoulders are taped down, tilt head up
- Midline skin incision at occipitocervical junction; incision from below occipital protuberance to C3
- Fascia divided – access occiput and spinous process of C2
- Sharp dissection of muscle/ligamentous attachments
- Laminae and facet joints are exposed
- Proximally avoid greater occipital nerve

Postgraduate Orthopaedics: The Candidate's Guide to the FRCS (Tr & Orth) Examination, Ed. Paul A. Banaszkiewicz, Deiary F. Kader, Nicola Maffulli. Published by Cambridge University Press. © Cambridge University Press 2009.

- C1 exposed avoiding vertebral artery, venous plexus and the nerve
- Lower cervical spine – incision from C2–C7, followed by midline division of fascia
- Muscles dissected and retracted – expose laminae and lateral masses

Complications

- Poor positioning – problems with ventilation
- Eyes and axillae can be compressed orbital/brachial plexus injuries
- Neurological injury – head movement, instruments or haematoma
- Vertebral artery also at risk, particularly at C1

Thoracic spine: posterior approach

Background information

- Deformity correction
- Resection/stabilization of posterior tumours and fracture fixation, (partial) laminectomy, arthrodesis, instrumentation and costoplasty
- Vertebral size increases down thoracic spine
- Nerve foramina just behind/above rib heads
- Flexion – nerve root sheaths move up above T6 and down below T6
- Canal relatively narrow in thoracic region

Technique

- Patient prone – abdomen free (minimize blood loss)
- Midline incision, curved to convex side (scoliosis)
- Skin infiltration with adrenaline – reduces bleeding
- Spinous process periosteum or apophysis split longitudinally – repair later
- Muscles dissected off posterior elements subperiosteally
- Avoid pressure on eyes, brachial plexus, chest or breasts, ears and iliac crests
- If deficient laminae, use transverse process hooks
- Midthoracic spinal cord and muscles are relatively poorly vascularized so avoid excessive traction

Technique for vertebroplasty

- Percutaneous approach

Thoracic spine: posterolateral approach (costotransversectomy)

Uses

- Perivertebral abscess drainage (TB)
- Thoracic disc prolapse
- Unilateral body resection for small tumours

Technique

- Patient in prone position for bilateral approach or in lateral position for unilateral approach
- Longitudinal incision lateral to spinous process/curved incision – lateral apex
- Dissect through trapezius and latissimus dorsi lateral to the paraspinal muscles
- Detach muscles from rib and retract
- Transverse process and medial rib removed
- Costotransverse ligament/joint capsule dissected subperiosteally, extrapleurally
- Protect root, follow pedicle to vertebral body
- Pleura dissected off anteriorly

Complications

- Avoid damaging neurovascular bundles especially the artery of Adamkiewicz on the left from T8 to L1

Thoracic spine: transthoracic (anterior) approach

Uses

- Corpectomy – tumours, interbody fusion, anterior release deformity correction, disc excision and epiphysiodesis for deformity
- Double approach – extensive multilevel access
- Avoid damage to lung, great vessels and liver
- Avoid ligating more than three contiguous segmental vessels

Technique

- Patient in lateral decubitus position, table flexed
- Incision one to two levels above affected level, extending from paraspinal muscles to midaxillary line
- Trapezius and latissimus dorsi dissected superficially
- One level – remove rib; several levels – remove proximal rib
- Rib dissected subperiosteally and removed preserving intercostal bundles
- Parietal pleura incised
- Lung retracted to expose vertebra
- Nutrient arteries ligated and divided/preserved
- Anterior longitudinal ligament can be elevated
- Can expose/remove pedicle
- Disc removed to posterior longitudinal ligament
- Rib for graft or replaced
- Right side – exposure better, usually use left (vascular control easier)

Lumbar spine: posterior approach

Uses

- Disc enucleation
- Exploration of nerves
- Excision of tumours
- Instrumentation for fusion or fracture fixation

Technique

- Patient's position: prone, kneeling or on supports/cushions (abdomen free) or lateral with supports, affected side up and knees and hips flexed
- Approach: spinous processes palpable; iliac crest – L4/5 disc space
- Start at sacrum and work up or mark level with needle and radiographs
- Midline longitudinal incision over spinous processes; length of incision determined by levels approached
- Dissect between paraspinal (erector spinae) muscles – internervous plane. Two layers – sacrospinalis superficially, multifidus and rotators deep

- Supply – lumbar posterior primary rami. Incise lumbar fascia longitudinally – one or both sides of midline; reflect muscles from spinous processes – Cobb elevator. Apophysis of spinous process split (young patients)
- Dissect laterally across lamina ±facet joints
- Continue down lateral border of facet joint and mammillary process to transverse process – posterolateral fusion. Dissection anterior to intertransverse membrane risks nerve root damage
- Segmental vessels run in angle between transverse processes posteriorly around facets close to posterior primary rami. Cauterize – avoids bleeding
- Clear interlaminar space, expose ligamentum flavum, remove or detach peripherally to expose epidural fat and bluish dura. Blunt dissection laterally to floor of canal; retract dura and roots medially to expose posterior annulus of disc
- Increase exposure – laminotomies and partial undercutting facetectomy to decompress lateral recess
- Careful retraction of roots/dura – prevents nerve root injury, dural tears and CSF leaks
- Abdomen free to reduce venous engorgement and minimize bleeding, free veins carefully from roots/dura, cauterize with bipolar diathermy. Bleeding controlled with patties/thrombin paste or cellulose sponges/gauzes
- Clear nucleus with pituitary Rongeurs – avoid breaching anterior annulus which may be torn. This avoids injuring the aorta, inferior vena cava and iliac vessels
- Can extend (C1 to sacrum) for extensive deformity correction

Lumbar spine: anterior approach

- Upper and middle lumbar spine
- *Uses*: scoliosis, tumours and anterior decompression and fixation of thoracolumbar burst fractures

Thoracolumbar (Hodgson)

- Patient in lateral decubitus position with their limbs and trunk supported. The table should be flat and open at the sides to allow access. Side of approach depends on pathology: approach scoliosis from the convexity; approach an infection from the side of the abscess. Usually left-sided, so avoid IVC and liver

- Resect rib one level above highest vertebra; for example, for L1 or L2 resect the 10th/11th rib
- Make a skin incision over the rib, curved distally and longitudinally. Dissect serratus anterior, external oblique and latissimus dorsi. Remove the rib. Incise the pleura, open the chest and site rib spreaders. Split the costal cartilage to enter the retroperitoneum. Sweep away Gerota's fascia and peritoneum with swabs. Divide the abdominal muscle layers. Divide the diaphragm 2 cm from its origin down to the vertebrae. Make a distal extension for access to S1
- Divide psoas from vertebrae, avoiding nerves. Preserve or ligate segmental vessels; avoid the ligation of three or more vessels because of ischaemia
- Closure – close the diaphragm using marker sutures to help. Suture the costal cartilage anteriorly ±retroperitoneal drain. Close abdominal muscles separately. Place a chest drain before rib approximation. Close pleura, periosteum and intercostal muscles. Suture serratus anterior and latissimus dorsi separately

Lower lumbar spine

Uses

- Anterior discectomy and fusion or disc replacement
- Corpectomy and cages for tumour, trauma and infection

Technique

- Pararectal retroperitoneal approach
- Patient supine with their hips/knees slightly flexed
- Make a skin incision in the midline. Incise the linea alba, lift the left rectus and retract it laterally (preserve segmental nerve supply). Incise the

posterior rectus sheath laterally above the arcuate line. Find the peritoneal edge. Extend the sheath incision proximally/distally. Avoid entering the peritoneum. Enter the retroperitoneal space and sweep away the peritoneum with a swab; expose psoas (nerves on surface), ureter and iliac vessels. For **L5/S1** dissect the lumbosacral plexus with a pledget. Avoid injury (risk of retrograde ejaculation in males). Ligate/divide the median sacral vessels and expose the disc (retract vessels in bifurcation). For **L4/5** retract the aorta/IVC to the right. Ligate and divide segmental vessels at L5 and the iliolumbar vein/ascending lumbar vein

- Closure: close the rectus sheath, being careful to prevent hernias. This procedure should only be done by surgeons familiar with the anatomy (general or vascular surgeon recommended)
- For patients who have had previous surgery, who have scarring or who are having revision surgery, use the transperitoneal approach for L5/S1. Patient's position should be supine and Trendelenburg. Incision: lower midline/Pfannenstiel. Divide the linea alba and peritoneum at the midline. Retract the mesentery/small bowel superiorly, sigmoid to the left. Incise the posterior peritoneum longitudinally 2 cm to the right of the midline. Dissect fat/hypogastric plexus bluntly, and ligate/divide the median sacral vessels if they are intact. Expose the disc by retraction of vessels. Close the posterior peritoneum, avoiding torsion of the mesenteric root. Close the peritoneum and rectus sheath separately

Pathology of the spine

The ageing spine and degenerative disc disease

- Age-related changes affect particularly the intervertebral discs in the spine
- Normal intervertebral disc has an outer portion (annulus fibrosus) and a central portion (nucleus). The annulus is composed mainly of type I collagen fibres (strong cross-links) and resists compression/

hoop stresses well. Nucleus: a loosely arranged collection of type II collagen with a high content of hydrophilic glycosaminoglycans

- In young normal adults: the nuclei are well hydrated (hydrophilic properties) and show up as white on T_2-weighted MRI images. With age the annulus changes, and there is less type I and more type III collagen. The bonds become less strong with age and the discs cannot withstand forces as well as they used to. The annulus splits and the nucleus can prolapse/herniate, which can lead to sciatica. The annulus is thinnest posterolaterally, such that posterolateral disc prolapses are common. The nucleus also degenerates: the water content drops such that its appearance is dark or black on T_2-weighted MRI images
- There are secondary age-related changes in the facet joints, e.g. arthrosis (osteophytes or cysts). This can lead to root irritation or compression
- Modic endplate changes occur, which show up as increased uptake on various MRI sequences

Paediatric spine

Cervical spine

Anatomy

- Congenital anomalies – failure of fusion or of segmentation
- C1 has two posterior ossification centres – synchondrosis
- Two anterior synchondroses appear at 6–24 months. They fuse by 4–6 years of age (space for cord defined at this age)
- Posterior bifid arches in 5%
- Dens – two ossification centres – fuse by 3 months. At 8–10 years the ossiculum terminale forms, and fuses to rest at 10–13 years
- Facet orientation changes as the spine develops
- In a young child, the cervical spine can stretch without injury but the cord can be injured without bony injury, so-called SCIWORA
- Ligamentous laxity/shallow facet angles – translation (pseudosubluxation) usually at C2/3

- Normal motion must be differentiated from pathological motion: a line is drawn from the posterior arch of C1 to the posterior arch of C3. The posterior arch of C2 lies on or behind the line if normal
- The large head results in a higher fulcrum, i.e. at C2/3 rather than at C5/6 as seen in adults

Congenital disorders

Basilar impression

- Lateral radiographs show indentation in the skull base made by the upper cervical spine
- Diagnosis – CT and MRI
- Signs – odontoid peg compresses the brainstem and obstructs CSF flow. The dens is below the foramen magnum so neurological compromise is rare
- Associations
  - Vertebral anomalies, Klippel–Feil syndrome, achondroplasia, spondyloepiphyseal dysplasia and Morquio syndrome
- Secondary impression can be caused by conditions that soften bone. It is often of little consequence
- Management
  - Surgery can help the possible associations, i.e. syringomyelia, Arnold-Chiari malformation, atlantoaxial instability and cord compression
- Prognosis – often little consequence
  - Hydrocephalus due to CSF flow obstruction
  - Cord compression can lead to weakness/ spasticity

Occipitalization of the atlas

- May be an incidental radiographic finding. C2 and C3 are also fused, which leads to atlantoaxial instability with neurological compromise
- Half of cases have basilar impression
- Diagnosis is difficult in younger children because their bones are not ossified; dynamic radiographs and CT and MRI scan are helpful
- Treatment – an arthrodesis is required for those with instability. Reduction is dangerous so fixation in situ is recommended: craniectomy and

posterior arch excision with fixation have good results

Odontoid anomalies
- Types
  - Aplasia, hypoplasia and os odontoideum formation
  - Aplasia is rare
  - Hypoplasia accompanies dysmorphic conditions. Can all cause atlantoaxial instability or vertebral artery compression
- Diagnosis – dynamic radiographs/CT are helpful
- Management – surgery is performed for significant instability (for those children with an atlanto–dens interval >5 mm)

Klippel–Feil syndrome
- Congenital failure of segmentation of any part of the cervical spine
- Occurs at 3rd to 8th weeks of gestation
- Associations – Sprengel's shoulder and other congenital anomalies
- Signs – low posterior hairline, short neck and reduced ROM seen in 50%; often flexion/extension well preserved; scoliosis in 60%, half require treatment; 14% have heart disease; 30% have deafness. Most are normal and symptoms develop in adulthood
- Management – most do not require surgery, only if they have neurological symptoms

Congenital muscular torticollis
- Signs
  - Painless for the first 2 months of life
  - Sternocleidomastoid contracts and the head tilts to that side and the chin to other
  - Palpable mass; often resolves by 1 year. Fibrosis can compromise the accessory nerve making the deformity worse
- Aetiology – ? muscle ischaemia – an isolated phenomenon
- Differential diagnosis – tumours, congenital bony deformities of cervical spine
- Associations – unless it resolves plagiocephaly develops, 20% have hip dysplasia

- Treatment – 90% respond to physiotherapy (passive stretches); start before 1 year; surgical resection required if not responding to physiotherapy

Developmental problems
- Atlantoaxial instability
- Associations
  - Morquio syndrome, spondyloepiphyseal dysplasia, Larsen's syndrome and achondroplasia
  - 25% of children with Down's syndrome
- Diagnosis – atlanto–dens interval >5 mm is diagnostic
- Management
  - Patients with >10 mm interval and neurological symptoms require surgery
  - Down's – frequent complications
  - Fixed dislocation not reduced – decompress and fix in situ
  - Decompress and fix in situ if there is pharyngeal infection or Grisel's syndrome
  - Torticollis can result
  - Most resolve – if not they require posterior fixation

Cervical kyphosis
- Aetiology – post-laminectomy or congenital, traumatic, metabolic conditions or tumours
- Early intervention prevents problems

Juvenile rheumatoid arthritis
- Can affect cervical spine
- Atlantoaxial instability – less common than in adults
- Stiffness, widespread X-ray changes seen
- Little pain unless fracture or infection

Vertebral disc calcification
- Uncommon in childhood – often at C6/7
- 30% trauma, 15% previous infection
- Pain, stiffness and torticollis; 25% have a fever
- Most resolve rapidly – neurological deficits settle in 90% patients with conservative management

Neoplasms

- Primary neoplasms are rare
- Benign lesions include osteochondromas, hae-mangiomas and osteoblastomas. Eosinophilic granulomas – vertebra plana
- Wedging with infection or Ewing's sarcoma
- Neurofibromatosis can cause extensive bone loss
- Diagnosis – imaging or biopsy by treating surgeon

Trauma

- Cervical spine fracture rare in children. Under 8 years of age, fracture of occiput to C2 is the commonest
- Older children have same pattern as for adults. High index of suspicion with head injury
- Juvenile spine boards have recesses to accommo-date the patient's head size and so avoid flexing the cervical spine
- Atlanto-occipital injury is usually fatal
- Diagnosis is important, avoid traction
- Power's ratio is important
- SCIWORA – in up to 20% of cases. Odontoid frac-tures are most common around 4 years and may have associated epiphyseal injuries. Non-surgical treatment usually successful
- Follow-up of fractures is important to avoid late angulation
- Compression fractures are rare. Older children – vertebral endplates are not ossified and so can be injured. Discs are rarely involved

Thoracolumbar spine

Congenital scoliosis

- Prognosis depends upon deformity type, location and age at onset
- Block vertebrae seldom cause severe deform-ity. Hemivertebrae can cause severe deformity unless incarcerated. Fully segmented have open discs either side. These have the highest chance of progression. Double hemivertebrae can progress unless on opposite sides when they can balance each other out. Unilateral unsegmented bars usually lead to progression. Early arthrodesis pre-vents severe deformity. MRI is recommended as part of pre-operative assessment (can have asso-ciated neurological anomalies)
- Treatment
  - Posterior bilateral arthrodesis – with anterior arthrodesis as this avoids the crankshaft phe-nomenon (continued anterior growth after posterior fusion) especially with lordosis. With hemivertebrae, hemiepiphysiodesis can be effective with post-operative casting
  - Excise hemivertebrae. Correction with instru-mentation is relatively risky

Congenital kyphosis

- Failure of formation or segmentation. Anterior failure of formation is the worst form and can lead to paraplegia. Posterior correction can be required for <55°
- Larger curves – a combination of anterior/poste-rior approaches is best. An interbody arthrodesis is performed to arrest growth using a strut graft close to the vertebral body. Correction is among the most risky of spinal operations

Adolescent idiopathic scoliosis

- Curves >10° in 2%–3% of all children and >20° in 0.2%–0.3%. Much more common in females than in males: ratio = 4–6:1. In 20% the parent is affected
- Aetiology – unknown. Numerous theories exist:
  - In some there is a genetic component, with sev-eral affected family members
  - Gene probes are used to map the genome of these families
  - Balance abnormalities or muscular imbalance
  - Sagittal imbalance important
  - Often lordosis
  - Most cases involve thoracic rotation to the right; most left thoracic curves are not idiopathic
  - MRI scan can show cord tethers, Arnold–Chiari malformation or syrinx formation even with normal neurological examination

- Screening advocated. Most patients requiring surgery present before age 10 (Risser sign of 0 or 1)
- Risk of progression
  - Higher for those with large curves, thoracic and double curves and for those who are premenarchal at presentation
  - With curves of 20°–29°, 68% of those who are Risser 0 or 1 and 22% of those who are Risser 2–4 progress
  - Follow-up every 6 months is recommended
  - Males stop growing later than females so later progression is possible
  - Larger curves can affect vital capacity
- Radiographs
  - Cobb angle measurement error 5°–10°
  - The end vertebrae are carefully selected
  - Large X-ray doses are incurred in longer-term surveillance so take PA radiographs to reduce thyroid/breast exposure
  - MRI quick scan surveillance methods are being developed
- Management
  - Bracing
    - Controversial for curves 20°–40° in immature spines
    - Compliance a problem
    - Stressful for patient/family
    - Lung function can be affected
    - Various braces used: underarm braces for curve apices below T8
    - Continue until skeletal maturity
    - Some progress after bracing
    - Compensatory curves can increase with bracing
  - Exercise programmes alone – no value
  - Transcutaneous electrical stimulation – no proven benefit
  - Surgery
    - The mainstay was posterior correction for many years using Harrington rods with a neurological complication rate <1% but a pseudoarthrosis rate of up to 10%
    - Hook constructs such as C-D and TSRH were more effective

- Now there are many pedicle screw systems, which are more powerful and improve and maintain the correction better
- De-rotation aids cosmesis and improves rib hump
- No prolonged immobilization postoperatively
- Often correct hypokyphosis. Severe, fixed curves are fixed through anterior release and fixation with rods and screws. This aids de-rotation and allows shorter instrumentation. However, this can be kyphogenic
- With King II curves (thoracic curve larger), usually only the thoracic curve needs to be instrumented. Extend the bottom of the instrumentation to Moe's stable vertebra. Extend to sacrum only if absolutely necessary
- The lower the level of the arthrodesis, the higher the risk of back pain. Avoid overcorrection of the main curve as this can exacerbate compensatory curves
- Surgery should only be carried out in selected centres, with full PICU and neurophysiological monitoring expertise
- Note risk of Crankshaft phenomenon, which can occur in skeletally immature patients who have had arthrodesis of just the posterior spine. Avoid by combining with anterior arthrodesis in younger/less skeletally mature patients
- Neurological injury occurs in <1% and SEPs during surgery minimize risk. MEPs are used in many centres. The Stagnara wake-up test is still used in some centres. The rib hump is not always corrected satisfactorily – costoplasty with rib resection can help

Infantile and juvenile scoliosis (early onset)

- Presentation – infantile <3 years; juvenile 4–10 years. Infantile curves are more common in the UK than in the USA
- Aetiology – is there a role for the positioning of babies?

- Prognosis – related to rib vertebral angle difference (RVAD):
  - Infantile – RVAD >20° is significant
  - Juvenile – >10° is significant
  - Thoracic hypokyphosis can cause progression
- Treatment
  - Bracing/serial casting forms the first-line treatment
  - More severe progressive curves present real management problems
  - Growing rods can control curves until the patient is old enough for definitive surgery

Neuromuscular scoliosis

Cerebral palsy
- Scoliosis is rare in ambulators, common in sitters or those with total involvement
- Bracing and customized wheelchairs can help
- Decision to operate is multidisciplinary
- Instrumentation – upper thoracic spine to sacrum. Rods are secured to the pelvis (Galveston technique). Severe curves require a combined approach
- Aim is to maintain function

Myelodysplasia
- Scoliosis (congenital or paralytic) secondary to spina bifida
- Associated problems – syringomyelia, hydromyelia and tethered cord can cause progression (investigate with MRI scan)
- Correction of cause may reverse curve
- In most cases with a severe kyphosis it can be resected
- Skin problems arise from previous closure of myelomeningoceles
- VP shunts may need revision
- Treat urinary tract infections aggressively

Spinal muscular atrophy
Three types:
I – Werdnig–Hoffman: presents from birth to 6 months; prognosis guarded

II – chronic Werdnig–Hoffman: presents at 6 months to 5 years
III – Kugelberg–Welander: mildest form; presents at 2–17 years. Autosomal-recessive disease in which patients lose anterior horn cells
Many require surgery for scoliosis. Bracing not well tolerated. Growing rods do not work well.

Duchenne muscular dystrophy
- Sex-linked recessive disease
- Relentlessly progressive: patients stop walking at 12–14 years; 50%–80% then develop scoliosis that affects sitting and breathing. Bracing not well tolerated
- Early surgery can prevent progression. Preoperative chest physiotherapy may avoid problems. Stop instrumentation at L4 or 5

Neurofibromatosis
- Dystrophic and non-dystrophic deformities
- Dystrophic deformities include: rib pencilling, vertebral scalloping and dural ectasia
- Management
  - Dystrophic curves do not respond to bracing, non-dystrophic can
  - Kyphoscoliosis – combined approach
  - Severe curves – vascularized rib graft can help
  - Preoperative MRI scanning aids planning
- Neurological deficits can arise from the deformity or tumours

Other secondary scoliosis

Marfan's syndrome
- Monitor scoliotic curves <25°
- Bracing tends not to work
- Arthrodesis for curves >45°
- Thoracic lordosis can affect pulmonary function
- Posterior arthrodesis is usually effective
- Anterior discectomy for rigid curves

Spinal cord injury
- Children with spinal cord injury have a 95% chance of developing scoliosis

- Two-thirds of those occurring before the growth spurt require arthrodesis
- Combined (anterior and posterior) approach best

Dwarfism
- Kyphosis improves in most patients
- Monitor and brace if progressing
- If worsens offer surgery: anterior release and graft with posterior arthrodesis and postoperative casting
- Hip flexion contractures can be exacerbated
- Foramen magnum stenosis can cause respiratory problems
- Lumbar stenosis is common and often progresses with age
- MRI avoids the risks of myelography

Osteogenesis imperfecta
- Scoliosis in over 50%
- Early arthrodesis recommended

Bone tumours

- Osteoblastomas and aneurysmal bone cysts are usually posterior. Request MRI to assess aneurysmal bone cysts
- Giant cell tumours are uncommon in the spine but do affect the body. Excision and grafting are recommended. Irradiation can cause sarcoma
- Eosinophilic granuloma – can cause vertebra plana but is often self-limiting. Observe unless there is neurological deterioration, in which case decompression/arthrodesis is recommended
- Laminectomy for compression – L2–S2. Decompress the canal, lateral recess and foramen. Laminectomy above L2 or when excessive can worsen kyphosis. Leave 50% of facet joints to avoid this. Kyphosis can occur after a dorsal rhizotomy procedure has been carried out for cerebral palsy
- Irradiation can cause a scoliosis after tumour treatment (convexity on the side of irradiation). Requires careful monitoring

Infection
- Aetiology – usually septic discitis caused by *Staphylococcus aureus*
- Presentation – begins in the vertebral endplate. Child cannot flex their spine but is not usually systemically unwell. They are rarely febrile and their bloods are normal except for a raised ESR. CRP can be high but not always. Late changes – disc space narrowing/blurred endplates on radiographs
- Investigation – CT and bone scans for diagnosis; MRI is best as it shows oedema and abscess formation. Aspiration biopsy is often negative
- Treatment – prolonged high-dose antibiotic is the mainstay of treatment with/without bracing. In adolescents, other bacteria are implicated

Osteomyelitis
- Much less common than discitis
- Presentation – patient is usually unwell with a fever and high WCC
- Often caused by *Staphylococcus aureus* infection
- Management – long-term antibiotics and surgical stabilization for deformity/instability. Vascularized grafts can avoid sequestra

Spinal tuberculosis
- Affects bone early and discs late
- Relatively rare
- Neurological deficit not common in children
- Early antituberculous treatment can suffice with cast immobilization
- Later disease – surgical abscess removal and fusion, accompanied by anti-tuberculous treatment
- Conservative management – kyphus and pain can be a problem

Disc prolapse

- Epidemiology – 2% in children/adolescents; 5 times more common in those with a family history
- Presentation – fewer neurological deficits in children than in adults. Usually nerve root tension signs. Often severe sciatica but no back pain
- Treatment – surgery good if early but the results tail off with longer duration of symptoms

Table 19.1 Classification of spondylolisthesis

I	Dysplastic
II	A Spondylolysis
	B Isthmus elongation
	C Acute fracture
III	Traumatic
IV	Degenerative
V	Pathologic
VI	Iatrogenic

- If there are posterior apophyseal avulsions, sciatica is usually cephalic. CT scanning shows this
- MRI disc changes are rare in children

Spondylolysis

- If presents early – aged <8 years – there is usually a family history
- Most cases are in adolescents. It is thought to be due to microtrauma or a hormone imbalance during the growth spurt
- It is common in gymnasts and other athletes
- Spondylolysis often causes degenerative disc disease in those <25 years of age
- Treatment is controversial
  - Conservative measures – bracing and activity modification often works
  - Hot spots as shown by bone scan or SPECT scanning. Stress fractures may heal
  - Surgery after 6 months for persistent pain: posterolateral arthrodesis with disc degeneration. With normal discs, the pars defects are repaired with bone grafting (techniques include Scott wiring or Buck screw fixation and various specific implants such as DOS)

Spondylolisthesis

- Classification – given in Table 19.1 (Wiltse and Newman 1976)[1]

- Management depends on pain and degree of slip
  - Meyerding[2] classification Grades I–IV – 25% divisions of vertebral body diameter
  - Meyerding classification Grade V – spondyloptosis
- Surgery or conservative management can lead to slip progression
- Conservative treatment for Grade I – rest and bracing and then resume activity when pain free
- Pain, slip progression and neurological symptoms require surgery: posterolateral fusion at L5–S1 for Grade I–II slips and at L4–S1 for Grade III–IV slips
- Reduction of slip and kyphosis by in situ fusion for progression with a slip angle >35°. Cosmesis and hamstring tightness are improved
- The commonest complication of reduction is L5 root injury; extensive damage to the plexus is less common
- Fusion in situ rarely leads to cauda equina syndrome. Management by removal of posterior S1 and reduction

Scheuermann's disease

- Normal thoracic kyphosis is 20°–45°. At T1–T5 it is difficult to see – a kyphosis of >33° at T5–12 should alert suspicion
- Scheuermann's disease is signified by a Cobb angle of >45° for the kyphosis; wedging of >5° of three adjacent vertebrae and vertebral endplate irregularities
- Epidemiology – 1% of population has hyperkyphosis; male: female ratio is 1:1.4
- Aetiology – unknown; cartilage endplates are abnormal
- Presentation – Schmorl's node formation is common. Kyphosis is rarely painful
- Management
  - >50° curves should be braced until patient is skeletally mature

[1] Wiltse LL, Newman PH (1976) Classification of spondylolysis and spondylolisthesis. *Clin Orthop Relat Res* **117: 23–9.**

[2] Meyerding HW (1932) Spondylolisthesis. *Surg Gynecol Obstet* 54: **371.**

- Curves progressing to >75° or those that are cosmetically unacceptable – anterior release and posterior osteotomies with fusion
- Thoracolumbar curves of only 30° can be cosmetically unacceptable and painful. Anterior vertebral body defects
- Pain often settles with rest or bracing. Surgery is for cosmesis
- Lumbar Scheuermann's is a separate identity of limited and doubtful clinical significance. Radiological diagnosis – pain but no deformity. Rest helps the pain

Trauma

Cervical spine

Recent advances in the safety of cars and the compulsory wearing of helmets for motorcyclists have improved the survival of patients with cervical spine injuries, who often died previously. Careful assessment/management is required for patients with potential cervical spine injuries – it is essential to prevent spinal cord injury. Assess according to ATLS principles. CT and MRI scanning help assessment.

Assessment

ABC. Life-threatening conditions take priority – cervical spine needs to be controlled and protected until cleared. Use tape/sandbags with a hard collar and immobilize the patient on a spinal board initially. A high index of suspicion is mandatory with head or facial injuries and an altered level of consciousness.

Hypovolaemic shock can be difficult to distinguish from neurogenic shock: 20% of spinal-cord-injured patients are hypotensive and 75% have neurogenic shock. Bradycardia is suggestive of neurogenic shock, and diaphragmatic breathing suggests a cervical cord injury. The aims of resuscitation are to restore cord perfusion without causing oedema.

Symptoms and signs are transient but can suggest more serious underlying injury. Repeat the neurological assessment – trends of improvement or deterioration should be noted.

Table 19.2 The Frankel grading system

A	complete paralysis
B	sensory preservation below level of injury – no voluntary motor function
C	sensory preservation below level of injury – useless motor function
D	sensory preservation below level of injury – useful voluntary motor function
E	Normal function

Examination

- Make an overall assessment with specific cranial nerve and neurological examination
- Cranial nerve deficit indicates vertebral artery injury or high cervical fractures/dislocations. Neck tenderness is not always present
- A full neurological assessment of trunk and limbs is mandatory. Sensory changes (body parts not dermatomes) show variability between individuals: 10% have another spine injury
- Sacral sensory sparing – very important – this indicates that the patient has potential for improvement
- Spinal shock is different from neurogenic shock. Definition of spinal shock is that there are absent reflexes which subsequently recover. The bulbocavernosus reflex recovers first. This makes the prediction of recovery difficult, especially in terms of bowel and bladder function. If total deficit persists for more than 24 hours after spinal shock recovers the potential for recovery is limited but subtotal deficits can recover almost fully
- Assessment is according to the Frankel grading system (Table 19.2). Other systems of grading are available, e.g. ASIA (American Spinal Injury Association)

Investigation

- Important – cannot rely solely on examination – many patients will not or cannot comply. Correlation between X-rays and neurological examination is not good. You need good-quality radiographs that must be interpreted accurately

- Radiographs – lateral, AP, oblique, peg views. CT and MRI are useful adjuncts
  - Lateral view (trauma series) picks up most significant injuries: cervicothoracic junction (pull down shoulders or swimmer's view); soft-tissue swelling, alignment (4 lines), canal size and integrity of bones; canal size 0.8 times body diameter or above (there is a greater likelihood of injury if it is smaller)
  - AP view – useful for lateral mass fractures or sagittal splits. Altered spinous process spacing with flexion injuries. Open mouth view – C1 and C2 (peg view). If poor, alter the angle more caudal or cephalad
  - Trauma oblique views – beam at 45°. Patient supine, cassette on far side. Shows pedicles and facet joints well. This provides more information about facet joints than CT or MRI
  - Flexion/extension radiographs. Flexion views are the most useful. Patient must be supervised if instability suspected. Flex the neck – support it with lead-gloved hand or pillow. Compare motion at adjacent levels. More useful later when the muscle spasm/splinting has subsided
- CT scan – adjunct to plain radiographs. Shows laminar fractures better than X-rays
  - C1/2 level – rotatory subluxation. Use to view the cervicothoracic junction if it is not seen on radiographs
- MRI
  - Advantages are that neural structures/discs can be seen. Good for haematomas and syringomyelia. Can see some posterior ligament/muscle injuries, but not all
  - Disadvantages – fractures not as well visualized
  - Special equipment and anaesthetist needed for paralysed, ventilated patients
- Tomography – used for lateral masses and facet joint visualization – angle beam. Shows peg fracture lines well
- Myelogram – seldom used; with patient in prone position, extend their neck; dangerous in acute injury

- Bone scanning – technetium 99 can be useful in patients with pre-existing changes/old injury

Classification – neural and osteoligamentous

Neural

- Complete and incomplete
- Incomplete – nerve root injury, anterior cord syndrome, central cord syndrome and Brown–Sequard (hemi cord) syndrome
- Evaluation of recovery is made using the Frankel grading system
- Quantitative systems for evaluation of extent – points are given for motor and sensory sparing. This is time consuming. Level is determined by the distal-most normal level

Osteoligamentous

- Based on presumed mechanism of injury. Much information gained from biomechanical cadaveric studies
- Three-column theory – anterior, middle and posterior. Instability is a widely used term but there is no consensus on definition or best management

Treatments for spinal cord injury

Drug treatments

Early studies[3] indicated that corticosteroids prevent oedema and improve outcome. The results were encouraging, although the complication rate rose. Later studies[4] (NASCIS II) looked at even higher doses and it was found that the outcome was better if treatment started within 8 hours of injury. More recent studies did not confirm this, so most centres in the UK no longer use steroids. Check policy with local spinal injuries unit.

---

[3] NASCIS 1 (1984) Efficacy of methylprednisolone in acute spinal cord injury. *J Am Med Assoc* **25**(1): 45–52.

[4] NASCIS II (1990) A randomized, controlled trial of methylprednisolone or naloxone in the treatment of acute spinal-cord injury. Results of the Second National Acute Spinal Cord Injury Study. *N Engl J Med* **322**(20): 1405–11.

Management aims
- To minimize neck pain, stiffness and the risk of re-injury
- In terms of neurology the aim is to prevent deterioration and promote recovery – the recovery of just one nerve root can affect independence
- To realign displaced fractures/dislocations – a solid union minimizes the risk of re-injury
- **Neural recovery** – realign (decompress) and immobilize to allow recovery of function. Remember – disc material can encroach on nerves and the cord even when bones are realigned
- **Avoid laminectomy** unless fixing as it promotes instability
- **Realign quickly** – reduction in less than 4 h is best but is often not possible (for geographical/logistical reasons)
- Consider the various options and choose the best one on a case-by-case basis
- **Surgical treatment** – demands fewer resources but superior skills required

Methods
- **Bed rest with traction** – this is time consuming/ risky
- **Skeletal traction**
  - Gardner–Wells tongs are best. Halo rings need time and expertise
  - The advantage of skeletal traction is that it can be used throughout the whole treatment period
  - Questions to address include: how much weight should be applied during traction? How quickly should the weight be increased? Is muscle relaxation useful?
  - Do not apply skeletal traction without a prior MRI scan as the cord can be damaged by an extruding disc fragment
- **Manipulation** – this can be used in a few selected cases but only by someone who can decompress the cord/stabilize the neck surgically
- **Open surgical realignment** – required for irreducible cases. This is the only option with locked facets/delayed presentation

- **Ligamentous disruption** – internal fixation (anterior interbody grafting and posterior screw and rod constructs or wiring)
- **Ligament injury** – grafting, autogenous bone or bone substitutes are useful for ligament injury. Many different substitutes available including tantalum trabecular metal cages for interbody fusion
- **Immobilization** to prevent loss of alignment and allow healing
  - Rest, brace or reconstruct surgically
  - Orthoses – soft collars, firmer collars with occipital mandibular cervical control, occipital mandibular thoracic (Philadelphia, Miami J or Aspen)
  - SOMI braces with lower thoracic control and craniothoracic braces (halo vest)

Types of injury according to site

Upper cervical – occiput to C2
- Different from sub-axial cervical spine
- Synovial joints are transversely orientated
- There are no discs between the vertebrae – head impact
- Cord diameter: canal diameter is small in this area and most survivors have no neural injury. If patients are paralysed they often die before they reach the hospital

Occipital condyle fractures
- Rare – usually axial compression of laterally flexed neck or avulsion injury
- Treat conservatively in a Philadelphia-type collar
- Can be associated with cranial nerve palsies

Atlanto–occipital joint
- Rare – subluxations reduce themselves, dislocations are usually fatal
- Power's ratio is helpful (lateral radiographs): this is the distance from the basion to the posterior arch of C1 divided by the distance from the opisthion to the anterior arch of C1. Normal value

is 1; a value >1 suggests anterior dislocation, and a value <1 indicates posterior dislocation
- Avoid traction as this carries a risk of over-distraction. Immobilization in a halo vest is best
- Occiput–C1 fusion can prevent late displacement

Atlas (C1) fractures
- Posterior arch – can be bilateral. Seen on lateral radiographs. If present, there is a 50% chance of other neck injury. Soft collar or firmer collars are indicated for isolated fractures
- Combined anterior and posterior (Jefferson) fractures – axial compression. X-rays reveal two-, three- or four-part fractures. Take AP open mouth peg radiographs. Lateral mass displacement is a common finding. Anterior soft-tissue swelling is seen on lateral radiographs
- Rotatory subluxation – apparent lateral mass displacement
- By definition the transverse atlantal ligament is intact if the sum of displacement is less than 7 mm. A CT scan will show ligament avulsion. Flexion/extension lateral radiographs will reveal disruption with >3 mm of atlanto-dens interval. Management aims at preventing late subluxation and cord damage
- Cranial traction is better than a halo vest to reduce lateral mass displacement although the relationship with outcome and long-term pain is not clear
- Undisplaced injuries – use a collar. Displaced injuries – usually require prolonged traction and a halo vest
- Avulsion of longus colli from the anterior arch – use a collar

Atlanto axial (C1/2) injuries
- **Rotary** injury within normal ROM – Fielding and Hawkins Type I. This comprises partial capsular ligament disruption with an intact transverse atlantal ligament. Atlanto-dens interval is no greater than 3 mm. Asymmetry is seen on AP open mouth radiographs and CT scan

- **Unilateral anterior subluxation** – unilateral capsular and transverse atlantal ligament tear. Rotation about intact opposite side (Fielding and Hawkins Type II). Atlanto-dens interval is 3–5 mm
- **Bilateral anterior subluxation** – transverse atlantal ligament and unilateral or bilateral capsular ligament disruption. No rotation if symmetrical (Fielding and Hawkins Type III) and the atlanto-dens interval is >5 mm. Wink sign (AP radiographs) – C1 lateral mass rides over C2. C1 can rotate in three planes. The cause is usually a blow to head, e.g. a fall onto the occiput or an RTA. Management – gentle traction with/without manipulation of the locked joint. Late cases may be irreducible. Because of the joint shape – posterior bone graft and screws/wiring can be required (halo may not control)
- **Posterior subluxation** – rare (Fielding and Hawkins Type IV). Damage to dens allows posterior migration. Address as part of management

Atlas (C2) fractures
Dens or odontoid peg fractures. There are three types, based on level at which fracture occurs:
- **Type I fractures** – avulsion of alar ligaments off one side of tip (connect dens to occiput)
  - Flexion/extension lateral radiographs – looking for anterior subluxation of C1 ± atlanto–occipital dislocation
  - Treat symptomatically – cervical collar
- **Type II fractures** – transverse fracture at base of dens. Displacement with C1 dens ligaments usually intact. This is the most common and most problematic type of atlas (C2) fracture. The highest rate of non-union is seen in the elderly
  - Other risk factors – amount, direction of displacement (posterior worse), delay in diagnosis and re-dislocation in halo vest
  - Accepted management – halo vest, posterior wiring with arthrodesis of C1–C2 (Brooks, Griswold, Gallie), posterior screw arthrodesis of C1–C2 (Magerl or Harms) and anterior C2 fixation (Apfelbaum)

- Care with posterior displacement to avoid further displacement with wiring
- Halo vest for 3 months if displacement <5 mm and the patient is younger than 50 years old
- Posterior screw fixation better if the C1 anterior arch is also fractured; this is technically demanding and requires expertise. Avoid fusion to occiput in order to preserve motion
- **Type III fractures** are through the vertebral body; they can angulate and translate
  - Management – halo vest for 12 weeks ± prolonged traction to maintain alignment until "sticky". Collar is better for elderly patients with stable fractures

Bilateral pars (Hangman's) fracture/traumatic spondylolisthesis

This does not always involve C2/3 disc. Most do not occur following longitudinal traction (hangings). They occur because of the extension or axial compression of an extended neck or because of flexion of a flexed neck (on lateral radiograph).

There are four subgroups:

- **Type I** – minimally displaced; manage with Philadelphia-type collar
- **Type II** – significant angulation or translation; manage with halo vest for 12 weeks
- **Type IIA** – posterior widening of C2/3 disc space with traction; treat with halo vest, avoid over-distraction; treatment is difficult and may need ORIF
- **Type III** – angulation and translation with unilateral or bilateral facet dislocation at C2/3

Lateral mass compression fracture

This is uncommon and occurs following placement of an axial load to a laterally flexed neck. C2 lateral mass can be comminuted. Treat symptomatically – possibly in a halo vest if the fracture is comminuted. Late fusion to C1 may be necessary for pain and degenerative change.

C3 to C7 injuries

Fairly uniform and different to C1 and C2. Ratio of cord to canal diameters is less in the subaxial spine and there is decreased intervertebral mobility.

There are three types:

Type 1: Minor compression/avulsion fractures, no facet joint injuries or ligament disruption

Type 2: Facet joint injuries – displaced, disc can be disrupted with risk of cord injury

Type 3: Complex fractures with loss of anterior load bearing and compromise of canal. For example, burst and teardrop fracture/dislocations

Type 1 – spinous process fracture – C7 (clay shoveler's fracture) commonest. Single sudden overload. Avulsion of ligamentum nuchae (C6 and7). Non-union common but treatment symptomatic.

Transverse process fracture – uncommon – muscle avulsion – symptomatic treatment.

- Teardrop avulsion fracture – anterior inferior corner of body
  - Much less severe than teardrop fracture/dislocation
  - Hyperextension – flexion/extension views rule out hypermobility
  - Treatment – collar and activity modification (few weeks)
  - Late subjacent disc degeneration
- Wedge compression fracture – loss of anterior vertebral height. Posterior wall intact
  - Posterior ligament taut with 25% loss of anterior height (with >50% compression – this suggests posterior ligament disruption and it becomes a complex or type 3 injury)
  - For compression fracture with <25% loss of height, treat with collar. If flexion/extension views suggest instability then carry out a posterior fixation

Type 2 – facet joint injuries – frequently missed. Trauma oblique radiographs are important

- Subluxation (unilateral or bilateral)
- Partial tearing – posterior ligaments and/or disc
  - Lateral radiographs looking for anterior subluxation of vertebra and soft-tissue swelling. Articular processes may overlap more. Supervised flexion/extension views looking for possible hypermobility
  - Tomography can show fractures. If there is minimal displacement place patient in a Philadelphia-type collar for 6 weeks. Regular

review. Posterior wiring/grafting for progressive displacement

- Unilateral facet dislocation
  - Forward rotation of one side around the other side, which is fixed. Body subluxes forwards by 25% of the AP diameter. Lateral masses of displaced vertebra overlap on lateral view, "bowtie sign"
  - AP radiograph looking for spinous processes deviated to the affected side. An articular process can cause nerve root compression. Seen in trauma oblique X-rays. Delays in diagnosis are not uncommon – patient can have torticollis
  - Treatment is controversial – traction and/or open reduction. Some authors use closed reduction with gentle traction under X-ray control
  - Pain and neurological recovery are better with reduction. Open reduction using the posterior approach, unless the disc can be extruded in which case use a combined approach
  - Extrusion is more common with bilateral facet dislocation and can cause devastating neurological injury if not removed before reduction. MRI is mandatory. Treat the patient in a halo vest for 3 months after reduction or use open reduction and wiring/grafting. With lateral mass or articular fractures, additional stability may be needed
- Bilateral facet dislocation
  - High incidence of associated cord injury. Can be seen as a 50% anterior slip of body above on lateral radiograph. Almost all ligaments and the disc are disrupted. Associated with disc herniation; investigation with MRI is important. Any disc prolapse must be removed before reduction in order to avoid paralysis. Traction often reduces dislocation. The force required for reduction can be high – up to one-third of the body weight. The safe upper limits are unknown – up to 30 kg is used. Re-dislocation is uncommon. Realignment can allow neurological recovery. Spinous process wiring can aid stability
  - Articular process fracture – often accompanies facet dislocations. Can allow anterior displacement

after reduction. Posterior wiring alone may not prevent slip. Look carefully at lateral and oblique radiographs. Apical fractures are associated with transient high-grade slip and cord injury

- Small fractures – patient rest can prevent slip. There is a risk of root and cord injury with basal superior process fractures. They are often caused by flexion of the superior vertebra. With basal inferior process fractures there is no associated nerve injury or vertebral flexion
- Treat small apical fractures with orthoses. Larger fractures require posterior wiring/grafting. Posterior screw/rod fixation is more stable than spinous process wiring

- Type 3 – complex fractures
  - Involve canal. Complex fractures of the vertebral body are commonest followed by fractures of the lamina and pedicles
  - Complex fractures of the vertebral body alone tend to be caused by axial compression
  - There are three subgroups of increasing severity
- Sagittal plane fracture
  - Vertical compression, sagittal not coronal. Associated with other fractures/extensive ligamentous injury and/or paralysis. AP radiographs (lateral radiographs can be normal)
- Burst fracture
  - Retropulsion of fragments into canal – superior endplate, inferior body. Variant of teardrop fracture dislocation
  - Management – prolonged traction until uniting or anterior graft/cage. Traction may not decompress canal and open decompression can be required. Anterior plating improves support with posterior ligament disruption
- Teardrop fracture-dislocation
  - This often involves major compressive forces with anteroinferior and posteroinferior fragments. A posteroinferior fragment whether or not associated with a facet fracture can lead to cord injury. Manage with anterior strut and/or plate
  - Body fracture and facet/laminar fracture

- Combination determined by posture of neck when injured
- Most severe mechanical insufficiency – anterior and posterior reconstruction
- Others – bilateral laminar fractures and bilateral facet dislocation
  - Treatment – posterior wiring or screw fixation
- Floating lateral mass fracture
  - Often with associated injuries such as disc disruption which allows anterior subluxation
  - Internal fixation is usually required
- Ankylosing spondylitis with cervical fracture
  - Rare; most patients have a cord injury. Difficult to see on radiographs and you need a CT scan
  - Management – halo traction, orthoses or internal fixation; surgery but there is associated morbidity. Pseudoarthrosis is not uncommon with all treatments
- Open wounds and gunshots
  - Rarely the cause of severe osteoligamentous injury. Antibiotics are as good for infection. Removal of the missile does not lead to improved recovery

Internal fixation

- Anterior plates – locking plates are good with little screw loosening. Unicortical screws are sufficient except for severe posterior ligament injury, in which case posterior fixation or SOMI brace is also required
- Posterior rods and lateral mass or pedicle screws can be used from occiput to sacrum if needed. Precise placement is required in the neck in order to avoid the vertebral artery

Injury without fracture or subluxation

Sprains/strains

These are associated with pain and localized tenderness. There is stiffness with slight loss of lordosis and can cause chronic pain. Treat as for sprains elsewhere – rest, NSAIDs and mobilization. Causes include RTA and acceleration or deceleration injuries (whiplash-associated disorder). Hugely controversial area and usually involves medico-legal claims. It is not well studied or understood. There are a plethora of symptoms, of which pain and stiffness are only two features. Many report persistent symptoms. Most patients who settle do so in the first 3 months. Outcome is very difficult to predict and many factors are associated with a worse outcome. Most need conservative management and only very few need surgery for disc prolapse. Cord or root dysfunction is unusual.

Hyperextension injury in the elderly with spondylosis can cause central cord syndrome. Sensory loss is variable whereas motor loss is worse in the arms than in the legs. Treatment is with orthoses although recovery is often poor.

Thoracolumbar spine trauma

The thoracolumbar spine is the commonest site of spinal injury. The aims of treatment are to preserve life, to protect neurological function, to minimize risk of further injury and to maintain or restore alignment and stability. Spinal fractures involve several structures, including facets, ligaments and discs. Restoring alignment is not always necessary for union and function and neurological recovery are unpredictable despite surgical decompression/stabilization.

Pre-hospital care

A high index of suspicion at the scene is advised and the mechanism of injury can predict the likelihood of fracture. For example, if the patient was wearing a lap seatbelt suspect a flexion distraction injury.

A shoulder harness prevents many thoracolumbar injuries but can increase the risk of cervical spine injuries.

Patients who have been ejected from a vehicle often present with a spinal injury. If they are unconscious treat them as though they have a spinal injury until proven otherwise.

Early hospital care

Immobilize the patient on a spinal board until they have been fully assessed. In cases of neurological injury or instability placing the patient on a spinal bed is best as it protects pressure areas until the patient has been stabilized. Thoracolumbar fractures often occur with abdominal trauma. There is a 10% chance of other spinal injury so evaluate the whole spine.

These types of injuries are often missed initially in obtunded patients.

History and examination

- Take a complete history and make sure that it is well documented
- Complete a full neurological assessment
  - Elucidation of sensory sparing is important; its presence improves the chance of recovery
  - If there is sensory sparing (i.e. incomplete cord injury) recovery can be remarkable
  - The bulbocavernosus reflex is mediated via the spinal cord at S1–S3; an absent bulbocavernosus reflex worsens prognosis
  - The bulbocavernosus reflex is the first to recover following spinal shock, i.e. within 48 h. If the reflex returns but there is no other recovery (i.e. there is complete cord injury), any other recovery is unlikely
- Assess the patient for other injuries
  - 10%–15% of those with spinal injuries also have significant visceral injuries
  - 10%–15% of those with a head injury have missed fractures and nerve injury
- Investigations
  - Radiographs – AP and lateral radiographs of the spine
  - CT best for delineating fractures, canal encroachment and posterior element involvement. Cannot pick up subtle horizontal fractures. Reformatting can help
  - Spiral CT has superseded tomography
  - Spikes of bone can tear the dura

- MRI is best for neural elements and ligaments and it can show cord injury (signal changes differentiate oedema from infarction). Limitations with pacemakers and claustrophobia, etc.
- Myelography is seldom used

Classification of fractures

Holdsworth's two-column theory has been replaced by the three-column theory (Denis):

Anterior column – anterior two-thirds of the vertebral body and the anterior longitudinal ligament

Middle column – posterior body and posterior longitudinal ligament, posterior annulus and cord/cauda equina

Posterior column – posterior elements

Columns fail alone/together by:
- Compression
- Distraction
- Rotation
- Shear

There are four types of fracture:
- Compression
- Burst
- Flexion distraction (seatbelt)
- Fracture dislocations

Compression fractures
- Fracture of the anterior vertebral body (anterior column)
- Middle column remains intact
- Posterior column can fail in tension
- The anterior height of the body is diminished by <40%
- The posterior height remains normal
- No translation
- Stable – rarely involves neurological injury

Burst fractures
- Disruption of middle column
  - Often causes retropulsion of bone into the canal
  - Variable amount of disruption

- CT scan required: interpedicular distance may be increased
- AP radiograph
- Posterior elements involved
  - 50% have neurological injury
  - Entrapment in laminar fracture ±dural laceration
- Five groups identified by Denis
  - A – both endplates with retropulsion
  - B – superior endplate
  - C – inferior endplate
  - D – combination of A with rotation
  - E – lateral fracture with retropulsion and end-plate fracture

Flexion distraction injuries
- Chance (1948)[5] – upper half spinous process and pedicles through to superior vertebral body. Stability variable depends on anterior longitudinal ligament. Can be bony, mixed or purely ligamentous
- Bony lesions unite but ligamentous lesions may remain unstable. AP and lateral radiographs show increased interspinous distance. Posterior vertebral height can be greater than the anterior height on lateral radiographs. Seldom associated with neurological injury unless translation occurs

Dislocations
- Unstable – all three columns involved
- Multiple forces
- Some reduce spontaneously
- Often accompanied by neurological deficit, dural tears and other visceral injuries

Extension injuries
- Tensile force to anterior longitudinal ligament and anterior annulus
- Compression of posterior elements ±anterior vertebral avulsions and posterior element fractures
- Usually stable

[5] Chance GQ (1948) Note on a type of flexion fracture of the spine. *Br J Radiol* **21**: 452–453.

Transverse process fractures
- Blunt trauma or contraction of paraspinal muscles
- If L5 and more proximal levels are fractured, consider:
  - Vertical shear pelvic disruption (haemorrhage and visceral injuries)
  - Neurapraxia of roots – typically L3 and L4

Spinous process avulsions
- Rare in lumbar spine unless due to direct trauma
- Stable unless accompanied by dislocation

Facet fractures
- Uncommon – previous laminectomy
- The more proximal/displaced the fracture, the worse the injury
- Neurological injury occurs within seconds and management depends on
  - Level of injury (cord, conus or cauda equina)
  - Amount of displacement/canal reserve and degree of canal encroachment
- Vascular compromise affects the extent of neurological injury
- Treatment
  - Aims to maintain cord microvasculature to prevent deterioration
  - Many drugs tried but there is little evidence of good clinical efficacy
  - As with cervical cord injury give a high dose of corticosteroids in the first 8 h although this is controversial and most UK centres have stopped this because of serious side-effects
  - Check the policy with your local spinal injuries unit

Management of fractures

Compression fractures
- These are stable and rarely involve neurological compromise. Symptomatic treatment is advised: bed rest, analgesia and mobilization
- Bracing is controversial

- Avoid compressive forces on the spine for 12 weeks
- The fractures are potentially unstable if there is >50% height loss anteriorly, >20° of kyphosis or multiple adjacent fractures. Manage with bracing and/or internal fixation (anterior or posterior) – again this is controversial
- Some can present with increased kyphosis at up to 4 months so close follow-up is needed
- Increased kyphosis is a relative indication for fixation

Burst fractures
- Management depends on stability and neurological injury
- Conservative management (Guttman) is advised for neurologically intact patients
- Long-term back pain is usually mild and is not associated with neurological deterioration
- Kyphotic deformity is not related to pain
- Retropulsed bone can be reabsorbed/remodelled
- Posterior fixation is adopted by many surgeons and has shown some improvement in kyphosis and a reduction of retropulsed bone
- There are complications with surgery
- A kyphotic deformity can recur unless the anterior column is grafted
- Early posterior devices such as Harrington rods (three-point fixation) involved the fixation of a relatively long segment
- Pedicle screw constructs (four-point fixation) involve the fixation of a shorter segment
- There is an associated risk of nerve injury with pedicle penetration when using screws
- If there is three-column failure over-distraction is possible
- Posterior instrumentation is indicated if there is a >50% loss of height, >20° of kyphosis or significant canal compromise. This decompresses the canal in most cases
- If there is neurological injury consider anterior decompression
- Laminectomy is seldom indicated, except where neural elements are trapped in posterior elements in which case stabilization is indicated

Flexion distraction injuries
- Bone and/or soft tissue is involved
- If bone alone is involved, manage the patient with an extension brace
- If posterior ligaments are disrupted, restore the tension band (posterior instrumentation is used in compression unless the middle column cannot load bear)

Fracture dislocations
- This is usually associated with neurological injury
- Treatment aims to realign and stabilize the column, followed by early mobilization
- Posterior instrumentation needs distraction to control the rotation

Extension injuries
- These are often stable injuries that can be managed using flexion orthoses for 8–12 weeks

Timing of surgery
Emergency decompression is required for cauda equina syndrome or progressive neurological deficit. If there is complete cord injury, delay surgery until the oedema settles: early decompression does not improve results.

Late anterior decompression can improve outcome. In neurologically intact patients with an unstable injury, operate once other conditions allow.

Decompression
- Indirect – posterior distraction
- Direct – anterior exploration

The posterior longitudinal ligament needs to be intact for ligamentotaxis. Indirect decompression is not possible if surgery is delayed until the fracture is "sticky". It is difficult to assess the reduction intra-operatively. The posterior approach for anterior decompression works in the lumbar spine and thoracolumbar junction. It is dangerous in the thoracic spine because there is less space. The anterior approach is best for visualization but it is demanding and the reduction of kyphosis obtained may be less. Use grafts or cages to restore the anterior column. The newer, expanding cages are easier to use. Patients still require posterior fixation in many cases. Removal of implants is difficult at the front.

Hook systems

These were originally used for deformity correction. They allow the facility to distract and compress, which avoids the need for sublaminar wires that can risk further injury and are time consuming to insert. Allows the instrumentation of shorter segments using double claws at either end.

Pedicle screw systems

- Improve sagittal correction and secure bony fixation
- Minimize the number of levels that need to be instrumented
- Best for Tl2–L5 but can be used from occiput to sacrum
- Screws can cause neural and vascular injury or break and dislodge in up to 15% of cases
- Screw breakage is less with anterior grafting

Cervical degenerative conditions and reconstruction

Cervical spondylosis and radiculopathy

Neck pain has many causes, of which muscle strain and degenerative disc disease are the commonest. It is common for patients to have local tenderness on palpation and stiffness.

Neurological examination can be normal without radicular pain. Radiographs can be normal or show spondylosis. Treatment involves short-term rest and analgesics, traction and collars followed by gentle physiotherapy. Manipulation rarely causes neurological injury. Facet joint injections can help in selected cases. Unless there are neurological symptoms or signs, scanning is of little benefit: 25% of normal controls have MRI abnormalities and this increases with age. The commonest levels are C5/6 and C6/7 followed by C4/5 – analogous to the

lumbar spine. Discography and discometry are controversial. Some report good pain relief with anterior cervical discectomy and fusion for single-level spondylosis.

Radiculopathy

Radiculopathy is often a consequence of cervical disc prolapse. Usually one dermatome is affected. C5/6 prolapse and C6 radiculopathy is the most common presentation. Posterolateral prolapse is commonest although central and anterior prolapses can occur.

Small prolapses can be asymptomatic, whereas large central prolapses lead to myelopathy and cord signal change. Early treatment as for neck pain is advised. Most settle over a few weeks. If there is no improvement at 6–12 weeks, consider imaging and surgery.

If scan findings fit the clinical picture, surgery can help. Results of anterior cervical discectomy and fusion show that 80%–95% of patients have an excellent or good outcome. With adjacent level disease the success rate is 60%–65%. During surgery, the central disc and protruding fragments and osteophytes are removed to decompress the cord and roots. The posterior longitudinal ligament is left, or removed in order to see the dura. Posterior foraminotomies are carried out for lateral soft prolapse or foraminal stenosis. This avoids fusion. Not fusing risks long-term kyphotic deformity. Fuse with iliac crest graft with or without plate fixation or with cages with or without graft and plating. Cervical disc replacement also avoids fusion and kyphosis although longer-term results show that many fuse anyway.

Cervical spondylotic myelopathy

Degenerative changes causing cord compression, especially in the mid-cervical spine. Compression is multifactorial: osteophytes, disc bulges, facet hypertrophy and a thickened bulging ligamentum flavum impinge on the cord. Ossification of the posterior longitudinal ligament (OPLL) is common in the Far

East. Myelopathy becomes more common with age. Small canals predispose to the condition.

Loss of lordosis exacerbates compression because the cord becomes relatively ischaemic. Anterior column problems are common, whereas posterior column function is often normal. Lower motor neurone problems affect the upper limbs with upper motor neurone features (weakness, spasticity and ataxia) in the lower limbs. The onset is insidious unless the cause is a large disc prolapse. MRI is the investigation of choice, with lesions shown as signal change. CT myelography is recommended in cases of compression. Electrophysiological studies show cord damage. SSEPs can be used to monitor cord activity during surgery.

The natural history of the condition is unclear. Conservative treatment has mixed results. Surgery is required when there is progressive deterioration, the aim being to halt progression and, in some cases, to reverse dysfunction. Anterior decompression is achieved by corpectomy or partial corpectomy (anterior trench) with cage or rib or fibular graft reconstruction. In cases of extensive disease or posterior compression the posterior approach is better. When deciding whether to perform a laminectomy or laminoplasty, remember that the latter preserves stability and some motion, whilst avoiding screw and rod stabilization. Skip laminectomy is sometimes chosen as it gives comparable results to laminoplasty with lower morbidity. This is important in the elderly.

For a kyphosis the anterior approach produces better correction of the deformity. The results are worse if there are established cord changes.

Rheumatoid arthritis

Signs and symptoms

- The cervical spine is frequently affected, notably the proximal and sub-axial cervical spine
- Pain and neurological compromise, compounded by pannus
- Erosion of bone and soft tissue leads to instability
- Atlantoaxial instability common

- Translation >10 mm indicates that the transverse, alar and apical ligaments are involved. This often leads to myelopathy
- Cranial settling occurs later and compresses the upper cord and brainstem (monitor Ranawat's line on lateral radiographs)
- Lower cervical spine – facet joint involvement allowing subluxation

Assessment – history/examination

- Flexion/extension radiographs are useful for assessing instability
- CT myelography has been superseded by MRI as it shows soft tissues/cord better
- Most have pannus around the odontoid peg
- Electrophysiological tests – cord signal change in flexion not extension
- Cord compression is indicated by an AP diameter <13 mm

Management and prognosis

- Conservative management – rheumatological treatment and braces
- The disease is unpredictable and can regress
- Surgery is indicated in cases of progressive instability or neurological deterioration (severe pain)
  - Mobile subluxation should be reduced before surgery
  - Problems – wound healing and pseudoarthrosis
  - Usually approach posteriorly ±cord monitoring
  - Anterior decompression is required in cases of anterior compression but can destabilize the spine further
- Disease at C1–C2 is managed by posterior wiring with bone grafting. This prevents cranial settling from progressing
  - Occasionally occipito–cervical fusion is carried out for cranial settling
  - Fixation can allow pannus to shrink
  - Postoperative stabilization with a halo vest is often needed
  - In cases of subaxial disease fuse the affected level(s)

Ankylosing spondylitis

The cervical spine is fixed in flexion (chin-on-chest deformity if severe). Flexion can also affect the thoracic and lumbar spine plus hips. Patients cannot see ahead. Address the hip and lumbar deformities first. A cervicothoracic osteotomy helps but is risky. In cases of acute pain suspect a fracture of the ankylosed spine close to the cervicothoracic junction. A translation or haematoma can injure the cord. Stabilize the patient using a halo vest or surgery. Spondylodiscitis is sometimes described. This is usually a combination of instability and an inflammatory mass. It is thought to be an old fracture with non-union.

Infection

Osteomyelitis is relatively uncommon. If it is suspected on clinical grounds then order the following investigations: blood tests, bone scan and MRI. Needle aspiration may allow the culture of the causative organisms.

Surgery is required only for abscess drainage, to correct deformity or in cases of progressive neurological deterioration. Most operations are carried out via the anterior approach. Bone grafting is usually acceptable if the patient is on antibiotics although instrumentation is controversial. Often bracing/antibiotics suffice. Postoperative infections are treated similarly. Rarely the patient can contract meningitis, with devastating consequences.

Tumours

Most are metastatic and can cause instability and deformity. Cord compression can result from tumour, deformity or a pathological fracture. Conservative treatment is appropriate for limited disease, with bracing and radiotherapy or chemotherapy. Surgery is indicated for more extensive disease and involves anterior corpectomy and reconstruction with bone graft; cages or cement is often employed. Limited life expectancy is not a contraindication unless it is <6 weeks. Neurological compromise can recover after decompression and stabilization. Posterior surgery gives similar results to surgery using the anterior approach. C1/2 lesions are rare and are managed with surgery or halo vest stabilization and radiotherapy.

Primary tumours are rare in adults. Chordoma can occur at the top and bottom extremities of the spine. Plasmacytomas and myeloma are the commonest tumours. Aim for complete resection if possible.

MRI is most often used in cervical spine ± motor evoked potential testing where the level is in doubt.

Autogenous bone grafts are better than allograft when performing a multilevel fusion. Expandable cages are used as an alternative, i.e. interbody cages, such as metal or PEEK (trabecular metal cage avoids the morbidity associated with graft harvest). Anterior locking plates are used for fusion – unicortical screws decrease the risk of cord damage. Posterior wiring is still used although biomechanically; lateral mass or pedicle screws and rods are stronger.

Fibular grafts are stronger than other autogenous grafts.

Anterior plates are strong enough to stand alone. For C1–C2 lesions, the Magerl screw technique is more robust than Gallie wiring.

Complications

Anterior approaches
- Recurrent laryngeal nerve injury (2% incidence)
- Airway and oesophageal injury (but there are fewer root and cord injuries)

Halo vest complications
- Infection
- Pin loosening
- Meningitis (the worst complication)

Thoracolumbar reconstruction

Aims

To preserve function, maintain/restore stability, maintain motion and relieve pain.

Assessment

- Plain radiographs – AP and lateral (±coned views); occasionally oblique radiographs
- Lateral bending films – flexibility of deformities. Traction or forced fulcrum bending films assess correction possible
- CT scans – bony structures
- MRI scanning – gold standard
  - Shows soft tissues and neural elements well
  - Best for disc prolapses, spinal stenosis, infection or tumours with/without gadolinium enhancement
  - Difficult to interpret with deformity
  - Claustrophobics cannot tolerate MRI scans – open scanners avoid this, as does CT myelography
- Bone scanning is seldom used except in young patients with pain or if osteoid osteoma is suspected

Deformity

Adult scoliosis has four causes: idiopathic, congenital, neuromuscular, and degenerative.

Idiopathic scoliosis

This is the most common form of adult scoliosis and has a prevalence of 5%. Pain is often a major feature. The cause is difficult to diagnose and may be: disc prolapse, facet arthrosis, spinal stenosis (central or lateral recess) or the disc itself. Normally cosmesis is not the biggest issue. Role in the cause of pain is controversial. The prevalence is as for age-matched controls.

Deformity can progress after skeletal maturity (thoracic curves over 50° and if L5 is above the iliac crest at a rate of 1° per year). Lateral translation at the lower end increases disability. If there are later degenerative changes, there may be spinal stenosis requiring decompression. Decompression should be combined with fusion in order to prevent worsening the deformity or spondylolisthesis. Associated kyphosis can cause myelopathy.

Neuromuscular curves

Pelvic obliquity is a problem. The curves can be hyperlordotic or hyperkyphotic. Plan surgery carefully. Assess pulmonary function and look for associated cardiac and renal problems. The functional status of the patient can influence the treatment. Remember that surgery can exacerbate hip subluxation.

Indications for surgery include: pain, progressive deformity, neurological compromise and worsening respiratory function.

Degenerative adult scoliosis

This occurs in older adults in their fifth and sixth decades. The finding is often incidental – patients present with acute backache with/without trauma and radicular symptoms. They have a Cobb angle of 15°–50°.

Often there is lateral translation and/or degenerative spondylolisthesis. Surgery is indicated for pain, progression, neurological compromise and respiratory compromise.

Operate for stenosis not deformity. Decompress and fuse with instrumentation. Results very unpredictable.

Harrington rods are not very good for adult degenerative scoliosis. Problems include instrument failure in up to one-third of patients, pseudoarthrosis and degenerative changes above or below instrumentation.

Fusion to sacrum increases failure, pseudoarthrosis and flat back syndrome. In cases of rigid curves carry out multilevel osteotomies and/or rib releases with or without anterior release. Combined surgery is very major surgery and has a high morbidity. Osteopenia leads to failure of fixation and complications in 25% of cases. Pain may be helped in only 33%. Newer systems are better but problems remain. Pedicle screw insertion requires specific training and X-ray guidance.

Conservative management
- NSAIDs and exercises
- Females – assessment/management of osteoporosis

- Braces can help the pain
- Bed rest for acute exacerbations (few good studies)
- With fusion for scoliosis in teenagers, extension below L3 can cause chronic low back pain. The lower the fusion the higher the likelihood
- Problems: loss of correction, pseudoarthrosis, flat back syndrome and failure of fusion

Postlaminectomy deformity

Laminectomy is rarely indicated. If more than 50% of the facets are excised, biomechanical stability can be lost. This leads to progressive kyphosis. Prevention: avoid wide laminectomy or stabilize as well. Preserve at least half of the facet joint.

Post-traumatic kyphosis

A fixed deformity often does not need correction. Surgery is indicated for late progression, pain or progressive neurological deficit. Casting/bracing may not prevent progression. Anterior impingement requires anterior decompression and later posterior instrumentation. Multiple posterior closing wedge osteotomies are technically demanding. They are usually carried out on the lumbar spine (below the cord). Anterior release is important with complete discectomy before the vertebral body resection and cage/graft insertion.

Kyphosis

Symptomatic kyphosis is rare in adults. In cases of ankylosing spondylitis thoracic osteotomy has a very high risk. Lumbar osteotomy is most common, followed by cervical osteotomy. L2/3 is the commonest site, below conus medullaris. The facets are resected at 45° to the axis of the spine. Maximum correction is 45° at one level. Pedicle screws can improve correction although there is a high failure rate in cases with osteoporosis. Functional status is improved but the risks are significant.

Spinal tumours

Metastatic tumours are relatively common; primary tumours are rare. They start in the pedicles and spread.

The commonest sites of the primary tumour are: breast, lung, prostate, kidney, colon, bladder and head and neck. Over 50% of patients with bony metastases have spinal involvement. Twenty percent of patients have neurological involvement.

Radiotherapy

Although surgery has an increasing part to play, the mainstay of treatment for many tumours remains radiotherapy. Radiotherapy alone can be used for neurological compromise unless there is significant vertebral collapse. The initial neurological status determines outcome: 70% remain ambulatory, but those who were not ambulatory before treatment rarely walk after radiotherapy alone.

Tumour type and radiosensitivity also determine outcome. Prostate and lymphoreticular tumours respond best. Seventy percent of breast tumours are radiosensitive.

GI and renal tumours are often resistant to radiotherapy.

Surgery

Staging helps to determine the outcome of surgery for spinal metastases (Tokuhashi grading widely used[6]). Patients can often expect functional improvement, pain relief and, in a few cases, cure.

- Vertebral body resection can aid tissue diagnosis. It is also useful for reconstruction for pathological fracture dislocation or for neurological deterioration during/after radiotherapy
- Decompression leads to functional improvement even with prolonged paraplegia. Majority of patients with incomplete neurology continue

---

[6] Tokuhashi Y *et al.* (1990) Scoring system for the preoperative evaluation of metastatic spine tumour prognosis. *Spine* **15(11):** 1110–3.

walking; over 90% have bowel and bladder control
- Laminectomy is rarely indicated and has worse results than anterior surgery
- Renal metastases can cause catastrophic bleeding. Embolize preoperatively and operate within 48 h of embolization as the tumour circulation quickly re-establishes itself
- The approach taken and the results achieved depend on the site and extent of tumour
- Anatomic classification
  - Site: A – intraosseous, B – extraosseous, C – metastases
  - Zones I–IV
  - IA–IVA – intraosseous lesions within cortical boundaries
  - IA – spinous processes to pars and inferior articular processes
  - IIA – transverse processes, superior articular processes and pedicles to body
  - IIIA – anterior three-quarters of vertebral body
  - IVA – posterior and medial quarter of body
  - IB–IVB – extraosseous lesions beyond margins of appropriate zone
  - IC–IVC – intraosseous or extraosseous lesions with regional or distant metastases

Primary tumours

Primary tumours are rare. Chordoma and osteoblastoma are often in the spine. Seventy-five percent of vertebral body tumours are malignant, and 35% are found in the posterior elements.

In children and adolescents one-third of tumours are malignant; 80% of tumours in those aged over 18 years are malignant.

The 5-year survival is 86% for benign tumours, and 24% for malignant tumours. Surgery can improve function and outcome. Multiple myeloma is the commonest and has mixed results in response to chemotherapy and surgery. Solitary plasmacytomas can be cured by excision and reconstruction plus adjuvant systemic therapy.

Infections

Spinal infections are relatively common. Granulomatous infection (TB) varies in incidence compared to pyogenic infection geographically. Consider socioeconomic factors in TB. In pyogenic infections there may be a septic focus elsewhere and risk factors to consider, i.e. intravenous drug abusers and the immunocompromised. Brucellosis, *Candida* and coccidiomycosis occur in certain occupational groups.

Paralysis has an increased incidence in diabetes, rheumatoid arthritis, older age groups and proximal infections.

Normally an anterior abscess is approached from the front. This allows access to associated psoas abscesses. Arthrodesis is controversial: some advocate bone graft in infection and some use metalwork after aggressive debridement and with antibiotic cover.

Diagnosis is often late: there can be a 90-day delay or more. Delay is multifactorial: often there is little systemic response. Pain is vague and poorly localized.

Often there are other infections and normal blood indices. Technetium bone scans are 90% sensitive. MRI scanning is even more sensitive and specific in discitis (in one series it was 96% sensitive, 93% specific and 94% accurate). It is also non-invasive.

In MRI of discitis there is a low signal on T_1-weighted images in the disc and adjacent endplates, and a loss of endplate definition. There is increased signal on T_2-weighted images, which show loss of the intranuclear cleft.

Needle or open biopsy results are often negative. Indirect culture of urine/blood may help.

Conservative management includes rest/bracing with intravenous antibiotics.

Surgical debridement is carried out if the patient shows no improvement on antibiotics, has progressive vertebral collapse and deformity or progressive neurological deterioration. Debridement is carried out with or without autograft with antibiotic cover. Anterior decompression is carried out unless there is a posterior epidural abscess. Large deformities may need instrumentation although this is controversial.

Early diagnosis/treatment can avoid the neurological deterioration seen in 3%–40% of cases (more common with virulent infections). *Staphylococcus aureus* is the commonest organism, and early decompression and antibiotics are indicated.

Non-operative management does not usually improve neurology.

TB mimics other infections but affects the disc late in the course of disease. Vertebral collapse is common and the anterior longitudinal ligament is lifted off adjacent vertebrae. Extensive debridement and reconstruction are then indicated, especially if there is paraplegia. Cover with antituberculous therapy or treat with antituberculous therapy alone if there is no deformity or neurological compromise. Patients can recover as late as 9–12 months post-decompression.

Thoracic disc prolapse

Thoracic disc prolapse is rare (1 per million population per year) and accounts for less than 1% of all disc surgery. Asymptomatic prolapse is probably more common. Diagnosis is very late due to a low index of suspicion. MRI has increased the pick-up rate. Neurological symptoms are nebulous and vague. They can include lower limb spasticity, weakness, ataxia, numbness and bowel/bladder dysfunction.

Differential diagnosis: infection, neoplasia, cord infarction and demyelination.

Surgery can be anterior or posterior (costotransversectomy). Neurological recovery is often very good. Fusion is not carried out routinely.

Spinal cord monitoring

It is very important to carry out spinal cord monitoring during complex spinal surgery, especially deformity correction, in order to prevent cord injury. Monitoring must be sensitive, accurate, and relatively quick and risk free. It needs to identify reversible signal changes. The wake-up test is cumbersome. Electrophysiological testing has limitations. SSEPs are widely used and test the posterior sensory columns. Motor tract status can be inferred from the results.

Motor evoked potential monitoring is a good alternative and allows a better gauge of motor function.

Lumbar spine

Low-back pain is very common and has a 70% lifetime incidence (making it the commonest musculoskeletal problem). Fifty percent of episodes start to settle within 1 week and 90% within 3 months. It is hugely costly in terms of lost days at work and treatment. The majority of cases experience chronic, disabling low-back pain. It is only in the last decade that psychological illness has overtaken back pain as the leading cause for claiming disability benefit in the UK.

Epidemiology

Point prevalence is 7%–17%. The lifetime prevalence of chronic low-back pain is 5%.

The incidence varies between studies and some occupations pose more of a risk than others.

Sciatica

Lifetime incidence is up to 70%. At any time approximately 1 in 8 of those with low-back pain will have sciatica.

The natural history of sciatica is very similar to that of acute low-back pain – almost all have normal function within 6 months. Surgical intervention for lumbar disc prolapse is on the increase but there is great variation between countries; the rate is low in the UK compared to the USA. This is related to the number of spinal surgeons per head of population rather that to widely differing incidences.

Diagnosis

The conundrum is that studies have shown that many asymptomatic patients can have abnormal imaging, myelography, CT scanning and MRI. The incidence of degenerative changes rises with age – 20% at 20–30 years of age, 45% over 40 years and the majority are over 60 years old. The incidence of spinal stenosis also rises with age.

Interpret abnormal scans cautiously in light of clinical examination findings. Findings are only significant if the level of abnormality fits with the history/examination.

History

This is the most important aspect of assessment, followed by examination and imaging.

Pain is the usual symptom (low back or lower limb). Ascertain the predominant site. Is the leg pain radicular or referred? Referred pain – posterior (buttocks and thighs occasionally calf). Distribution is very variable reflecting the origin of tissues from sclerotomes. Radicular sciatic pain can be excruciating and below the knee or dermatomal. The site of back pain is important because treatment for lumbar pain is different from treatment for coccydynia.

The distribution of pain depends on the nerve root affected: L4, anterior knee and medial calf; L5, lateral calf/ankle, dorsum of the first web space on the foot; S1, lateral foot, sole and heel; L3, distal anterior thigh pain (hip pain and retroperitoneal tumours present with similar symptoms). Night pain is sinister and should raise suspicion of infection or neoplasm.

Cauda equina syndrome is a relative surgical emergency. Symptoms include perineal numbness, bilateral sciatica or lower limb numbness and urinary retention or incontinence with or without muscle weakness. Weakness alone does not require urgent surgery. Progressive weakness can respond if the cause of compression is found.

Mechanical low-back pain has a vague and intermittent onset, becoming more frequent and severe. Pain may be from a degenerating disc, which can prolapse causing sciatica.

Only 50% of disc prolapses occur after injury or heavy lifting. The results of treatment for injury/compensation claims are often poor. When taking the history note the exacerbating or relieving factors.

Sciatica is exacerbated by sitting and relieved by standing or lying. Pressure in the disc is greatest when sitting down (50% higher than when standing).

Mechanical low-back pain is worse with activity. Lifting, bending and twisting all exacerbate the problem.

Low-back pain/stiffness in young men – consider ankylosing spondylitis.

Psychosocial factors are important in chronic low-back pain and greatly affect the outcome of surgery, which is worse in certain social settings and with litigation claims. Even if claims are settled successfully the results tend not to improve.

Depression can affect perception of low-back pain. Waddell's inappropriate signs can indicate emotional distress.

Previous lumbar surgery is important: if it was unsuccessful then further surgery is unlikely to help unless it is strongly indicated.

Results: a first operation has a 70% success rate; second-time surgery, 50%; <30% for third operations. Sciatica not helped – prolapse missed. If the patient returns after a few months they are likely to have scarring that may be worsened by further surgery. Scarring may be prevented by barrier gels (expensive). If the pain returns later a recurrent herniation is more likely as the cause. The risk of recurrence after surgery is 8%–10%. Gadolinium-enhanced MRI scans show increased uptake in scar tissue and can differentiate this from a recurrent disc. If there is a prolapse at another level the pain has a different distribution.

Lumbar spinal stenosis

Lumbar spinal stenosis produces neurogenic claudication. The patient's history is likely to reveal back and buttock or leg pain that is worse on standing or walking and relieved by sitting bent forward. Patients walk bent forward over a shopping trolley. No symptoms are present when cycling (use the Van Gelderan cycling test to distinguish neurogenic

Table 19.3 Differentiating neurogenic from vascular claudication

Symptom	Type of claudication	
	Neurogenic	Vascular
Pain site	Thigh	Calf
Standing	Painful	Painless
Relieving factors	Bend forward	Stand
Walking distance	Variable	Fixed
Worse going	Downstairs	Upstairs

from vascular claudication; Table 19.3). The cause is partly mechanical. The canal and lateral recesses and neural foramina are narrowed by extension of the spine when upright. Venous obstruction is caused by the narrowing around the roots leading to relative ischaemia.

Examination

- Refines information gained from the history
- Inspection, looking for deformity (fixed or postural), scoliosis or list
- Palpation and percussion, noting tender areas. If there is superficial skin tenderness assess Waddell's non-organic signs
- Assess lumbar ROM. Assess flexion by seeing how far the patient can reach: shin, ankle, toes? Assess composite movement including hip flexion. Estimate the angle of the back from horizontal or excursion of skin marks (Schober's method)
- If flexion is painful this can indicate a disc prolapse; painful extension indicates spinal stenosis. Often the only finding in stenosis is a mildly positive femoral stretch test
- Root tension signs are important. A positive sciatic stretch test is seen in almost all L4/5 and L5/S1 disc prolapses. This decreases slightly with age. Crossover pain is uncommon (20% with proven disc prolapse) and is a strong indicator of nerve root tension
- The femoral stretch test is equivalent to the sciatic stretch in L2/3 and L3/4 herniation (less common)

- Check peripheral pulses in all patients
- Remember that back pain can be caused by abdominal pathology – aortic aneurysms, peptic ulcer disease, gallstones, retroperitoneal abscesses or tumours; it can also be caused by hip pathology

Investigation

- Plain X-rays – rarely abnormal, can show spondylosis, pars defects (spondylolysis), transitional segments, Schmorl's nodes and spondylolisthesis or spina bifida occulta
- Myelography seldom used – reasonably sensitive/specific for disc prolapse but is invasive
- CT myelography can be used if the patient is not suitable for MRI. It is more sensitive, as specific and slightly more accurate than non-contrast CT in lumbar disc prolapse
- CT shows bones well as well as lateral lesions (foraminal stenosis and osteophytes). 3D CT reconstruction may help although the radiation dose is high
- CT scanning after stress discography – delineates herniation well
- MRI scanning – gold standard, avoids ionizing radiation. Orthogonal images – sagittal and axial views are standard. Best for soft tissues. Delineates disc annulus from nucleus. "Degenerative disc disease" is shown as loss of nuclear hydration and changes in vertebral endplates. Gadolinium diethylenetriaminepentaacetic acid is helpful in postoperative imaging. Degenerative disc disease is not a disease but part of the natural ageing process of the body
- Discography is controversial. It can be used to assess the morphology of the disc during an attempt to reproduce typical pain. Normal subjects can get pain on discography, but some have no pain and yet abnormal disc morphology. Look for concordant pain in planning disc replacement surgery
- Role of EMG is limited. It can reveal root dysfunction that does not arise from compression. Diabetes can mimic disc prolapse through nerve

fibre infarction. EMG distinguishes peroneal neuropathy from L5 radiculopathy. It can also differentiate plexus from nerve lesions, tumours and polyneuropathy

- SEPs are used to evaluate sensory fibres of central and peripheral nerves, but they have many limitations

Other tests

Local injections can localize and treat the source of pain. Nerve root infiltrations are used for multilevel spondylosis and root entrapment at two levels. Facet injections can localize the site of pain and treat painful facet arthrosis. Facet syndrome is a controversial diagnosis. It is characterized by pain on exertion/lumbar extension, tenderness away from the midline over the facets and pain lying flat in bed at night (patient cannot get comfortable).

Rhizotomy is also used to localize the source of pain.

Acute low-back pain

Most resolve spontaneously with or without treatment. Many studies are difficult to interpret. There is no evidence that traction, corsets or bed rest are effective. There is limited evidence that flexion exercises help. Manipulation can help temporarily but not in the long term. It is best to use drugs with the fewest side-effects. Two days of bed rest followed by mobilization is as good as a longer rest and patients return to work sooner.

Chronic low-back pain

Defined as pain for >6 months. This accounts for the majority of the social/economic burden of back pain. There are many causes, and a structural cause is often not found. Often there is a significant psychological element. Endogenous opioid levels may be lower in those with chronic pain. Substance P levels in the CSF are lower in those with chronic pain.

Treat the physical and psychological factors. Biofeedback training as part of a functional restoration programme can be extremely effective.

Surgery for low-back pain

This is a very controversial topic. The exact source of the pain is often unknown. The intermediate outcome is often good. The surgeon needs to localize the source as well as possible. Discography has limited uses, with high false-positive and false-negative rates.

Fusion is done to abolish the painful movement of one or more motion segments. Patients can have a solid fusion with pain and a pseudoarthrosis with no pain. Despite its problems this remains a popular procedure for want of a better solution.

The type of fusion carried out depends on the surgeon's experience and training. Options include posterolateral instrumented fusion with pedicle screw constructs, anterior interbody fusion in addition, or anterior fusion alone. Scores of pedicle screw systems are available. Interbody fusion can be carried out from the back (PLIF), using cages (metal or PEEK) or by using a graft or from one side via the foramen (TLIF) using cages and/or graft or from the front. Recently devised, minimally invasive techniques have minimized morbidity and improved the speed of recovery. Non-fusion technology has been introduced and there are several total and partial (nuclear) disc replacements available with variable results. There is controversy over whether motion should be preserved. Some advocate that pain relief is better than fusion. Intermediate and longer-term results are similar despite the more physiological theory. Few studies show higher success rates than 70% good or excellent results.

Total disc replacements of various types are available: UHMWPE, ceramic or metal-on-metal bearings.

Partial disc replacements can be mechanical or comprise bags filled with hydro gel; there were problems of extrusion with early designs. This could lead to devastating complications such as cauda equina syndrome.

Soft-tissue ligament stabilization has been popular over the last 15 years. Global (SEM) ligament stabilization had promising results in the early stages but many failed at 2 years. The early results of Dynesys (Zimmer, Swindon, UK) were similar. Recently launched newer devices include Wallis ligament (Abbott Spine, Bordeaux, France) and Diam (Medtronic, Tolochenaz, Switzerland). These are interspinous devices.

Radicular pain

Degeneration of the disc occurs as part of normal ageing with the end result of disc prolapse causing sciatica. The majority of younger patients with lumbar disc prolapses are symptomatic. Many older patients are asymptomatic despite disc bulges. Not all disc bulges cause sciatica and there are other factors involved. Chemicals can cause pain, e.g. substance P, VIP, calcitonin gene related peptide and several cytokines. The presence of disc material in the canal causes an intense inflammatory response and this contributes to radicular pain.

The dorsal root ganglion appears to modulate pain and can cause persistent pain.

One study of disc prolapses over 10 years treated conservatively or surgically showed favourable results for surgery at 1 year, and no significant difference at 4 or 10 years.

Surgery relieves symptoms quickly but does not alter the outcome. The natural history is favourable anyway.

Conservative management methods: rest, analgesia, epidural steroid injections, physiotherapy, braces, traction and manipulation. Short-term rest, analgesics and anti-inflammatories are commonly advocated.

Prognosis – >90% resolve spontaneously, <10% require surgery. Initial results of surgical discectomy are generally good with relief of radicular pain in over 90%. Remove only extruded or sequestrated fragments to preserve the disc for the future. One-third of patients can experience back pain after discectomy although few require further surgery.

Microdiscectomy allows good illumination but has a higher risk of complications than open discectomy. Mini-open discectomy has little morbidity with fewer complications.

Chemonucleolysis is almost as effective as discectomy and less invasive. However, the results are not as good but many studies are biased and flawed.

Anaphylaxis with chymopapain is overemphasized and is virtually eliminated by preoperative antihistamines. Patients can get back pain that settles in a few weeks. Neurological complications have also been reported.

Percutaneous lumbar discectomy is less invasive but is not suitable for extruded or sequestrated prolapses because the results are not as good as open discectomy in these cases.

Spinal stenosis

This is more common than prolapse in older patients. Cause is multifactorial and involves disc and facet joints. The disc degenerates placing abnormal loads on the facet joints. This leads to facet arthrosis. There is loss of disc height and over-riding of the facets, which narrows the lateral recess and foramen. The facet capsule and PLL bulge in with ligamentum flavum (thick/less elastic) and this narrows the central canal. Lordosis exacerbates foraminal narrowing. Ischaemia is caused by venous outflow obstruction/altered CSF flow and contributes to the pain.

Spinal stenosis can be due to compression in the central canal, the lateral recess or foramen or a combination of all three. A congenitally narrow canal (achondroplasia) predisposes patients to spinal stenosis. Scoliosis or spondylolisthesis can narrow the canal. Epidural lipomatosis can compress the thecal sac in a normal canal.

Natural history is unknown and the condition can settle with time/activity modification. Conservative treatment – anti-inflammatory medication. Cycling is encouraged to keep active. Steroid epidurals offer temporary relief.

The diagnosis and extent can be determined by MRI scan. Decompression surgery is required to remove the compressing elements. Remember to leave >50% of the facet joint in order to avoid destabilizing the spine, necessitating fusion.

Preserve disc as this aids stability. Thankfully in the UK there are now fewer laminectomies and more laminotomies.

Spinous process osteotomy can aid access for multi-level decompression. It has less morbidity as the paraspinal muscles are dissected on one side only.

Short-term success rates: 70%–85% but there is deterioration with time. More extensive decompression has worse results.

Fusion improves results (extensive decompression or spondylolisthesis with or without reduction of the slip).

Recent developments include interspinous spacers. They give an indirect decompression by opening the lateral recess and foramen at the level of insertion. Early results are promising, but a longer follow-up is required. Best results if the patient is unfit for major open decompression; less effective for severe central canal stenosis.

The hand oral

20. Syllabus and general guidance   273
Paul A. Banaszkiewicz

21. Hand oral core topics   276
Paul A. Banaszkiewicz and
John W. K. Harrison

Syllabus and general guidance

Paul A. Banaszkiewicz

Hand surgery syllabus for the FRCS (Tr & Orth) examination

"The hand" covers the hand and forearm and the structures anatomically contained within. Knowledge of the structural anatomy and the biomechanics of joint and tendon function is required.

Pathology

A working knowledge of the acute conditions and trauma of the hand is required, i.e. injury to the bones, joints, tendons, nerves, skin and vessels of the hand and infective processes.

Knowledge of the non-acute congenital, degenerative, inflammatory (rheumatoid) and neoplastic conditions as well as benign tumours, e.g. ganglions, is also required.

Training in operative hand surgery

For the purpose of the examinations, the trainee should have gained experience in the operative management of:
- The acutely injured hand
- Fractures, including scaphoid non-union
- Dislocations
- Nerve injuries
- Tendon injuries and common tendon transfers

- Skin grafts
- Infections

In elective surgery, the candidate must have sound knowledge of the procedures appropriate for carpal tunnel syndrome, trigger finger, Dupuytren's contracture, benign tumours, degenerative conditions of the carpometacarpal joint and wrist joints and surgery of the rheumatoid hand.

Long cases

- Brachial plexus injuries
- Peripheral nerve injuries
- Rheumatoid shoulder/hand and wrist

Short cases

- Brachial plexus lesions
- Carpal instability
- Carpal tunnel syndrome
- Basal thumb osteoarthritis
- Duplicated thumb
- Dupuytren's disease
- Kienböck's disease
- Median nerve injury
- Ulnar nerve injury (high and low)
- Perilunate dislocation
- Radial nerve palsy
- Rheumatoid hand and wrist
- Ulnar collateral ligament injuries

Postgraduate Orthopaedics: The Candidate's Guide to the FRCS (Tr & Orth) Examination, Ed. Paul A. Banaszkiewicz,
Deiary F. Kader, Nicola Maffulli. Published by Cambridge University Press. © Cambridge University Press 2009.

Basic science

- APB wasting
- Flexor tendon sheath/vinculae
- Brachial plexus
- Name muscles in deep flexor compartment of forearm
- Extensor compartments of the wrist
- Identify EPB, APL, EPL and EDQ tendons
- Label a diagram of the brachial plexus
- Ulnar nerve anatomy at wrist
- Seddon's classification of nerve injury
- Factors influencing outcome in nerve repair

Children

- Camptodactyly
- Clinodactyly
- Congenital bands
- Delta phalanx
- Enchondromata
- Radial club hand
- Syndactyly
- Congenital absence of thumb

Trauma

- Bennett's fractures radiograph (name deforming forces)
- Carpal instability
- Compartment syndrome
- Digital nerve injury
- DRU joint injury
- Fingertip injuries
- Finger amputations
- Flexor tendon injuries: repair, rehabilitation and late reconstruction
- Frykman classification
- "Mangled hand"
- Pathoanatomy of MCP joint dislocation
- Phalangeal fractures (classification)
- Scaphoid injuries/periscaphoid injuries
- Scaphoid non-union

- UCL injuries/Stener lesion
- Volar Barton's fracture

Rheumatoid

- Boutonnière
- Elbow replacement
- MCP joint replacements
- Rheumatoid thumb

Others

- Dupuytren's disease: associations, management of PIP joint contracture, treatment options
- Kienböck's
- RSD
- TB dactylitis
- Tumours
- Tourniquets
- Radial nerve palsy and tendon transfers

MCQ paper

- Ganglions
- Trigger finger
- Management principles for the rheumatoid hand
- Causes of loss of extension in the rheumatoid finger

General guidance

The hand oral can be tricky and it is best to bat safe with this one. There is a large amount of material that candidates can be asked. In addition the standard and general flow of the oral are known to vary from one table of examiners to the next.

One particular style of oral is very straightforward and basically consists of a series of clinical photographs and radiographs of common hand conditions that the average trainee would have no difficulty in recognizing. It is a case of describing what you see, the diagnosis, differential diagnosis and management options. Another style of oral can be extremely difficult with a small number (three or four) of esoteric topics that examiners seem to dwell on for far too long.[1] Candidates were never very sure of how they were doing throughout the oral. The examiners were typically old school and did not provide much feedback.

It is a combined oral with paediatrics, both orals lasting 15 min each. There are usually one or two paediatric hand trauma questions thrown in at some stage from either the hands or paeds examiner.

Working with an experienced hand surgeon for 6 months should prime you up with the necessary knowledge needed to get through this oral. A thorough, practical, safe knowledge of hand surgery is required rather than textbook minutia. Before the exam it helps greatly if you can have practice orals with an experienced hand surgeon. Some topics are fairly predictable but it is still surprising how they can catch you out.

---

[1] Comparison of Kutler double lateral V-Y advancement flap with the volar V-Y flap of Atasoy.

21

Hand oral core topics

Paul A. Banaszkiewicz and John W. K. Harrison

Anatomy

Physes

In the hand these are located distally in the 2nd to 5th metacarpals, and proximally in the thumb metacarpal and phalanges.

Flexor pulleys

Fingers

In the fingers the flexor pulleys facilitate sheath collapse and expansion during digital motion. There are five annular pulleys: A2 and A4 pulleys originate from bone and it is critical to preserve them to prevent bowstringing of the flexor tendons; A1, A3 and A5 originate from the volar plates. A1 pulley is released in trigger finger.

Three cruciate pulleys are not critical for flexor function. C1 is distal to the A2 pulley over the proximal phalanx; C2 and C3 are either side of the A4 pulley over the middle phalanx.

Thumb

In the thumb there are two annular pulleys and one oblique pulley. The oblique pulley is most important. A1 overlies the MCP joint, attached to the volar plate. A2 overlies the IP joint, attached to the head of PP. The oblique pulley overlies the shaft of PP. The tendon of adductor pollicis attaches to the A1 and oblique pulleys.

Vinculae

The vinculae are folds of mesotendon carrying blood supply to both tendons from transverse branches of the digital arteries. There is a short vinculum (vinculum brevis) and a long vinculum (vinculum longus) to each FDP and FDS tendon. The vincular system is supplied by the transverse communicating branches of the common digital artery. Nutrition of the tendons is also derived from diffusion through the synovial fluid.

Anatomy of the intrinsic muscles

The intrinsic muscles have their origins and insertions within the hand. These are the thenar muscle group, hypothenar muscle group, adductor pollicis, lumbricals and interossei.

Lumbrical muscles (4)

The lumbrical muscles are the workhorse of the hand. They are the only muscles to originate on a tendon (FDP) and insert on a tendon (radial lateral band of the extensor expansion). The radial two lumbricals are innervated by the median nerve and the ulnar two lumbricals by the ulnar nerve. Median-nerve-innervated lumbricals are unicipital. Ulnar-nerve-innervated lumbricals are bicipital (arise by two heads from adjacent FDP tendons). Action is MCP joint flexion and IP joint extension. Laceration of FDP distal to the lumbrical origin leads to lumbrical plus finger.

Postgraduate Orthopaedics: The Candidate's Guide to the FRCS (Tr & Orth) Examination, Ed. Paul A. Banaszkiewicz,
Deiary F. Kader, Nicola Maffulli. Published by Cambridge University Press. © Cambridge University Press 2009.

Interosseous muscles (7)

Four dorsal interosseous muscles abduct away from the axis of the middle finger (Dorsal ABducts, or DAB). Three palmar interossei adduct the index, ring and little fingers towards the axis of the middle finger (Palmar ADducts or PAD).

The interosseous muscles arise from the metacarpal bones: the larger dorsal interossei from two adjacent metacarpals, the smaller palmar interossei from the metacarpal of the finger to which each passes.

The dorsal interossei insert into the lateral sides of the index and middle fingers and to the medial sides of the middle and ring fingers. The palmar interossei insert into the medial side of the index finger and to the lateral sides of the ring and little fingers. All are supplied by the ulnar nerve. An occasional variant is for the 1st dorsal interosseous muscle to be supplied by the median nerve.

Anatomy of the extrinsic muscles

The extrinsic extensor muscle bellies of the hand overlie the dorsum of the forearm and their tendons pass over the dorsum of the wrist to insert in the hand.

Dorsal extensor compartments of the wrist (6)

There are 6 fibro-osseous tunnels through which the extensor tendons pass and they are numbered from the radial side to the ulnar side.

1. **APL/EPB**. Located on the radial surface of the radial styloid. Chronic tenosynovitis here is known as De Quervain's disease. Both tendons are in separate synovial sheaths.
2. **ECRL/ECRB**. ERCL inserts onto the base of the 2nd metacarpal, and ERCB onto the base of the 3rd. Intersection syndrome.
3. **EPL**. Lister's tubercle separates the 2nd from the 3rd compartment. Delayed rupture following distal radius fractures.
4. **EIP/EDC**. Extensor tenosynovitis and ruptures. Contains the posterior interosseous nerve.

5. **EDM**. Double tendon. Floor is dorsal capsule of DRUJ. Vaughan Jackson rupture in rheumatoid arthritis.
6. **ECU**. Lies over the head of the ulna. Snapping ECU.

Extensor tendons and hood

The extensor tendon broadens before dividing into three slips over the dorsal surface of the proximal phalanx. The central slip inserts into the base of the middle phalanx. The two lateral or marginal slips receive attachments from the lumbrical and interossei tendons to form a broad extensor expansion or hood, which overlies the metacarpal head and the proximal part of the PP. Over the middle phalanx the lateral slips are held dorsally by the **triangular ligament** and volarly by the **transverse retinacular ligaments**. Imbalance of the lateral bands results in a swan neck or boutonnière deformity. The transverse retinacular ligaments attach to the volar plate.

Oblique retinacular ligament (ORL)

Bilateral strong narrow bands that originate from the periosteum of the PP and A2 pulley and insert into the extensor tendon at the base of the DP. Active extension of the PIP joint tightens the volarly placed ORL, leading to passive extension of the DIP joint (tenodesis effect).

Sagittal band

Connects the extensor tendon to the volar plate of the MCP joint to extend the MCP joint. In hyperextension of the MCP joint the IP joints fall into flexion because the extensor tendon distal to the sagittal band becomes lax. In this position the IP joints can only be extended by the intrinsics.

Boundaries of the anatomical snuffbox

The "snuff box" is a hollow area distal to the radial styloid on the dorsal–radial aspect of the wrist.

Floor: scaphoid

Radial border: extensor pollicis brevis (and abductor pollicis longus)
Ulnar border: Extensor pollicis longus
Proximally: Radial styloid
Distally: Base of thumb metacarpal

The radial artery courses through the snuffbox on its way to the dorsal first web space. Part-origin of the cephalic vein overlies the ASB.

Cleland's ligament (C in Cleland's and ceiling, i.e. dorsal)

A fibrous ligament between the phalanges and the dermis (skin) that is dorsal (posterior) to the neurovascular bundle. These fibrous bands are located between the middle of the PP and the DIP joint.

Grayson's ligament (G in Grayson's and ground, i.e. more volar)

A very fine membrane, which lies in front of the neurovascular bundle. Originates from the anterior layer of the fibrous flexor tendon sheath and inserts into the skin.

FDS of the small finger

Absent in 30% so remember that it may be absent in flexor tendon injury of the little finger. Comparison with the opposite side is essential when evaluating for an FDS laceration in the small finger.

EDC of the small finger

EDC may be absent in half of people in whom extension is achieved by the EDM.

Nail anatomy

The nail plate is supported by the nail bed. This consists of the germinal matrix (lunula is the visible portion) that produces the nail, and the sterile matrix that produces keratin to thicken the nail. The eponychium is the proximal nail fold and the paronychium is the lateral nail fold.

Blood supply of the hand

The hand has a generous blood supply.

Superficial palmar arch

Lies 2 cm distal to the deep arch. Surface anatomy is the distal palmar crease. The superficial arch is the curved continuation of the ulnar artery and is incomplete in 80% as there is no anastomosis with the superficial palmar branch of the radial artery.

From its convexity a palmar digital artery passes to the ulnar side of the little finger and three common palmar digital arteries run distally to the web spaces between the fingers where each vessel divides into proper palmar digital arteries that supply adjacent fingers. The arteries lie superficial to the nerves in the palm and deep to the nerves in the digits.

Deep palmar arch

Surface anatomy is Kaplan's line (from the hook of hamate to the base of the first web space). The deep palmar arch is an arterial arcade formed by the terminal branch (deep branch) of the radial artery anastomosing with the deep branch of the ulnar artery and is complete in 98%. Lies deep to the long flexor tendons and superficial to the interosseous muscles.

From its concavity three palmar metacarpal arteries pass distally and join with the common palmar digital branches of the superficial arch.

Radial artery

The radial artery passes into the hand between the two heads of the first dorsal interosseous muscle. Lying between the first dorsal interosseous and adductor pollicis muscle it gives off two branches.

The *radialis indicis artery* passes distally between the first dorsal interosseous and adductor pollicis muscles to supply the radial side of the index finger.

The *princeps pollicis artery* passes distally along the metacarpal bone of the thumb and divides into the two palmar digital branches of the thumb at the metacarpal head.

The main trunk of the radial artery passes into the palm between the oblique and transverse heads of adductor pollicis to form the deep palmar arch.

Examination corner

Hand oral 1

Photograph straight out of "Interactive hand",[1] of the volar aspect of the wrist – asked to identify various anatomical structures.

Hand oral 2

Similar to oral 1 with an interactive photograph of the back of the wrist – asked to identify labels to various anatomical structures.

[1] McGrouther DA, Colditz JC, Harris JM, Stoller DW. *Interactive Hand Therapy*, 2nd edn. London: Primal Pictures.

Anatomy of the median nerve

Nerve roots

Formed by the joining of the lateral and medial cords of the brachial plexus in the axilla (C6, C7, C8, T1).

Course

- Lies lateral to the brachial artery in the arm, then crosses anteriorly to lie medial to the artery in the antecubital fossa, passing beneath the bicipital aponeurosis
- No branches before the elbow
- It descends between the two heads of pronator teres and is separated from the ulnar artery by the deep head of pronator teres

- Then passes beneath the fibrous arch of FDS in the proximal third of the forearm
- About 5–6 cm distal to the elbow it gives off the anterior interosseous branch (motor to FPL, FDP index finger and pronator quadratus)
- In the forearm it descends between FDS and FDP roughly in the midline
- It becomes superficial just above the wrist where it lies between the tendons of FDS and FCR
- Palmar cutaneous branch (sensory to thenar skin) arises 5 cm proximal to the wrist joint, ulnar to FCR and passes over the flexor retinaculum
- Main nerve passes deep to the flexor retinaculum, to the radial side of the tendons of FDS
- The recurrent motor branch to thenar muscles arises at the distal end of the carpal tunnel (see below)
- The median nerve finally ends by dividing into medial and lateral branches to supply the radial 3½ digits

Branches

Near the elbow

- PT
- FCR
- PL
- FDS

In the forearm (anterior interosseous branch[1])

- FPL
- Radial half of FDP
- PQ

In the hand

- Motor – the "LOAF" muscles of the thenar eminence:
  - **L**ateral two lumbricals
  - **O**pponens pollicis
  - **A**bductor pollicis
  - **F**lexor pollicis brevis

[1] Descends on the interosseous membrane to the wrist.

Sensory

- Flexor surfaces and nails of the radial 3½ digits
- Skin thenar eminence supplied by the palmar cutaneous branch, which is given off 5 cm above the wrist

Carpal tunnel anatomy

Fibro-osseous tunnel formed by the concavity of the anterior surface of the carpus and roofed over by the flexor retinaculum. Knowledge of the anatomy of the carpal tunnel is essential in order to undertake carpal tunnel decompression.

Boundaries of the carpal tunnel

- Radial wall: scaphoid tuberosity, ridge of trapezium
- Ulnar wall: pisiform, hook of hamate
- Floor: carpus, proximal metacarpals
- Roof: flexor retinaculum

Contents (10)

Nine flexor tendons and the median nerve.
- FPL – the most radial structure
- Median nerve (just deep to the flexor retinaculum and lateral to FDS)
- FDS – lies on the profundus tendons arranged 2-by-2 (middle and ring lie superficial to index and little). *Remember, 34 (third and fourth) over 25 (second and fifth)*
- FDP – all together on a deeper plane (lie side-by-side on the floor of the carpal tunnel)

The FCR tendon lies in a separate fibro-osseous tunnel deep to the flexor retinaculum.

Flexor retinaculum

Attachments

The flexor retinaculum is attached to the pisiform and hamate on the ulnar side and to the ridge of the trapezium and the tuberosity of the scaphoid on the radial side. There is also a deep slip, which

is attached to the medial lip of a groove on the trapezium.

Functions

- Prevents bowstringing of the long flexor tendons
- It gives partial insertion to some muscles (PL, FCU)
- It gives partial origin to some muscles (thenar and hypothenar muscles)

Variations of the motor (recurrent) branch of the median nerve

A key surgical landmark and major surgical danger in carpal tunnel release. Surface landmark is the intersection of the flexed middle finger tip with Kaplan's line.

There are three main variations to the motor branch in the palm and several other much less common variations:

1. **Extraligamentous branch** (50%) arises from the volar radial aspect of the median nerve distal to the transverse carpal ligament and recurrent to the thenar muscles. The nerve hooks radially and upwards to enter the thenar muscle mass between the FPB and APB muscles
2. **Subligamentous branch** (30%) arises from the anterior surface of the nerve within the carpal tunnel, emerging distal to the flexor retinaculum and recurrent to the thenar muscles
3. **Transligamentous branch** (20%) arises from the anterior surface of the nerve within the carpal tunnel and pierces the flexor retinaculum

There are other rarer divisions described: ulnar side of the nerve, anterior surface of the nerve, double motor branches and high division. Patients with rare variations usually have a large palmaris brevis muscle.

Variants of the palmar cutaneous branch of the median nerve

The course of the palmar cutaneous branch of the median nerve may vary in four important ways:

1. Normally the nerve is given off 5 cm proximal to the wrist and runs along the ulnar side of FCR

before crossing the flexor retinaculum. The nerve divides into two major branches, medial and lateral, whilst crossing the flexor retinaculum

2. There are two distinct branches, which travel separately across the wrist
3. The nerve enters the carpal tunnel and penetrates flexor retinaculum
4. Nerve may be replaced by a branch from the radial or ulnar nerve

Kaplan's cardinal line

Kaplan described an anatomical guideline for locating the recurrent motor branch of the median nerve. Kaplan's line is a line drawn from the distal border of the abducted thumb to the hook of hamate.

The recurrent motor branch of the median nerve entering the thenar muscle mass is estimated by the intersection of Kaplan's line and a vertical line from the radial border of the middle finger.

The hook of hamate lies at the intersection of the ulnar border of the ring finger and Kaplan's line. The deep palmar arch lies deep to Kaplan's cardinal line. The superficial palmar arch lies 2 cm distally, deep to the distal transverse palmar crease.

Examination corner

Hand oral

Clinical photograph of a recent surgical scar over the thenar crease suggestive of carpal tunnel decompression. The scar however was placed far too radial, over the thenar muscle mass, and extended straight across the wrist cutting perpendicular to the flexor crease.

Candidate 1

Examiner: This woman has had recent surgery to her hand. What do you think of the scar and its position?

Candidate: There is a recent longitudinal mid-palmar scar over the thenar crease, which extends proximally across the distal wrist crease into the distal forearm (long pause). (The scar looked like one used for a carpal tunnel release but slightly atypical and the candidate was not entirely sure if he/she should mention carpal tunnel release.)

Examiner: (who was expecting the candidate to continue talking and therefore ended up prompting the candidate) What do you think of the scar itself?

Candidate: The scar extends straight across the wrist.

Examiner: What surgery do you think she has had?

Candidate: Carpal tunnel decompression.

Examiner: Do you normally extend the incision for decompression proximally above the wrist joint?[1]

Candidate: (who was aware of the controversy but was unsure what to say, hesitant, and trying to second guess the examiner) No, I generally do not go above the wrist with my initial skin incision for a straightforward carpal tunnel.

Examiner: I can't think of any particular reason why you should extend the skin incision above the distal wrist crease. What do you think of the scar?[2]

Candidate: The scar looks as though it is still maturing, suggesting that surgery was only recently performed.

Examiner: Don't you think the scar is a bit too medial and also crossing the flexion crease at 90°? With this incision important structures may be damaged and in addition a contracture may develop over the wrist joint.

Candidate: Yes.

Examiner: Show me on my hand the incision you would use when performing a carpal tunnel release. Hands candidate a pen.

The candidate draws the incision on the examiner's palm.

Examiner: What structures pass through the carpal tunnel?

Candidate: The carpal tunnel contains the flexor digitorum superficialis and profundus tendons to all fingers, flexor pollicis longus and the median nerve.

Examiner: (not particularly happy with the candidate[3]) What structures can be damaged during a carpal tunnel release?

Candidate: The palmar cutaneous branch of the median nerve and the recurrent motor branch to the thenar muscles.

Examiner: Where are these nerves given off?

Candidate: The palmar cutaneous branch of the median nerve is given off 5 cm above the wrist joint and the recurrent motor branch to the thenar muscles just distal to the flexor retinaculum.

Examiner: Show me where exactly these nerves travel – trace them out on my hand. (Offers outstretched hand to candidate.)

On reflection the candidate thought that they should have picked up straight away that the scar was way too far radially into the thenar muscle bulk and then gone on to mention the structures placed at risk with this incision; this, despite numerous promptings by the examiner as to what they wanted the candidate to say.

The vital components to this oral scenario were immediate recognition of the misplaced surgical incision and the surface anatomy of various anatomical structures at risk from carpal tunnel decompression.

Candidate: I never recovered from not immediately recognizing the fairly obvious misplaced surgical scar. I also thought there was some catch in the questions being asked.

Normally when performing carpal tunnel decompression I extend the skin incision slightly above the distal wrist crease. I was unaware that this was slightly controversial. Instead of defending my practice to the examiner I second-guessed what they wanted me to say but I didn't sound convincing in my reply. I was only vaguely familiar with Kaplan's cardinal lines, which I should have mentioned when discussing the surface anatomy of the various nerves at risk.

[Fail]

[1] Controversial. Some authorities recommend extending your incision above the distal wrist crease to make sure the fascia of the distal forearm is released as this can cause tight compression of the nerve. Others feel that this structure can be adequately decompressed with a smaller incision using scissors and retractors to protect the median nerve. Still others feel that decompressing the transverse carpal ligament is sufficient. However, you should not cross perpendicular to a flexion crease.

[2] The third occasion on which the examiner had prompted the candidate with this particular question but the candidate still didn't pick it up.

[3] The candidate's answer was reasonable but the examiner wasn't particularly happy. I think the examiner had given up on the candidate at this stage.

Candidate 2

The candidate immediately picked up that the position of the scar was sub-optimal and explained the structures at risk.

Candidate: I am concerned the scar has been placed too radially for a carpal tunnel decompression.

The case was fairly straightforward; the crucial element was that you had to immediately spot that the incision was far too radial.

[Pass]

Carpal tunnel syndrome

Incidence

- 1% in the general population (14% in diabetics)

Causes

The acronyms PRAGMATIC or ICRAMPS help you to remember the causes of carpal tunnel syndrome:

P – Pregnancy
R – Rheumatoid arthritis
A – Arthritis (degenerative)
G – Growth hormone (acromegaly)
M – Metabolic (hypothyroidism, gout, diabetes mellitus)
A – Alcoholism
T – Tumours
I – Idiopathic (most)
C – Connective tissue disorders (amyloidosis, haemochromatosis)

or

I – Idiopathic
C – Colles', Cushing's
R – Rheumatoid
A – Acromegaly, amyloid
M – Myxoedema, mass (diabetes) mellitus
P – Pregnancy
S – Sarcoidosis, systemic lupus erythematosus

Symptoms

- Paraesthesia in radial 3½ digits
- Worse at night
- Weakness in the hand, dropping things
- Pain
- 40% bilateral involvement
- M: F 1:6
- Not always classical

Signs

- Examine neck movements
- Swelling over volar aspect of the wrist

- Wasting of thenar muscles
- Trophic ulcers
- Sensation (light touch, two-point discrimination)
- Power (APB)
- Provocative tests
  - Median nerve compression test (Durkin's) – apply direct pressure with your thumb over the nerve, with the patient's elbow extended and wrist flexed 60° (86% sensitivity, 83% specificity)
  - Tinel's sign (74% sensitivity, 90% specificity)
  - Phalen's test (positive if signs <60 s) (61% sensitivity, 83% specificity)
- **Sensitivity**: The proportion of patients with carpal tunnel syndrome testing positive
- **Specificity**: The proportion of patients without carpal tunnel syndrome testing negative (this assesses how effective the test is at excluding those patients without carpal tunnel syndrome)

Nerve conduction studies (NCS)

Abnormal if:
- Sensory conduction is prolonged >3.5 ms (demyelination)
- Increased distal motor latency >4.0 ms
- Decreased amplitude (axonal loss)
- Accurate 85%–90%
- False-negative rate 10%–15%

On which patients do you perform NCS? – Safe answer is to say all patients in whom carpal tunnel syndrome is suspected but who have negative carpal tunnel provocation tests.

Differential diagnosis

- Cervical disc disease
- Peripheral neuropathy – alcohol, diabetes
- Pronator syndrome
- Spinal cord lesions – tumour, syrinx, MS
- Thoracic outlet syndrome
- Collagen vascular disorders
- Raynaud's disease
- RSD

Management

Non-operative

Indicated in those with mild intermittent symptoms without neurological impairment, who have had symptoms <1 year, and who have no muscle wasting. The classic indication is a temporary, reversible carpal tunnel syndrome (pregnancy). Splintage in neutral (extension increases tunnel pressure), NSAIDs, short-term diuretics, steroid injections (80% transient relief, 20% symptom free at 12 months).

Surgical

Indicated in those with progressive persistent symptoms with neurological defects.

1. **Open carpal tunnel decompression:** 95% good or excellent results. Allows good visualization of the median nerve and the contents of the tunnel. Physiological state of the nerve can be assessed.

   Incision – a safe incision is offered (Figure 21.1): longitudinal from the distal wrist crease and just ulnar to palmaris longus,[2] in line with the radial border of the ring finger, and distally to Kaplan's line. It is not routinely recommended to cross proximal to the wrist crease.

   Adjunctive surgical procedures – no demonstrable benefit of additional synovectomy or internal neurolysis following carpal tunnel release and may lead to adhesions.

2. **Endoscopic carpal tunnel release:** introduced to reduce the incidence of pillar pain but this has not been demonstrated. Use either the Agee (one incision) or Chow (two incisions) technique. Steep learning curve with increased early complication rate including actual injury to the median nerve. Pain less at 3 months compared to open release, but no difference at a year.[3]

---

[2] To find palmaris longus, oppose tip of thumb to radial side of the distal phalanx of the little finger, with the wrist flexed.

[3] Atroshi I, Larsson GU, Ornstein E, Hofer M, Johnsson R, Ranstam J (2006) Outcomes of endoscopic surgery compared with open surgery for carpal tunnel syndrome among employed patients: randomised controlled trial. *Br Med J* **332**(7556): 1473.

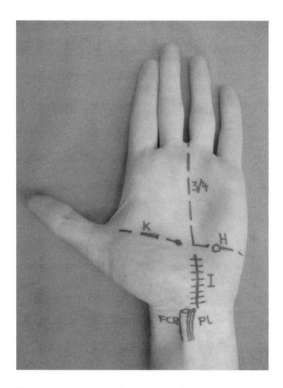

Figure 21.1 Landmarks for open carpal tunnel decompression. 3/4, Space between the 3rd and 4th digits; I, incision; H, hook of hamate; K, Kaplan's line; black spot, motor branch; Pl, palmaris longus; FCR, flexor carpi radialis

Complications of carpal tunnel release

Infection: <1%.

Tender scar: Due to division of very fine terminal branches of the palmar cutaneous nerve.

Haematoma: Major bleeding rare if observe safe anatomical landmarks.

Dehiscence: Sutures removed too early.

Damage to nerves: Recurrent motor branch of the median nerve, palmar cutaneous branch median nerve, ulnar nerve.

Pillar pain: Pain felt when pushing down on the base of the hand following carpal tunnel release. Aetiology uncertain, possibly due to gradual stretching of intercarpal ligaments, which are no longer de-tensioned by the flexor

retinaculum. Others suggest that division of the flexor retinaculum disturbs the alignment of the pisotriquetral joint, which is the source of pillar pain.

Complex regional pain syndrome: Rare but always mention in consent.

Weakness of grip: Returns to preoperative levels in 3 months.

Bowstringing of flexor tendons: More a theoretical complication than a practical one.

Failed carpal tunnel release

Recurrent or persistent symptoms in up to 20%. Most problems are due to inadequate release. Other differential diagnoses include cervical radiculopathy at C5/6, compression of the upper trunk brachial plexus and proximal median nerve compression. Double crush phenomenon relates to more than one site of compression that if isolated would not cause symptoms, but together cause symptoms. Perform NCS after at least 3 months.

Symptoms unchanged: Wrong diagnosis, inadequate decompression, postoperative fibrosis, double crush phenomenon

New symptoms: Normal structures damaged at surgery, new diagnosis

Re-exploration is indicated if:

• Positive Phalen's test
• Nocturnal symptoms
• Positive NCS after 3–6 months
• Relief of symptoms after steroid injection

Examination corner

Hand oral 1

Carpal tunnel syndrome

• Symptoms
• Signs
• Tests
• NCS (principles, findings)
• Open versus endoscopic

Hand oral 2

Carpal tunnel syndrome

Examiner: Who would you perform nerve conduction studies on?

Examiner: Show me in my hand how you would do a carpal tunnel decompression (examiner wearing a glove).

Examiner: What nerves are in danger?

Examiner: If you extend your incision distally what structure is in danger (deep palmar arch)?

Examiner: What are the surface markings of the deep palmar arch?

Examiner: What would you do if you found a space-occupying lesion of the nerve at an open carpal tunnel release?

Candidate: I would close the wound as the decompression has been performed, and refer the patient to a surgeon with microscopic skills.

Examiner: How would you manage a patient with thenar wasting and weakness (explain to the patient that muscle will not return, and consideration for tendon transfers – see later)?

Pronator syndrome

Background

Essentially a high median nerve entrapment. The median nerve is vulnerable to compression at a variety of sites around the elbow.[4] A rare clinical condition.

Sites of entrapment

- Ligament of Struthers – 1% population (supracondylar process)
- Bicipital aponeurosis (lacertus fibrosis)
- Origin of the pronator teres (abnormal anatomy, tight fibrous bands)
- Proximal arch of FDS

---

[4] Although it is called pronator syndrome, it is not only compression of the median nerve when it passes between the two heads of the pronator teres – the compression may occur at various sites.

Clinical

- Pain or ache in the volar proximal forearm and tender to palpation
- Paraesthesia of the median-nerve-innervated digits and thenar eminence (palmar cutaneous branch)
- Usually no night symptoms of paraesthesiae or tingling
- Weakness of the forearm or clumsiness of the hand. Phalen's test generally negative, as the site of compression is proximal to the transverse carpal ligament. Tinel's test negative at the wrist but may be positive at the proximal anterior aspect of the forearm

Provocative tests

- Resisted elbow flexion with forearm supination (bicipital aponeurosis)
- Resisted forearm pronation with elbow extended (two heads of pronator teres)
- Isolated long finger PIP joint flexion (FDS origin)

Investigations

- NCS usually unhelpful
- EMG may show evidence of reduced innervation of muscles

Management

- Usually responds to non-operative treatment – modification of activities, NSAIDs, heat and massage
- If not settled after 6–12 months, surgical decompression of all potential sites of compression

---

Examination corner

Hand oral

Clinical photograph demonstrating operative release of the nerve. Name potential sites of compression.

Anterior interosseous syndrome

Background

Purely motor entrapment – no sensory disturbance. AIN supplies FDP to index and middle fingers, FPL and PQ.

Tests

- Direct pressure over the nerve may elicit symptoms (Tinel's sign negative)
- Symptoms occur acutely with sudden onset of dull non-specific pain in the proximal third of the volar forearm
- Weakness of flexion at the DIP joint of the index finger and IP joint of the thumb (OK sign)
- The middle finger profundus may have some weakness but usually has some function because of cross-over innervation from the ulnar nerve
- Mild weakness of pronation
- OK sign – tip-to-tip pinch. Tests FDP to the index finger and FPL. If patient makes a square instead of a circle this is called the Kiloh–Nevin sign
- To isolate PQ – test resisted forearm pronation with the elbow maximally flexed (elbow flexion eliminates pronator teres)

Differential diagnosis

- Parsonage–Turner syndrome (bilateral AIN syndrome – viral brachial neuritis, motor loss preceded by intense pain in the shoulder region)
- Mannerfelt–Norman Syndrome (FPL rupture)[5]

Sites of constriction

- Deep head of the pronator teres muscle (most common site of compression)

---

[5] Occasionally only the thumb or index finger is involved generally indicating a more distal compression of the nerve and one must be careful not to confuse this with an isolated tendon rupture of either FPL or FDP of the index finger.

- FDS arcade
- Enlarged bicipital bursa
- Gantzer's muscle (accessory head FPL)

Investigations

- NCS usually unhelpful

Management

Non-operative management

Elbow splinting in 90° of flexion, NSAIDS, etc. Many symptoms and signs will gradually resolve in time.

Surgical decompression

This is indicated following the failure of conservative treatment for 6 months. Surgery involves complete exposure of the AIN from its origin from the median nerve. Results are unpredictable.

Examination corner

Hand oral

Clinical photograph of the OK sign – patient making a square instead of a circle.
Spot diagnosis
- Possible causes
- AIN-innervated muscles
- Management

Anatomy of the ulnar nerve

Nerve roots

The nerve arises from the medial cord of the brachial plexus (C8, T1).

Course

- Passes through the medial intermuscular septum at the mid-point of the arm

- Passes through the arcade of Struthers (band of fascia from the medial head of triceps to the medial intermuscular septum) approximately 8 cm proximal to the medial epicondyle
- Passes through the cubital tunnel behind the medial epicondyle
- Enters the forearm between the two heads of FCU
- Passes distally on the medial side of the forearm on FDP and deep to FCU
- Gives off the dorsal cutaneous branch 5 cm proximal to the wrist
- At the wrist lies between FCU tendon and ulnar artery (artery–nerve–tendon or ANT)
- Passes through Guyon's canal between the pisiform and the hook of hamate and divides into superficial and deep branches at the distal end
- Superficial branch supplies palmaris brevis and is sensory to the ulnar 1½ digits
- Deep (motor) branch passes ulnar to the hook of hamate and then deep between the heads of origin of flexor and abductor digiti minimi

Branches

Motor

- FCU
- FDP to little and ring fingers
- All small muscles of the hand except LOAF (see "Anatomy of the median nerve" above)

Sensory

- Ulnar 1½ digits
- Medial skin palm

Examination corner

Basic science oral

- Describe the course of the ulnar nerve
- Explain the ulnar paradox and its cause
- Explain differences between a high and a low ulnar palsy

Ulnar nerve compression

Aim to diagnose whether the patient has a high or a low lesion. Cubital tunnel syndrome is far more common.

Symptoms

- Paraesthesia of the ulnar 1½ digits (±ulnar dorsal aspect of the hand)
- Difficulty in fine motor activities
- Weakness of pinch grip (adductor pollicis)
- Vague, ill-defined dull ache of the forearm

Signs

- Ulnar claw hand
- Wasting of the small muscles of the hand (hypothenar eminence, metacarpal guttering, first dorsal interosseous)
- Wasting of the ulnar border of the forearm (FDP and FCU)
- Decreased sensation in the ulnar 1½ digits (±dorso-ulnar hand)
- Weakness of the interossei and lumbrical muscles
- Positive Froment's test
- If there is a high lesion, there will be weakness of FDP to the ring and little fingers (Pollock's test) and FCU
- Tenderness over the ulnar nerve at the elbow
- Positive Tinel's test behind the medial epicondyle of the elbow

Ulnar paradox[6]

There is less clawing of the hand the more proximal the nerve lesion, as a more proximal lesion will cause weakness of FDP thus reducing the amount of flexion at the IP joints of the little and ring fingers.

---

[6] Very common examination question – "What is the ulnar paradox?"

Cubital tunnel syndrome

Sites of entrapment

Arcade of Struthers[7]

Formed by a band of deep fascia from the medial head of triceps to the medial intermuscular septum.

Cubital tunnel

Fibro-osseous tunnel posterior to the medial epicondyle. Proximally the nerve lies within a groove on the dorsal aspect of the medial epicondyle and the canal is completed superficially by a fibrous aponeurotic arch (Osborne's ligament/cubital tunnel retinaculum[8]). Distally the tunnel is formed by a fibrous arch connecting the two heads of FCU and then between the two heads of FCU (flexor carpi ulnaris aponeurosis).

Other causes of compression

- **Bony abnormalities**. Osteophytes, cubitus valgus
- **Anconeus epitrochlearis muscle** (accessory muscle). Vestigial muscle originating from the medial border of the olecranon and inserting into the medial epicondyle, and crossing over the cubital tunnel. Is an uncommon cause of ulnar nerve compression at the elbow, which may be bilateral
- **Constricting fascial bands**
- **Tumours, ganglions**
- **Scarring**
- **Recurrent subluxation nerve around medial epicondyle**

Differential diagnosis

Suspected cubital tunnel syndrome may be mimicked by other disorders including:

- Cervical disc disease
- Spinal tumours

---

[7] Not to be confused with his ligament, which arises from a supracondylar spur and may compress the median nerve.
[8] Confusingly the names of various retinaculum/fascia around the elbow seem to be interchanged/different depending on which textbooks are read. Remember in the exam to keep things simple.

- Thoracic outlet syndrome
- Apical lung tumour (Pancoast's)
- Post-radiotherapy brachial plexopathy

Oral question

How do you differentiate a T1 nerve root lesion from an ulnar nerve palsy?

A patient with a T1 root lesion may have a Horner's syndrome, paraesthesia over the medial aspect of the forearm and weakness of all small muscles of the hand with clawing of all four fingers.

Management

Conservative management

- Conservative treatment may relieve symptoms of ulnar nerve dysfunction at the elbow in as many as 50% of patients
- Patients should be given general instructions on posture, avoiding prolonged elbow flexion
- Night splints (in degrees of extension)
- Corticosteroid injections are avoided due to risk of injury to the ulnar nerve

Surgery

Operations used include:

1. **Simple decompression** (release of the cubital tunnel retinaculum)
2. **Decompression with medial epicondylectomy:** theoretical advantage of a more extensive decompression than simple release without the disturbance in blood supply of the nerve
3. **Anterior transposition** of the ulnar nerve, which may be to the subcutaneous, submuscular or intramuscular positions. Anterior transposition risks devascularization of the nerve. It is best indicated when either:
   - A bony deformity is present in the groove behind the medial epicondyle
   - Or the nerve exhibits a tendency to sublux or dislocate with elbow flexion and extension

Transposition of the ulnar nerve can be to the subcutaneous tissues above the fascia of the flexor pronator group, within the musculature of the flexor pronator group itself with the fascia repaired, or beneath the flexor pronator group with the origin repaired to the medial epicondyle.

In most straightforward cases there is very little difference in outcome whether the nerve is treated by simple decompression, medial epicondylectomy, subcutaneous transposition or submuscular transposition. A satisfactory outcome is achieved in approximately 80% of patients using any of these techniques and function generally returns within 6 months.

There are several surgical options available to treat this condition, my preference would be … because …

It is important to ensure that the ulnar nerve is mobilized and decompressed fully for some distance both proximal and distal to the elbow joint.

Complications from surgery
- Infection
- Scar tenderness
- Neuromas (medial antebrachial cutaneous nerve)
- Complex regional pain syndrome
- Failure to relieve symptoms following decompression due to either the presence of severe intraneural fibrosis or inadequate decompression
- Disruption of blood supply to nerve
- Irritation of superficially placed nerve

Following the failure of a previous decompression of the ulnar nerve at the elbow treatment generally consists of some form of anterior transposition most commonly utilizing a submuscular or intramuscular technique. Success in improving symptoms and function is reported in as many as three out of four patients.

Froment's sign. FPL (anterior interosseous nerve) compensating for weakness of adductor pollicis

Jeanne's sign. Hyperextension of the thumb MP joint (involvement of FPB)

Pollock's test. Resisted flexion of DIPJs of ulnar two digits testing FDP

Wartenberg's sign (little finger escape). Abduction of the extended little finger from unopposed action of EDM due to weakness of 3rd palmar interosseous muscle

Positive elbow flexion test. Maximally flexing the elbow produces pain and paraesthesiae in the ulnar nerve distribution within 60 seconds

Ulnar tunnel syndrome

Due to ulnar nerve compression in Guyon's canal. Much less common than entrapment of the nerve at the elbow. Pain is usually less significant when compared to ulnar nerve compression at the elbow or carpal tunnel syndrome.

Signs

- Local tenderness, Tinel's test, Phalen's sign, severe ulnar clawing, weakness, atrophy, paraesthesia of the ulna 1½ digits (Figure 21.2)
- Dorso-ulnar sensory branch spared[9]

Anatomy of Guyon's canal

- Roof: volar carpal ligament
- Ulnar wall: pisiform
- Radial distal wall: hook of hamate and ADM
- Floor: transverse carpal ligament and pisohamate ligament

The ulnar nerve and artery lie beneath the volar carpal ligament on top of the transverse carpal ligament in Guyon's canal.

Causes of compression

The causes of compression are numerous and include:
- Tumours, ganglion, lipoma (soft-tissue masses)
- Thrombosis/pseudoaneurysm of the ulnar artery
- Pisiform instability
- Pisotriquetral arthritis
- Fractures distal to the radius/ulna, hook of hamate, pisiform

[9] The following differentiate low lesions from high lesions:
Involvement of the dorsal sensory branch of the ulnar nerve
Weakness of FDP of the little finger
Weakness of FCU
(Localization of Tinel's test to the cubital tunnel)

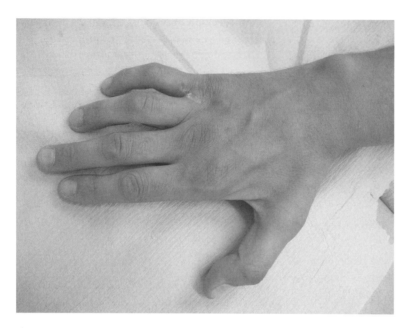

Figure 21.2 Ulnar nerve palsy

- Palmaris brevis hypertrophy
- Muscle anomalies

Symptoms

Symptoms may be pure motor, sensory or mixed based on the location of compression within the tunnel. The tunnel is divided into three zones:

Zone 1

Area proximal to the bifurcation of the nerve. Combined motor and sensory symptoms.

Zone 2

Surrounds the deep motor branch and has pure motor symptoms only. Ganglions and hook of hamate fracture are the most likely aetiology in zones 1 and 2.

Zone 3

Surrounds the superficial sensory branch of the ulnar nerve and has sensory symptoms only. Thrombosis or aneurysm of the ulnar artery is the most likely aetiology in zone 3. Allen's test and Doppler studies are useful in making the diagnosis.

Differential diagnosis

- Cubital tunnel syndrome
- Cervical disc disease
- Thoracic outlet syndrome
- Motor neurone disease (motor signs greater than sensory)

Management

The key to management is identifying the aetiology:
- NCS
- MRI for ganglions
- CT for hook of hamate fractures
- Doppler US for ulnar artery thrombosis

Conservative

Wrist splinting, avoidance of repetitive trauma.

Surgical

Decompression of both motor and sensory branches ±excision of the pisiform/hook of hamate. Release of the volar carpal ligament, isolating the ulnar nerve proximal to the wrist initially with a longitudinal incision radial to FCU.

Occasionally patients are seen who have carpal tunnel and Guyon's canal compression syndrome simultaneously. The volume of Guyon's canal increases after carpal tunnel release, and ulnar compressive symptoms improve in approximately one-third of patients following carpal tunnel release alone.

Examination corner

Hand oral 1

- Describe the picture
- Sites of compression
- Cause of clawing

Hand oral 2

Ulnar claw hand

The examiner held out their hand like they had Dupuytren's contracture in the little and ring fingers flexed at MCP and IP.

Examiner: What do you call this deformity: is there a specific name to it?

Candidate: Finger in palm deformity (although the little finger was not fully into the palm).

Examiner: NO!

Candidate: A claw hand.

Examiner: Yes! What are the causes of claw hand?

Examiner: What is ulnar paradox?

Radial nerve compression

Anatomy

- Arises from the posterior cord of the brachial plexus (C5, 6, 7, 8)

- Passes through the triangular space to enter the spiral groove where it lies on the medial head of triceps
- Pierces lateral intermuscular septum ~7 cm proximal to lateral epicondyle
- Passes deep to the mobile wad in the radial tunnel giving off a superficial branch
- Becomes the posterior interosseous nerve (PIN) as it passes deep to the superficial head of supinator

Sites of entrapment

- Axilla (Saturday night palsy)
- Humeral shaft fracture – it was thought that this has a higher incidence with a Holstein–Lewis fracture (middle and distal third humerus), but recent meta-analysis[10] showed that it is more likely with a shaft fracture

Posterior interosseous nerve compression

Introduction

- Pain at the lateral elbow
- Weakness of wrist extension with radial drift (ECRL innervated higher than PIN take off)
- No sensory loss

Clinical features

- Onset often insidious
- Dull aching of the proximal forearm
- Difficulty extending fingers and thumb
- Wrist extension is still possible (ECRL not affected) but it is weak plus there is an element of radial deviation (ECRB)
- Able to extend the IP joints due to interossei

---

[10] Shao YC, Harwood P, Grotz MR, Limb D, Giannoudis PV (2005) Radial nerve palsy associated with fractures of the shaft of the humerus: a systematic review. *J Bone Joint Surg Br* **87**(12):1647–52.

PIN innervates (9)

- ECRB, supinator, EIP, ECU, EDC, EDM, APL, EPB, EPL

Sites of compression/entrapment

- Thickened fascia at radiocapitellar joint
- Radial artery (recurrent leash of Henry)
- Edge of ECRB
- Arcade of Frohse (tendinous proximal border of supinator)
- Distal edge of supinator

Unusual causes

- Chronic radial head dislocation
- Fracture of the radial head or neck
- Synovitis of the radiocapitellar joint
- Mass lesion (lipoma, ganglion) at the elbow

Differential diagnosis

- C7 radiculopathy
- Lateral epicondylitis

Management

Conservative initially as many patients will spontaneously improve. Avoidance of aggravating activities, NSAIDs, etc. Full surgical decompression of all potential compression sites if no improvement.

Radial tunnel syndrome

Introduction

Entrapment of the superficial branch of the radial nerve. Pain is the only problem without motor or sensory dysfunction. This is essentially a clinical diagnosis. Due to the close proximity of the nerve to the lateral epicondyle the condition can be difficult to differentiate from a "resistant" tennis elbow (coexists in 5% of patients).

Anatomy of the radial tunnel

- Medial: biceps tendon and brachialis
- Lateral: brachioradialis, ECRL and ECRB
- Roof: brachioradialis
- Floor: radiocapitellar joint capsule and supinator muscle

Clinical features

History

Deep-seated dull aching/pain in the extensor muscle mass often radiating to the wrist.

Examination

1. **Localized tenderness** directly over the PIN distal to the lateral epicondyle
2. **Middle finger extension test** – each finger is tested under resisted extension. Testing the middle finger (firm pressure over the dorsum of the PP) increases the pain. Due to ECRB inserting into the base 3rd metacarpal. Test is positive if it produces pain at the edge of the ECRB in the proximal forearm. Performed with the elbow and middle finger completely extended and the wrist in neutral position
3. **Resisted active supination test** – the radial tunnel begins at the radial–humeral joint and extends to the end of the supinator muscle. In radial tunnel syndrome the maximal tenderness is distal to the radial head in a line from the lateral epicondyle through the radial head to a point 2–3 cm more distal over the radial tunnel

Causes

As for PIN syndrome but not usually any mass lesions:
1. **Fibrous bands** tether nerve to the radiocapitellar joint capsule
2. Radial **R**ecurrent leash of vessels (the leash of Henry)
3. Fibrous medial edge along ECRB

4. Fibrous **A**rcade of Frohse (proximal superficial edge of supinator)
5. **S**upinator (distal border)

Investigations

- Diagnostic injection of local anaesthetic into the radial tunnel
- NCS not particularly helpful, as they are usually normal, which is in contrast to the PIN compression syndrome

Management

Non-operative

- Long non-operative approach warranted
- Activity modification
- Temporary splinting
- NSAIDs

Surgical

- Operative release is often disappointing with only 50% satisfactory results
- Co-incidental undiagnosed tennis elbow can lead to failure of radial tunnel decompression

Wartenberg's syndrome (cheiralgia paraesthetica)

Neuritis/compression neuropathy of the superficial sensory branch of the radial nerve. This is a relatively uncommon condition.

Causes

- Entrapment beneath the tendinous insertions of brachioradialis and ECRL (by a scissor-like action between the tendons)
- Anomalous fascial bands
- Tight jewellery
- Watchbands
- Thrombosis of the radial recurrent vessels
- Haemorrhage in the proximal forearm

Clinical features

Burning, numbness or pain in the distribution of the superficial radial nerve (outer aspect of the distal forearm). Tenderness along the course of the nerve proximal to the wrist. The most useful sign is a positive Tinel's test directly over the nerve as it exits from beneath brachioradialis.

Dellon's sign

Active forceful pronation of the forearm and ulnar deviation of the wrist with the elbow extended by the side for 60 s may provoke symptoms of numbness or tingling in the territory of the sensory branch.

Management

Conservative

- Local steroid injection, NSAIDs, avoidance of watch straps crossing the area, removal of compressing garments or jewellery at the wrist, wrist splints
- Approximately 50% of patients respond to conservative treatment

Surgery

- Surgical exploration and release of constricting tissue
- Considered after a 6-month period of non-operative treatment
- Results of surgical exploration are unpredictable
- Careful release of the nerve using a "no touch technique"

Examination corner

Short case

Lipoma in the forearm causing pressure neuritis of the superficial radial nerve

Clinical findings: numb over the dorsum of index finger and first web space

Dupuytren's disease

This is an absolutely must-learn topic for both the clinical short cases and hands oral.

Definition

Proliferative fibroplasia of the palmar and digital fascia forming nodules and cords with secondary flexion contracture of the finger. Dupuytren described the disease in Paris in 1831 (although he was not the first to do so).

Risk factors for Dupuytren's disease

- Positive family history
- Northern Europeans
- Male
- Alcohol excess
- Diabetes
- Chronic lung disease
- Smoking

Epilepsy not now thought to be a risk factor.[11]

Dupuytren's diathesis

This is an aggressive disease that is likely to recur in some patients, with early onset of disease, multiple areas of involvement, positive family history and bilateral disease.

It is associated with:
- Ledderhose's disease – plantar fibromatosis
- Peyronie's disease – penis
- Garrod's pads – nodules over the dorsal surface of the PIP joints

Epidemiology

More than 25% of men of Celtic origin over 60 years of age have evidence of DD. The male-to-female reported ratios vary from between 4:1 and 10:1. Those of Oriental origin and diabetics tend to have palmar

disease but not joint contracture. There is no reported predilection for side or dominance. Unilateral disease is more commonly a sporadic finding without a family history and is usually less severe. In females DD is seen later and is usually less severe.

Aetiology

The aetiology of DD is essentially unknown. There are two main theories on the mechanism of pathological change:
1. **Intrinsic theory** – metaplasia of the existing fascia
2. **Extrinsic theory** – a subdermal origin for the diseased tissue that attaches itself to and grows on underlying fascial bands

The myofibroblast is the key cell and contains actin allowing active contraction. These cells produce fibronectin, to link to other myofibroblasts, and increased amounts of type III collagen.

Oxygen free radicals that occur in hypoxic tissue are thought to play a role via fibroblast stimulation. Cytokines (transforming growth factor-β, platelet-derived growth factor, fibroblast growth factor) are also probably involved, and stimulate transformation of fibroblasts into myofibroblasts resulting in fibrous hyperplasia of palmar fascia.

Genetic link is autosomal dominant with variable penetrance. Genetic studies have yet to identify the relevant genes.

Interestingly it has been noted recently that patients given treatment for gastric cancer developed a Dupuytren-like disease. The treatment decreased the ratio of systemic matrix metalloproteinase (MMPs) to tissue inhibitory metalloproteinases (TIMPs).

Symptoms

- Progressive digital deformity as a result of cord formation
- Difficulty washing face, combing hair, putting the hand in a pocket or a glove
- Decreased manual dexterity at work
- Pain (synovial sarcoma) or paraesthesia are rarely seen

---

[11] Geoghegan JM, Forbes J, Clark DI, Smith C, Hubbard R (2004) Dupuytren's disease risk factors. *J Hand Surg* **29**: 423–6.

History

- Hand dominance
- Family history
- Rate of progression
- Diabetes
- Alcohol
- Foot/penis involvement
- Smoking
- Trauma

Examination

- Sex
- Previous scars
- Skin pits
- Digits involved and cord type
- MCP angle (measure with PIPJ fully flexed as cord can cross both joints)
- PIP angle (measure with MCPJ fully flexed)
- Garrod's pads over the dorsal PIP joint
- Sensation
- Digital Allen's test
- Mention Ledderhose's and Peyronie's

The combination of PIP joint in a fixed flexion deformity with the MCP joint in flexion signifies a severe deformity and a poor prognosis.

Normal digital fascia

- Pretendinous bands
- Spiral bands
- Natatory ligaments
- Lateral digital sheet
- Transverse palmar fibres (Skoog's)

Named cords

- Central/pretendinous (MCP contracture)
- Spiral (pre-tendinous cord, spiral cord, lateral digital sheet and Grayson's ligament) – PIP joint contracture
- Lateral
- Natatory (adduction contracture)
- Abductor digiti minimi

Bands are normal fascial structures, cords are diseased.

Grayson's ligament on the volar surface of the finger is involved, whilst Cleland's ligament is usually spared. The spiral cord pushes/displaces the neurovascular bundle superficially and towards the midline of the finger where it is at risk of damage during the distal palmar dissection.

Three stages of Dupuytren's disease (Luck)

1. **Proliferative**. Large myofibroblasts, very vascular, minimal extracellular matrix, random cell proliferation
2. **Involutional**. Dense myofibroblast network, increased amounts of type III collagen fibres compared to type I
3. **Residual**. Myofibroblasts disappear replaced by fibrocytes

Indications for surgery

- MCP joint contracture >30°
- PIP joint contracture >15°
- First web space contracture

Even a severe MCP joint contracture will correct with excision of the Dupuytren's cord as the collateral ligaments are not in a shortened position. A PIP joint contracture leads to a stiff joint as the volar plate shortens.

Excision of an early nodule may cause a flare-type reaction causing an early return of the disease.

Hueston's tabletop test – involves placing the hand and fingers prone on a tabletop. The test is positive when the hand will not go flat. This test rarely alters management decisions, but is of value as a screening test for general practitioners to identify those patients requiring referral.

Informed consent

- Aims – excision of the diseased tissue to restore full movement
- General/regional anaesthetic

Complications:

- Recurrence rate 30%–50% at 10 years.[12] Majority do not require further surgery
- Incomplete correction of PIP joint contracture
- Wound healing delay
- Temporary or permanent digital nerve impairment (1.5%)
- Splinting regimen postoperative (night splints up to 6 months)
- Amputation

Surgical options

1. Fasciotomy

Indicated only for a well-defined pretendinous palmar cord causing an MCP joint contracture. Quick and can be performed under local anaesthetic. It may also be used in severe multiple digital contractures if the palmar skin is macerated to allow the fingers to be opened away from the palm. Risk of digital nerve injury and recurrence. Percutaneous needle fasciotomy is controversial and should only be undertaken by an experienced surgeon.

2. Partial fasciectomy

The digital neurovascular bundles are identified proximally and traced distally. Only the longitudinal contractile cords and nodules that are responsible for a joint contracture are excised, or segmental fasciectomy.[13]

3. Complete fasciectomy

McIndoe popularized this technique using a transverse palmar incision to excise the entire palmar fascia. The procedure has now been abandoned as it is impossible in practical terms to excise the entire palmar fascia and attempting to do so does not necessarily prevent recurrence. Secondly the extensive

dissection is a major assault on the hand resulting in swelling, joint stiffness, haematoma formation and possibly skin necrosis.

4. Dermofasciectomy

Indicated for recurrent disease with skin involvement. Involves excision of overlying skin and diseased tissue. The defect is replaced with a full-thickness skin graft from the forearm or groin (hair free). The skin graft acts as a firebreak to recurrence. DD does not recur deep to full-thickness grafts. Recurrence rate is 8% at 5.8 years follow-up.[14]

5. Staged distraction and fasciotomy followed by fasciectomy

First described by Messina, this is usually reserved for severe PIP joint involvement. It is a two-stage procedure, which involves applying an external fixator to provide tension along the cord. The DD regresses under stretch and then a planned fasciectomy is performed after a few weeks.

6. Amputation

Consider for severe recurrent disease.

Incisions

A good incision should provide well vascularized skin flaps, extensile exposure and access for identification and preservation of the digital nerves and arteries.

1. Bruner

Zigzag with apex made at each finger flexor crease. Allows excellent exposure laterally. Raised skin flaps should be full thickness and flap apex

[12] Bulstrode NM, Jemec B, Smith PJ (2005) The complications of Dupuytren's contracture surgery. *J Hand Surg* **30**: 1021–5.
[13] Moermans JP (1991) Segmental aponeurectomy in Dupuytren's disease. *J Hand Surg Br* **16**: 237–9.

[14] Armstrong JR, Hurrens JS, Logan AM (2000) Dermofasciectomy in the management of Dupuytren's disease. *J Bone Joint Surg Br* **82**: 90–4.

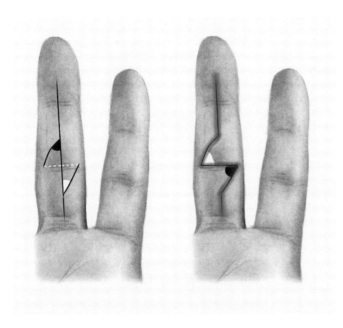

Figure 21.3 How to draw a z-plasty. 1. Draw perpendicular (white dotted line) to longitudinal incision. 2. Mark flaps (white and black angles are at 60°). 3. Cross over flaps as shown

angle >60° to prevent tip necrosis. Take care at the apex to avoid damage to the underlying neurovascular bundle.

2. Straight longitudinal incision closed with z-plasties

Midline incision with z-plasty of the flaps at closure (Figure 21.3). It has the advantage of lengthening the wound.

3. McCash open technique

Transverse palmar incision with digital extension, either Bruner or z-plasty, along the digit. The wound provides excellent access to the diseased tissue and is left open at the end of the procedure. Good technique in elderly patients, as it causes less oedema and haematoma formation, it is useful if you are short of skin, and it causes less pain and stiffness

postoperatively; however, it takes a relatively long time to heal (6–8 weeks).

Oral question

Discuss the different surgical approaches and techniques used for DD.
    Describe a postoperative rehabilitation programme.
    Why use a midline dorsal incision to a digit? (Causes less damage to dorsal veins.)

PIP joint release

- Release the check rein ligaments (proximal attachment of the volar plate that normally prevents hyperextension)
- Release of accessory collateral ligament
- Incise fibrous flexor sheath
- Volar plate release (contentious)

- Full collateral ligament release is not recommended
- ±Trans-articular k-wire (4 weeks)

A full release of the volar plate may cause excessive scarring and result in loss of flexion, which is more disabling than a flexion contracture.

Postoperative management

Apply volar splint with digits extended for 2–4 days. Then actively mobilize and apply a night splint for up to 6 months.

Postoperative complications

Intra-operative

- Digital nerve injury (1.5%)
- Digital artery injury (actual incidence not known as there are good anastomoses to compensate if one artery is damaged)

Overstretching of the finger and spasm in the digital arteries may lead to digital ischaemia. Positioning in flexion, patience and application of warm saline usually return the perfusion.

Early postoperative

- Haematoma (release tourniquet before closure)
- Skin flap necrosis
  - Small areas of skin loss will heal spontaneously but healing of larger areas is slow and may result in scar contracture
- Finger loss
  - More common in revision surgery with prior damage to a unilateral digital vessel, hence the need to assess sensation and perform a digital Allen's test preoperatively to identify potential hazards
- Infection

Late postoperative

- Stiff hand
- Loss of grip strength 6/52

- Complex regional pain syndrome type 1 (4% males, 8% females)
  - Rare but serious complication. Cardinal features are excessive pain, stiffness and vasomotor instability
- Inadequate release
- Scar-related problems
- Recurrence of disease
- Flare reaction (combination of tenderness, shiny redness of the wound, swelling)

Examination corner

Hand oral 1

Clinical picture of severe DD affecting the little and ring fingers

Candidate: This is a clinical picture, which demonstrates severe DD affecting the ring and little fingers. The fingers are almost into the palm with almost a 90° contracture of the PIP joint of the little finger.

Examiner: Who gets DD?

Candidate: Male, Northern Europeans, positive family history, excessive alcohol intake, diabetes, a chronic lung disease, chronic pulmonary tuberculosis. Possibly a history of previous hand trauma, though this is disputed.

Examiner: So what will you tell the patient about the surgery involved?

Candidate: I would tell the patient that surgery is not curative, and that the disease can recur. I would mention that he has severe contractures of his fingers and we may not be able to get them fully straight.

I would also mention the risk of digital nerve injury and vascular injury that in the worst-case scenario may result in amputation.

Hand oral 2

Clinical picture of DD affecting the PIP joint of the little finger

Examiner:
- What is the diagnosis?
- Consent me for the surgery
- How would you manage?
- Discuss the complications of surgery

- Why may a contracture of this joint not correct fully?
- Where would you start?

Candidate: In the palm.

Examiner: Why?

Candidate: To dissect the nerve as it is more easily identified here.

Hand oral 3

Clinical picture of severe DD affecting the PIP joint of the little and ring fingers

Candidate: This is a clinical picture, which shows a severe contraction of the PIP joint of the little and ring fingers. There appear to be cords present in the palm extending into the digits.

Examiner: (interrupting) You know what it is, it's DD. What will you tell the patient before surgery?

Candidate: I would say that surgery is not curative, that recurrence can occur. I would also mention that we are unlikely to achieve full correction of the deformity.

Examiner: Is there anything which may guide you clinically as to how much correction can be obtained?

Candidate: It is important to access the PIP joint with the MCP joint fully extended as well as flexed. The PIP joint deformity often improves with MCP joint flexion by relaxing the MCP joint deformity and the intrinsic muscles. In addition, there is a high likelihood of midline displacement of the neurovascular bundle (spiral cord) and I would estimate 1–1½ h for the surgery when planning my list.

Examiner: What incision will you use?

Candidate: I would use a Bruner's incision.

Hand oral 4

Clinical picture of DD

- Details on aetiology and presentation
- What tissue is involved
- What structures are involved
- What are the named cords
- Surgical indications
- Revision options

Kienböck's disease

Most surgeons have radiographs showing Kienböck's disease and they often show them during the hand oral for the FRCS Orth. This leads on to the usual questions about classification and treatment.

Introduction

Avascular necrosis of the lunate. First described by the Viennese radiologist Robert Kienböck in 1910. Usually unilateral although bilateral cases have been reported.

Aetiology

The aetiology of Kienböck's disease is unknown. Several theories have been put forward. It may occur as a result of a definitive single, though forgotten and trivial, wrist injury or be due to repeated minor trauma. No strong evidence to support either theory – probably multifactorial.

More common in wrists with ulnar-negative variance (the ulna is shorter than the distal radius). This can lead to abnormal loading of the lunate. Ulnar variance is measured on standard PA views of the wrist (shoulder flexed/internally rotated 90°, elbow flexed 90°, wrist neutral).

Classification (Lichtman)

This is a radiographic classification.

Stage I Normal. May be a linear or compression fracture

Diagnosed by MRI/bone scan

Stage II Sclerosis but no collapse

Stage III Collapsed and fragmentation

IIIA Carpal collapse

IIIB Carpal collapse plus fixed scaphoid rotation

Stage IV Generalized wrist osteoarthritis

Blood supply

- Extraosseous supply (Lee)
  - Single volar or dorsal vessel
  - Two vessels, no intraosseous anastomosis
  - Two vessels, anastomose
- Intraosseous (Gelbermann)

- There are three described patterns: I (10%), X (31%) and Y (59%). With each the proximal subchondral bone is poorly supplied

Clinical presentation

- Asymptomatic
- Insidious onset of mild wrist pain, slight restriction of wrist movements
- Tender over the dorsal lunate
- Weakness of grip strength

The conundrum – surgical management is controversial as the natural history is uncertain.[15] The severity of symptoms and radiological appearances do not correlate well. In planning treatment one needs to thoroughly assess the patient's pain and disability.

Management

Initial management includes rest, splintage and analgesia. Surgery is indicated if symptoms do not settle. There are numerous operations as there is no consensus. Important factors are relative ulnar length, and the stage of the disease. An additional posterior interosseous neurectomy to these procedures will reduce pain.

Joint levelling procedures

Indicated for stage I, II or IIIA disease if ulnar minus. Radial shortening preferred due to the increased risk of non-union with ulnar lengthening.

Radial osteotomy

Angular distal radial osteotomy to reduce the radial inclination of the distal radius has been suggested to reduce lunate pressure in stage I, II or IIIA disease if ulnar neutral. However, any effect may be due to the resulting hyperaemia from the osteotomy.

[15] Very likely one will be asked what type of skin incision to use for excision of a ganglion. Transverse skin incisions are more cosmetic. Longitudinal skin incisions are technically easier and more extensile but may damage the germinal matrix of the nail.

Vascularized bone grafts

Indication for stage I, II or IIIA disease if ulnar neutral. Good short-term results for: extensor compartments 2, 3 – intercompartmental supraretinacular artery (ICSRA); extensor compartments 4, 5 – extensor compartment artery (ECA).

Partial wrist fusion

Scaphotrapeziotrapezoidal (STT) or scaphocapitate fusion to maintain carpal height, to transfer load to the scaphoid fossa and to decrease loading on the lunate.

Capitate shortening has been shown to reduce load on the lunate by 66% but increases scaphotrapezial load by 150%.

Proximal row carpectomy has shown no benefit to an STT fusion for stage IIIB disease possibly because of pre-existing damage to the lunate fossa, which will articulate with the head of the capitate.

Total wrist arthrodesis

Effective pain-relieving procedure for stage IV disease or for patients who have failed other surgical treatments.

Examination corner

Hand oral 1

Radiographs demonstrating Kienböck's disease

The diagnosis was obvious.

Examiner: A 42-year-old businessman comes to your clinic complaining of mild left wrist pain. These are his wrist X-rays. What do you see?

Candidate: The AP radiograph shows marked sclerosis of the lunate. There are no osteophytes present and the lunate is not collapsed. The architecture of the wrist is well preserved.

Examiner: What do you think of his MRI scan?

Candidate: The MRI scans show decreased signal intensity consistent with the avascular necrosis of Kienböck's disease.

(I did not mention if the scan was a T_1- or T_2-weighted image which would have scored brownie points.)

Examiner: How do you classify Kienböck's disease?

Candidate: Kienböck's disease is usually diagnosed and staged on plain radiographs. Lichtman graded the disease into 4 stages radiographically.

Stage I has a normal lunate. Stage II sclerosis. Stage III is subdivided into A and B. The lunate is collapsed and fragmented but in IIIA there is no carpal collapse while in IIIB there is associated carpal collapse. Stage IV is generalized arthritis of the wrist.

The examiner suddenly became bored and switched off as I started to go through the Lichtman classification.

Examiner: How do you manage Kienböck's disease?

Candidate: Kienböck's disease can be treated in a number of ways such as shortening the radius. If there are more advanced changes present then a limited wrist fusion with or without excision of the lunate can be useful.

The decision to treat this man really depends on how many symptoms he is getting.

Feedback

The candidate's answer in print seems reasonable enough. The examiner felt that he/she had given a very poor reply with no proper structure or order to the question.

Candidate–examiner dialogues may be sometimes difficult for the reader to fully appreciate. They are taken out of context and unless the reader was actually in the oral himself or herself they will not fully appreciate the flow, the non-verbal communication and the drama of the whole event. The examiner was looking (I think) for an answer more along the lines of "My concern with Kienböck's disease is that radiographic appearances do not correlate well with clinical symptoms. I would need to more fully assess this patient with regards to functional disability and expectations from treatment."

Examiner: Come on now – how are you going to manage this gentleman? *The examiner was irritated at the poor answer to the previous question.*

Candidate: Has he got much pain?

Examiner: He is working as a manager with intermittent pain in his wrist that is not interfering with work.

Candidate: The X-ray appearances do not always correlate with symptoms.

Examiner: Exactly. That is the key point to all of this. Kienböck's disease can cause very little disability. The X-ray changes do not correlate well with symptoms. A patient may have severe radiographic changes of Kienböck's disease but only minimal symptoms. Furthermore the natural history of the disease is not well known, it does not always progress from stage I to stage IV. Surgery has not been shown conclusively to prevent progression of the disease.

Candidate: I would manage him conservatively.

Examiner: Yes – you have to have a very good reason to operate on a wrist with Kienböck's disease.

[Candidate fail]

Post mortem

Although the candidate was quick enough off the mark with the Lichtman staging of the disease s/he required prompting to emphasize the lack of correlation between radiographic findings and clinical symptoms. This point should have been mentioned fairly early on by the candidate.

In addition the candidate did not talk or allow himself/herself the opportunity to talk about conservative management of the disease. This should have been the first thing to point out when discussing management options. Indeed conservative management was the examiner's preferred method of management for this patient.

Candidate: I got caught out in this oral. I knew the subject reasonably well enough but I did not know what the examiner wanted or was looking for. The key fact about Kienböck's disease is that the radiographic appearance does not always correlate with symptoms *(and all the rest – see above)*. Although I knew this fact I did not fully appreciate its importance and this was exposed by the examiner who wanted me to come out and say this to them.

The message here is that there are certain key points or practical facts that you must know for a topic but they are not always emphasized particularly well in textbooks.

Hand oral 2

Management of Kienbock's stage II disease

Hand oral 3

Radiograph of Kienböck's disease

- What stage?
- How do you mange this?
- Indications for joint levelling procedures

Hand oral 4

Radiograph of Kienböck's disease

- What do you know about this?
- Classification
- Management options

Ganglion

Introduction

A cyst-ganglion is the commonest soft-tissue swelling of the hand and is not a true cyst as it is does not have an epithelial lining. It is a fibrous swelling usually attached to an underlying synovial cavity of a joint or tendon sheath. It contains clear mucinous fluid, which is a mixture of glucosamine, albumin, globulin and hyaluronic acid. It is unclear if ganglion fluid is simply synovial fluid, which has escaped from the joint, or if it is formed by cells in the synovium at the origin of the ganglion.

Pathology

The pathogenesis of ganglia is uncertain but theories of mucoid capsular degeneration and joint capsule synovial herniation have been proposed. They consist of compressed collagen fibres with no true epithelial or synovial lining membrane. There is no good evidence to support a traumatic or inflammatory aetiology.

Most common sites

- Dorsal wrist ganglion (from scapholunate ligament)
- Volar radial ganglion (radioscaphoid or trapeziometacarpal joints)
- Flexor sheath ganglion (appears in the A1 or A2 pulleys)

Clinical presentation

- Cosmesis
- Pain

- Variation in size, especially a reduction in size
- Wrist weakness
- Extrinsic compression of adjacent nerves (ulnar nerve in Guyon's canal, median nerve in the carpal tunnel)

Management

Non-operative management

Reassure the patient. This is a harmless swelling, which is not cancer and may resolve spontaneously in time. Useful to mention the bible was used as an old-fashioned treatment method and that surgery would be exchanging a swelling for a scar, etc.

Aspiration ±steroid injection

Commonly recurs after aspiration but useful to confirm diagnosis to patient.

Surgical excision

Excise for cosmesis, pain or functional disability. Recurrence rate 5%.

Dorsal wrist ganglion

Most common ganglion type (70% of all ganglions) arising from the scapholunate ligament. Occult ganglions may only be identified with wrist flexion. Transverse skin incisions preferred. Success depends on identification of the pedicle connecting the ganglion to the joint and excision of the surrounding capsule. The joint capsule should not be closed after surgical excision.

Volar radial wrist ganglion

Second most common ganglion (20%). Two-thirds arise from the radiocarpal joint at the scapholunate interval and one-third from the scaphotrapezial joint. Lie under the volar crease between the FCR and APL. An Allen's test before surgery is mandatory as the ganglion is often intimately adherent to the radial artery and requires careful dissection from it. Inadequate collateral circulation from the ulnar artery may contravene surgery. The recurrence rate is higher than for dorsal wrist ganglia.

Flexor sheath ganglion

Also known as a volar retinacular or seedling ganglion.

Third most common ganglion in the hand (~10%). Firm swelling felt at the base of the finger in the web space that can cause discomfort when gripping objects. Small, firm, hard and tender mass 2–5 mm in diameter. Arises between the A1 and A2 pulleys and does not move with finger flexion, unlike the flexor tendon nodule seen with trigger finger. Excise through a small Bruner's type incision with a margin of tendon sheath. Protect the neurovascular bundle. Recurrence after excision is very uncommon.

Mucous cyst

A mucous cyst is a dorsal digital ganglion arising from an osteoarthritic distal interphalangeal joint. The cyst tends to lie to one side of the extensor tendon. A dorsal osteophyte is commonly present and must be excised. May present as ridging of the nail plate or recurrent infection with discharge.

A transverse incision should be used to protect the germinal matrix of the nail bed. A horseshoe ganglion may grow either side of the extensor tendon. The ganglion is mobilized and traced back to the joint with trimming of any dorsal osteophytes present. Skin closure is either primary, a local rotation flap or a full-thickness skin graft.

Examination corner

Short answers/notes

Write short notes on the management of a 21-year-old woman who presents with a wrist ganglion.
Confirm the diagnosis of a ganglion.

History

- Usually painless swelling
- Examination

- Exclude worrisome features
- Transillumination

Management options

- Reassurance
- Especially if asymptomatic
- "You haven't got cancer"
- Aspiration (±steroid injection)
- Can be performed as an outpatient procedure and repeated if necessary
- Excision
- Indications would include a persistent, painful or enlarging ganglion
- Inform the patient that they would be substituting a scar for a swelling, that the scar may be painful, and that there may be an area of numbness around the scar
- Can be performed under either local or general anaesthetic
- Recurrence can occur ~ 10%
- Do not close the defect in the joint capsule after surgical excision of the ganglion
- Trace the pedicle down to the joint capsule and excise part of the joint capsule

Hand oral

Clinical photograph of either a dorsal or palmar wrist ganglion

Spot diagnosis
Usual questions about management

Osteoarthritis of the base of the thumb

Background

Peritrapezial osteoarthritis commonly affects post-menopausal women with 80% having radiographic changes although many have few symptoms.

Anatomy

The thumb carpometacarpal (or trapeziometacarpal) joint is saddle shaped allowing flexion-extension, abduction-adduction and rotation.

Opposition is a composite movement involving flexion and pronation.

Three main ligaments stabilize the joint:

- Lateral ligament
- Dorsal ligament
- Volar-ulnar or beak ligament

The beak ligament is the most important. It is extremely strong and the primary static stabilizer of the joint. It is thought that degeneration of this ligament leads to joint instability and early disease.

History

- Constant dull pain at the base of the thumb, worsened with use
- Pain at the MCP joint from compensatory hyperextension
- Night pain unusual
- Difficulties with ADLs (undoing screw top jars, doing up buttons, writing)
- Carpal tunnel symptoms

Examination

Look

- Squaring-off of the base of the thumb (shoulder sign – dorsal subluxation of the thumb's metacarpal base)
- Adduction contracture of the first web space
- Thenar muscle wasting
- Compensatory hyper-extension of the MCP joint to increase span due to the adduction contracture
- Look for trigger fingers and carpal tunnel syndrome (43% association)

Special tests

Painful and unlikely to be performed in the exam.

Grind test – pain with axial loading of the thumb metacarpal and rotation of the CMC joint; positive if pain disappears with repeat test with distraction of the joint. May feel crepitus.

Crank test – axial loading of the thumb with passive flexion and extension of the metacarpal.

A further test consists of longitudinal traction and pressure over the base of the thumb metacarpal to reduce the subluxed joint. Reproduction of pain strongly suggests disease at the thumb CMC joint.

Radiographs

AP and Robert's views (AP view with the thumb fully abducted and the forearm fully pronated).

Differential diagnosis (radial-sided wrist pain)

- De Quervain's
- Scaphoid non-union
- SNAC/SLAC wrist
- Kienböck's

Classification (Eaton and Littler)[16]

Radiological classification that corresponds poorly to clinical symptoms. Ask for Eaton views (stress X-ray examination) – thumbs against each other in resisted abduction, palms flat.

Stage 1

- Radiographs demonstrate widening of the joint space
- Synovitis and joint effusion
- Pre-arthritis stage

Stage 2

- Slight narrowing of the joint space
- Mild subluxation
- STT joint normal

---

[16] Staging of the disease was first described by Eaton and Littler in 1973. Further work led to combining of stages III and IV and the introduction of a new stage IV to give the classification system used by Eaton and Glicker in 1987. The problem is that most examiners (and candidates) are not familiar with this fact and refer to this new classification system by the old name.

Table 21.1 Surgical treatment options for osteoarthritis of the trapeziometacarpal joint

Trapeziometacarpal arthroplasty without excision of the trapezium
Trapeziectomy
    ±ligament reconstruction and tendon interposition
    ±soft-tissue interposition
Osteotomy
Arthrodesis
Joint replacement arthroplasty

Stage 3

- Joint space markedly narrowed
- Often sclerotic and cystic change
- Moderate subluxation

Stage 4

- Pantrapezial arthritis
- Severe subluxation
- Joint space is narrow, cystic and sclerotic subchondral bone changes

Management

Non-operative

The first-line management: NSAIDs, intra-articular steroid/local anaesthetic injections, thumb splinting, physiotherapy to strengthen thenar muscles.

Surgery

The indications for surgery are disabling symptoms unresponsive to conservative treatment.

Early stages of the disease (stage 1)
A soft-tissue reconstruction of the beak ligament using half of FCR passed through a hole drilled across the base of the thumb metacarpal (Eaton–Littler procedure). Contraindicated if degenerative changes are present.

More recently an extra-articular 30° extension osteotomy of the thumb has been described as an alternative method of management.

Late stages of the disease
There are numerous surgical treatment options for OA of the base of the thumb (Table 21.1). The choice depends on three main factors: whether there is isolated CMC joint disease or pantrapezial disease, the patient's activity level and surgeon's preference.

Procedures that preserve the trapezium or aim to maintain thumb length will theoretically preserve function. However, loss of trapezial height has not been shown to correlate with thumb strength postoperatively.[17]

1. Osteotomy
   A number of osteotomies have been described at the base of the first metacarpal. Good results have been reported with an abduction-extension osteotomy for Stage II and early Stage III disease. Suggested as a more durable procedure than an arthroplasty and restricts motion less than an arthroplasty but has not gained widespread popularity

2. Trapeziectomy
   Generally provides reliable pain relief but may be accompanied by thumb weakness. A good option, not a technically demanding operation but protracted rehabilitation time (6 months). Requires 4–6 weeks in a thumb splint postoperatively.
   Instability of the base of the thumb metacarpal is a possible complication. Numerous modifications to simple excision have been devised to try to prevent this (haematoma distraction, APL sling)

3. Excision plus ligament reconstruction and tendon interposition (LRTI)
   Still a popular procedure despite the fact that it is time consuming and there is no evidence of a benefit over simple trapeziectomy.[18] Ligament

[17] Downing ND, Davis TR (2001) Trapezial space height after trapeziectomy: mechanism of formation and benefits. *J Hand Surg Am* **26**: 862–8.
[18] Davis TR, Brady O, Dias JJ (2004) Excision of the trapezium for osteoarthritis of the trapeziometacarpal joint: a study of

reconstruction using FCR is done to support the base of the first metacarpal and to prevent thumb shortening, and the remaining tendon is rolled up to act as a spacer

4. Trapeziectomy with Silastic® spacer

   Good early results but no longer recommended due to silicone synovitis

5. Arthrodesis

   May be indicated for young high-demand patients with isolated trapezometacarpal disease who require a strong and painless hand.[19] Provides stability and power at the expense of loss of some movement. A technically difficult procedure, there is only a small area available for fusion, and may go on to non-union.[20] Places increased demands on the triscaphe joint, which may become painful. The joint is fused in a clenched fist position (20°–30° radial and 20° palmar abduction). The arthrodesis can be stabilized with an AO compact hand set T-plate, k-wires or a tension band wire

6. Joint replacement arthroplasty

   Both cemented and uncemented designs. Total joint replacements generally have a constrained ball and socket design with the stemmed ball inserted into the metacarpal and the socket anchored to the trapezium. Results only short-term so far in small series

A variety of surgical options exist and none is clearly superior. Overall expect 80%–90% good results

the benefit of ligament reconstruction or tendon interposition. *J Hand Surg Am* **29**: 1069–77.

[19] Some surgeons believe it is probably the operation of choice for young and middle-aged men who perform moderately heavy manual work. This is a classic example of a very difficult aspect of the FRCS Orth exam – being familiar with general orthopaedic knowledge but not aware of practical issues. A hand surgeon will say fusion is not always a particularly good choice as it is a difficult procedure, the bony surface area available for contact is small and you may well end up with a non-union. This exposes you as having limited clinical experience (see footnote 20 for counter thrust).

[20] Arthrodesis of the thumb should certainly be mentioned as a possible treatment option for base of thumb arthritis. Quickly go on to mention the difficulties involved with the procedure. It demonstrates a working practical knowledge of hand surgery rather than theoretical book knowledge and gives more credit to your answer.

whatever procedure is used. Therefore, length of surgery and rehabilitation time are important. Patients should be warned that several months might be needed in order to gain the full benefit from the procedure. The procedure of choice depends partly on the stage of the arthritis, the demands placed on the hand and on the surgeon's experience and preference.

A large number of surgeons in the UK still perform simple trapeziectomy alone, and trapeziectomy with a ligament reconstruction is the most commonly performed procedure for arthritis at the base of the thumb worldwide.

MCP joint hyperextension

This may disappear with correction of the adduction contracture at the thumb metacarpal. However, surgical options include a volar capsulodesis if the joint surfaces are intact, or a fusion if there are painful degenerative changes.

Incision

Longitudinal incision over the anatomical snuffbox. Take care not to damage the branches of the superficial radial nerve. The dissection is taken down on to the capsule between EPB and EPL. The radial artery crosses the floor of the anatomical snuffbox and has to be carefully mobilized dorsally. A longitudinal capsular incision is then made and before subperiosteal dissection of the trapezium, which can be removed whole or piecemeal.

Examination corner

Hand oral 1

Clinical photograph of hand demonstrating shoulder sign

- Usual questions about symptoms and management options
- Surgical incision and structures at risk

Hand oral 2

- Trapeziectomy for CMC osteoarthritis
- Silastic® replacements
- Recent literature[1]

[1] Davis TR *et al.* (1997) Trapeziectomy alone, with tendon interposition or with ligament reconstruction? *J Hand Surg Br* **22**(6): 689–94.

Small joint arthritis

History for this should cover any skin, eye or bowel problems.

Osteoarthritis

- Involves base of thumb and distal interphalangeal joints mainly
- Heberden's (DIPJ) and Bouchard's (PIPJ) nodes are painful dorsal osteophytes

Systemic lupus erythematosus (SLE)

- Chronic inflammatory disorder with joint involvement in 75%. Malar rash, fever, pericarditis. In the hand there is similar deformity to rheumatoid deformity with joint subluxations and dislocations but normal joint spaces and no erosions. Soft-tissue procedures are unsuccessful, and require arthrodesis (or arthroplasty)

Gout

- Urate crystal deposition due to various causes (idiopathic, thiazide diuretics, renal failure, malignancy). Causes acutely inflamed joints and characteristic punched-out lesions. Gouty tophi and kidney stones may occur. Crystals are negatively birefringent (yellow) on polarized light microscopy

Psoriasis

- Arthritis present in 20% psoriatics. HLA-B27 in 50%. Other manifestations include extensor and scalp plaques, and nail pitting. In the hand, there is asymmetric arthritis with marked deformity ("pencil in cup")

Haemochromatosis

- With osteoarthritic changes to the metacarpal heads this should be considered as a rare cause and a full blood count performed

Rheumatoid arthritis of the wrist and hand

Introduction

Rheumatoid arthritis is a chronic inflammatory symmetrical polyarthropathy and systemic disease of unknown aetiology.

The main structures requiring treatment are painful, arthritic joints, tendon rupture and subluxation, and nerve compression.

Although the wrist is seldom the first joint affected by rheumatoid arthritis it ultimately becomes involved in over 90% of patients. One-quarter of all rheumatoid surgery is on the hand. More proximal disease must be corrected first and this includes shoulder and wrist problems, before wrist and hand, otherwise corrective surgery will be difficult and recurrence probable.

Rheumatoid factor (IgM autoantibody to IgG) is present in 80%.

Pathophysiology

Inflammation and synovitis lead to stretching of ligaments and capsule. Volar subluxation and supination of the carpus occur due to laxity of the strong extrinsic volar carpal ligaments. This, with distal radioulnar joint disease, leads to prominence of the ulnar head (caput ulnae). There is radial deviation of the metacarpals altering the line of pull of the EDC tendons. This, combined with capsular laxity from synovitis, leads to volar-ulnar subluxation of the MCP joints. Tightness of the ulnar intrinsics causes imbalance of the digits leading to swan-neck and boutonnière deformities.

Rheumatoid nodules are present in 25% and consist of a collagen capsule, and fibrous and central necrosis if large.

History

- Pain
- Weakness
- Loss of function (it should be noted that, despite advanced disease, patients maintain an excellent level of function)[21]
- Swelling
- Cosmetic deformity
- Hobbies

Clinical

Pan-carpal disease

Synovial proliferation and inflammation involve the whole wrist joint causing pain, stiffness and swelling. The inflammatory synovitis causes ligament laxity and destruction of articular cartilage, and invades bone causing cyst formation and bone destruction. The end stage is either spontaneous fusion of the wrist joint or palmar dislocation and ulnar translocation of the radiocarpal articulation.

Peri-scaphoid disease

Synovitis disrupts the radiocarpal and intercarpal ligaments leading to rotatory instability of the scaphoid and carpal instability (DISI pattern). The intercarpal ligaments and wrist capsule become stretched and weakened. The scaphoid assumes a flexed position leading to loss of carpal height, the carpus drifts into radial deviation and there is volar subluxation of the radiocarpal joint. The carpus ultimately dislocates in a volar and ulnar direction. Power grip is weak; the wrist is no longer stable.

[21] ADLs – washing, dressing, feeding.

Distal radio-ulnar joint instability

The ulnar subluxates dorsally (caput ulnae syndrome). Prominence of the ulnar gives rise to the piano key sign[22] due to destruction of the TFCC.

MCP joint

Volar-ulnar subluxation. Synovitis causes capsular laxity. Compensatory ulnar deviation at MCPJs from longitudinal pull of extensor tendons with radial deviation of metacarpals. Ulnar intrinsics then shorten.

Extensor tenosynovitis

Attrition over the prominent ulnar head causes extensor tendon ruptures initially affecting the little finger (Vaughan Jackson syndrome).[23] EPL can rupture around Lister's tubercle.

Flexor tenosynovitis

Pain and volar swelling. FPL can rupture in the carpal tunnel from synovitis of osteophytes over the scaphotrapezial joint. An anterior interosseous nerve syndrome is the differential.

Carpal tunnel syndrome

Secondary effect of swelling at the wrist joint.

Assessment

Looking is the most important part as these patients commonly have marked pain

Quickly screen neck, shoulder and elbow movements. Place hands on a pillow

Swellings – nodules, MC heads, caput ulnae

Obvious deformity – subluxed ulnar head/carpus, deviation metacarpals, z-deformity of

[22] You press down on the ulnar head like a piano key and you get a note from the patient.
[23] Differential diagnosis of "dropped fingers": extensor tendon ruptures, subluxed MCP joints, ulnar subluxation of the extensor tendons, PIN palsy and trigger finger.

the thumb, swan-neck/boutonnière, dropped fingers

Scars (three most common rheumatoid patient scars: dorsal midline from wrist arthrodesis, transverse over MC heads from MCP joint arthroplasty and longitudinal over thumb from MCP joint fusion)

Muscle wasting

Feel any obvious swellings over joints for synovitis and along subcutaneous border of ulna for nodules

Active movement – forearm rotation for DRUJ (loss of supination as the ulnar head is subluxed dorsally), prayer position for wrist extension, back of hands together for wrist flexion, global screening finger movements – "can you make a fist then straighten out your fingers?"

Functional assessment – different grips

Power – "squeeze my fingers"

Tripod – "hold a pen"

Key – pulp to pulp

Precision – tip to tip, "pick up a coin"

Radiographs

PA and lateral wrist radiographs plus PA of the whole hand to assess the severity of arthritis throughout the hand. Rheumatoid wrist disease can be staged using either the Larsen (Stage 0–5) or Wrightington classification (Grade 1–4).

Planning treatment

Surgery is indicated for pain, deformity and loss of function. Treatment should be individualized based on the type and severity of the local destructive process, the involvement of other joints in the upper and lower extremities, the overall status of the patient's disease and the patient's background and expectations from surgery.

In the rheumatoid patient lower limb problems should in general be treated before upper limbs. Retention of walking ability is of overriding importance and periods of crutch walking following lower

limb surgery are best avoided after reconstructive procedures on the upper limbs.

More proximal joints (shoulder and elbow) should be treated before distal joints (wrist and hand) – the hand has to be positioned to carry out appropriate tasks that require good function at the shoulder and elbow. Urgent procedures – in the hand there are some procedures that should be carried out urgently. These include tenosynovectomy to prevent tendon ruptures or to release nerve compression.

Operative management

Wrist joint

Synovectomy ±Darrach's for early disease (rarely in isolation). Performed through a dorsal approach and both the wrist and distal radioulnar joints are cleared of inflammatory synovium.

Wrist arthrodesis

In the rheumatoid wrist arthrodesis provides excellent stability and relief of pain. It is performed through a straight longitudinal dorsal skin incision and the dorsal halves of the carpal bones and the distal radius are fragmented with bone nibblers.[24] The bone fragments are then packed into the wrist joint which is stabilized with a Steinmann or Stanley intramedullary pin. This is normally inserted through the head of the third metacarpal and passed down the metacarpal shaft across the wrist joint and into the distal radius. Alternatively damage to the MCP joint can be avoided by introducing the pin between the bases of the second and third metacarpals but this gives less secure fixation.

In general plate fixation is avoided in the rheumatoid patient. The porotic bone does not take screws well and there are concerns about wound healing.

---

[24] In the rheumatoid patient there is a natural tendency to bony ankylosis of the wrist. Some surgeons insert the pin without operating on the dorsal aspect of the wrist and this is sufficient to encourage wrist fusion. (The position of wrist fusion is in some ways pre-determined by this technique.)

Wrist arthrodesis is a good surgical procedure. There is a high rate of fusion with few operative or postoperative complications. If a pseudoarthrosis develops it is rarely symptomatic. If bilateral wrist fusion is performed the dominant wrist should be fused in slight flexion to facilitate perineal care. Ideally both wrists should not be fused; if possible one should be replaced to allow retention of some movement.

Wrist arthroplasty

The aim is for active wrist motion with an arc of movement ~30°–40°. Prerequisites for a wrist arthroplasty include good bone stock; the deformity must not be too severe (contraindicated if the wrist joint is subluxed or dislocated); and functional extensor tendons. A relative contraindication is previous sepsis.

The Swanson Silastic® interposition arthroplasty essentially functions as a spacer. It has a high failure rate with fracture and synovitis but many survive well in the long term (little movement). Implants using conventional materials (metal on polyethylene) mainly fail in the short to medium term due to distal component loosening. Improved results have been reported with the Universal II total wrist replacement.

Prostheses are inserted through a dorsal approach. It is generally only appropriate in the very low-demand patient with a well-balanced wrist.

Salvage of failed arthroplasties remains difficult because of loss of bone stock.

Distal radio-ulnar joint

Darrach's procedure (plus synovectomy)
Dorsal approach through the floor of the 5th extensor compartment leaving a cuff of capsule on the radius for the repair. Osteotomy through the metaphysis conserving as much length as possible. Main complaint is painful impingement of the ulnar stump on the radius. Any pre-existing ulnar carpal translation is a contraindication as this may progress.

Ulnar head replacement
Some good short-term results and avoids the complication of impingement seen with Darrach's. Essentially a hemiarthroplasty presently and some erosion of the sigmoid notch may occur.

Sauve–Kapandji procedure
Arthrodesis of the DRUJ and resection of a segment of proximal ulna to allow forearm rotation through the resulting pseudoarthrosis. Instability of the proximal ulnar stump may cause troublesome impingement against the shaft of the radius.

Radio-lunate fusion (Chamay procedure)
For ulnar translocation of the carpus.

MCPJ replacement

Silastic replacement (Swanson® and NeuFlex®). Transverse or longitudinal skin incisions. Protect dorsal veins. Longitudinal capsulotomies to radial side of extensor tendons. Capsule and ulnar intrinsics released. Cut metacarpal heads just distal to the collateral ligaments. Ream and insert the implants. At closure, suture lax radial capsular flap under the extensor tendon to the ulnar capsule, to correct radial deviation. This can be carried out with or without intrinsic transfer.

Methotrexate

RA is often treated by the cytotoxic drug methotrexate. Continuing methotrexate during elective surgery has caused concern about whether there is an increase in the risk of postoperative infections and surgical complications. Suddenly stopping the drug often results in a flare-up of the disease, making movement painful and rehabilitation difficult. Recent published work suggests that the continuation of methotrexate treatment does not increase the risk of either infections or early surgical complications in rheumatoid patients.[25] Current practice

---

[25] Grennan DM, Gray J, Loudon J, Fear S (2001) Methotrexate and early postoperative complications in patients with rheumatoid arthritis undergoing elective orthopaedic surgery. *Ann Rheum Dis* **60**(3):214–17.

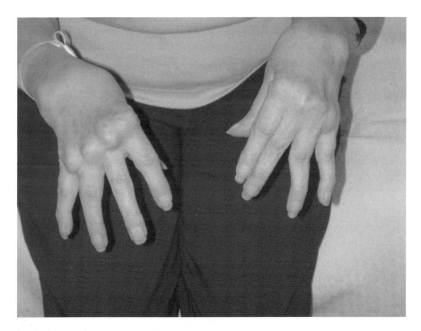

Figure 21.4 Clinical picture of severe rheumatoid hands

is to continue methotrexate treatment throughout elective orthopaedic surgery.

Examination corner

Adult elective orthopaedics oral 1

AP radiographs of a severely deformed rheumatoid wrist

Description of radiograph
   Principles of management
   Be careful when mentioning synovectomy in this particular instance – the bony changes are too advanced to preclude any useful benefit from synovectomy but if the wrist was less severely affected synovectomy may be useful.
   A fairly lengthy discussion on the relative merits of arthrodesis versus arthroplasty of the wrist took place. I was fine with wrist arthrodesis ("talk me through how you do a wrist arthrodesis") but got cornered on wrist arthroplasty, which I knew next to nothing about.

Hand oral 1

Rheumatoid hands

- Generalized wrist synovitis – management
- Tendon rupture (EIP) – aetiology and management

Hand oral 2

- Rheumatoid hand with caput ulnae
- How would you manage this patient?
- Vaughan Jackson syndrome

Adult elective orthopaedics oral 2

Radiograph of rheumatoid hands

- Describe the radiograph
- Discussion on the aetiology of the condition

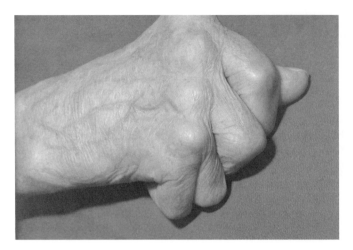

Figure 21.5 Clinical picture of a rheumatoid hand

Hand oral 3

Clinical picture of rheumatoid hands (Figure 21.4)

- Describe the types of deformities present
- What are the causes of these deformities?
- Brief discussion on management

Hand oral 4

Clinical picture of a rheumatoid hand (Figure 21.5)

- Describe the abnormalities present (describe the picture)
- Can you explain why they occur and how they progress once present?
- What are the causes of loss of finger extension in rheumatoid arthritis?
- What are the reasons for extensor tendon rupture?
- How would you mange extensor tendon ruptures?

Hand oral 5

Extensor tenosynovitis in the rheumatoid hand

- Diagnosis
- Differential diagnosis

- Complications
- Tendon rupture and caput ulnae
- Principles of tendon reconstruction in the rheumatoid hand

Rheumatoid arthritis: flexor and extensor tendons

Introduction

Tenosynovitis in the rheumatoid hand is more obvious on the extensor surface of the wrist and hand but one should not neglect to also examine the flexor side of the hand and wrist for its presence.

Symptoms

If flexor tenosynovitis is present in the **carpal tunnel** it can cause
- Carpal tunnel syndrome
- Tendon rupture

Palm and fingers

- Triggering
- Loss of active finger flexion or passive finger extension

The consequences of flexor tenosynovitis are pain, stiffness (restricted active motion) and tendon rupture. Inevitably flexor tenosynovitis can co-exist with any related joint problems in the hand.

Examination

Examination for flexor tenosynovitis can be difficult as swelling is sometimes minimal, but restriction of active movement and crepitus as bulky tendons move beneath pulleys are common.

Look

- Overall posture of the hand
- For evidence of tendon ruptures, isolated swan-neck deformities (isolated rupture of FDS)
- Swelling is seldom visible (or palpable) beneath the flexor retinaculum, but appears in the palm, distal forearm and digits

Feel

- Puffy thick feel to the rheumatoid hand
- Pinch test
  - Normally you can pinch between your finger and thumb two thicknesses of skin in front of the proximal phalanx. Thickened tenosynovium bulges out through defects in the fibrous sheath and creates a wodge of tissue instead
- A thickened sensation around the distal palmar crease area at the entrance to the A1 pulley may indicate the presence of synovitis
- Palpation of the fingers may indicate the presence of nodules or diffuse synovitis

Move

- Examination of tendon function for both FDS/FDP
- Crepitus over the tendons

Inability to flex the DIP joint

- Tendon rupture
- Adherence of FDP to FDS

- Triggering caused by nodules

Tendon rupture results from invasive synovitis, infarction secondary to vasculitis, attrition from bony prominences and pressure under the unyielding extensor or flexor retinaculum.

Management

Acute synovitis

Conservative

- Splintage and drugs
- Steroid injections into the carpal tunnel or tendon sheath (may itself cause tendon rupture)

Surgery

Surgery is indicated by:

- Failure of conservative treatment at 4 months and the presence of persistent and painful tenosynovitis
- Median nerve compression in the carpal tunnel
- Triggering
- Tendon rupture

Timely tenosynovectomy is vital in preventing tendon rupture and preserving the function of the hand. When there is doubt it is better to perform a tenosynovectomy to prevent tendon rupture than to persist with medical treatment. The surgeon should adopt an aggressive approach towards rheumatoid tenosynovitis and be prepared to intervene surgically on a prophylactic basis.

Chronic synovitis

Synovectomy – three sites:

- Carpal tunnel (floor of the carpal tunnel is inspected for bony spicules and excised if present)
- The palm at the level of the mouth of the A1 pulley
- Fingers at the level of the PIP joint just distal to the A2 pulley

Make a Bruner's incision. Remove diseased synovium and intertendinous nodules, and repair any tendon defects. Release of the A1 pulley in rheumatoid arthritis is controversial as it may allow ulnar

Table 21.2 Options for reconstruction

Tendon ruptured	Salvage procedure
FDS	None
FDP – wrist	Suture to adjacent FDP tendon or tendon graft
FDP – finger	DIP joint fusion
FDP + FDS finger	Tendon graft or FDS transfer from another finger
FPL	Synovectomy and fusion IPJ

migration of the flexor tendons and aggravate ulnar drift deformity at the MCP joint. The annular pulleys should be preserved (including the A1 pulley) and the tendon sheath is opened between the annular pulleys. Postoperative stiffness can be a problem and early mobility is essential.

Tendon rupture

- Primary tendon repair – primary repair is generally not possible due to poor tissue at the tendon ends
- Primary tendon graft – fraught with difficulties and results are usually poor; in a young patient this should at least be considered
- Tendon transfer – limited availability on flexor side (palmaris longus, brachioradialis)
- Side-to-side suture – good in older patients, should be considered for ruptures at the wrist level
- Arthrodesis (DIPJ – ruptured FDP but intact FDS)

Full synovectomy should be performed simultaneously with any tendon reconstruction (Table 21.2), as re-ruptures are not uncommon.

Loss of both tendons within the digital sheath is disabling but reconstruction is difficult. Transfer of the FDS from another finger can be used if a healthy distal FDP stump is present otherwise tendon grafting may be necessary despite its unpredictable outcome.

Vaughan Jackson syndrome

Rupture of EDC of ring and little fingers due to attrition from prominent ulna (caput ulnae) and DRUJ synovitis.

Differential diagnosis of dropped fingers

- Ulnar subluxation of extensor tendons
- Volar subluxation of MCP joints
- PIN palsy
- Locked trigger finger

Management

- Synovectomy ±Darrach's for pre-rupture
- Above + tendon transfer (EIP to EDM) for rupture

Mannerfelt–Norman syndrome

The most common flexor tendon to rupture in rheumatoid arthritis. FPL rupture due to scaphotrapezial synovitis.

Management

- Prompt exploration of the carpal canal and removal of diseased synovium and osteophytes (scaphotrapezial joint)
- IPJ arthrodesis preferred – gives a stable thumb with good power transmitted from the short muscles
- Transfer FDS of the ring finger – a possible option but the range of motion gained is small. It is difficult to get the tension right
- A free tendon graft could be used to bridge the gap

Oral question

Describe the typical manifestations of rheumatoid disease at the hand and wrist

---

Rheumatoid thumb

Introduction

More than two-thirds of rheumatoid patients have some involvement of the thumb. All three joints can be affected. The thumb is used in almost all daily activities and the presenting complaint is usually of painful loss of function.

Classification (Nalebuff)[26]

This classification is not sequential and only describes different patterns of deformity.

Type 1: Boutonnière-like deformity

MCP joint flexion and IP joint hyperextension. The basal joint is not affected. This is the most common pattern of deformity in the rheumatoid thumb. The primary disease is at the MCP joint where synovitis bulging dorsally causes attrition of the EPB insertion and extensor hood damage with loss of MCP joint extension. The EPL subluxes ulnarly and in time starts to act as a flexor of the MCP joint. The IP joint gradually hyperextends because all the muscles are now extending the IP joint. In the early stages both the MCP joint flexion and IP joint hyperextension are passively correctable. However, relatively rapid fixed deformities develop initially of the MCP joint and later of the IP joint as well.

Type 2: with CMC joint subluxation

A combination of the type 1 boutonnière deformity with subluxation or dislocation of the CMC joint. This is rare. The treatment is similar to that for type 1 deformity but the addition of trapeziectomy or CMC joint arthroplasty is nearly always necessary.

Type 3: Swan-neck deformity

The reverse of the boutonnière type deformity. This is the second most common rheumatoid thumb deformity. The disease starts at the CMC joint and

leads to subluxation of that joint. Deformity is CMC joint subluxation/dislocation leading to an adduction contracture. It is impossible to get the thumb out of the palm without hyperextending the MCP joint, which in turn causes IP joint flexion. Mobility is needed at the basal thumb joint so that the thumb can be positioned appropriately and therefore this precludes fusion.

Type 4: Gamekeeper's thumb

Disease is confined to the MCP joint and is similar to a UCL rupture. The ligament is stretched rather than ruptured and this often results in a secondary adduction contracture of the web space. The CMC joint and IP joint are usually normal. Surgical treatment is aimed at stabilizing the MCP joint. In the early stages this is achieved by synovectomy and repair or reconstruction of the UCL. In more advanced cases where joint destruction is present arthrodesis of the MCP joint with or without a web space release is indicated.

Type 5: Hyperextension of the MCP joint

This is rare. The deformity is caused by isolated hyperextension of the MCP joint due to slackening and lengthening of the volar plate. There is no adduction of the metacarpal, which distinguishes it from the swan-neck deformity. As this hyperextension increases there is compensatory flexion of the IP joint due to FPL tightness. Treatment is with some form of tenodesis or if necessary arthrodesis. The aim is to provide stability to the MCP joint in extension.

Type 6: Arthritis mutilans

Severe destruction of all joints with gross instability and shortening of the thumb. This is difficult to manage and treatment usually involves fusion to maintain or gain length.

General rules

- Primary joint indicates the deformity and other joint collapses into a particular instability pattern

---

[26] For simplicity we have combined Nalebuff's classification with management options. A word of caution is needed though: different treatment options are recommended by different authors for the various types and stages of the rheumatoid thumb. We do not claim to be experts in this difficult area of surgery and only offer a suggested guide to possible treatment options available for the purposes of passing the exam.

- Second joint deformity can become fixed and require treatment
- It is impossible to consider the primary joint in isolation and the effect of treatment on one joint must be considered in relation to its effect on other joints
- Is the joint deformity flexible or fixed?
- The thumb collapses into a zigzag pattern in both the flexion/extension and abduction/adduction planes
- Instability in the thumb particularly at the MCP and IP joints is more disabling than loss of flexion and extension

---

Examination corner

Hand oral 1

Clinical photograph of a rheumatoid hand

- Describe the deformities present
- What classification systems are used for the deformities seen?
- Describe the management of the boutonnière thumb

Hand oral 2

Clinical photograph of a rheumatoid thumb

- Describe Nalebuff's classification
- Describe the management options
- Describe the management of web-space contracture

Boutonnière deformity of the finger

Introduction

PIP joint flexion and **DIP joint hyperextension.** Boutonnière is the French word for buttonhole, and is used in this context because the head of the PP buttonholes through the extensor hood secondary to rupture of the central slip.

Pathology

It is caused by central slip attenuation or rupture due to synovitis. Volar subluxation of the lateral bands occurs due to disruption of the triangular ligament. The lateral bands become converted from an extensor to a flexor of the PIP joint. The functional loss with a boutonnière deformity is a lot less than with the swan-neck deformity, especially if some flexion is possible at the distal joint.

Acute injury

This is usually traumatic and can be difficult to diagnose. Treatment is conservative using a "Capener splint" which allows active DIP joint flexion/extension.

Elson's test for acute central slip disruption[27]

The PIP joint of the finger is bent 90° over the edge of a table. With resisted middle phalanx extension, the DIP joint either:

- Goes into rigid extension (positive test – disruption of the central slip) because all the forces in the finger are distributed to the terminal tendon through the intact lateral bands, or
- Remains floppy (negative test)

Classification (Nalebuff and Millender)[28]

Based on the degree of deformity, the presence of passive correctability and the state of the joint surfaces:

    Mild – PIP joint lag of 10°–15° in extension
    Moderate – PIP joint lag of 30°–40° in extension
    Severe – PIP joint in fixed flexed position with joint involvement

---

[27] Acute test for central slip disruption before deformity is evident. A surprising number of candidates get mixed up and end up talking about Elson's test for a chronic deformity.

[28] To be on top of your game for the FRCS Orth hand oral you should aim to be able to reel off this classification system ad verbatim and similarly be able to discuss the various treatment options. The same criterion applies to the swan-neck deformity and the rheumatoid thumb deformities. It is easy to get overload fatigue if you go through large amounts of complex hand stuff in a single night. This information takes a little while to sink in and usually needs at least two reads before the material begins to make sense.

Management options for chronic deformity

Many operations have been described for the management of this deformity but often the results from surgery can be highly variable and unpredictable. A word of caution – great care is needed when deciding to operate on the PIP joint as although extension may be regained, one can easily lose flexion and end up either no better off or worse off than before surgery. Moreover correction of a mild boutonnière deformity is often associated with minimal functional improvement and the re-occurrence rate is high. The results of soft-tissue reconstruction of rheumatoid boutonnière deformity can be unsatisfactory and if surgery is required fusion of the PIP joint in a functional position may be a safer option.

Terminal tendon release

Release of the extensor mechanism at the junction of the middle and proximal thirds of the middle phalanx, which leaves the ORL intact. The lateral bands slide proximally, increasing extensor tone at the PIP joint and the intact ORL provides extensor tone to the DIP joint. Or more simply there is less hyperextension stress on the DIP joint and the flexion of the PIP joint is lessened.

Secondary tendon reconstruction

- Excision of scar tissue and direct repair of central slip
- Free tendon graft (central slip reconstruction)
- Lateral band transfer procedure

These are only carried out after passive joint motion has been restored.

Littler

Divide lateral bands at different levels. Suture shorter to stump of central slip, and longer to the longer distal lateral band stump.

Matev

The radial lateral band is divided over the middle phalanx and the ulnar lateral band more distally. The proximal stump of the radial lateral band is passed through the central slip and anchored at the dorsal base P2 centrally. The ulnar lateral band is sutured to both lateral bands at their insertions.

Arthrodesis

Arthrodesis should be performed in varying degrees of flexion depending on which finger is being fused.

Arthroplasty

Unpredictable functional benefit.

Examination corner

Hand oral 1

Clinical photograph of a rheumatoid boutonnière finger deformity

Spot diagnosis
- What is a boutonnière deformity?
- How are boutonnière deformities classified?
- What are the management options for a boutonnière deformity?

Hand oral 2

Clinical photograph of a rheumatoid hand

- General description of the picture
- Questions on various deformities including boutonnière deformity

---

Swan-neck deformity

Introduction

PIP joint hyperextension and DIP joint flexion.

Pathology

The deformity is caused by an **imbalance of forces** at the PIP joint and a lax volar plate. Unlike the boutonnière deformity the condition can be secondary to problems at either the MCP joint or DIP joint. The condition most commonly occurs in rheumatoid disease although there are other rarer causes (mallet finger, laceration or transfer of FDS). The deformity can only occur if hyperextension is possible at the PIP joint.

Causes

- Intrinsic tightness secondary to MCP joint disease
- Intrinsic contracture
- FDS rupture
- Volar plate insufficiency
- Mallet deformity
- Extrinsic spasticity

The chief complaint is a loss of flexion of the PIP joint.

Classification (Nalebuff types 1–4)

1. Flexible hyperextension deformity of the PIP joint
2. PIP joint flexion is limited when the MCP joint is maintained in extension. Intrinsic muscle tightness is present
3. Limited PIP joint flexion in all MCP joint positions but the PIP joint surface is still preserved
4. PIP joint is stiff and there is destruction of the articular surface of the joint

Management

1. Extension restriction splint (if the PIP joint is a problem) or fusion DIP joint (if the DIP joint is a problem)
2. Intrinsic release plus some form of tenodesis on the volar aspect of the PIP joint
   - Oblique retinacular ligament reconstruction
   - FDS tenodesis
3. Either a soft-tissue procedure or arthrodesis. Prerequisites for a soft-tissue procedure are full flexion of the PIP joint before soft-tissue reconstruction, which may require MUA, sometimes the release of the dorsally contracted skin and then intrinsic release, if appropriate, and some form of tenodesis
4. Arthrodesis is probably the procedure of choice in this advanced stage

FDS tenodesis

Through a volar incision one limb of the FDS tendon is divided proximally and passed either dorsally through the middle phalanx or around the A2 pulley and sutured onto itself, to provide a volar tether to hyperextension. K-wires are placed across the joint for 4 weeks.

Examination corner

Hand oral 1

Clinical photograph of rheumatoid swan-neck finger deformity

- What is the swan-neck deformity?
- What is it caused by?
- How do you manage it?
- How do you classify them?

Hand oral 2

Clinical photograph of rheumatoid hand swan-neck deformity

- Describe Nalebuff's classification
- What are the operative options for this patient?

Scaphoid fractures

The scaphoid is the most commonly fractured bone in the carpus. Knowledge is required of the diagnosis and management of acute fractures and the complications of non-union and AVN.

Blood supply

The blood supply of the waist and proximal pole of the scaphoid (70%) is derived from the dorsal branch of the radial artery entering distally on the dorsal ridge through ligamentous and capsular attachments. The proximal pole is the region with the most tenuous blood supply, owing to the distal to proximal (retrograde) intraosseous supply. The distal scaphoid and tuberosity (30%) are supplied by branches of the superficial palmar branch of the radial artery.

Mechanism

Fall onto an outstretched hand resulting in forced dorsiflexion of the wrist.

Examination

- Fullness in the ASB (effusion in wrist)
- Tenderness in the ASB and scaphoid tuberosity
- Reduced range of motion (but not dramatically)
- Pain at extremes of motion
- Pronation followed by ulnar deviation will cause pain

Investigation

Radiographs (scaphoid series)

Four standard radiographs
- PA in ulnar deviation (extends scaphoid)
- Lateral
- Two oblique views

Bone scanning

- Sensitive but not specific

CT

- Sensitive (reported 100%) but low specificity (75%)
- More accessible than MRI

MRI

- Excellent sensitivity and specificity
- Fracture line will be visible on T_2-weighted sequence as a line of high signal, which represents marrow oedema
- Changes present on MRI scan after 12 hours

Displacement

Defined as:
- Displacement >1 mm
- Angulation >10°
- SL angle >45°
- CL angle >15°

Fracture location

- Proximal pole (25%)
- Waist (65%)
- Distal pole and tuberosity (10%)

Classification (Herbert 1990)

- Type A: Stable fractures
  - Tuberosity and incomplete fractures
- Type B: Unstable fractures
  - All complete fractures
- Type C: Delayed union
- Type D: Non-union

Management

Undisplaced

- Scaphoid cast or percutaneous fixation
- Percutaneous fixation allows earlier mobilization in active patients but has no proven increased union rate or decreased time of healing
- If cast, remove and X-ray again at 8 weeks
- If still tender then treat in cast for a further 4 weeks
- At 12 weeks leave free regardless of whether there is tenderness or not

There is no proven benefit of plastering above or below the elbow, or of including the thumb or not.

Displaced

ORIF
- Headless compression screws (differential pitch on screw to provide compression) e.g. Herbert,

Herbert–Whipple (cannulated), Acutrack (cannulated), Kompressor

- K-wires – good ease of insertion but they do not provide compression. Use if there is marked comminution

Surgical technique

Volar

Indicated for waist fractures as it does not damage the dorsal blood supply and can correct a humpback deformity. Surface landmarks are the scaphoid tuberosity and FCR tendon. Skin incision is longitudinal along the radial border of FCR curving radially at the distal wrist crease. Divide the superficial branch of the radial artery and dissect through the bed of the FCR tendon sheath. Incise and reflect the capsule and the radioscaphocapitate and radioscapholunate ligaments. Screws are placed distal to proximal, 45° to the horizontal and 45° to the long axis of the forearm. A piece of trapezium may need to be excised to gain access to the distal pole of the scaphoid.

Dorsal

Use for proximal pole fractures as it provides access with the wrist hyperflexed. Care is needed to avoid damage to the dorsal blood supply. The incision is distal to Lister's tubercle. The approach is between the third and fourth extensor compartments (EPL and EDC). Transverse capsulotomy. Flex the wrist 90° to expose the proximal pole and reduce the fracture with flexion and traction. The entry point for the guide-wire is just radial to the scapholunate ligament and aim along the thumb metacarpal.

Scaphoid non-union

Incidence

- Distal pole <10%
- Waist 10%–20%
- Proximal third 30%
- Proximal fifth 100%

Poor prognosis

- Delay in treatment
- Displaced fractures
- Proximal pole fractures
- AVN
- Smokers

Management

The aim is to achieve a union and prevent early degenerative changes from developing (SNAC wrist). Some form of graft is required in the treatment of scaphoid non-union unless degenerative changes are present, in which case salvage surgery should be offered. Studies suggest an overall union rate of 66% with surgical treatment.

Inlay (Russe) graft

Corticocancellous inlay graft set in a cavity made in the proximal and distal fragments of the scaphoid through a volar approach. The graft is slightly longer than the defect. The graft does not need internal fixation as the natural shape of the scaphoid clamps down on this graft and keeps it stable.

Interposition (Fisk) graft

Corticocancellous opening wedge graft placed through a volar approach and designed to restore scaphoid length and correct angulation. Preferred option for a humpback deformity and carpal instability (DISI).

Vascularized bone graft

Studies have shown union rates of 100% with a vascularized bone graft, and therefore should they be used for all non-unions? There are excellent arterial anastomoses around the distal radius. Various pedicle grafts can be used and are either volar (e.g. pronator quadratus or Mathoulin graft) or dorsal (e.g. 1,2 – intercompartmental supraretinacular artery (ICSRA) – Zaidemberg graft).[29]

[29] Zaidemberg C, Siebert JW, Angrigiani C (1991) A new vascularized bone graft for scaphoid nonunion. *J Hand Surg Am* **16**: 474–8.

Oral question

Why treat a scaphoid non-union?

- To decrease pain
- To decrease the risk of secondary OA
- To correct carpal kinematics
- To increase function

Note that 30%–50% will still develop OA of the wrist despite union of the fracture.

Non-union with AVN

AVN of the proximal pole is an important predictive factor in the success of surgery to treat non-unions. The incidence varies widely from 9% to 40% following waist fractures. Radiographs may show increased density of the proximal scaphoid fragment (due to decreased bone turnover). Gadolinium-enhanced MRI may correlate with outcome but the gold standard is punctuate bleeding at surgery.

The present management for AVN is a vascularized bone graft.

Oral question

Discuss the nature and treatment of non-union and AVN

Examination corner

Hand oral 1

Radiograph of a waist of scaphoid non-union

Approaches to the scaphoid – both dorsal and volar

Examiner: Demonstrate Kirk Watson's test to me.

Hand oral 2

Radiograph of a scaphoid non-union post screw fixation

Discuss your management now.

Hand oral 3

- Scaphoid fracture

- Management options
- Acute fixation versus cast: arguments for and against
- Type of cast you would use and for how long
- Evidence in the literature supporting use of this cast

Hand oral 4

Radiograph of a waist of scaphoid non-union

Only three topics were covered in the hand oral but there was detailed probing in each topic.

Examiner: This is a radiograph of a 24-year-old joiner who fell onto his right outstretched hand.

Candidate: The candidate has a fracture of the waist of the scaphoid.

(There was a large cystic area and bone sclerosis and resorption associated with the fracture, and the radiograph didn't look quite right for a simple fracture.)

Examiner: For a start this is not a fresh fracture. The gentleman sustained only a wrist sprain. The radiograph shows a scaphoid non-union – can't you see the large cystic area associated with it? You do not get these cysts after a straightforward scaphoid fracture. Anyway the give away was that the mechanism of injury for a scaphoid fracture was all wrong. Most scaphoid fractures occur after a fall onto the radial aspect of the palm with extreme dorsiflexion and radial deviation, not just falling onto an outstretched hand.

You should have picked this up in the history because if you treat it as a fresh fracture you are doomed to failure.

Examiner: Do you know of any classification systems for scaphoid non-unions?

Candidate: I am not completely familiar with it but I believe the classification system is from A to D.

Examiner: What you are talking about or have mentioned is a classification system for scaphoid fractures but not for non-union.

(Crossed wires here – I was not aware of a specific classification system for scaphoid non-unions. The problem was that I did not know Herbert's classification system very well. This system includes acute fractures, delayed unions and non-unions. Thinking through afterwards I am sure we were both talking about the same thing.)

Examiner: So how are you going to treat this injury?

Candidate: I would fix it with a Herbert screw and bone graft.

Examiner: What do you do if your boss has left you this case and you get no bleeding whatsoever from the freshened ends of the scaphoid?

Do you just fix it, not tell anybody and hope for the best?! What are you going to do in this situation?

Candidate: I am not sure.

Examiner: Have you heard of a vascularized bone graft or a proximal row carpectomy? It is a difficult situation but you shouldn't just fix it. The patient should have had an MRI scan before surgery.

Hand oral 5

Radiograph of a complete waist of scaphoid fracture (Herbert B2)

Examiner: How would you manage this fracture?

Candidate: This is a Herbert B2 fracture. Its management is controversial. Some surgeons would fix it and others would manage it conservatively. There are advantages and disadvantages of each option.

Examiner: You choose to fix it with a Herbert screw but it goes onto a non-union – what would you do?

Candidate: This is a difficult situation. I would first get a bone scan or MRI scan to rule out AVN. Assuming AVN was excluded I would re-fix it with a Herbert screw and bone graft. If this failed I would bail out at this stage and refer on to an experienced hand surgeon who may want to consider a vascularized bone graft harvested from the distal radius.

(The examiners were very happy with this answer.)

Hand oral 6

Scaphoid non-union

- Demonstrate Kirk Watson's test
- Approaches to the scaphoid – dorsal and volar
- Bone grafts
- Fixation techniques

Hand oral 7

Radiograph of displaced waist of scaphoid fracture

- Diagnosis obvious
- Undisplaced versus unstable displaced scaphoid fracture
- Discussion of carpal instability – various angles, etc.
- SNAC wrist

SNAC wrist

With a non-union of the scaphoid, arthritis is likely to develop at 5–10 years. The proximal pole behaves like a ball and socket joint and does not develop degenerative changes, but the distal pole flexes and OA develops initially at the volar lip of the radial styloid.

Patients commonly present after minor trauma with wrist pain having been previously asymptomatic. Radiographs show a non-union with longstanding degenerative changes.

Classification

1. Arthritic changes between the radial styloid and distal scaphoid
2. Degenerative process affecting the whole scaphoid fossa of the distal radius
3. Capitolunate arthritis (radiolunate joint spared)
4. Whole carpus involved

Management

Stage 1

- Radial styloidectomy and limited carpal fusion (SC or SLC)
- If the scaphoid proximal pole is necrotic it may be removed after performing a limited arthrodesis between the distal scaphoid and capitate and styloidectomy

Stage 2

- Scaphoid excision and four-corner fusion (if no radiolunate arthritis)
- Proximal row carpectomy is another option (if no arthritis of the head of the capitate)

Stage 3

- Scaphoid excision plus four-corner fusion is probably the procedure of choice as the head of the capitate is involved

Stage 4

• Wrist arthrodesis

Examination corner

Hand oral 1

SNAC wrist

• Diagnosis
• Classification and management options in a young manual worker

Hand oral 2

SNAC wrist grade I in an asymptomatic man

How would you manage this patient?

Carpal instability

Introduction

Complex area and not yet fully understood but for the FRCS Orth exam you should be familiar with carpal row anatomy, extrinsic and intrinsic ligaments, simple carpal biomechanics and common injury patterns.

Definition

Carpal instability is a term used to describe abnormal carpal biomechanics under physiological loading due to disruption of the complex ligament system that controls the relative motion of the bones that form the carpus.

Carpal anatomy

The biomechanics of the wrist joint are difficult to understand without first understanding some anatomy. The carpus is composed of two rows of bones: the proximal row and the distal row. There are four main joints at the wrist: DRUJ, radiocarpal, midcarpal and carpometacarpal.

Distal row

The bones in the distal row are: trapezium, trapezoid, capitate and hamate. They are bound together by strong interosseous (intrinsic) ligaments and move together as a single unit.

Proximal row

The bones in the proximal row are: scaphoid, lunate and triquetrum. The proximal row moves as an intercalated segment. It has no direct muscle attachments and is linked by strong intrinsic ligaments. It moves as a result of forces applied to the distal carpal row causing relative movement at the midcarpal and radiocarpal joints.

Intrinsic ligaments

The intrinsic ligaments have their origin and insertion within the same carpal row. They are short stout structures, which are not amenable to surgical repair. The distal row firmly binds all the distal carpal bones together so that they move as one. The most important proximal row ligaments are the scapholunate ligament (SLL) and the lunotriquetral ligament (LTL). Both these ligaments allow some (but not excessive) movement between the proximal carpal bones and transmit forces along the row to ensure adaptive motion.

Extrinsic ligaments

The extrinsic ligaments connect the carpal bones to the radius or metacarpals. They are stronger volarly. The dorsal aspect ligaments are weaker and consist of radiolunotriquetral (RLT) and transverse ligaments (basis for the Berger flap[30]).

---

[30] Berger RA *et al.* (1995) New dorsal approach for the surgical exposure of the wrist. *Ann Plast Surg* **35**(1): 54–9.

Space of Poirier

There are no ligaments running from the centre of the distal end of the radius to the capitate and this leaves an area of weakness over the front of the lunocapitate joint. A lunate dislocation or perilunate fracture dislocation is associated with a transverse capsular rent through this inherently weak region.

Kinematics

Kinematics involves the study of movements of a body without reference to the forces that are acting to cause that movement. The proximal carpal row flexes in radial deviation and extends in ulnar deviation.

Row theory

The proximal carpal row is interlinked by the interosseous ligaments and moves independently of the distal carpal row.

Column theory

The wrist consists of three longitudinal columns: the lateral column (scaphoid), which is mobile; a central column (capitate, lunate), which provides flexion/extension; and a medial column (hamate, triquetrum), which allows carpal rotation. Each column provides a different type of wrist stability.

There has been disagreement between the various supporters of each theory but it would appear that some wrists function more like rows and others more like columns.

Terminology

Elements of the official terminology for instability are complex but it is critical to grasp them; they include:

- **Static** – Constant
- **Dynamic –** Intermittent
- **Dissociative –** Between bones of the same carpal row (e.g. DISI/VISI)

- **Non-dissociative** – Between the proximal and distal rows or between the proximal row and distal radius (e.g. midcarpal)

No universally accepted system exists for classifying carpal instabilities. Generally speaking four patterns of instability are described.

Carpal instability dissociative (CID)

Relates to instability between (or through) carpal bones of the same row (either proximal or distal).

Carpal instability non-dissociative (CIND)

Relates to instability between carpal rows or transverse osseous segments and can be caused by ligament injury or bony fracture (or both).

Carpal instability complex (CIC)

Combination of CID and CIND lesions.

A CIC is most often seen as a perilunate fracture/dislocation and the volar lunate dislocation. The Mayfield Classification of this injury has four stages progressing from radial to ulnar.[31] They can be lesser arc (ligamentous) or greater arc (radial styloid, scaphoid or capitate fracture):

- Stage I – Rupture of the scapholunate and radioscaphocapitate ligaments
- Stage II – Dislocation of the capitolunate joint
- Stage III – Rupture of the lunotriquetral interosseous ligament
- Stage IV– Dislocation of the lunate

In 95% of cases the capitate dislocates dorsally off the lunate. In a volar lunate dislocation it passes through a weakness between the volar extrinsic ligaments – space of Poirier.

Carpal injury adaptive (CIA)

Another type of carpal instability is called adaptive and is the consequence of deformity in

---

[31] Mayfield JK (1980) Mechanism of carpal injuries. *Clin Orthop Relat Res* **149**: 45–54.

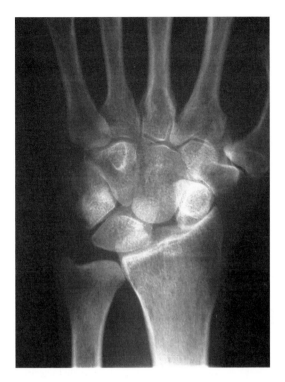

Figure 21.6 Radiograph showing marked scapholunate dissociation with flexed scaphoid (ring sign), loss of carpal height and loss of the radioscaphoid joint space (SLAC wrist)

the distal radius from a fracture. Therefore, it should correct with anatomical reduction of the fracture.

Clinical features

History

- Mechanism of any injury (e.g. history of a sprained wrist which fails to resolve)
- Aim to localize symptoms
- Pain with loading activities and weakness
- Click or clunk on wrist movement
- Swelling
- Loss of function

Examination

- Swelling
- Localized tenderness (scapholunate ligament found just distal to Lister's tubercle)
- Active and passive range of motion

Special tests

Specific provocative manoeuvres should be performed based on the patient's symptoms:

Pseudostability test – for midcarpal instability

Kirk Watson's test – assesses scapholunate ligament competence[32]

Reagan's ballottement test – for lunotriquetral instability. Trap the lunate between the thumb and index finger of one hand and the triquetrum in the other as the bones are moved independently and in opposite directions to each other

Kleinman shear test – the examiner's thumbs are placed on the dorsal aspect of the triquetrum and lunate and the bones are translated in an opposite direction with respect to each other

Investigations

X-rays

Carpal instability series:

- PA/lateral view of the wrist (wrist in neutral)
- Clenched fist PA view

Scapholunate instability (Figure 21.6):

- Scapholunate angle >60°
- Scapholunate gap >3 mm (Terry Thomas sign)
- Ring sign (end-on view of distal pole of flexed scaphoid)
- Step in Gilula's lines

Static instability:

- If present will show up on the X-ray

Dynamic instability:

- May not be seen even on the clenched fist view

---

[32] This test is known by various names such as the "Kirk Watson test", the "Watson test" or the "scaphoid shift test". For some reason examiners seem to be particularly fond of asking candidates to demonstrate this test in the hand oral.

If you clinically suspect a ligament injury but the Kirk Watson's test and/or radiographs are negative, book the patient for either an MR arthrogram or an arthroscopy depending on your level of suspicion.

Arthroscopy

Allows direct visualization of the radiocarpal and midcarpal joints, and intrinsic ligaments (Geissler classification for scapholunate instability). Dynamic stress tests can also be performed (although not with physiological loading). Arthroscopy allows the assessment of:

- Cartilage surfaces
- Synovium
- Intrinsic and extrinsic ligaments
- Relative stability/motion of the carpal bones to each other
- Presence of anomalous structures, entrapped or mechanically interfering tissues, scar and/or other blocking tissue

The acronyms DISI and VISI refer to the static posture of the lunate seen on a true lateral radiograph of the wrist. Comparison radiographic views of the contralateral wrist are essential because these findings may be noted in an asymptomatic wrist and may represent a normal variant.

Dorsal intercalated segment instability (DISI)

When the lunate is extended or rotated dorsally in relation to the long axis of the radius and capitate the situation is called DISI. The scapholunate angle is >60° (normal 30°–60°, average 47°).

Causes include:

- SLL injury
- Scaphoid fracture
- Kienböck's
- Perilunate injury

Volar intercalated segment instability (VISI)

When the lunate is flexed and the scapholunate angle is less than 30° the situation is called VISI. It is much less common than DISI and is most commonly caused by lunotriquetral ligament injury.

Management

Scapholunate ligament injury

Acute

Early open repair through a dorsal approach by direct suture, pull through sutures or suture anchors. Supplemented by K-wire stabilization of the scapholunate and scaphocapitate joints. Delayed open repair can be performed up to 6 weeks after acute injury.

Chronic

Surgical procedures are classified as either bony or soft tissue:

- Soft tissue: Excellent results have been reported for a modified Brunelli procedure (FCR tenodesis).[33] Dorsal capsulodesis (Blatt capsulodesis) has fallen out of favour
- Bony procedures: Limited wrist fusion such as the scaphotrapeziotrapezoid fusion (STT), to correct DISI. These procedures can be technically difficult and demanding

Lunotriquetral ligament injury

Rarely recognized acutely but if so then perform acute open repair of the ligament. The scaphoid and lunate are both flexed leaving the triquetrum extended. VISI due to CID. Chronic symptomatic lunotriquetral instability should be treated by either lunotriquetral fusion or FCU tenodesis.

Acute perilunate dislocation

Emergency treatment is closed reduction with open repair of the ligaments possibly when the swelling has settled.

Closed reduction

- Dorsal perilunate dislocation – hyperdorsiflex the wrist, apply traction and try to hinge the capitate

[33] Talwalkar SC, Edwards AT, Hayton MJ, Stilwell JH, Trail IA, Stanley JK (2006) Results of tri-ligament tenodesis: a modified Brunelli procedure in the management of scapholunate instability. *J Hand Surg Br* **31**(1):110–17.

head onto the lunate before flexing the wrist. Likely to reduce due to extensive soft-tissue injury

- Volar lunate dislocation – hyperdorsiflex the wrist, apply pressure on the lunate to reduce and flex the wrist. May not reduce in a closed procedure. Open reduction is required for volar lunate dislocation through an extended carpal tunnel incision

ORIF

- All injured structures (radial styloid/scaphoid fracture, scapholunate ligament injury) can be repaired through a dorsal approach although a carpal tunnel release may be required
- K-wires are used for bony stabilization

Examination corner

Hand oral

Radiographs demonstrating perilunate and lunate dislocations

These are really quite common in either the hand or trauma oral. This is a spot diagnosis that you really must be able to recognize without any prompting from the examiners. Even in the heat of the exam you should not miss these injuries as you are not a junior casualty officer but a candidate sitting a specialist exit exam. Go away and practise pattern recognition of these injuries. Mention that you need to see two views, AP and lateral, and be prepared to discuss surgical approaches and treatment options.

Examiner: You are called down to the accident and emergency department because a motorcyclist has come off his motorbike at high speed and landed on his right wrist. The casualty officer has asked you to look at this X-ray to see if there is a fracture present.

Candidate: This is a PA radiograph of the right wrist. The most obvious feature is a break in Gilula's lines about the wrist, the carpus is foreshortened with overlapping of the proximal capitate and distal lunate margins. There is radial displacement of the fractured scaphoid with the distal carpal row. I would want to get a lateral radiograph to confirm my suspicion.

Examiner: This is his lateral X-ray.

Candidate: The lateral radiograph confirms a dorsal trans-scaphoid perilunate dislocation of the carpus. The lunate lies in a neutral position within its lunate fossa, in line with the radius. The distal poles of the scaphoid and triquetrum have

---

displaced dorsally. The longitudinal axis of the capitate lies dorsal to the longitudinal axis of the radius.

(Or if the lunate is displaced there is a spilled teacup sign. The lunate is volarly rotated and displaced resembling a spilled teacup.)

Examiner: You must always get a lateral X-ray in these situations.
- How will you manage this injury?
- What surgical approach will you use?

Candidate: After a thorough neurological examination the patient needs to be taken urgently to theatre for reduction of this injury. Internal fixation can be performed at a later stage when swelling has settled, using a dorsal approach to visualize the scapholunate ligament, but a volar incision may also be required. Plaster immobilization is necessary for 6 weeks while the ligaments heal. Long term I would be concerned about avascular necrosis of the proximal pole of the scaphoid.

Mayfield *et al.* (1980)[1] defined four stages of lunate instability – a reproducible pattern of progressive perilunate instability:

1. Instability limited to the scapholunate joint (SL)
2. Plus instability of capitolunate (SL+CL)
3. Plus triquetrolunate (SL+CL+TL)
4. Dorsal disruption of the radiocarpal ligament leaving the lunate totally unstable. Massive swelling. Check for median nerve symptoms; 8% are open injuries

---

[1] Mayfield JK, Johnson RP, Kilkoyne RK (1980) Carpal dislocations: pathomechanics and progressive perilunar instability. *J Hand Surg Am* **5**(3): 226–41.

Scapholunate advanced collapse (SLAC wrist)

Background

Progressive arthritis due to scapholunate interval disruption with a flexion deformity of the scaphoid.

Pathology

SL ligament disruption allows the lunate to extend and the scaphoid to flex, thus reducing carpal height. Arthritis develops initially between the radial styloid process and the distal scaphoid, and then progresses to involve the whole radio-scaphoid joint. The capitate migrates proximally through the widened scapholunate interval (loss of carpal height), leading to capitolunate arthritis. The radiolunate joint is spared as it is a ball and socket joint and lunate extension still allows concentric loading of the lunate fossa of the distal radius.

Scapholunate interval – >3 mm

Carpal height ratio – Used to assess carpal collapse. Ratio of carpal height to the length of the third metacarpal determined on a PA radiograph. The normal value for carpal height is >0.54 (0.46–0.61)

Ring sign – Cortical silhouette of the flexed scaphoid tuberosity seen on PA view

Scapholunate angle – Long axis of the scaphoid in relation to the long axis of the lunate. Average 47°

Capitolunate angle – 0°–15°

Classification of SLAC wrist

Watson has classified SLAC wrist into four stages:

Stage 1. Arthritis between the scaphoid and radial styloid

Stage 2. Arthritis between the scaphoid and entire scaphoid facet of the radius

Stage 3. Stage 2 plus arthritis between the capitate and lunate

Stage 4. Generalized arthritis

Management of SLAC wrist

Non-operative

Indicated if symptoms are minor/minimal. Advice, analgesia, wrist support, etc.

Surgical

Options for surgical treatment are based on the stage of the disease:

Stage 1

- Radial styloidectomy ±scaphoid stabilization (STT fusion) ±capitolunate fusion
- Technically demanding; must adhere to strict surgical details (Kirk Watson); results can be unpredictable; excessive resection can result in wrist instability and ulnar translocation

Stage 2

- Scaphoid excision and four-corner fusion
  - If it unites (non-union 7%) a good result is maintained in the long term and preserves some wrist movement (50% normal). Performed through a midline dorsal incision and scaphoid used as the bone graft. Incomplete reduction of the dorsiflexed lunate may result in limitation of wrist extension. The Spider plate was introduced to improve results over K-wires/screws. However, studies have not yet shown this
- Proximal row carpectomy
  - Best motion (60% normal), worst grip strength and pain relief, technically less difficult

Stage 3

- Scaphoid excision and four-corner fusion

Stage 4

- Wrist fusion
  - Best pain relief, good grip strength but loss of motion. Immobilize the wrist for a couple of weeks in plaster beforehand to see how the patient gets on. Position of wrist fusion is slight extension (20°)

Examination corner

Hand oral

PA and lateral radiographs demonstrating scapholunate dissociation with obvious Terry-Thomas sign

Discussion on various radiographic features of carpal instability.

Widening of the scapholunate interval >3 mm (Terry-Thomas sign is so-called because of the comedy actor who had a large gap between his two front teeth). Increased scapholunate angle (> 45°) in the lateral view. Cortical ring sign of the scaphoid in the PA view – due to a volarflexed scaphoid. V sign of Taleisnik – refers to the volar silhouette of the palmar flexed scaphoid and radius seen on the lateral view. Discussion on management followed.

Flexor tendon injuries

Types of injury

The position of the hand at the time of injury determines tendon retraction.
- Flexed fingers – distal tendon retracts
- Extended fingers – proximal tendon retracts

Biology of healing

Intrinsic healing is the formation of collagen bundles directly across the injury site. Extrinsic healing involves the formation of a layer of scar tissue surrounding the injury site and can lead to adhesions. Aim for "no-touch" technique to prevent damage to tendons and adhesions.

Repair weakest at 6–12 days. There are three stages of healing:

Inflammatory (cellular)	0–5 days
Fibroblastic (collagen)	5–28 days
Remodelling (cross-linking)	>28 days

Contraindications to repair

- Wounds liable to infection
- Uncooperative patient

Zones

Kleinert and Verdan classified flexor tendon injuries according to the anatomical zone of injury:

Zone 1. Distal to FDS insertion

Zone 2. Bunnell's "no man's land". From A1 pulley to FDS insertion. FDS and FDP tendons are enclosed in a flexor sheath

Zone 3. Distal edge of flexor retinaculum to A1 pulley

Zone 4. Within the carpal tunnel

Zone 5. Proximal to the carpal tunnel

There are similar but less specifically described zones for the thumb, prefixed by T:

Thumb T1. FPL insertion to A2 pulley

Thumb T2. Zone 1 to distal part of the A1 pulley

Thumb T3. Zone 2 to carpal tunnel

Management

Primary repair should be carried out as early as possible after the injury. Apply a tourniquet and regional anaesthesia or a general anaesthetic. Make a Bruner's incision and use windows between pulleys. For retracted tendons try to milk the tendon with the wrist/digits flexed. If this fails make a small transverse incision at the level of the distal palmar crease just proximal to the A1 pulley. Pass a Silastic® cannula from the distal wound through the sheath to the proximal wound. Attach a catheter to the proximal end tendon and pull through to the distal wound. Multiple core suture techniques are described (Modified Kessler technique, cruciate, Bunnell, Tsuge, etc.). Use 3/0 non-absorbable sutures. Strength of repair is related to the number of core strands crossing the repair site, but repair becomes more difficult to perform the higher the number of strands. A circumferential epitenon suture (6/0 monofilament) is used to reduce gapping of the tendon ends and increases strength by 20%. Close the sheath, if possible. For zone 2 injuries it is recommended to repair both tendons.

Rehabilitation

Aim to mobilize early (48 h postoperatively) to prevent adhesions.

There is debate over the advantages and disadvantages of the Belfast (active) and Kleinert (passive) regimes. Kleinert has a lower re-rupture rate (5%) than Belfast (10%), but is complicated and has an increased rate of contractures. Belfast – dorsal thermoplastic splint with flexion wrist 20° and MCP 70°. Kleinert – elastic band sutured/glued to the nail and attached proximally to the splint across the volar side of the wrist to allow active extension but passive flexion.

Complications

- Re-rupture
- Infection
- Adhesions

- Joint contractures – too tight a repair or from prolonged splintage
- Bow stringing – from damaged pulleys

There is debate over whether surgeons should perform a double or a single-only (FDP) tendon repair.

Reconstruction

Defined as a delayed primary repair performed >3 weeks after injury. Contracture of the muscle-tendon unit has usually occurred and a tendon graft is often required. It can be carried out as a one-stage or two-stage procedure.

Prerequisites for tendon reconstruction:
- Motivated patient
- Adequate skin and soft-tissue cover
- Full passive range of movement of joints
- Adequate sensation and circulation of finger

Methods

- Delayed direct repair
- Single-stage flexor tendon grafting
- Two-stage grafting
- Tenodesis or arthrodesis
- Amputation

Two-stage flexor tendon reconstruction

First stage

Aims
- Tenolysis and release of joint contractures
- Digital nerve repair or grafting
- Provide healthy skin (may require a flap)
- Full flexion on traction of the Silastic® rod at the wrist
- Preserve A1, A2 and A4 pulleys

Second stage

Carried out 2–3 months after first stage. Tendon graft options include:
- Palmaris longus
- Plantaris – medial to tendo Achilles

- Long toe extensors – 2nd, 3rd or 4th toes
- EIP
- Fascia lata

FDP avulsion injuries

Due to forced extension of a flexed DIPJ

Classification (Leddy)

I – Tendon end in palm. Rupture of vinculae
II – Tendon held at level of PIPJ by long vinculum
III – Held at A4 pulley by avulsed bony fragment
IV – Profundus avulsed off bony fragment

Management

In types I and II, extensive trauma and complications of adhesions and the quadriga effect are seen. DIP joint fusion should be considered. Type III requires ORIF and the fragment can be held with sutures that are passed through the distal phalanx and then tied on to a button on the nail.

Examination corner

Hand oral 1

Examiner: What order of structures do you repair with a deep laceration at the level of the wrist with nerve and tendon damage?

Candidate: My order of repair would be to repair the median nerve first because it is the most difficult and time-consuming structure to repair followed by the flexor tendons, which are easier.

[Fail the whole oral]

A candidate giving this answer has never seen a zone 5 injury repaired let alone performed one and is not experienced enough to practise independently as a consultant. The median nerve is a superficial structure at the wrist. One repairs the median nerve beautifully but how can you then hope to move it out of the way adequately (without pulling this delicate repair apart) to get to the deeper flexor tendon structures for repair? This candidate shows a total lack of basic orthopaedic understanding.

Hand oral 2

Clinical photograph of laceration over the volar surface of the middle phalanx index finger with pointing finger sign (Zone 2 flexor tendon injury)

Candidate: There is a laceration over the volar surface of the middle phalanx index finger and the attitude of the finger suggests a flexor tendon injury.

Examiner: Your SHO thinks it is just a simple finger laceration.

Candidate: It is ironic you mention this because I have come across this situation on two separate occasions recently where a serious flexor tendon injury has been misdiagnosed as a simple laceration by a junior colleague. I always examine every patient preoperatively myself so that I know for sure if I am dealing with a flexor tendon injury.

Examiner: How do you test for FDS and FDP function – demonstrate it on my hand. Why do you keep the remaining fingers extended when testing for FDS function in an individual finger?

Examiner: Which postoperative regimen do you use and why?

Candidate: I use the Belfast regimen, which is early, controlled active mobilization. This gives good results.

Examiner: What do you mean by good results?

Candidate: With modern rehabilitation recovery of range of movement should be about 90% of what can be expected in about 80%–90% of cases.

Examiner: There is also the Kleinert regimen that is an extension block splint with a rubber band to passively flex the fingers. In the Duran programme passive flexion is used for the first 4 weeks, protecting the repair with an extension block splint and active flexion is introduced over the next 2 weeks. Grip strengthening exercises and lifting are avoided for 3–4 months.

[Pass]

Hand oral 3

Zone I flexor tendon injuries

• Incisions
• Methods of repair

Hand oral 4

Clinical photograph of a hand with a 3- to 4-cm horizontal laceration over the ulnar side of the distal palm

• I was asked to draw how I would extend the wound for exploration
• I was also asked what structures might be damaged
• I was asked about the principles of, and my own practice of, tendon repair and postoperative rehabilitation
• I was asked about the principles and my own practice of nerve repair
• I was asked about the clinical signs of re-innervation of a nerve – Tinel's sign, etc.

Hand oral 5

Flexor tendon laceration

• Surgical technique, sutures

Hand oral 6

Flexor tendon injuries

• Show me how you examine an injured hand
• What are the results of flexor tendon repairs?
• Discuss the rehabilitation regimes: Kleinert, Duran and Belfast
• Are there any particular problems with Kleinert rehabilitation? (PIP joint stiffness)

Thumb amputation

Examination corner

Hand oral

Clinical photograph of thumb amputation

A patient arrives in casualty with this injury. What is your management?

History

- Age, occupation, hand dominance
- Mechanism of injury
- Pre-existing hand problems
- Ischaemia time (warm – 6 h hand/12 h digit, cold – 12 h hand/24 h digit)
- Current medication
- Previous medical history
- Hobbies
- Smoking
- Tetanus status

Examination

- Level of injury
- Amputated part
- Degree of crush/avulsion
- Quality of skin and soft tissues
- Degree of contamination

Investigations

- Radiographs of the hand and injured part

Management

Absolute contraindication for re-implantation include:
- Life-threatening concomitant trauma
- Severe premorbid disease
- Severe injury to the digit – extensive degloving, gross contamination

Relative contraindications:
- Lengthy warm ischaemia time
- Elderly with microvascular disease
- Uncooperative patient

Surgical options

Refer to experienced hand surgeon or the plastic surgeons if not experienced in dealing with this type of injury.[1, 2]
- Primary closure
- Re-implantation
- Thumb reconstruction:
  - Wrap around procedure
  - Great toe transfer
  - Second toe transfer procedure

[1] In the FRCS Orth exam play it safe and start your discussion of surgical options with this statement. This may be all that the examiners are looking for, namely that you are willing to refer on complex cases out of your area of expertise rather than take on a case you are not experienced enough in dealing with.
[2] After making this general statement although the examiners will still probably wish to discuss the various surgical options available they will generally make allowances if you do not know them in particularly great detail; in reality you have covered yourself beforehand. If however you have implied that you would take the case on yourself then you look stupid if your technical knowledge is then found to be vague.

Ring avulsion injuries

This is a topic that under normal circumstances one would briefly skip over during the course of preparation for the FRCS Orth exam. You need to be reasonably familiar with this one as it tends to be asked more often than you would normally expect.

Background

- Underestimated injury

Urbaniak classification

Class 1

- Circulation adequate, circumferential laceration
- Standard bone and soft-tissue management

Class 2

- Circulation inadequate
- A – No additional bone, tendon or nerve injury
- B – There are additional injuries present
- Vessel repair (microvascular) is required
- In general class 2B injuries may be better treated with amputation

Class 3

- Complete degloving of skin ±amputation through the DIPJ. These injuries are unlikely to gain

adequate function and amputation is usually required
- The most common complication following surgical reconstruction is cold intolerance

---

Examination corner

Hand oral

Clinical photograph of ring finger ring avulsion injury

Classification and prognosis

Mallet finger

This is another favourite FRCS Orth question in either the hand or trauma oral.

Definition

A mallet finger deformity is a loss of extension at the DIP joint. Mostly closed but may be caused by a laceration. Either soft tissue or bony.

Tendinous mallet finger

Mechanism of injury is thought to be forced flexion of the DIP joint (e.g. a ball striking the tip of an extended finger).

Management

Non-operative management generally, consisting of splintage of the DIP joint in extension for 6 weeks. Plastic off-the-shelf mallet (Stack) splints lead to skin maceration so use custom-made splints from short lengths of zimmer splint and change them regularly. The results of both non-operative and operative treatment are not always satisfactory, with only 30%–40% of patients regaining full extension of the DIP joint. Surgery can lead to a loss of flexion and is not recommended.

Bony mallet deformity

Bony avulsion of the insertion of the extensor tendon to the distal phalanx. Management depends on the size of the fragment, any displacement and whether the distal phalanx is subluxed (volarly). If it is undisplaced, treat in a mallet splint for 6 weeks (X-ray again at 1 week). If it is displaced, place in mallet splint and X-ray. If it is now undisplaced treat as above; if it is still displaced, book the patient for ORIF. If the joint is subluxed the patient will need ORIF.

Operative technique

ORIF is performed through a transverse incision dorsally over DIP joint with v-extensions laterally. A single screw for a large fragment or a pull through 3/0 PDS Kessler suture is placed into the bony fragment. The suture is passed through onto the volar surface of the finger and tied over a button. If the joint is subluxed, reduce it and hold with a longitudinal K-wire across the DIPJ for 4 weeks.

Chronic mallet finger

Initially treat with mallet splint for 6 weeks. If the deformity persists and the patient is requesting treatment, book for DIP joint fusion.

Fingertip injuries

Either soft tissue or bony. Principle is to achieve a well-healed fingertip and to preserve length. If there is no exposed bone these heal well with Tegaderm dressings changed weekly and moulded over the tip of the finger, especially in children. If there is exposed bone this needs soft tissue coverage. Either shorten the bone end and perform primary closure or local flap coverage (Atasoy, Cutler, cross-finger), or perform terminalization. This is indicated for a severely crushed distal phalanx, and is made through the DIPJ with trimming of the condyles of the head of the middle phalanx.

The nail plate lies beneath the nail and is responsible for its growth. If there is a crush injury possibly involving the nail bed, the nail should be removed and the nail bed explored and repaired as appropriate.

High-pressure injection injuries

These are rare but severe injuries that should be treated as a surgical emergency. There is a history of severe pain with use of high-pressure equipment. The non-dominant hand is more commonly affected. Paint is thought to be more toxic than grease. Extensive soft-tissue necrosis occurs despite an often small entry wound. The extent of spread depends on the site of entry, anatomical barriers and the volume and pressure of the substance injected. Material readily passes along tendon sheaths as these offer the pathway of least resistance. This requires urgent exploration, fasciotomy and removal of as much of the injected material as possible. The wound is excised and extended proximally and distally until the full extent of spread is revealed and as much material and non-viable tissue as possible is removed. Repeat debridement at 48 h should be done. Broad spectrum antibiotics are given, tetanus status checked and the hand is splinted and elevated in the position of safety. Aggressive treatment has reduced the amputation rate, with most patients returning to their original work. Digital injections are, however, followed by high rates of necrosis and amputation, and of long-term morbidity in surviving digits.

Examination corner

Hand oral

Clinical slide of a pressure injection

Management

Compartment syndrome

Decreased tissue perfusion in a myofascial compartment leading to muscle necrosis and contractures. Presents with severe pain. Due to crush injury, burns and multiple fractures. Treat by prompt decompression through two dorsal incisions (over the 2nd and 4th metacarpals for interossei), carpal tunnel release ±midlateral incisions over the hypothenar and thenar eminences, and midlateral release to digits.

Tendon transfers

In the oral just relax, take a deep breath in and answer the question.

Definition

A tendon transfer is the use of a functioning muscle–tendon unit to restore function in a non-functioning muscle or tendon.

Indications

- Permanent nerve injury
- Ruptured or avulsed tendon or muscle
- Neuromuscular disease

Principles of tendon transfers

- Motivated patient
- Full passive range of movement of joints
- Sacrificable – donor tendon must be expendable so as not to lead to functional loss
- Sufficient amplitude – determined by the amount a muscle can be stretched from its resting position, plus the amount it contracts. This is the same as excursion. Wrist flexors/extensors – 33 mm; finger extensors – 50 mm; finger flexors – 70 mm. The transferred muscle–tendon unit needs amplitude to produce the movement required
- Adequate strength – force is proportional to the cross-sectional area of the muscle. Power is force × distance. The power of a donor muscle will reduce by one MRC grade after transfer and if a weak donor is chosen it may be too weak for useful function after transfer
- Synergistic action – the transferred muscle must be under good voluntary control. This is best if it was synergistic with its desired action after the transfer, as it will be more readily integrated into normal hand use and easier to rehabilitate

- Straight line of pull – best if the tendon runs in a straight line, which permits it to exert its maximal effect. This is not always possible and some transfers need to go through a pulley or through the interosseous membrane in the forearm. This can weaken the action of a tendon transfer
- Only one transfer for one function per motor unit

Operative technique

- Multiple short transverse incisions
- Careful tendon handling
- Correct tension

Joining the tendons

- End-to-end anastomosis
- End-to-side
- Side-to-side
- Tendon weave procedures (Pulvertaft weave)

All methods can be used.

Classic transfers

Median nerve – low lesion (wrist)

Deficit – weakness of thumb abduction and opposition. "Simian (monkey-like) hand."
   Transfers:
- Ring finger FDS is transferred to APB via pulley in the FCU tendon
- Huber – abductor digiti minimi to APB insertion
- Camitz – if thenar wasting is noted at carpal tunnel decompression, transfer palmaris longus and a strip of palmar aponeurosis to APB
- ±MCP or IP fusion

These tendon transfers allow the thumb to be placed in a more functional position with some dynamic control.

Median nerve – high lesion (elbow)

Deficit – as for low lesion plus loss of flexion of the index and middle fingers.
- FDP tendons to the index and middle fingers and sutured to little and ring fingers

- Brachioradialis to FPL (flexes IPJ of the thumb)
- EIP or EDQ to APB for thumb adduction

Ulnar nerve – low lesion

Deficit – weak pinch (first DI and adductor pollicis), ulnar claw hand.
   Transfers:
- ECRB or brachioradialis to adductor pollicis
- EIP to first DI
- Zancolli capsulodesis (correction of clawing ring/little fingers)

Radial nerve

Deficit – wrist extension, finger extension (at MCPJ) and EPL.
- Pronator teres to ECRB (wrist extension)
- Palmaris longus to EPL (thumb extension)
- FCR/FCU (through interosseous membrane) to EDC (MCP joint extension)

Examination corner

Hand oral 1

- What are the important principles of a tendon transfer?
- What is a tendon transfer?

Hand oral 2

- What are the indications for a tendon transfer?
- What are the prerequisites for a tendon transfer?
- Are there any tendon transfers you are familiar with?
- Describe EI to EPL

Trigger finger

Background

Also known as digital tenovaginitis or stenosing tenosynovitis. Swelling of the superficial and deep flexor tendons adjacent to the A1 pulley at a metacarpal head. The ring and middle fingers are the most commonly affected in adults, although occasionally the thumb is affected and rarely the index finger. Commonly seen in diabetics.

Clinical features

- Pain
- Clicking
- Swelling
- Unable to straighten finger

Pain on both active and passive movements of the digit. The patient may voluntarily demonstrate triggering. Persistent locking of the finger may lead to a fixed flexion contracture at the PIP joint. A tender nodule can be sometimes felt at the A1 pulley.

Aetiology

Exact aetiology is unclear. Whether tightness of the fibrous tendon sheath results in inflammation and narrowing of the sheath or degeneration of the tendon results in tendon enlargement and nodule formation remains unclear. Indeed both may occur in response to inflammation. Often follows trauma or unaccustomed activity.

Management

Steroid injection – inject around the tendon sheath (not into the tendon itself)

Open surgical release – day case under local anaesthetic and tourniquet. Warn about digital nerve injury and recurrence

Open surgical release

- Make a transverse incision over the distal palmar flexor crease or an oblique incision over the MC head
- Blunt dissection
- Identify the proximal edge of the A1 pulley and release the first 1 cm of the pulley
- If the A2 pulley is released this can result in bowstringing tendons

The most common complication of open release is digital nerve injury. Diabetes is a poor prognostic indicator for non-operative treatment. Multiple digits may be affected. These patients may also be especially prone to developing stiffness following surgical release.

Oral question

How does the management of a trigger finger differ in a rheumatoid patient?

Causes of a flexor contracture

- Congenital – camptodactyly
- Skin – scar contracture
- Fascia – Dupuytren's disease
- Flexor tendon sheath – fibrous contracture
- Tendon – FDP avulsion/rupture, adhesions, extensor tendon rupture
- Capsular structures – volar plate shortening
- Block to extension – osteophytes, loose bodies

If the finger is locked in flexion exclude:

- Infection
- Arthritis

Examination corner

Short notes

A right-handed woman aged 60 presents with catching of her dominant ring finger when making a fist. What are your differential diagnosis and management?

Hand oral 1

Clinical photograph of a hand with one of the fingers flexed into the palm (ring or middle)

Spot diagnosis
- What is the diagnosis?
- What is the differential diagnosis?
- What conditions are associated with trigger finger?

• What is the management?
• When would you perform open release?

Brachial plexus

Common exam case as there are good signs and it is an excellent test of functional anatomy. Do not be confused by patients who have had reconstructive surgery (i.e. have scars) and therefore possibly have had nerve grafting or transfers which lead to unexpected findings. Need to diagnose pre-ganglionic (poor prognosis) from post-ganglionic lesions.

Anatomy of the brachial plexus[34]

The brachial plexus is formed from the ventral primary rami of C5–T1. It is organized into five components: roots, trunks, divisions, cords and branches (remember the mnemonic **R**ob **T**aylor **D**rinks **C**old **B**eer).

There are:
• 5 roots
• 3 trunks (upper, middle, lower)
• 6 divisions (2 from each trunk)
• 3 cords (posterior, lateral, medial)
• Multiple branches

Branches

The 3 branches from the roots are:
• Long thoracic nerve
• Dorsal scapular nerve
• Nerve to subclavius
There is 1 branch from the trunks:
• Suprascapular nerve
  • There are no branches from the divisions.
  • The branches from the cords (3–5–5 rule) are:
  • There are 3 branches from the lateral cord:

---

[34] Some examiners ask you to draw out the brachial plexus. Needless to say practise several times beforehand. Some candidates were absolutely spot on with this one and had perfected a special routine for this.

• Musculocutaneous nerve
• Lateral pectoral nerve
• Lateral head of median nerve
There are 5 branches from the medial cord:
• Ulnar nerve
• Medial pectoral nerve
• Medial cutaneous nerve of the arm
• Medial cutaneous nerve of forearm
• Medial head of median nerve
(The ulnar nerve is the most important branch and the rest of the branches begin with the word medial)
• **5** branches of posterior cord are:
  • Subscapular nerves – upper
  • Subscapular nerves – lower
  • Thoracodorsal nerves
  • Axillary nerve
  • Radial nerve
(Acronym: 2 STAR – 2 **S**ubscapular nerves, **T**horacodorsal nerve, **A**xillary nerve and **R**adial nerve.)

The roots of the brachial plexus lie between the scalenus anterior and medius muscles. The trunks lie in the posterior triangle of the neck. The divisions of the trunks lie behind the clavicle and at the outer border of the first rib; the divisions form the cords, which come to lie in the upper axilla.

Aetiology

• RTA (particularly motorcyclists)
• Birth trauma (shoulder dystonia, large infants, maternal obesity, diabetes and forceps delivery)
• Shoulder girdle trauma
• Gunshots
• Iatrogenic (accessory nerve)
• Perioperative causes: poor positioning of the patient

Classification

Leffert – four types of brachial plexus lesion (Table 21.3)

Infraclavicular injuries have a better prognosis than supraclavicular injuries.

Table 21.3 Leffert classification

I	Open
II	Closed
IIA	Supraclavicular
	Pre-ganglioma
	Post-ganglioma
IIB	Infraclavicular
III	Radiotherapy
IV	Obstetric
IVA	Erb's (upper root)
IVB	Klumpke's (lower root)
IVC	Mixed

Pre-ganglionic injury (root avulsion)

• Horner's syndrome. Proximally innervated muscles are affected – rhomboids and serratus anterior (from roots). Severe pain in an anaesthetic limb. Constant crushing/burning pain down the limb. Paralysed diaphragm (phrenic nerve C3/4/5) may be seen on chest X-ray (inspiration and expiration views). Phrenic nerve palsy is most likely to indicate avulsion of the C5 root. Fractures of the transverse processes of the cervical vertebrae or a fractured first rib indicate a high-energy injury with likely intradural injury of the lower two roots. Scapulothoracic dissociation is often associated with root avulsion and major vascular injury

Investigations

• Key radiographs are chest and C-spine
• MRI of the C-spine or CT-myelography
Findings consistent with a severe injury include pseudomeningocele (T_1-weighting), empty root sleeves (T_2-weighting) and cord shift away from the midline.

Neurophysiology is not usually helpful in the acute situation and indeed may be misleading unless both neurophysiologist and surgeon are familiar with the interpretation. With a post-ganglionic lesion the sensory nerve action potential is intact as the dorsal root ganglion is in continuity with the nerve.

Management

The priority is severe life-threatening injuries – head, chest or viscera. Immediate surgery is indicated if there is penetrating injury or iatrogenic trauma.

Methods of management

• Neurolysis
• Nerve repair
• Nerve graft
Donor nerves include the sural, medial brachial and antebrachial cutaneous nerves.
• Nerve transfer[35]
  • T3/4 intercostal nerve to the musculocutaneous n.
  • Spinal accessory nerve to the suprascapular n.
  • Contralateral C7 nerve root to median n.

Early versus late exploration of the brachial plexus

Advantages of early versus late exploration include:
• No scar tissue, therefore making for an easier dissection
• Able to define the injury at an early stage
• Possibly a better outcome in terms of relief from neuropathic pain and function

Priorities of surgery

• Shoulder stability
• Shoulder external rotation
• Elbow flexion
• Wrist extension

Horner's syndrome

This is due to a lower plexus root avulsion and interruption to the sympathetic supply to the eye from damage to the stellate ganglion at the level of T1. Causes ptosis of the upper eyelid, miosis of the pupil

---

[35] Neurotization refers to transfer of a healthy nerve to re-innervate a more important nerve and is used in the same way as nerve transfer.

(smaller diameter), anhidrosis (loss of sweating on one half of the face) and enophthalmos. Usually shows up 3–4 days after injury and correlates with a C8 or T1 root avulsion.

Surgical approaches

- Transverse supraclavicular incision
- Transclavicular approach

After a complete lesion surgery gives a chance of a modest return of hand function in children and young adults.

Management of adult brachial plexus injury

Open injuries

Early surgical exploration and nerve repair are usually essential. The exact timing will depend on the overall condition of the patient, haemorrhage and availability of an appropriate surgeon. A similar policy should be pursued when injury to the brachial plexus or other nerve, e.g. accessory, has occurred as a complication of surgery. Where the wound is untidy, e.g. shot gun injuries, delayed exploration may be more appropriate. If transfer to a specialist unit is required then it must be arranged urgently.

Closed injuries

Low-energy injuries

Low probability of nerve disruption and most cases will recover spontaneously. Therefore, manage conservatively initially. Perform neurophysiology if there is no clear clinical evidence of improvement. Only consider surgery if complete absence of function of all/part of the plexus remains at 2–3 months.

High-energy injuries

1. **Combined with vascular injury.** These cases present a logistical problem for management. Early surgical exploration is mandatory preceded by arteriography. The degree of urgency depends on:
   - The overall condition of the patient
   - Blood loss from the arterial injury

- Limb ischaemia – this may not be critical for the upper limb; in which case some delay, allowing for planning of an appropriate surgical team/transfer to another unit, is possible. If possible, skeletal, vascular and nerve reconstruction should be carried out at one operation. However, if this is not possible and vascular reconstruction is performed initially, a second operation for the nerves must be arranged within days as further delay may make it technically impossible

2. **Without vascular injury.** Since there is a high probability of nerve disruption, early referral to a specialist unit should be considered. The indications for early surgical exploration are:
   - Complete absence of function of any part of the plexus
   - A patient who is fit for operation
   Very early operation (within days), before scar tissue has formed, is attractive. This is particularly the case if surgery is required, in any case, for fracture fixation. However, if other factors, such as multiple injuries, preclude early operation, then it should not be delayed more than 2–3 months, as there is clear evidence of deterioration in the results of repair after that time

Late treatment

- Shoulder stability
  - Arthrodesis
- Shoulder external rotation
  - L'Episcopo procedure – latissimus dorsi transferred dorsally to infraspinatus insertion for external rotation in an upper trunk lesion
- Elbow flexion
  - Pectoralis major/latissimus dorsi transfer to biceps insertion for elbow flexion, or
  - Steindler flexorplasty – transfer of the medial epicondyle and flexor muscle origin to the anterior humerus through brachialis for elbow flexion

Examination corner

Hand oral 1

- Early versus late exploration of brachial plexus injuries
- Advantages and disadvantages of each
- Current literature on the subject

Hand oral 2

- Upper trunk: Pre- and post-ganglionic injury, Erb's point, weakness patterns
- Operations described: transfers, cable grafts

Tumours of the hand

Differential

- Ganglion (see earlier)
- Giant cell tumour of tendon sheath (pigmented villonodular synovitis, xanthoma)
  - Second commonest soft-tissue tumour of the hand. Firm swelling on volar aspect of the digits. Twenty percent arise from joints, and bony erosions are seen in 10%. Treat by excision, with a recurrence rate of 10%
- Epidermal inclusion cyst
  - Generally seen on the volar aspect with a small wound on close inspection. Painless
- Enchondroma
  - Benign cartilage tumour. Cause of pathological fracture and bone graft once fracture is united
- Lipoma
- Neurilemmoma
  - Schwann cell origin and encapsulated so can be shelled out of nerve
- Glomus
  - Painful lesion in cold temperatures as this is a tumour of perivascular temperature-regulating bodies. Fifty percent are under the nail. MR can be useful. Treat by excision
- Sarcoma
- Acrometastasis
  - Metastasis to a digit. Very rare

Squamous cell carcinoma of the skin over a finger digit

This is one of those esoteric hand oral questions that regularly appear in the FRCS Orth hand oral. They always seem so straightforward afterwards (when discussing them with colleagues) but for the unprepared candidate in the heat of the exam you can certainly struggle with them.

A clinical photograph in the hand oral is essentially a spot diagnosis. You may be asked a list of likely causes, investigations and management.

Examination corner

Hand oral 1

Clinical photograph of lesion on finger

Diagnosis: Squamous cell carcinoma
Further assessment and management

Hand oral 2

Clinical photograph of squamous cell carcinoma at the tip of a finger with ulceration, necrosis and skin breakdown

Spot diagnosis

Examiner: The elderly gentleman is seen in your clinic with the lesion on his finger. How will you manage it?

Candidate: There is an ulcerating lesion with skin breakdown and necrosis over the DP of the ring finger. I would want to get a radiograph of the finger to look for bony involvement.

Examiner: The bone is not involved. The radiograph is normal. What do you think the diagnosis is?

Candidate: Some form of soft-tissue tumour. Possibly infection.

Examiner: How are you going to mange it?

Candidate: Probably by an amputation.

[fail]

The candidate did not know the lesion was a squamous cell carcinoma of the skin. As a result the candidate appeared unsure and hesitant. Although the definitive treatment might well be amputation there was no mention about staging the lesion.

Congenital hand deformities

Introduction

The examining board is very conscious of its responsibility to provide a fair examination as well as a rigorous one.

In the FRCS Orth examination hand oral any congenital abnormality is fair game for the examiners to show. There is an opportunity to discuss Swanson's classification of congenital deformities. If you are very unlucky there will be an opportunity to discuss the development and function of the hand. Likewise any congenital abnormality may also appear in the short cases (cleft hand, syndactyly, polydactyly).

Background

About 1 in 600 children is born with a congenital upper limb deformity.

Swanson's classification

1. Failure of formation
   a Transverse arrest – amelia
   b Longitudinal arrest – radial club hand, cleft hand
2. Failure of differentiation
   a Soft tissue involvement
   b Skeletal involvement
3. Duplication (polydactyly)
4. Overgrowth (macrodactyly)
5. Undergrowth – Madelung's deformity
6. Congenital constriction hand
7. Generalized skeletal anomalies

Radial hemimelia

Absence or hypoplasia of pre-axial structures: radius, radial carpus and thumb. Bilateral in up to 75% of cases. In unilateral cases the opposite thumb is hypoplastic. The ulna is bowed and thickened and only 60% of its normal length.

Heikel's classification of radial club hand (how much of the radius is present)

1. Short radius
2. Hypoplastic radius
3. Partial absence of the radius
4. Absent radius

Radiographs

- Humerus is short
- Ulna is curved and thickened and only 60% of normal length
- Radius hypoplastic or absent
- Carpal bone fusion or absence
- Absence of digits

Associated conditions with radial club hand

- Fanconi's syndrome (aplastic anaemia)
- Thrombocytopenia absent radius
- Holt–Oram (cardiac septal defects)
- VATER (**V**ertebral anomalies, imperforate **A**nus, **T**racheo-o**E**sophageal aplasia, **R**enal anomalies)

Management

- Counselling
- Search for associated congenital abnormalities
- Observe initially
- Centralization and thumb reconstruction
- Pollicization, provision of a thumb
- Transfer, shortening and rotation of the index finger (Buck–Gramcko method)

Abnormal distribution of nerves and arteries must be appreciated prior to surgery.

Contraindications to surgery

- Severe neurovascular anomalies
- Stiff elbow
- Good function
- Surgery can be dangerous if there are other congenital conditions

Ulnar club hand

Less common than radial club hand. No associated cardiac or haematological problems. Wrist is stable but the elbow is a problem. Ulnar digits are often absent and, if present, syndactylized.

Swanson's classification of ulnar club hand

1. Hypoplastic ulna
2. Total absence of the ulna
3. Humeroradial synostosis (congenital fusion of the elbow joint)
4. Deficient ulna and absent wrist

Pre-axial polydactyly (thumb duplication)

- Occurs 0.8 per 1000 live births. Approximately 50% are Wassel type 4
- Usually sporadic and unilateral and not associated with syndromes unless Wassel 7
- Wassel 7 associated with:
  - Holt–Oram
  - Fanconi's syndrome
  - Blackfan–Diamond syndrome

Classification (Wassel)

Based on the complete or incomplete duplication of each phalanx:
1. Bifid DP
2. Duplicate DP
3. Bifid PP
4. Duplicate PP
5. Bifid metacarpal
6. Duplicate metacarpal
7. Triphalangism

Principles of management

Forming one thumb out of two

1. Preserving the skeleton of one thumb and augmenting this with soft tissue from the second thumb. Nearly all of one digit is retained and augmented with tissues from the other digit. Tissues from the "spare part" duplicate that are not used are excised. This allows for obtaining a good size match and tendon and ligament balance. This is the favoured option.
2. The other option is removing the central composite tissue segments from each thumb and combining the two into one (Bilhaut-Cloquet procedure). There are significant problems with stiffness, size, angular deformities, nail scarring and function. This procedure is generally avoided unless there is no other way to obtain a thumb of sufficient size.
3. Segmental digital transfer. This is occasionally performed when there is a clearly superior proximal segment on one digit and a clearly superior distal segment on the other digit. Bring the best distal segment of one duplicate onto the best proximal segment of the other.

Wassel 4–6

Retain ulnar thumb so that integrity of the UCL is maintained.

Excision

Appropriate where duplication is rudimentary without skeletal elements or the accessory thumb is widely separated from a normal thumb.

Hypoplasia of the thumb

Commonly requires pollicization of the index finger in the first year of life.

Classification of thumb hypoplasia (Buck–Gramcko)

Type I: Minor hypoplasia. Normal skeleton and musculature but all hypoplastic (just a small thumb)

Type II: Hypoplasia. Reduced volume or absence of thenar muscles. First web space in adduction contracture

Type III: Absence of thenar muscles. Severe first web space contracture. Metacarpophalangeal joint instability. May have absence of trapezium and scaphoid

Type IV: Pouce flottant (floating thumb). Rudimentary appendage attached by a small skin bridge. No metacarpal, trapezium or scaphoid. Neurovascular pedicle within the skin bridge

Type V: Total aplasia (absent thumb). No skeletal or soft tissue elements

Blauth's classification of thumb hypoplasia (5 types)

Thumb hypoplasia has also been classified by Blauth:

Type I: Short thumb, hypoplastic thenar muscle

Type II: Adduction contracture, UCL instability, normal skeleton with respect to articulations

Type IIIA: Extensive intrinsic and extrinsic musculotendinous deficiencies, intact CMC joint

Type IIIB: CMC joint not intact

Type IV: Floating thumb

Type V: Complete absent of thumb

Type 1 requires no treatment. Types IIIB–V are treated with pollicization. Types II and IIIA are treated with reconstruction addressing the following issues:

- Stabilization of the MCP joint
- Ulnar collateral ligament
- Web deepening
- Opponens transfer if opposition is insufficient
- Extrinsic flexor and extensor exploration with correction of any anomalies

Principles of thumb reconstruction

- Allow opposition
- Must be sensate
- Must have good circumduction at the carpometacarpal joint
- Joints must be stable to allow pinch grip

Camptodactyly

Congenital digital flexion deformity. Usually occurs at the PIP joint of the little finger. Affects <1% of the population. Can be familial. No functional significance in the majority. Can be static or progressive. There are two types:

- Type 1 infantile type
  - Seen in infancy, affects both sexes equally
- Type 2 adolescent type
  - Adolescent type more common in females, frequently bilateral but not symmetrical, familial deformity, increases during adolescent growth spurt

Aetiology

The deformity has been attributed to the following abnormalities:

- General absence of development of all tissues of the digit
- Abnormal lumbrical origin
- Contracture of the collateral ligaments of the digits
- Flexor and extensor tendon imbalance
- Abnormal FDS origin or insertion

Management

Reassurance and stretching, avoid surgery if at all possible. Surgery may be indicated for patients with a flexion contracture of >60°. Release skin, fascia, tendon sheaths, intrinsics, collateral ligaments and volar plate. Lengthen the FDS tendon.

Clinodactyly (lateral plane deformity)

Radioulnar curvature of the little finger. More common in males. Usually bilateral. There are three types:

I – Minor angulation, normal length (very common)

II – Minor angulation, short phalanx, associated with Down's syndrome

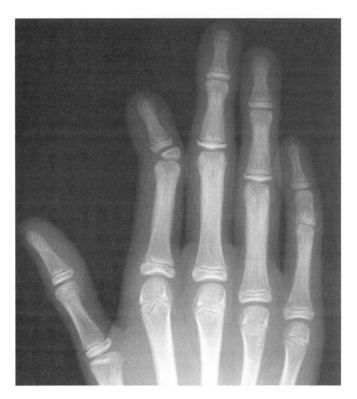

Figure 21.7 Delta phalanx

III – Marked deformity, associated with delta phalanx

A delta phalanx is a wedge-shaped phalanx with a C-shaped physis.

Management

If a delta phalanx replaces a normal bone manage by an opening reverse osteotomy. If delta phalanx is an extra bone then excise it (Figure 21.7).

> Clino has C and "L"= lateral plane, Campto has C and "A"= AP deformity

Kirner's deformity

May be mistaken for clinodactyly. Volar and radial curvature at the distal phalanx of the little finger. Usually inherited as an autosomal-dominant trait. Frequently bilateral.

Management

Surgery is generally for cosmetic reasons only. Avoid when the growth plate is open – corrective osteotomy.

Examination corner

Hand oral 1

Clinical photograph of duplicated thumb

- Diagnosis
- How do you classify duplicated thumb (Wassel)?
- Principles of treatment and treatment of type shown

Hand oral 2

Clinical photograph of syndactyly

- Asked for a classification system for congenital hand deformities (Swanson's)

Hand oral 3

Clinical photograph of camptodactyly

Usual questions
- What is this deformity?
- What causes the deformity?
- How is it managed?

Hand oral 4

Clinical photograph of syndactyly

Asked for classification of congenital hand deformities.

Hand oral 5

Clinical photograph of a radial club hand

Examiner: You are called to the paediatric ward because a newborn baby has the above condition. What is this deformity?
  Spot diagnosis.
Examiner: OK – how do you manage it?

I thought I answered the questions fairly well but the discussion seemed to be going around in a bit of a circle. The examiner seemed a bit unhappy and eventually came out with what they really wanted. Somewhere along the way I should have mentioned that there was a high incidence of other congenital deformities with this condition and I might want to consider arranging a renal and cardiac ultrasound! [Candidate pass]

Hand oral 6

Clinical photograph of radial club hand

Examiner: What is the diagnosis and how do you manage it?

Candidate: This is a clinical picture, which is suggestive of bilateral radial hemimelia. Both forearms are short; there is radial and volar deviation at the wrist and hypoplastic thumbs. The fingers also appear poorly developed.

There is no point in beating around the bush as the diagnosis is obvious. However after you have given the diagnosis continue to describe the clinical features on the photo.

Work through an answer of the management options beforehand rather than jumping about with this one as I did: I first mentioned that it will be very upsetting to the parents and one would need to spend time with them.

I did not mention a search for associated congenital abnormalities, which the examiners pressed me about. I suggested observing the condition initially.

For mild cases manipulation and control with strapping may be all that is required.

I mentioned the words "*centralization of the wrist/forearm deformity*" and "*thumb reconstruction*" and the examiners were happy with this and were not interested in any further details whatsoever.

When discussing management options try to avoid jumping straight in with surgery. [Candidate pass]

Hand oral 7

Clinical photograph of radial club hand

What is the diagnosis and how do you manage it?

  Spot diagnosis and very quick. The examiners were not looking for a detailed answer. The whole thing took less than 30 s maximum before we moved on to another clinical photograph.

Hand oral 8

Radiograph of obvious radial club hand

Spot diagnosis.

Infections of the hand

It is essential to diagnose these early and manage them promptly or they will likely lead to devastating loss of function.

Background

Most infections are due to *Staphylococcus aureus*, but 50% of infections are due to multiple organisms and 30%–40% grow anaerobic organisms.

Other common causative organisms include:

- Streptococci
- Enterobacter
- *Klebsiella*
- *Pseudomonas*
- Enterococci
- *Proteus*
- *Bacteroides*

Rare causative organisms include:

- *Mycobacterium marinum* (fish tank granuloma)
- *Gonococcus*
- *Pasteurella multocida* (in cat bites)
- *Eikenella corrodens* (in human bites)
- *Erysipelothrix rhusiopathiae* (abattoir workers)
- *Haemophilus influenzae* (in children from 2 months to 3 years)

Classification

- By infecting organism
- Anatomical location

History

- Penetrating injury, fight bite – note where
- When
- Pain
- Loss of function
- Medical history – diabetes
- Tetanus status

Examination

- Temperature, pulse and respiration
- Examine for puncture wounds
- Swelling
- Posture of the hand
- Warmth
- Tenderness
- Test motor and sensory function
- Examine the arm for spreading lymphangitis
- Epitrochlear lymph nodes drain the ring and little fingers, axillary nodes drain the radial digits
- Cellulitis resolves with antibiotics only and elevation

Investigations

- FBC, ESR, CRP
- Blood cultures
- Wound swab/pus sample
- Radiographs

Anatomical site

Paronychia/eponychia

Most common infection of the finger. It is an infection of the nail fold. Usually *S. aureus* following a minor local injury. If on one side (paronychia) drain by incision with blade angled away from nail bed to avoid damaging it. If extending around both sides of the nail and migrating under the nail, the so-called horseshoe abscesses, treatment involves removing the nail to drain the infection, and replacing it to prevent adhesions under the nail fold.

Felon

A subcutaneous abscess of the distal pulp of the finger. The abscess is situated in one of the small compartments of the finger pulp formed by the vertical fibrous septa. Drain through a vertical midline incision distal to the skin crease taking care to break down all containing septa.

Web space infection

The subfascial web space is a fat-filled space situated on the palmar surface of the hand and interdigital area. The limits of the web space are the natatory ligaments distally, the deep attachment of the palmar fascia proximally and its attachment to the tendon sheath laterally. The infection arises from a wound to the skin between the fingers. Web space infections may lead to a collar stud abscess.

Management
Two longitudinal incisions, one dorsally and one ventrally, but the web should not be incised.

Flexor sheath infection

This is a surgical emergency as it can cause tendon adhesions or rupture.

Anatomy
The flexor sheaths of the index to the ring fingers start from the proximal edge of the A1 pulley. The little finger flexor sheath connects to the ulnar bursa (contains flexor tendons 2–5 deep to the flexor retinaculum). The thumb sheath connects with the radial bursa. The radial and ulnar bursae can communicate through the Space of Parona (proximal to the carpal tunnel) causing a "horseshoe abscess".

Clinical features
Kanavel's four cardinal signs:
- Finger held in a flexed position
- Sausage digit (symmetrical swelling)
- Severe tenderness along the tendon sheath
- Pain on passive extension of the finger

Management
Intravenous antibiotics and prompt surgical drainage. Make a transverse incision over the distal finger crease or a midlateral incision at the level of the middle phalanx, and open the tendon sheath and pass a cannula. Make a second transverse incision at the level of the distal palmar crease and the sheath just proximal to the A1 pulley and flush through till clear.

Infections of the radial and ulnar bursae

These arise following spread from the little finger or thumb flexor tendon sheaths.

To drain the radial bursa, make a lateral incision over the proximal phalanx of the thumb and enter the sheath. Introduce a probe and push it towards the wrist. Make a second incision where it is palpable just proximal to the wrist. Irrigate with a cannula. To drain the ulnar bursa, open it distally on the ulnar side of the little finger, and through a transverse incision just proximal to the wrist and lateral to FCU. Beware of the ulnar nerve and artery. Irrigate.

Deep palmar space infections

The mid palmar and thenar spaces are potential fascia spaces in the palm. The two spaces are situated deep to the flexor tendons and lumbrical muscles in zone 3 and superficial to the interossei and adductor pollicis. The two spaces are separated by a vertical septum from the middle finger metacarpal.

Mid palmar space infections

Infections here cause a severe systemic reaction, generalized swelling of the hand and fingers, which resemble a rubber glove, and loss of active motion of the middle and ring fingers.

Drain through a curved incision beginning at the distal palmar crease, extending ulnar-ward to just inside the hypothenar eminence.

Osteomyelitis

General principles are the same as for larger bones. However, if amputation is necessary, it should be done at the joint proximal to the infected bone or the infection will not clear. Infection of the finger pulp may erode the distal phalanx, but may improve when the overlying abscess is drained.

Human bite ("fight bite") injuries

These are common. The patient presents with a history of punching someone and a wound over the MCP joint. Fracture of the metacarpal should be excluded by radiographs. Assume the patient to have a septic arthritis and all need a formal arthrotomy and wash out under general anaesthetic. Pathogens include the normal flora of the mouth, which includes 42–190 different organisms. The most common infecting organism is still *S. aureus*, other common organisms include *Streptococcus*, *Eikenella corrodens*, *Enterobacter*, *Proteus* and *Serratia*. The average delay in presentation is 2.5 days.

Examination corner

Short notes

Description of a fight bite injury scenario over the index MCP joint presenting 3–4 days later. It is now infected. What is your management?

Hand oral 1

Clinical photograph of chronic paronychia

Management

Hand oral 2

Clinical photograph of fight bite injury to the MCP joint of the index finger

Management

Tuberculous dactylitis

Inflammation of the phalanges or the metacarpals. The bone becomes enlarged, spindle shaped and in the case of tuberculous dactylitis is painful. The skin overlying the affected bone appears smooth and shiny. With further progress the skin may become red, tender and frequently an abscess forms.

In syphilitic dactylitis the swelling is painless. Sickle cell disease causes dactylitis due to infarction of bone secondary to thrombosis of the nutrient artery.

Radiographs in tuberculous dactylitis

- Soft-tissue swelling
- Cortical thinning
- Medullary destruction
- Periosteal reaction

Management

Curettage for culture material followed by antituberculous chemotherapy and splinting.

Differential diagnosis

- Pyogenic infection
- Syphilis
- Enchondroma
- Mycetoma (Madura hand)
- Multiple xanthomatosis
- Sickle cell disease

Diagnosis can be confirmed by biopsy. In spina ventosa there is grossly swollen, spindle-shaped bone.

Examination corner

Hand oral

Clinical photograph of tuberculous dactylitis (spina ventosa)

This is a clinical photograph of a swollen, sausage-shaped left index finger digit suggestive of dactylitis.

The overlying skin is shiny and red.

The usual cause is tuberculosis; other causes could include syphilis or sickle cell disease.

Triangular fibrocartilage complex lesions

There are several topics that you are extremely unlikely to ever be asked about in the FRCS Orth exam. It is always risky saying "never" and that's why one learns these topics on the off-chance that they in fact turn up. Although I doubt very much you will be asked about TFCC lesions, one should know about the anatomy of the TFCC, the two subgroups

Table 21. 4 Classification of TFCC lesions

Class 1:Traumatic injuries	
1A	Central perforation or tear
1B	Ulnar avulsion with or without ulnar styloid fracture
1C	Distal avulsion (origins of UL and UT ligaments)
1D	Radial avulsion (involving the dorsal and/or volar radio-ulnar ligaments)
Class 2: Degenerate TFCC tears	
2A	TFCC wear (thinning)
2B	2A plus lunate and/or ulnar chondromalacia
2C	TFCC perforation plus lunate and/or ulnar chondromalacia
2D	2C plus LT ligament disruption
2E	2D plus ulnocarpal and DRUJ arthritis

of TFCC lesions (Table 21.4) and the various management options available.

Introduction

The TFCC is important in loading and stabilizing the DRUJ. Tears are a relatively rare cause of ulnar-sided wrist pain and are classified according to their location.

Anatomy of the TFCC complex

- Dorsal and volar radio-ulnar ligament
- Articular disc
- Meniscus homologue
- Ulnar collateral ligament
- ECU subsheath
- Origins of the ulnolunate and lunotriquetral ligaments

The periphery is well vascularized whereas the radial central portion is relatively avascular, thin and prone to degenerative changes. Peripheral tears are usually traumatic whilst central tears are generally degenerative and are often found in association with ulnar-positive variance.

Clinical presentation

- Ulnar-sided wrist pain
- Tenderness over triangular fibrocartilage
- Pain with ulnar deviation of carpus and compression

Investigations

Radiographs

- TFCC is not visualized on plain radiographs
- May show ulnar-positive variance
- Localized subchondral defect of the lunate due to impaction on the distal ulnar

Arthrography

- Leakage of dye distally

MRI

- Offers improved accuracy in the diagnosis of TFCC tears

Diagnostic arthroscopy

- Gold standard

Management

Traumatic injuries

All acute traumatic lesions of the TFCC are initially managed non-operatively with immobilization and NSAIDs.

In general:

1A – Arthroscopic resection of the torn portion
1B – Arthroscopic repair
1C – Arthroscopically assisted limited open repair
1D – Partial excision or direct repair with ulnar shortening

Degenerative tears

The abnormalities involve a pathological progression of disease associated with ulnar-positive variance and impaction between the ulnar head and the proximal pole of the lunate. Non-operative treatment is tried first with rest, immobilization and steroid injections.

Surgical treatment is aimed at decompressing the ulnocarpal articulation. Traditionally surgery involved diaphyseal ulnar shortening with the added advantage of tightening the ulnocarpal ligaments and is particularly recommended when concomitant LT instability is present.

Other options include the wafer (2A-2C) or arthroscopic wafer (2C) resection of the ulnar head. Positive ulnar variance greater than 2 mm is a contra indication to wafer resection and is best managed with diaphyseal shortening. Class lesions are managed with a limited ulnar head resection such as a Suave-Kapandji procedure (arthrodesis of the DRUJ and creation of a pseudoarthrosis at the level of the ulnar neck).

Darrach's resection of the distal ulna is considered a salvage procedure because of the concerns regarding impingement and instability of the residual ulnar stump.

Examination corner

Hand oral

Management of TFCC lesions

Most TFCC tears respond to conservative management – splintage, steroid injections, and restriction of activities.

Peripheral tears may be repaired arthroscopically or at open operation, although this procedure is not easy as the TFCC is small and exposure is limited.

Large central flap tears will not heal; they may be debrided arthroscopically but this is ineffective if there is ulnar impaction as the ulna will still abut on the lunate.

Ulnar impaction is treated with ulnar shortening, either a shaft osteotomy or trimming of the distal end of the ulna beneath the TFC (wafer procedure of Feldon). The ulna needs only to be shortened 1–2 mm and it is not necessary to repair or resect the TFCC tear.

Wrist arthrodesis

Indications

A painful or unstable wrist joint with advanced destruction due to:
- Osteoarthritis
- Rheumatoid disease
- SNAC/SLAC wrist
- Salvage of failed wrist arthroplasty
- Salvage in Kienböck's disease

Contraindications

- Infection
- Lack of soft-tissue coverage

This procedure is more beneficial for young, active patients or middle-aged patients but not for elderly patients.

Preoperative considerations

In the rheumatoid wrist the application of a dorsal plate increases the chances of a dorsal wound dehiscence.

Range of movement of other joints

Remember that the elbow and shoulder joints will have to compensate for loss of wrist motion.

Surgical details

Dorsal approach in the wrist

With a severe deformity, consider a wider exposure to the first dorsal compartment in order to allow excision of the radial styloid. The individual carpal bones and distal radius are exposed with the wrist in hyperflexion. Articular cartilage is removed with a Rongeurs. It is important to treat the long finger CMC joint in the arthrodesis or a painful non-union may occur, whereas most surgeons usually prefer to spare the index CMC joint in order to allow its participation in power grip.

Ulnar head

In RA consider resection of the ulnar head, and then using it for a bone graft.

Position of arthrodesis

With a non-RA wrist
Place in 20° of dorsiflexion because this position allows for power gripping. Maximum grip is generated in 35° of dorsiflexion but this interferes with ADLs.

In the rheumatoid wrist
A neutral or a flexed position is more desirable. In the frontal plane a position of 5°–10° of ulnar deviation is preferred in order to counterbalance the zigzag collapse and ulnar drift. Despite the usual recommendations, some patients will prefer slightly more flexion or extension in the wrist. If possible, consider casting the wrist before surgery in extension and the neutral position to determine which position is more comfortable for the patient.

Methods of fixation

Steinmann pin fixation
Through the third metacarpal into the radius or via the second or third web space of the hand. Plaster for 8 weeks to prevent rotation.

AO wrist fusion plate
This is an 8-hole titanium plate with 2.7-mm screws inserted into the distal four holes and 3.5-mm screws in the proximal four holes. In order to have the wrist in 20° of dorsiflexion, a contoured plate is necessary. Lister's tubercle will have to be removed in order to achieve a flat bed for plate application and use as a bone graft. Excise all cartilage and insert bone graft (do not forget the third carpometacarpal joint). Most often the plate is applied to the long metacarpal so that three cortical screws can be inserted into the metacarpal and four screws into the radius (often a screw will also be inserted into the capitate).

Postoperative routine

- Volar splint for 6 weeks
- Union is usually achieved by 3 months
- Plate is not removed unless it causes symptoms

Complications

- Extensor tenosynovitis is the most common complication and is related to a prominent dorsal plate and screws
- Skin necrosis
- Infection
- Transient nerve palsy
- Persistent pain (exclude non-union)

Complex regional pain syndrome

Definition

An abnormal reaction to injury characterized by pain, swelling, stiffness, vasomotor instability and osteoporosis of the affected part.

Classification

CRPS type I

Clinical findings that occur after a noxious event include:

- Regional pain
- Sensory changes
- Alloying
- Abnormalities of temperature
- Abnormal sudomotor activity
- Oedema
- Abnormal skin colour

CRPS type II (causalgia)

Includes all the above features with a peripheral nerve lesion.
    Four cardinal signs:

- Disproportionate amount of pain
- Swelling

- Stiffness
- Discoloration

Clinical features

Complex regional pain syndrome is a biphasic condition characterized by early oedema with late muscle contracture and joint stiffness. The sites of predilection are the hand and foot, with the syndrome now being increasingly recognized in the knee. Complex regional pain syndrome begins up to a month after the precipitating trauma. As the direct effects of injury subside, a new diffuse, unpleasant, neuropathic pain arises. Pain is the most significant feature and is out of all proportion to that expected from the initial injury. Characteristically it is a severe, constant, unremitting burning and/or deep aching pain. It worsens and radiates with time.

The following are also common but not universal:
- Allodynia – pain due to a stimulus that does not normally provoke pain (noise, emotion)
- Hyperalgesia – increased pain to a normally painful stimulus
- Hyperaesthesia – increased sensitivity to a stimulus
- Hyperpathia – excessive perception of a painful stimulus
- Dysaesthesia – abnormally perceived unpleasant sensation, spontaneous or provoked

Vasomotor instability and oedema dominate the early picture. In the classic presentation the limb is initially dry, hot and pink but soon becomes blue, cold and sweaty. Pitting or hard (brawny) oedema develops, which is usually diffuse and localized to the painful and tender region. Loss of joint mobility (stiffness) occurs due to swelling and pain. Passing into the later phase the oedema subsides and the limb atrophies. Hair becomes fragile, uneven and curled whilst the nails in the affected extremity become brittle, pitted, ridged and discoloured brown. The skin is thin and joint creases and subcutaneous fat disappear. The joint capsules and collateral ligaments become shortened, thickened and adherent causing joint contracture. Initially

symptoms are generally localized to the site of injury. As time progresses, the pain and symptoms tend to become more diffuse.

Duration

Variable. In mild cases it is usually several weeks followed by remission. In many cases the pain may continue for years and, in some cases, indefinitely. Some patients experience periods of remission and exacerbation.

Aetiology

A number of precipitating factors have been identified including:
- Trauma (often minor)
- Ischaemic heart disease and myocardial infarction
- Cervical spine or spinal cord disorders
- Cerebral lesions
- Infections
- Surgery

In some patients a definite precipitating event cannot be identified.

Investigations

Complex regional pain syndrome is a clinical diagnosis and there is no single diagnostic test.
- Radiographs
  - Radiographic features occur late and consist of rapid bone loss including visible demineralization with patchy, subchondral or sub periosteal osteoporosis, metaphyseal banding and profound bone loss
- Bone scan
  - Increased uptake of isotope in early complex regional pain syndrome. Later on the bone scan returns to normal. A normal bone scan without radiographic evidence of osteoporosis virtually excludes adult complex regional pain syndrome
- Diagnostic sympathetic block (stellate ganglion)

Management

- Good analgesia
- Physiotherapy
- Active range of movement exercises
- Sympathetic blockade
- Centrally acting analgesic medication (amitriptyl-ine, gabapentin or carbamazepine)

Early management gives optimal results whilst delay in diagnosis and management may contribute to a poor outcome.

Examination corner

Hand oral 1

Classification and management of RSD

Hand oral 2

RSD hand

Diagnosis, management

Splinting of the hand and wrist

A splint may appear in the clinicals or be used as a prop in the orals. Therefore a basic understanding of principles of use, materials and indications is needed.

Definition

- Type of orthosis (external device to support a body part)

Uses

- Immobilize, protect, control mobilization, prevent deformity

Types

- Static
- Dynamic

Materials

- Plaster/synthetic
- Thermoplastic – become malleable with heating (water bath)
- Examples
  - Capener – provides passive extension force (three-point loading) to PIPJ for boutonnière, but allows active flexion against resistance
  - Murphy rings – statically limit PIPJ hyper-extension and allow flexion for swan-neck deformities
  - Stack – static extension to DIPJ for mallet finger
  - Dynamic outrigger – for extensor tendon repair/MCPJ replacements; allows passive extension/active flexion

Miscellaneous oral questions

It is impossible to cover every possible hand oral topic that could be asked in the FRCS Orth exam in detail. Below, however, are some less well-known questions which candidates may be asked.

Hand oral 1

Clinical photograph of a large, well-circumscribed, lobu-lated, firm mass situated over the volar surface of the long finger (Figure 21.8). Painless but slowly enlarging. Radiographs show no bony abnormality.

What are the diagnosis and management?

Spot diagnosis of pigmented villonodular synovitis (giant cell tumour of tendon sheath).

After a ganglion this is the second most common tumour found in the hand and a classic favourite with examiners.

A benign lesion, radiographs are usually normal but may show soft-tissue swelling or may show local pressure effects on bone.

Localized form of PVNS that arises from a tendon sheath or adjacent joint. A diffuse form of giant cell tumour not seen in the hand that occurs in areas adjacent to large weight-bearing joints. This is synonymous with the extra-articular form of PVNS. Local complete excision is recommended but the condition has capacity for local reoccurrence (10%–20%).

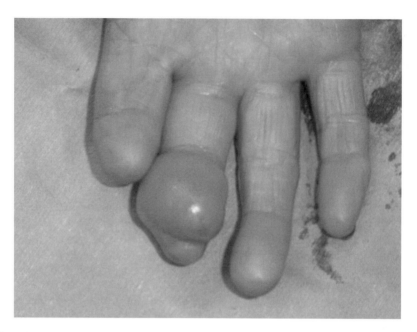

Figure 21.8 Clinical photograph of hand swelling

Must discuss differential diagnosis of a soft-tissue swelling of the digit.

Hand oral 2

Clinical photograph of subungual exostosis

A spot diagnosis, move on to it if you know it; if not, a safe approach is to describe what you see and then go through a differential diagnosis.

This is a bony diverticulum from the terminal phalanx and has the typical cartilaginous cap seen with exostosis elsewhere in the body. This elevates the nail plate with subsequent ridging if the germinal matrix is involved. It is thought the aetiology is probably traumatic but this is in dispute. The treatment is surgical excision. It is necessary to first remove the nail, then the nail bed is split and elevated, the exostosis removed and the nail bed can be sutured back into place.

Differential diagnosis includes:

- Glomus tumour (Masson's tumour) which presents as discoloured areas under the sterile matrix and has a vascular-neural origin

- Enchondroma
- Subungual inclusion dermoid cyst following an old penetrating injury (look for an overlying scar, which may be very small)
- Amelanotic melanoma, which usually presents as a granulation in the centre of the nail, but this diagnosis must be considered if there is swelling beneath the nail. The diagnosis may be delayed as it may mimic infection. Nodal involvement is present in 40% of patients at first presentation. A biopsy should be taken including sampling of the lymph nodes and then the tumour can be staged before definitive treatment, which usually consists of ray amputation and chemotherapy. A clinical picture of subungual melanoma is sometimes shown in the hand oral.

Hand oral 3

Pigmented lesion under nail bed

Differential diagnosis: melanoma, subungual haematoma, glomus tumour

Hand oral 4

Fingertip injury

Fingertip injuries of the distal phalanx
Management in a young, female non-smoker, dominant hand, tip available

Trauma oral 1

Skier's thumb

- Stener lesion
- Approach
- Complications

Trauma oral 2

Rugger jersey finger

- Classification
- Discussion of Bruner's incisions
- Pull out suture

Hand oral 5

De Quervain's disease

- Presentation
- Diagnosis
- Which tendons are involved and what is the appropriate surgical approach?

Hand oral 6

Bennett's fracture

- Why is it unstable (i.e. what is the deforming tendon)?
- Management
- What size of K-wire is used for fixation?

SECTION 6

The paediatric oral

22. Paediatric oral topics 359
Joseph Alsousou and Paul A. Banaszkiewicz

Paediatric oral topics

Joseph Alsousou and Paul A. Banaszkiewicz

Introduction

The paediatric oral topics section is a brief overview of some of the more important paediatric topics that tend to regularly appear in the examination.

The paediatric oral can be tricky as the examiners expect you to have both a comprehensive range and depth of paediatric knowledge. Candidates may struggle unless they have had a reasonable working exposure to paediatrics, ideally 6 months as part of a higher surgical training rotation. Some topics are very predictable – in the oral candidates will invariably get one of the big three (DDH, Perthes and SUFE), not infrequently all three.

The paediatric oral for the most part consists of clinical photographs and radiographs acting as props to lead you into a particular topic. Occasionally a video of gait analysis in a CP patient is thrown in at the end to stretch you.

In general candidates can come across two types of oral:

1. A series of rapid-fire clinical photographs and radiographs. A spot diagnosis of the topic and from this a fairly superficial/generalized discussion about management of the condition.

2. In the second oral type fewer topics are covered but there is a greater probing of paediatric knowledge, particularly management issues.

The key elements for success in the oral are:

- To have worked for 6 months in a paediatric orthopaedics higher surgical training job
- Correctly gauging the depth of paediatric knowledge required for the oral. Aiming too high can be a disaster; too low and you will fail
- Similar principles apply with your reading material. Some paediatric books are a little flimsy, whilst others are subspeciality textbooks that are difficult to revise from
- Go on a well recommended and established paediatric course. There has been some feedback suggesting that several courses may be a little too detailed for the exam but you will need to ferret this out yourself. The Alder Hey Paediatric course consists of 3 days of lectures. It is regarded as being a bit dry but goes through everything you need to know for the examination together with the latest treatments, etc. In addition there is the Bristol Paediatric FRCS (Orth) Revision Course, which is a 2-day interactive course in paediatrics consisting of viva practice, clinical examination and key clinical topics. The Birmingham Paediatric Orthopaedic Course is a 3-day course designed to prepare candidates for the paediatrics component of the exam. I have no personal experience with any of these courses but various candidates have given positive feedback about each of them
- Towards the end of your preparation for the exam get your local paediatric FRCS Orth examiner to viva you at least once, preferably on a couple of occasions
- Try to set up a study group of trainees about to sit the examination and regularly meet up to go through different areas/topics of revision

Postgraduate Orthopaedics: The Candidate's Guide to the FRCS (Tr & Orth) Examination, Ed. Paul A. Banaszkiewicz,
Deiary F. Kader, Nicola Maffulli. Published by Cambridge University Press. © Cambridge University Press 2009.

Developmental dysplasia of the hip (DDH)

It is almost certain that you will be asked about DDH in your children's orthopaedics oral. This in itself is not particularly helpful as it is a big, complex and controversial subject to learn. Virtually any area of DDH including peripheral side topics can be asked about. For starters it is very important to be able to recognize it on a clinical photograph or radiograph. Quite where the discussion will then go to is anybody's guess.

Definition

DDH comprises a wide spectrum of hip abnormalities ranging from mild acetabular dysplasia to complete dislocation of the hip.

Incidence

- Established dislocation 1–2 per 1000 live births
- Unstable hips at birth 15–20 per 1000 live births
- Left hip more than right hip (60% left, 20% right and 20% bilateral)[1]

Risk factors for DDH

- Family history, first born, females (80%), breech presentation (especially if knees extended), oligohydramnios and twins

Associated ("packaging") conditions

- Torticollis, plagiocephaly, metatarsus adductus, congenital recurvatum or dislocation of the knee, calcaneovalgus feet and clubfoot deformities[2]

---

[1] The examiners may ask you why the left hip is significantly more affected than the right. The left hip is adducted against the mother's lumbosacral spine in the most common intrauterine position (left occiput anterior). In this position less cartilage is covered by the bony acetabulum and instability can develop.

[2] In the exam, you may be asked about associated hip abnormalities in a child with one of these abnormalities.

Aetiology theories

Anatomy

Shallow acetabulum and capsular laxity often co-exist at birth, and improve hip range of movement to aid delivery. Femoral head is >50% uncovered at birth, which predisposes to subluxation/dislocation.

Primary acetabular dysplasia

The evidence is weak. If it does exist, it only becomes apparent in children who present late.

Genetic theory

The probability of having a child with DDH in at-risk families is 6% if there are normal parents and one affected child; 12% if there is one affected parent but no prior affected child; and 36% if there is one affected parent and one affected child.

Mechanical theory

Intrauterine malposition, which is supported by a high incidence in association with frank breech presentation with knees extended, twins and other postural deformities of the limbs.

Firstborn children are affected twice as often as subsequent siblings, presumably on the basis of an unstretched uterus and therefore tighter uterine space with less room for normal fetal motion.

Breech presentation is probably related to the strong hamstring forces on the hip that result from knee extension. The increased tension on the hamstrings pushes the femoral head out of the acetabulum.

Maternal hormone-induced DDH theory

Females may be affected more frequently because of the increased ligamentous laxity that transiently exists as the result of circulating maternal hormones and the additional effect of oestrogens that are produced by the female infant's uterus. This produces a temporary period of susceptibility in which abnormal positioning of the hip may result in instability.

Investigations

Clinical examination

Varies with age, may have:
- Asymmetrical groin folds or skin creases (not an accurate clinical sign)
- Limitation of abduction (on nappy changes) (>20° needs referral to the orthopaedic surgeon)
- Leg length discrepancy: positive Galeazzi's sign, the affected side is shorter when the knees and hips are flexed
- Ortolani's test (head **o**ut) (**o** for **O**rtolani and **o**ut). This test reduces a dislocated hip. There is a "clunk" or jerk when the head snaps over the posterior acetabular rim back into the acetabulum
- Barlow's test (provocative test). Identifies an unstable hip that can be dislocated by the examiner. There is an exit "clunk" when the hip is dislocated out of the acetabulum
- Limp (unilateral dislocation) or waddling gait with hyperlordosis of the lumbar spine (high bilateral dislocations) evident after walking

---

Oral questions

What is developmental dysplasia of the hip?

What are the risk factors for DDH?

What other conditions are associated with DDH?

What is Ortolani's test?

What is Barlow's test?

Ultrasound examination of the hip

- Ultrasound examination for DDH is well established. It offers sensitivity and specificity >90% but it is not infallible. Images can be difficult to interpret, it can over-diagnose the condition, it

does not tell us who to treat and it poses logistical problems in organization
- The routine use of universal ultrasound screening has yet to be established. Reasons include resource implications, extra clinics and radiographers required, training implications, etc. Agreement is needed on who to treat and long-term outcome studies are required. As it is very sensitive there is concern about false-positive results, which may lead to over-treatment of hips (and its potential complications) that would otherwise stabilize spontaneously
- Selective ultrasound screening when there is clinical suspicion or in babies with risk factors is more cost-effective and has a high rate of detection. However, it does not prevent the appearance of late cases[3]

Graf hip angle measurements are based on three lines and two angles (Figure 22.1):
1. **Baseline** is drawn on the ilium to the junction of the cartilaginous roof and bony acetabular roof
2. **Bony acetabular roofline**
3. **Cartilaginous roofline**
4. The **alpha** (α) **angle** is formed by the bony acetabular roofline and the iliac line
5. The **beta** (β) **angle** is between the baseline and the cartilaginous roofline

In the normal hip $\alpha > 60°$, and the smaller the angle the greater the dysplasia. When $\beta > 77°$ the hip is subluxed and the labrum is everted.

The hip ratio measurement calculates the percentage of femoral head coverage under the bony roof.

Graf ultrasound classification

Based on the depth and shape of the acetabulum as seen on coronal image. Four types of hip are described:

Type I: Normal hip.

Type II: Shallow acetabulum with a rounded rim. Immature or somewhat abnormal. Immature

---

[3] Jones D (1998) Neonatal detection of developmental dysplasia of the hip (DDH) [Leading editorial]. *J Bone Joint Surg Br* **80**(6):943–5.

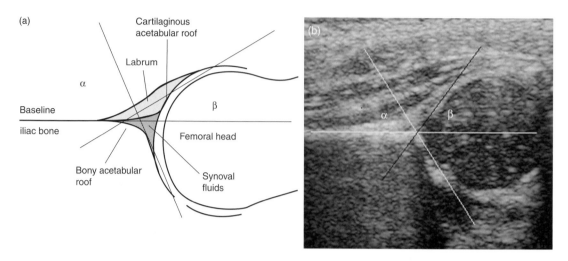

Figure 22.1 Graf (α) angle between baseline and bony acetabular roofline. Normal value >60°. Graf (β) angle between baseline and cartilaginous roofline. Normal value <55°

(physiological) hip spontaneously resolves in infants <3 months old. Mildly dysplastic in infants >3 months old persists without treatment.

Type III: Subluxated or low dislocation. Bony roof deficient, labrum everted.

Type IV: High dislocation. Flat bony acetabulum. Labrum interposed between femoral head and lateral wall of the ilium.

Natural history of untreated DDH

- **Muscles** about the hip contract and become shortened. Iliopsoas tendon becomes interposed between the femoral head and acetabulum blocking reduction
- The **hip joint** becomes more dysplastic and filled with fibrofatty tissue (pulvinar)
- The **capsule** becomes redundant and expanded. An arthrogram may show an hourglass constriction of the joint capsule caused by the contracted iliopsoas, which blocks hip reduction
- **Ligamentum teres** becomes lengthened, hypertrophied and redundant

- The **femoral head and neck** remain anteverted and in valgus position. Head becomes misshapen and flattened with delayed ossification of the epiphysis
- **Acetabulum labrum** becomes elongated and hypertrophied and may infold into the joint (inverted limbus) blocking reduction of the femoral head
- **Abnormal femoral head** and **false acetabulum** develop in the ilium wing
- **Transverse acetabular ligament** contracts and is a major block to a deep concentric hip reduction

Radiology

- Hilgenreiner's horizontal line through tri-radiate cartilage (Figures 22.2, 22.3)
- Perkin's vertical line from the outer edge of the acetabulum (AIIS)

The hip should be in the inner and lower quadrant between these lines. If **subluxed**, the femoral neck lies **lateral** to Perkin's line. When **dislocated**, the femoral neck lies **lateral** to Perkin's line and

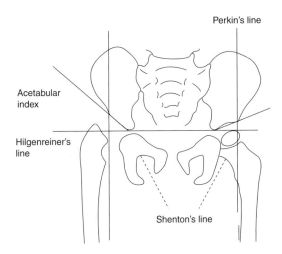

Figure 22.2 Assessing radiographs in DDH

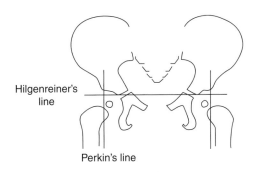

Figure 22.3 Radiographic assessment of DDH

superior to Hilgenreiner's line. Characteristic features include:

- Break in Shenton's line
- Increased acetabular index (normal is <25°; >30° indicates dysplasia, significant if >40°)
- Delay in appearance of the ossific nucleus of the femoral head
- Lateral and superior migration of the femoral neck
- Delayed ossification: U figure or teardrop of Koehler

Arthrogram (what to look for)

Whether the acetabulum is dysplastic
- Is the hip subluxed or dislocated? Can the hip be reduced?
- Is there soft-tissue interposition (pulvinar fat)?
- Is there pooling of the dye medially (normal ≤7 mm)?
- Is the ligamentum teres hypertrophic and redundant?
- If the labrum is normal or inverted (limbus), look for a rose thorn sign of an inverted labrum between the femoral head and acetabulum
- Is there an hourglass constriction of the capsule (by psoas tendon)?

How to perform an arthrogram
- Place patient in supine position, usually with GA, aseptic technique
- Use fluoroscopic control with careful placement of the needle through the adductor approach into the empty acetabulum
- Check the position of the needle using fluoroscopy and inject a small amount of diluted contrast medium
- Image in the position of dislocation and reduction. Note any obstacles to reduction and determine the stability of reduction
- Dangers include scoring of the femoral head cartilage with the needle, injection into the growth plate or the piercing of femoral blood vessels

Management

Pavlik harness

Dynamic flexion/abduction orthosis used in children up to 6 months old. It maintains the affected hip in 90°–100° of flexion and abduction (usually halfway between full abduction and dislocation, approximately 60°) and restricts extension and adduction.

The harness allows for motion within the range of reduced stability. It is used for 8–12 weeks and requires close observation. This is successful in managing DDH in 90% of cases before the age of 3 months.

The use of Pavlik harness is contraindicated when there is major muscle imbalance as in myelomeningocele, major stiffness as in arthrogryposis or ligamentous laxity such as Ehlers–Danlos syndrome.

Complications of Pavlik harness

- Femoral nerve palsy secondary to excessive hip flexion
- Brachial plexopathy due to compression from high-riding shoulder strap and knee subluxations from improperly positioned straps
- AVN occurs in as many as 2.4% of cases splinted in the safe zone
- Failure of hip reduction
- Fixed posterior dislocation with damage to the posterior acetabulum due to failure to detect persistent dislocation (Pavlik harness disease)
- Skin maceration

Closed reduction and application of a spica cast

- Usually indicated in children between 6 and 12 months old
- The hip is flexed and the thigh is lifted and abducted to bring the femoral head into the acetabulum
- The reduced hip must be maintained in a physiological position of flexion/abduction
- Intraoperative arthrogram is performed to confirm depth and stability of reduction and hip spica cast is applied
- An interposed labrum is often accepted as the limbus will remodel with time. If an adduction contracture limits abduction a percutaneous adductor tenotomy is usually necessary and will also increase the safe zone
- Cast is removed at 6 weeks under anaesthesia and second spica cast is applied with less flexion and abduction. If limbus interposition was present repeat the arthrogram to confirm concentric reduction
- At 3 months, the hip is again assessed under anaesthesia. A third spica cast is sometimes required
- If the quality of reduction is uncertain on an AP radiograph confirm reduction by a CT scan

Indications for open reduction

- Failure to achieve a concentric reduction, the femoral head is persistently above the tri-radiate cartilage or will not enter the acetabulum
- Position required to maintain reduction is extreme
- If arc of reduction and re-dislocation is <20° (small safe zone)
- Failed previous closed reduction
- Beyond 12 months, it is usual to attempt a closed reduction although certainly after the age of 18 months this is unlikely to be successful
- Primary management in children >2 years old

Medial approach hip

Before walking age (6–9 months). Several medially based approaches. The true medial approach described by Ludloff utilizes the interval between pectineus and adductor longus and brevis. Ferguson modified it to pass between adductor longus and brevis anteriorly and adductor magnus and gracilis posteriorly.

- **Advantages**
  - Small groin incision, minimal soft tissue dissection, avoids splitting the iliac apophysis, approaches the hip joint over the site of the obstacles to reduction
- **Disadvantages**
  - Poor exposure, poor visualization of joint interior, unable to reef redundant capsule, concerns regarding the completeness of removal of obstacles to reduction, risk of re-dislocation, increased rates of AVN
- **Technique (Ferguson)**
  - Supine with affected hip flexed, abducted and externally rotated
  - Make a longitudinal incision on the medial side of the thigh starting 3 cm below the pubic tubercle. Incision runs down over adductor longus
  - Develop a plane between gracilis and adductor longus; best done using finger dissection
  - Continue dissection between adductor brevis and adductor magnus to uncover the posterior

division of the obturator nerve. Feel the lesser trochanter. Iliopsoas is divided thus exposing the anterior, superior and inferior aspects of the hip joint capsule

- Hip joint capsulotomy and division of the transverse acetabular ligament
- Look out for the anterior and posterior branches of the obturator nerve. Also look out for the medial femoral circumflex artery if the iliopsoas tendon has not been isolated and cut under direct vision

Anterior approach hip (Smith–Peterson)

This is the most common approach. This approach should definitely be used if the patient is of walking age (1 year), if the hip is irreducible, if the child is >18 months old or if there is any doubt about the need for performing a secondary procedure.

- **Advantages**
  - Excellent exposure, exposure of choice in high dislocation, has a low risk of AVN, lends itself to additional operative procedures such as pelvic osteotomy
- **Disadvantages**
  - Large scar, large surgical approach, blood loss. Scar can be made more cosmetically acceptable by using a transverse incision rather than a curved iliofemoral incision. Damage to the lateral cutaneous nerve in the thigh and hip abductors, iliac wing deformity and postoperative stiffness
- **Technique**
  - Smith–Peterson approach with modified bikini incision
  - Patient is supine and is placed close to the edge of the table. Sandbag may be used to elevate the affected hip forwards
  - Iliac crest apophysis is split and abductors elevated. An interval is opened up between tensor fascia lata laterally and sartorius medially
  - Plane between rectus femoris and gluteus medius is opened up. Both heads of rectus femoris are detached and retracted medially.
  - Retract the gluteus medius laterally. The capsule of the hip joint should come into view

Proximal varus femoral osteotomy

Used to correct either anteversion or valgus deformity of the femoral neck in patients with dysplasia that reduces with abduction and internal rotation. Procedure is most useful when acetabular dysplasia is not severe. Benefits of femoral osteotomy decrease after 4–8 years of age. If the deformity is severe the procedure is combined with a pelvic osteotomy and functions primarily as a shortening osteotomy to facilitate reduction.

Pelvic osteotomy

Reconstruction procedures

1. Salter innominate osteotomy

   Prerequisite factors include a concentric, completely reduced femoral head, a congruent hip joint with good ROM and no fixed flexion (psoas) or adduction contractures

   Anterior approach hip is used. Innominate bone is osteotomized with a Gigli saw from the sciatic notch to the anterior inferior iliac spine. The entire acetabulum together with the pubis and ischium is rotated as a unit anteriorly and laterally with the pubic symphysis acting as a hinge. The displacement is maintained by a wedge of iliac bone crest fixed with pins. There is a risk of damaging the sciatic nerve and superior gluteal artery at the sciatic notch. Lengthens by approximately 1 cm

2. Pemberton osteotomy

   Indicated in child with more severe acetabular dysplasia that may not be completely corrected by the Salter osteotomy. Osteotomy starts approximately 10–15 mm above the AIIS, proceeds posteriorly, and ends at the level of the ilioischial limb of the tri-radiate cartilage (halfway between the sciatic notch and posterior acetabular rim). The acetabulum is hinged anteriorly and laterally on the flexible tri-radiate cartilage

3. Steel triple innominate osteotomy

   Indicated in an older child with severe acetabular dysplasia when the pubic symphysis is rigid (age >8 years). It consists of osteotomies of the ischium and pubic in addition to the Salter innominate osteotomy. The entire acetabulum is then rotated to a position that provides maximum acetabular coverage of the femoral head

4. Ganz osteotomy

Indicated for residual severe dysplasias in adolescents and young adults to improve congruency and containment of the hip. Technically challenging and difficult to learn. The osteotomy allows extensive acetabular reorientation, including medial and lateral displacement. Osteotomies are performed in the pubis, ilium, and ischium. The osteotomy crosses the tri-radiate cartilage and therefore must be done after skeletal maturity

Salvage procedures

1. Chiari osteotomy

Indications include severe acetabular dysplasia with inadequate femoral head coverage; dislocations that have been reduced but have later become subluxations; when other reconstruction options are not possible; and a symptomatic subluxed hip with early osteoarthritis to buy time (10 years, possibly 15 years)

The iliac osteotomy is angled from the sciatic notch to the ASIS. The acetabulum is displaced medially and vertically hinging on pubic symphysis. The hip capsule is interposed between the newly formed acetabular roof and femoral head. Relies on periarticular soft-tissue metaplasia for coverage. Complications include the cut being made too high or too low and sciatic nerve injury. Procedure will shorten the affected leg

2. Staheli's shelf procedure

Main indication is an aspherical dysplastic joint that is too deformed for a reconstructive acetabular realignment but is not deformed enough to necessitate a Chiari osteotomy

Thin strips of corticocancellous bone graft are slotted into the anterolateral aspect of the ilium between the reflected head of rectus femoris and the capsule. Dissection of abductor muscles off the side of the pelvis weakens them and worsens an abductor lurch if already present

---

Examination corner

Paeds oral 1

- DDH – late presentation and role of arthrogram
- Economics of preoperative traction before open reduction

Paeds oral 2

DDH in an 18-month-old child

- History and examination
- Arthrogram findings
- Management options

Paeds oral 3

- Clinical finding in a neonate with suspected DDH

Paeds oral 4

- DDH management
- Open reduction indications and approaches
- Which soft tissues should be released or excised to ensure reduction?
- Complications

Paeds oral 5

- An ultrasound image of DDH
- Anatomical structures and features on the USS

Paeds oral 6

Examiner: What radiographic features are present in DDH?
Candidate: The characteristic features include: break in Shenton's line, increased acetabular index, delayed ossific nucleus, development of a false acetabulum, proximal and lateral migration of femoral neck and centre edge angle <20°.
Examiner: What would you find by examining the child?
Candidate: On inspection, the child would have asymmetrical groin folds. They would have limited abduction

and a leg length discrepancy. Galeazzi's sign demonstrates this, where the affected side appears shorter when the knees and hips are flexed. If the hip is unstable but congruent, Barlow's test would be positive. Ortolani's test would be positive if the head is dislocated.

Examiner: The child is 8 months old. What would your management be?

Candidate: I would investigate this child's hip by ultrasound screening and an X-ray. To confirm the diagnosis I would perform an arthrogram under GA. On confirming the diagnosis I would manage this with close reduction and spica cast.

Examiner:
- How do you do an arthrogram?
- What can you see on the arthrogram?
- How do you check the adequacy of reduction?
- What are the complications of treatment?
- How do you reduce the incidence of AVN?

Paeds oral 7

- Management of DDH presenting at 2 years
- Smith–Peterson approach to the hip

Paeds oral 8

Clinical photograph of Ortolani's test

- How is it performed?
- Sensitivity
- Management at 8 months
- General discussion about screening

Slipped upper femoral epiphysis (SUFE)

Definition

A disorder in which a dehiscence occurs through the growth plate of the immature hip. The femoral head remains in the acetabulum; the neck displaces anteriorly and rotates externally.

Epidemiology

- Relatively rare, annual rate of 3/100 000 in whites and of 7/100 000 in blacks

- Bilateral in 30% of cases, with subtle changes of pre-slipping (minor femoral head tilting) seen in 70% of cases
- ♂:♀ 3: 1; male age 12–14 years, female age 11–13 years
- Obesity is a significant risk factor for the condition
- If the patient is <9 years or >16 years and has a retarded bone age or short stature, consider endocrinopathy
- Most patients have a varus deformity hip. Valgus deformity is rare (epiphysis slips superiorly in relation to the neck of femur)

Aetiology

Most cases are idiopathic. It may be associated with endocrine and metabolic disorders, be a complication of treatment with chemotherapy and radiotherapy or occur with administration of growth hormone for short stature.

A multitude of potential aetiological causes have been suggested, including:

- **Alteration in hip mechanical forces**: several anatomical features are thought to increase the risk of a slip
- **Retroversion of the femoral head** (>10° from normal) leads to increased shear stress across the growth plate
- **Slope of the growth plate** is significantly increased in patients with a unilateral slip
- Increased physeal height due to a widened hypertrophic zone
- **Maturation factors:** not usually seen in girls after the menarche. Imbalance between oestrogen and growth hormone increases the thickness of the physis while reducing its resistance to shear. Patients have a relatively uniform skeletal age. The slip appears to occur in a narrow skeletal age range
- **Ultrastructural defects of the physis** itself: widening and weakening of the hypertrophic zone with abnormal cartilage maturation, endochondral ossification, and perichondral ring instability and disorganization of the columnar cell arrangement.

Slip usually occurs in the hypertrophic zone of provisional calcification but can pass through multiple zones

- **Endocrine factors:** bilateral SUFE is seen in 70% patients with endocrine disease compared to 20%–40% of the normal population
- **Triggering traumatic event:** found in many cases

Clinical presentation

- Unexplained antalgic limp
- Poorly localized dull pain in the hip, thigh and knee of several weeks' duration
- Decreased range of hip movement (internal rotation, flexion and abduction), progressive external rotation deformity and shortening
- If the thigh is flexed it typically rolls into external rotation and abduction (figure 4 position)
- Children may present acutely with extreme pain, often after trauma

Classification

Old classification system for SUFE[4]

This is based on the duration of symptoms and does not consider the stability of the slip:

- Pre-slip: radiographic finding of irregularity, widening and fuzziness physis
- Acute slip: sudden onset of symptoms within 3 weeks. Usually follows trauma
- Acute-on-chronic slip (20%): symptoms for >3 weeks with sudden exacerbation of pain which may or may not be associated with acute trauma
- Chronic (60%): symptoms for >3 weeks

New classification system for SUFE (Loder)

Outcome-related classification of slips based on epiphyseal stability. This classification system is useful as it correlates with outcome and predicts the likelihood of AVN.

[4] Various classification systems have been proposed over the years based on displacement of the epiphysis, angular displacement of the epiphysis and the stability of the epiphysis.

1. **Stable slip.** The child is able to weight bear with or without crutches
2. **Unstable slip.** Child is unable to tolerate any kind of weight bearing on the affected hip:
   - Unstable hips have a 47% satisfactory prognosis compared to a 96% satisfactory prognosis in the stable-hip group
   - The incidence of AVN in the stable group is nil, whereas 50% in the unstable-hip group will develop AVN
   - Joint effusion is absent and the severity of slip is less in the stable-hip group

Severity of slip (Wilson)

Based on the portion of uncovered physis:

- **Grade I:** 0%–33% of the metaphysis is uncovered – mild slip
- **Grade II:** 33%–50% – moderate slip
- **Grade III: >50% –** severe slip

Carney's classification

Based on the slip angle of Southwick. This is important with regard to the long-term prognosis of the slip:

- Grade I: mild <30°
- Grade II: moderate 30°–60°
- Grade III: severe >60°

Investigations

Radiology (six radiographic features of SUFE)[5]

1. Kline's line (Perkin's sign). A line drawn on the superior border of the femoral neck transects the femoral head and does not pass through the femoral head = Trethowan's sign
2. Metaphyseal blanch sign of Steel. A crescent-shaped, dense area in the metaphysis on AP view represents superimposition of the posteriorly displaced epiphysis
3. Joint space increased inferiorly

[5] Classic oral question: "What are the six radiographic features of a SUFE?"

4. Widening and irregularity of physis (appears woolly, earliest sign)
5. Decreased epiphysis height (slipped posteriorly)
6. Remodelling changes of the neck (in chronic slips): smooth superior anterior portion and callus formation on inferior posterior portions

Frog lateral (Lauenstein view)

Physeal line: a line between the superior and inferior margins of capital physis
Femoral neck line: normally perpendicular to physeal line
Southwick angle: head-shaft angle of the affected side is subtracted from the head-shaft angle of the normal side (normal = 10°)
Capital physeal femoral neck angle: between physeal line and femoral neck line. In the normal hip it is 90°

Management

The primary goals of management are stabilization of the slip to prevent further progression, and promotion of physeal closure. Operative options include:
- Pinning in situ: with a single cannulated AO screw (for grade I and II slips)
- Bone graft epiphysiodesis (high complication rates: AVN, chondrolysis, HO bone formation)
- Primary osteotomy by experienced paediatric hip surgeon (for severe slip)

How do you check your screw is not in the joint?

- Serial radiographs
- Screening the hip with the image intensifier (moving the image intensifier around)
- Radiographic contrast medium injection through the cannulated screw

Osteotomies (not for the occasional surgeon)

The more distally chosen the site, the lower the rate of AVN and chondrolysis. In severe SUFE, the following osteotomies can be carried out at four levels:
- Subcapital osteotomy
  - Dunn procedure. A relatively high degree of deformity can be corrected by subcapital osteotomy but the growth plate must still be open. This is a cuneiform subcapital wedge resection with trimming posterior beak. This remains controversial due to the high reported rates of AVN (37%)
  - Fish and Cuneiform. Similar to Dunn with modification
- Basal cervical osteotomy. Offers a less precise correction but gives good results. Avoids dissection of the adjacent growth plate
- Intertrochanteric osteotomy (Kramer)
- Subtrochanteric osteotomies
  - Southwick triplanar osteotomy at the level of the lesser trochanter. Reasonably safe but technically difficult

Complications

- Chondrolysis. Rapid progressive loss of articular cartilage associated with pin penetration of the joint and multiple screw fixation. Diagnosis indicated by virtually nil range of hip movement, hip pain and a narrowed joint space. Confirm with MRI
- AVN. Related to unstable (50%) or severe (25%) slip
- Subtrochanteric fracture. Due to low screw placement at insertion or removal
- Degenerative joint disease. Can develop in well-treated moderate slips with no complications. Approximately 10% of patients with SUFE develop OA
- Residual leg length inequality and rotational deformity (severe slips that may require late corrective osteotomy)

Examination corner

Paeds oral 1

Severe unstable SUFE

- Outline your management, including AVN rates and types of corrective osteotomy

Paeds oral 2

SUFE: radiographic spot diagnosis
- Predisposition
- Management of severe grade III slip
- Fish and Dunn osteotomies: examiner wanted to hear the word "shortening". Subcapital osteotomy without shortening carries an unacceptably high risk of AVN due to stretching of the contracted posterior vessels as the head is reduced on the femoral neck

Paeds oral 3

Radiograph of severe SUFE
- Classification of slips, particularly the Loder classification system
- Incidence
- Management of severe slips: pin in situ versus osteotomy
- Discussion about various osteotomies and complications of each (higher incidence of AVN in more proximal osteotomies such as Dunn compared to the Southwick biplanar osteotomy)

Examiner: Do you know any papers in the last year about management of severe SUFE?
Candidate: I mentioned a review paper about management of SUFE.[1] This led on to discussion of another paper from Southampton concerning the timing of reduction and stabilization of an acute, unstable SUFE.[2] The examiner knew both papers very well and we discussed the second paper in a fair amount of detail.

Paeds oral 4

Lateral radiograph of SUFE with history of sudden onset of knee pain

Examiner:
- What is the diagnosis?
- What will you find on clinical examination?
- What radiographic changes are present to indicate this as being an acute-on-chronic slip?
- What will you do?
- What complications can occur?
- What is the incidence of chondrolysis?

Examiner: Would you pin this boy's other hip? (It looked normal on the radiograph.)

Candidate: No. But I will follow-up with serial radiographs into maturity with advice to come back if there is knee or hip pain.
Examiner: What does the recent literature say on this?
Candidate: There are papers that advocate fixing the normal side prophylactically. I would refrain except in situations of clinical need and (as he seemed to like the idea of prophylactic pinning, I added) in predisposed individuals.
Examiner: What are the predisposing conditions?

Paeds oral 5

SUFE

- Aetiology, clinical presentation and management

Complications

- Outline the principles of single AO screw fixation and how you would do it
- Would you reduce the slip or fix in situ?
- Would you take out the screw – what does the literature say?

[1] Uglow MG, Clarke NM (2005) The management of slipped capital femoral epiphysis. *J Bone Joint Surg Br* **86**(5): 631–5.
[2] Phillips SA, Griffiths WE, Clarke NM (2001) The timing of reduction and stabilization of the acute, unstable, slipped upper femoral epiphysis. *J Bone Joint Surg* **83**(7): 1046–9.

Perthes disease (coxa plana)

This is an A list topic. It is an extremely important subject and a favourite with examiners.

Background

It was originally thought that Legg–Calvé–Perthes disease was transient tuberculosis of the hip. The diagnosis only became apparent after the development of radiographs.

Definition

Non-inflammatory idiopathic AVN of the femoral head in a growing child produced by interruption of blood supply to the proximal femoral epiphysis.

Epidemiology

- 1 in 9000
- Most common age of presentation is 4–9 years (80% cases)
- ♂: ♀ 4: 1
- Bilateral 10%: asymmetrical and never simultaneous
- Susceptible child: usually a boy aged 4–9 years, social class 4–5. Child often has a short stature with delayed bone age (usually by 2 years). The child is often wiry, thin, very active, and noticeably smaller than his age group

Aetiology

Poorly understood, there are several theories:
1. **Repeated ischaemic episodes at the femoral epiphysis** (rather than a single event) lead to the disease syndrome. Following the ischaemic episodes, most of the epiphysis becomes avascular. While enchondral ossification temporarily halts, the articular cartilage continues to grow. This results in widening of the medial cartilage (joint) space and a smaller ossification centre in the involved hip. Revascularization occurs from the periphery. Therefore, resumption of enchondral ossification within the epiphysis begins peripherally and progresses centrally. New bone is deposited on avascular bone, producing a net increase in bone density. In subchondral area, bone resorption exceeds new bone formation. This becomes weak and is prone to collapse. Symptoms result from subchondral fractures.
2. **Hydrostatic pressure theory.** Epiphyseal arteries transverse the neck between bone and an inelastic capsule. This makes them vulnerable to pressure rise, e.g. reactive synovitis. The femoral neck venous drainage is disturbed with increased interosseous venous pressure. This leads to arterial or venous thrombosis.
3. **Fibrinolytic disorders** have received much attention recently. There is evidence to support the association between thrombophilic and hypofibrinolytic disorders. These include:

- Protein S and C abnormalities
- Leiden factor 5 mutation (active factor 5, which is not cleaved properly)
- Anticardiolipin antibodies
- Micro-trauma or passive smoking (effects fibrinolysis, possibly accounts for association with low socioeconomic class)

Clinical presentation

- Early phase: pain (groin, often knee pain) and decreased ROM (especially abduction and internal rotation) in both flexion and extension. There is also antalgic gait (due to pain)
- Late phase: Trendelenburg gait

Differential diagnosis

Unilateral Perthes disease

- Transient synovitis
- Infection (septic arthritis, tuberculosis and osteomyelitis)
- Blood dyscrasias (lymphoma, leukaemia)
- Juvenile chronic arthritis
- Rheumatic fever
- Sickle cell disease

Bilateral Perthes disease

- Hypothyroidism
- Multiple epiphyseal dysplasia
- Spondyloepiphyseal dysplasia
- Gaucher's disease

Imaging

Waldenstrom's radiographic staging

- **Necrotic stage (initial stage).** Changes include microfractures, dense sclerotic femoral head and overgrowth of the articular cartilage resulting in coxa magna, an increased joint space and crescent sign (Caffey's sign)
- **Fragmentation (resorption) stage**. The damage is done; this is a process of ongoing necrotic bone

resorption and new bone formation. This repair process produces the appearance of lateral fragmentation of the femoral epiphysis

- **Re-ossification (healing) stage**. Further re-ossification occurs and radiodensity becomes normal
- **Remodelling stage (residue stage)**. Femoral head is healed but continues to remodel until skeletal maturity. Residue deformity may be coxa magna, coxa plana or coxa breva

In general, necrotic and fragmentation stages last approximately 6 months each, the re-ossification stage 18 months, and the remodelling stage 3 years.

Catterall's head-at-risk signs (radiographic predictors)

Radiographic findings associated with poor prognosis include:

- Lateral subluxation (most important)
- Calcification lateral to the epiphysis
- Gage's sign: V-shaped defect laterally
- Metaphyseal cysts
- Horizontal growth plate

Classification systems

- Catterall has four groups
- Salter–Thompson has two groups
- Herring lateral pillar classification has three groups

Catterall's classification[6]

Based on amount of femoral head involvement on AP and lateral radiographs. It is determined during the fragmentation stage. The group may appear to change during the disease process. Catterall's classification has large inter- and intra-observer errors.

Group I: Central anterior head involvement
Group II: More than 25% head involvement but medial and lateral columns intact

Group III: 75% femoral head involvement but intact medial column
Group IV: Whole head involvement

Salter–Thompson classification[7]

Based on the crescent sign, due to the extent of subchondral fracture. The advantage over the Catterall's classification is that it provides you with an early means of predicting what is going to happen to the femoral head.

Group A: Less than half the femoral head is involved and intact lateral pillar
Group B: More than half of the head is involved and involved lateral pillar

Herring lateral pillar classification[8]

Much less inter- and intra-observer error than Catterall's (inter-observer agreement 85%). The classification is evaluated in the early fragmentation stage on AP radiographs of the pelvis. The height of the lateral epiphyseal pillar is compared with the height of the normal contralateral epiphysis.

Group A: Lateral pillar intact
Group B: Lateral pillar collapsed but less than 50% of the normal side
Group C: Lateral pillar collapsed more than 50% of normal height

Management options

1. Conservative (supervised neglect)

NSAIDs, painkillers, physiotherapy and crutches, traction, hospital admission for acute exacerbations and regular outpatient follow-up.

---

[6] Catterall A (1971) The natural history of Perthes' disease. *J Bone Joint Surg* **53**(1): 37–53.

[7] Salter RB, Thompson GH (1984) Legg-Calvé-Perthes disease. The prognostic significance of the subchondral fracture and a two-group classification of the femoral head involvement. *J Bone Joint Surg Am* **66**(4): 479–89.

[8] Herring JA, Neustadt JB, Williams JJ, Early JS, Browne RH (1992) The lateral pillar classification of Legg-Calve-Perthes disease. *J Pediatr Orthop* **12**(2): 143–50.

2. Ambulation abduction brace

Bracing is controversial. Two studies concluded that bracing had not changed the natural history of the disease.[9, 10] This is a difficult type of treatment and there are concerns about when to start and when to finish bracing.

3. Operative containment

The theory behind containment is that development of a congruent joint is dependent on maximal contact between the immature femoral head and acetabulum.

- **Proximal femoral varus osteotomy.** This is not a de-rotation osteotomy although it can be combined with de-rotation to reduce anteversion and extension. Technically it is easier than a pelvic osteotomy but it shortens the leg and produces a prominent greater trochanter
- **Innominate osteotomy.** Can increase pressure on the femoral head. It is usually performed at a stage when stiffness of the pubic symphysis is an issue. A triple pelvic osteotomy is an aggressive form of management for the condition

4. Salvage procedures

- **Shelf arthroplasty.** Indicated in the older child to prevent subluxation and increase acetabular coverage
- **Chiari osteotomy.** Performed in the older child with little remodelling potential to increase the load-bearing area. May buy several years of pain-free hip function before further surgery is required
- **Valgus osteotomy.** For hinge abduction when an enlarged head is laterally extruded and impinges against the lateral acetabular rim on abduction, causing pain

- **Epiphysiodesis of the greater trochanter.** Patients with Perthes disease often exhibit relative overgrowth of the greater trochanter and shortening of the femoral neck that may result in a Trendelenburg gait and pelvic instability

Treatment guidelines by Herring

- **Patients who are less than 6 years of age:** there is no evidence that any form of treatment alters either the growth potential of the physis or the outcome, so the principle is to treat the symptoms
- **Patients who are 6, 7 or 8 years of age:** Group A are recommended to have symptomatic treatment. Group B do better with containment – either medical or surgical (it is controversial to mention medical containment although Herring mentions this in his article). Evidence on the effect of any treatment in Group C in this age group is inconclusive
- **Patients who are 9 years or over:** Group A are recommended to have symptomatic treatment while for patients in Group B and C there is a strong case for operative containment

When considering surgery think about:
- What is the **grade** of the disease?
- What is the **stage** of the disease?
- Necrotic or early fragmentation stage: game on for surgery
- Advanced fragmentation or later: the boat has been missed
- What is the **age** of the patient?

Stulberg's rating system at maturity[11]

Class I: Completely normal spherical head

Class II: Spherical femoral head with either coxa magna, short femoral neck or abnormally steep acetabulum

Class III: Non-spherical (ovoid, mushroom or umbrella shaped)

9 Meehan PL, Angel D, Nelson JM (1992) The Scottish Rite abduction orthosis for the treatment of Legg-Perthes disease. A radiographic analysis. *J Bone Joint Surg Am* **74**(1): 2–12.

10 Martinez AG, Weinstein SL, Dietz FR (1992) The weight-bearing abduction brace for the treatment of Legg-Perthes disease. *J Bone Joint Surg Am* **74**(1): 12–21.

11 Stulberg SD, Cooperman DR, Wallensten R (1981) The natural history of Legg-Calvé-Perthes disease. *J Bone Joint Surg* **63**(7): 1095–108.

Class IV: Flat femoral head, flat acetabulum

Class V: Flat femoral head but normal acetabulum

Three types of congruency were recognized:

1. Spherical congruency (Class I and II hips): arthritis does not develop
2. Aspherical congruency (Class III and IV hips): mild to moderate OA develops in late adulthood
3. Aspherical incongruency (Class V hips): severe arthritis develops before the age of 50 in these hips

Stulberg's results showed that a lack of sphericity alone was not the only predictor of a poor outcome (congruency was more important).

Poor prognostic factors

- Children >6 years old
- Female: mature earlier with less remodelling potential
- Catterall's head-at-risk signs (clinical)
  - Obesity
  - Adduction contracture
  - Progressive loss of hip motion
  - Flexion with abduction
- Advanced stage of disease at diagnosis
- Advanced grade (loss of containment)
- Recurrent episodes of stiffness

Arthrogram

It is used to assess suitability for surgery in equivocal cases:

- Hinging or point loading acetabulum
- Good area of contact
- Will the hip medialize?
- Is containment possible?

Long-term consequences

- Coxa magna: enlarged head
- Coxa plana
- Coxa brevis: short neck and overgrowth of the greater trochanter as a result of premature femoral neck physeal growth arrest
- Hinged abduction

Examination corner

Paeds oral 1

AP radiograph of the pelvis with severe (obvious) Perthes disease

A spot diagnosis oral (learn to recognize pattern radiographs of particular conditions). Testing a candidate's ability to articulate the radiographic features of Perthes disease.

Candidate: This is an AP radiograph of a pelvis in a child. The most obvious features are at the right hip. There is fragmentation and lateral displacement of the femoral head, concentric widening of the joint space, areas of increased sclerosis and metaphyseal cysts. The appearances are very suggestive of Perthes disease.

Examiner: How do you manage Perthes disease?

Candidate: My initial management of Perthes disease would be conservative – analgesia and NSAIDs for pain relief. Regular review in clinic. Admission to hospital for bed rest and traction. Physiotherapy. Avoidance of activities that provoke pain.

Examiner: If the condition is not settling down what else would you do?

Candidate: I would perform an arthrogram.

Examiner: This is what we did; what can you see?

Candidate: This shows that there has been some lateral subluxation of the femoral head with pooling of the dye medially.

Examiner: So how will you proceed?

Candidate: If the patient is still having a lot of flare-ups and pain I would consider either a femoral de-rotation osteotomy or pelvic osteotomy. But it is very rare to need to do this. Most children with Perthes disease can be managed with supervised neglect.

Examiner: How many hospital admissions would it take before you would proceed towards surgery?

Candidate: About three.

Examiner: Humph, I would probably have a lower threshold for surgery.

Paeds oral 2

Similar AP radiograph of the pelvis demonstrating severe Perthes disease at the left hip

Examiner: Yes this patient has severe Perthes disease with gross flattening of the femoral head. You mentioned Gage's sign being a radiolucency of the lateral edge of the epiphysis, growth plate and metaphysis. What are the other Catterall's head-at-risk signs?

Candidate: We can see also see metaphyseal cysts, lateral sub-luxation of the femoral head, a horizontal growth plate and calcification of the lateral epiphysis on this radiograph indicating that the patient has severe Perthes disease.

Examiner: What clinical features are associated with a poor prognosis?

Candidate: A patient older than 6, who is female and has a marked restriction of hip movements with recurrent episodes of stiffness.

Examiner: So how do you treat Perthes disease?

Candidate: I would manage Perthes disease initially conservatively, so-called supervised neglect. Analgesia, regular follow-up in clinic, physiotherapy and hospital admission for severe exacerbations. In only very severe cases would I consider surgery, such as a femoral de-rotation osteotomy or pelvic osteotomy.

The management of Perthes disease is somewhat controversial. The literature is rather confusing as different authors have different indications for surgical treatment. In fact some surgeons are sceptical about whether surgical containment works at all. Other surgeons are much more aggressive. Walk the middle ground and stay away from controversy unless you know the subject very well. You are there to pass the examination not get the gold medal. Remember 50% of patients do well without treatment and the majority of the remaining 50% will do well into their 5th decade without treatment.

Paeds oral 3

Perthes disease

- Aetiology, classification and prognosis

Paeds oral 4

Radiograph of advanced Perthes disease of the hip

- Diagnosis
- Classifications: Catterall, Salter–Thomson, Herring

- Prognostic factors
- How would "you" manage this patient?

Coxa vara

Definition

Localized bone dysplasia characterized by decreased neck-shaft angle (<110°) due to a defect in ossification of the inferomedial femoral neck (Fairbank's triangle).

Epidemiology

- Incidence 1:25 000
- Bilateral in one-third to one-half of cases
- No clear pattern of inheritance has been established, but there are reports of positive family histories and of identical twins being affected

Aetiology

- Congenital (noted at birth). Often associated with a short femur or skeletal dysplasia. Nearly always unilateral
- Developmental (AD, progressive). Historically has been called infantile, develops over time
- Acquired (trauma, rickets, Perthes, SUFE)

A defect of enchondral ossification in a metaphyseal triangular fragment of the inferior femoral neck, where physiological shearing stresses cause fatigue of the local dystrophic bone, resulting in a progressive varus deformity.

Weinstein classification

- Coxa vara associated with hypoplastic femur or PFFD
- Coxa vara associated with congenital skeletal dysplasia
- Acquired coxa vara (trauma, metabolic diseases such as rickets, and Perthes)
- Adolescent coxa vara associated with SUFE
- Idiopathic infantile coxa vara

Clinical features

- In unilateral cases children present with a painless progressive limp. The limp is not antalgic, it is painless and the weight-bearing phase is not shortened. In bilateral cases a waddling gait is noted
- Examination reveals a prominent greater trochanter on the affected side and weakness of hip abductors
- Positive Trendelenburg test and gait
- In unilateral cases there will be a leg length discrepancy (2–3 cm) and the thigh and popliteal creases are uneven
- Decreased internal rotation of the hip is often present due to decreased femoral anteversion or true retroversion

Differential diagnosis

Congenital

- Proximal focal femoral deficiency
- DDH
- Achondroplasia
- Associated with fibula hemimelia
- Bone dysplasia

Acquired

- Rickets
- SUFE

Radiographic assessment

Hilgenreiner's epiphyseal angle (HEA): the angle between Hilgenreiner's line and a line drawn along the femoral capital physis. The normal angle <25° (Figure 22.4).

Weinstein *et al.*[12] found that if the HEA was:
- <45°, deformity corrects spontaneously
- 45°–60°, outcome is uncertain and unpredictable – observe
- >60°, all patients will progress and therefore require corrective surgery

[12] Weinstein JN, Kuo KN, Millar EA (1984) Congenital coxa vara. A retrospective review. *J Pediatr Orthop* **4**(1): 70–7.

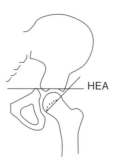

Figure 22.4 Measurement of Hilgenreiner's epiphyseal angle (HEA)

Management

The aim of surgery is to correct the neck shaft angle to 140°, HEA to less than 35°–40° and femoral anteversion (or retroversion) to a more physiological value.

Many types of osteotomy are described but the method is not critical as long as the aims of surgery are met. Among the intertrochanteric osteotomies the Pauwels Y-shaped and Langenskiöld valgus-producing osteotomies can give good results when the neck shaft angle is <80° (correction is difficult).

Limb length discrepancy

Definition

Leg length discrepancy (LLD) is a measurable difference in the overall length of the two legs, which can be true, apparent or functional.

Causes of leg length inequality (eight surgical sieves)

Congenital (small number but major difference in LLD)

- PFFD (inequality remains proportional to the length of the opposite limb)
- Congenital short femur
- Tibia/fibula hemimelia
- DDH
- Vascular malformations
- AV fistula
- Diffuse haemangioma

Trauma

- Diaphyseal fractures may lead to overlap and malunion. This is usually a static, non-progressive, small LLD
- Epiphyseal injuries can damage the growth plate. This may lead to partial (particularly Salter–Harris type 3 and 4) or complete growth plate arrest. If partial and the arrest is peripheral, it can cause a progressive angular deformity in addition to LLD

Infection

Growth plate arrest in septic dislocation (Tom Smith disease). Diaphyseal osteomyelitis can cause overgrowth due to bone hyperaemia.

Neurological

- Cerebral palsy, polio and spinal dysraphism

Neoplasms

- Neurofibromatosis, haemangioma

Skeletal dysplasia syndromes

- Hemihypertrophy and hemiatrophy syndromes
- Russell–Silver syndrome (shorter lower limb)
- Klippel–Trénaunay–Weber syndrome (asymmetrical limb hypertrophy)

Inflammatory conditions

- JCA (overgrowth)

Radiotherapy

Causes physeal damage and may lead to premature fusion of the growth plate.

Clinical evaluation

Standing

- Look for scoliosis, pelvic obliquity and joint contractures

- Stand on pre-measured blocks and reassess any scoliosis or pelvic obliquity
- Gait – short-leg gait. On the short side, stance stride is shorter and push-off reduced

Sitting

- Does the scoliosis correct? (If yes, then it is functional)

Supine

- Get a tape measure. True LLD measures the overall difference between the ASIS and the medial malleolus. Apparent LLD is measured between the umbilicus and xiphisternum to medial malleolus
- Galeazzi's test
- Thomas test to rule out flexion deformity of the hip
- Ankle – rule out equinus deformity
- Knee – flexion or hyperextension deformity
- Skin – previous operative scars, café-au-lait spots
- Temperature variation in the limb may indicate a haemangioma

Prediction of LLD

Green–Anderson tables

- Predict the remaining growth for the distal femur and proximal tibia according to skeletal age

Moseley straight line method

- Moseley converted the Green–Anderson tables into a straight line graph
- A logarithmic scale of predicting remaining limb growth along with expected discrepancy at maturity
- It assumes growth inhibition is constant and requires at least three scanogram measurements

White–Menelaus rule of thumb

- Used in the last few years of remaining growth (>10 years). This method assumes that:

- Distal femoral physis grows 9 mm per year (3/8 inch) (contributes 70% of femoral growth)
- Proximal tibial physis grows 6 mm per year (1/4 inch) (contributes 60% of tibial growth)
- Proximal femur grows 3 mm per year (1/8 inch)
- It further assumes that these physes fuse at the age of 16 in boys and 14 in girls
- Allows calculation of the discrepancy at maturity and the effect of epiphysiodesis. Reliable method as long as skeletal age is the same as chronological age

Eastwood and Cole method

- LLD measured using blocks or tape measure and the total discrepancy is plotted against chronological age. The points on the graph represent directly the pattern of increase in discrepancy
- Epiphysiodesis reference slopes are placed on the same graph

Bone age determinants (Greulich and Pyle atlas[13])

- AP films of the left wrist and hand are compared to radiographs in Greulich and Pyle atlas to determine skeletal age

Radiographic evaluation

Teleroentgenogram (grid films)

A single 3-foot radiograph of the entire lower limbs. Magnification distortion is minimal in small children, but it increases as the child grows bigger. Used in infants and young children.

Orthoroentgenogram

Also a 3-foot radiograph, but the radiographs are taken in three separate exposures centred exactly over the hip, knee and ankle to reduce magnification distortion.

[13] Greulich WW, Pyle SI (1959) *Radiographic Atlas of Skeletal Development of the Hand and Wrist*, 2nd revised edn. Stanford, CA: Stanford University Press.

Scanograms

Designed to avoid inaccuracies due to projectional errors. A series of radiographs of the hips, knees and ankles exposed separately to avoid magnification errors is taken with the child in the supine position with a metal ruler in between the extremities.

CT scanogram

Preferred method in patients with angular deformities or joint contractures. It measures the distance from the top of the femoral head to the medial malleolus. Allows a more accurate measurement of the whole limb length, and involves less exposure to radiation.

Management

It is widely accepted that LLD:
- <2 cm: managed conservatively
- 2–4 cm: epiphysiodesis is indicated in the longer limb
- >5 cm: lengthening ± epiphysiodesis is indicated

Epiphysiodesis (surgical growth arrest)

Open growth plate arrest (Phemister technique, 1933) has been replaced by percutaneous epiphysiodesis. Under radiographic control, a small window is cut in the peripheral part of the bone and the physis is curetted. This is usually performed 2–3 years prior to maturity on the distal femur or proximal tibial physis.

Staple epiphysiodesis is achieved by using 3 medial and 3 lateral staples. It is potentially reversible by removing the staples. It is less reliable than percutaneous epiphysiodesis, growth may not be retarded immediately and uneven inhibition may lead to condylar deformity. Attempts to correct more than 5 cm discrepancy may lead to miscalculation of limb growth potential or development of deformity due to uneven retardation of growth.

Lengthening procedures

Periosteal release

Useful adjuvant procedure particularly if a large LLD is anticipated. It can be repeated 4–5 years later although it is less effective. The procedure is performed by elevating and stripping the periosteal attachment adjacent to the growth plate.

Chondrodiastasis (physeal distraction)

Distraction force is applied progressively across the epiphyseal plate. The growth plate fractures, following which the bone is lengthened gradually and the distracted segment heals spontaneously. The operation is no longer widely used because initial lengthening is often followed by growth plate fusion. This has limited application and unpredictable results. Occasionally it is indicated for the correction of deformity sited at the level of the physis.

Diaphyseal lengthening

The diaphysis is divided and acutely lengthened by up to 3–5 cm. The lengthened bone is stabilized with a locked intramedullary nail. Supplementary bone graft is needed. The procedure remains unpopular because of a significant complication rate.

Diaphyseal osteotomy

The diaphysis is divided and followed by progressive distraction of 1.5 mm/day through an external skeletal fixation frame. Little new bone is formed within the gap and once the desired length is achieved the bone is fixed with a large plate with bone grafting across the callous bridge.

Ilizarov frame (circular)

The frame is formed by a series of full or half ring distractors and multiple small-diameter pins. The frame allows simultaneous correction of rotational and angular deformities as well as LLD. Corticotomy is performed at the lower metaphyseal level. Internal fixation and bone grafting are rarely required. The disadvantages of this frame are a steep learning curve, a long initial operating time and tethering of muscles.

De Bastiani Orthofix

A unilateral frame, which allows only distraction. Once attached it does not allow angular or rotational correction.

Complications

Many serious complications can occur with leg lengthening:
- Pin tract infection, loosening of pins
- Osteomyelitis
- Deformity of adjacent joints
- Nerve palsies
- Vascular injuries
- Muscle contractures and weakness
- Premature consolidation
- Malunion, delayed union and non-union
- Re-fracture after fixation removal
- Angular and rotational deformity

The safe limit of lengthening is 15% of the original bone length.

Examination corner

Paeds oral

Clinical picture of a child standing with one leg on a wooden block

- Causes of leg length discrepancy
- Causes of undergrowth
- Causes of overgrowth
- Pathology of osteomyelitis

Picture of CT scanogram

Discuss the potential pitfalls with this technique

Cerebral palsy

Definition

A permanent and non-progressive motor disorder due to brain damage before birth or during the first 2 years of life. The lesion is static but the clinical picture is not.

Incidence

- 2 per 1000

Aetiology

- Prenatal: placental insufficiency, toxaemia, smoking, alcohol, drugs, infection such as toxoplasmosis, rubella, CMV and herpes type II (TORCH)
- Perinatal: prematurity (most common), anoxic injuries, infections, kernicterus, erythroblastosis fetalis
- Postnatal: infection (CMV, rubella), head trauma

Classification

There is no universally accepted and satisfactory classification system for CP. It is best considered in terms of either physiology or anatomy.

Physiologic classification

- Spastic (pyramidal system, motor cortex)
- Athetoid (extrapyramidal system, basal ganglia)
- Ataxia (cerebellum and brainstem)
- Rigid (basal ganglia and motor cortex)
- Hemiballistic
- Mixed (combination of spasticity and athetosis)

Anatomical classification

- Monoplegia (one limb involved)
- Hemiplegia (one side of the body)
- Diplegia (lower limbs)
- Quadriplegia or total body involvement

Orthopaedic evaluation

The persistence of two or more primitive reflexes (Moro startle reflex, parachute reflex, tonic neck reflex, neck righting reflex and extensor thrust) usually means the child will be non-ambulatory.

Main problems with the musculoskeletal system are:

- Spasticity
- Lack of voluntary control

- Weakness
- Poor co-ordination
- Sensory impairment

Spasticity causes deformities that follow a staged pattern:

1. Dynamic contractures
   - Increased muscle tone and hyperreflexia
   - No fixed deformity of joints
   - Deformity is overcome during examination
2. Fixed muscle contractures
   - Persistent spasticity and contracture
   - Shortened muscle tendon units
   - Fixed deformity of joints: cannot be overcome
3. Fixed contractures with joint subluxation/dislocation and secondary bone changes

Gait disorders are the most common problem. The use of computerized gait analysis and force plate studies allows an individualized management plan.

Hoffer classification of ambulation potential

Ambulation is classified to four grades:

Grade 1   Community ambulator
Grade 2   Household ambulator
Grade 3   Therapeutic ambulator
Grade 4   Non-ambulators

General management

- A comprehensive assessment of a child with CP is essential in order to plan appropriate management. Because of the multiplicity of problems, a multidisciplinary team is required
- Evaluation and management plans should be organized for motor, sensory and cognitive problems such as: epilepsy, speech and hearing difficulties, visual defects, feeding difficulties, learning and behavioural problems
- Orthopaedics can only address spasticity problems and the deformity caused by the spasticity. The common sites of involvement are:
  - Spine deformity
  - Hip joint subluxation/dislocation
  - Flexion deformity of the knee

- Foot and ankle abnormalities
- Flexion deformity of the hand

The general interventional plan is to perform soft-tissue procedures early and bony procedures later.

Management options

- Dynamic contractures. Physiotherapy (stretching and casting), orthotic use, selective posterior rhizotomy, intramuscular *Botulinum* injection
- Fixed deformity. Tendon release or lengthening, muscle transfer, split tendon transfers
- Bony abnormalities. De-rotation osteotomy or joint arthrodesis

Clinical features

Spine

Scoliosis is the most common presentation. Requires surgical correction if curves are 50°–60° or there is worsening pelvic tilt. Custom moulded seat inserts allow better positioning but do not prevent curve progression. Bracing is controversial and is unlikely to stop curve progression but may be able to delay it.

Scoliosis curves are divided into Groups I (ambulators) and II (non-ambulators):

- Group I (double small curves with thoracic and lumbar involvement): managed with posterior fusion
- Group II (large lumbar or thoracolumbar curves): requires anterior and posterior fusion. If there is a significant pre-existing pelvic obliquity then fusion to the sacral joint is also needed to achieve adequate curve correction

Hip subluxation/dislocation

If hips dislocate they can be painful and make nursing difficult. Dislocation can contribute to pelvic obliquity and scoliosis.

Hip at risk

- Abduction <25°. Femoral head uncovered <50% (using Reimer's index on AP radiographs to give the migration percentage; Figure 22.5)

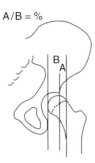

A/B = %

Figure 22.5 Hip migration index. The percentage of the femoral head that falls outside the acetabulum

- Managed with abductor tenotomy. Iliopsoas tenotomy can be performed at the same time but avoid in patients who can walk

Hip subluxation

- Head uncovered >>50%
- Femoral varus osteotomy (de-rotation and shortening)
- Additional pelvic (Dega's in a growing child and Chiari post maturity) osteotomy is occasionally necessary

Hip dislocation

- Early: open reduction, femoral shortening and varus de-rotation osteotomy
- Late: previously left out, now Girdlestone resection, excision with interposition
- In an older patient with complete dislocation consider valgus osteotomy with plate fixation. The proximal femur is shortened and placed in a marked degree of valgus to facilitate abduction and prevent articulation of the deformed femoral head against the pelvis

Windswept hips

- Characterized by abduction of one hip and adduction of the contralateral hip
- Adductor release
- Fixed deformity in an older child may need to be managed by a combination of varus osteotomy

on the abducted side and valgus osteotomy with shortening on the adducted side to create symmetry about the pelvis

Flexion contracture knee

- Spasticity of the hamstrings prevents the knee from fully extending at the end of the swing phase. As the hamstrings become tighter, knee extension is lost throughout the stance phase and the patient crouches. As the hamstrings become shorter, a fixed-knee-flexion contracture develops
- Spasticity of the quadriceps (co-spasticity) often co-exists. This may result in a stiff knee gait with impaired clearance (inadequate knee flexion) during the swing phase after lengthening (and therefore weakening) of the hamstrings
- If hamstrings alone are lengthened a stiff, flexed-knee gait becomes a stiff, extended-knee gait
- Indications for hamstring lengthening vary but guidelines are a popliteal angle of 90°–100° in non-ambulators and of 135° in ambulators
- Hamstrings are lengthened either proximally or distally, giving similar results
  - Proximal lengthening may increase lumbar lordosis
  - Distal lengthening may result in knee recurvatum if there is an uncorrected equinus contracture
  - Distal lengthening is preferred in ambulatory patients

Quadriceps contracture

- Rectus femoris distal tendon transfer to sartorius or iliotibial band is occasionally required to reduce quadriceps spasticity

Spastic crouch contracture

- Gait with flexed knees and hips, ankle dorsiflexion
- Either psoas or hamstrings or both are responsible
- May be precipitated by lengthening the Achilles tendon without addressing hamstring contractures

Foot and ankle

Ankle equinus

Caused by triceps surae contracture. Various surgical procedures are described for the correction of the equinus deformity:

1. **Baker's procedure**
   - An inverted U incision of the gastrocnemius aponeurosis is performed through a vertical midline incision in the middle one-third of the leg
   - Aponeurosis slides apart in a controlled and stable fashion
   - There is a high recurrence rate that makes re-lengthening virtually impossible
2. **Percutaneous Achilles tendon lengthening**
   - A triple hemisection technique, taking care to dorsiflex the foot only to the plantigrade position
   - Minimal scarring: the incisions are two lateral and one medial
   - The most unpredictable procedure especially in young children
3. **Technique for White sliding lengthening**
   - DAMP: **d**istal **a**nterior two-thirds, **m**edial two-thirds **p**roximal
   - Small risk of over lengthening
4. **Open Z-lengthening of Achilles tendon**
   - Neglected cases, severe deformity
   - Risk of over lengthening, calcaneus deformity and scar irritation (avoid placing incision to the side of the tendon)

If Achilles tendon lengthening is performed with tight hamstrings then a crouch gait occurs, and the child walks with their ankles maximally dorsiflexed and their knees flexed.

Hamstring tightness should be corrected at the same time as Achilles tendon lengthening.

Equinovarus

- Most often due to tibialis posterior spasticity although occasionally the tibialis anterior tendon is at fault
- Split tibialis posterior transfer involves rerouting half of the tendon dorsally to the peroneus brevis
- Split tibialis anterior tendon transfer to the cuboid is often combined with Achilles tendon and

tibialis posterior lengthening to manage a fixed equinovarus

Equinovalgus

- Spastic peroneal muscles pull the forefoot laterally
- Excessive valgus, external rotation and dorsiflexion of the calcaneus in relationship to the talus
- Management
  - **Grice arthrodesis**. Subtalar extra-articular arthrodesis performed through a lateral approach using a corticocancellous bone graft. Especially indicated in a growing child as it allows for full growth of the hind foot
  - **Subtalar fusion**
  - **Triple arthrodesis**. Operation of choice in children older than 12 years

Hands in cerebral palsy

- Surgery can achieve good cosmetic results but functional gains may be small
- Thumb in palm deformity is common but difficult to manage. Correction entails release of the adductor pollicis and first dorsal interosseous muscle, fusion of the MCP joint and rerouting of EPL
- Finger flexion contractures can be released by selective myotendinous lengthening in the forearm

---

Examination corner

Paeds oral 1

CP clinical photograph

Describe the diagnosis, classification, definition and management for hip problems in CP.

Paeds oral 2

Video clip of gait analysis in a child with scissors gait

Gait analysis in cerebral palsy includes:
1. Stability in stance phase
2. Foot clearance in swing

3. Normal initial contact
4. Step length
5. Energy conservation

Paeds oral 3

Video clip of scissors gait

Describe the gait.

Scissoring during gait is due to adductor spasticity. Legs are flexed slightly at the hips and knees, giving the appearance of crouching, with the knees and thighs hitting or crossing in a scissors-like movement. The typical features include:
- Rigidity and excessive adduction of the leg in swing phase
- Plantar flexion of the ankle
- Flexion at the knee
- Adduction and internal rotation at the hip
- Contractures of all spastic muscles
- Complicated assisting movements of the upper limbs when walking

Paeds oral 4

Examiner: What is cerebral palsy?

Candidate: CP is a permanent and non-progressive motor disorder due to brain damage before birth or during the first 2 years of life. The lesion is static but the clinical picture is not.

Examiner: How do you classify CP?

Candidate: CP can be classified either anatomically or physiologically. Physiological categories include spastic, athetoid, ataxia, and rigid or mixed varieties. The anatomical types include monoplegia, hemiplegia, diplegia and quadriplegia.

Examiner: What part of the brain is affected with athetoid CP?

Candidate: The extrapyramidal system, basal ganglia.

Paeds oral 5

Exactly the same questions as oral 4 (although I think it was a different examiner).

However, the examiner did not like the definition of CP, the sticking point being "non progressive". The examiner considered the disorder a progressive one. The candidate stuck to their guns and mentioned that although the lesion is static the clinical picture is not.

There was a bit of to and fro between the candidate and examiner about this point. [Pass]

Candidate: The examiner did not know the definition of CP particularly well and we spent a while arguing about whether the condition was progressive or non-progressive. It was a bit off-putting and was not the best way to start the oral off.

Paeds oral 4 and 5 highlight luck on the day. You may get one examiner who is happy with your answer or a different examiner who isn't and they will grill you and make things difficult and awkward for you.

Paeds oral 6

Clinical photograph of child with total-body-involvement CP

- Define CP
- Classify CP

Neurofibromatosis

Definition

Autosomal-dominant disorder of neural crest origin, which is often associated with neoplastic and skeletal abnormalities. There are two major types:
- Peripheral (Nf-1)
- Central (Nf-2)

Neurofibromatosis type 1 (peripheral neurofibromatosis or von Recklinghausen's disease)

- Incidence 1: 4500
- Autosomal-dominant gene mutation at chromosome 17
- The manifestations vary but all carriers will have some clinical features (100% penetrance)
- Neurofibromas are Schwann cell tumours

Diagnosis

Two or more of the following criteria are diagnostic:
1. At least five café au lait spots (5 mm child, 15 mm adult)
2. More than two neurofibromas or one plexiform neurofibroma
3. Axillary, groin and base of neck freckles
4. Optic glioma
5. Two or more Lisch nodules (benign iris hamartomas)
6. Osseous lesions: long bone cortex thinning with or without pseudoarthrosis, dystrophic scoliosis
7. Positive family history: first-degree relative with Nf-1

Musculoskeletal manifestations

- Scoliosis
- Extremity hypertrophy
- Pseudoarthrosis of long bones (tibia, ulna, humerus)
- Peripheral or spinal nerve tumour

Radiology

- Cortical bone defects: usually caused by neurofibromatosis tissue irritating the periosteum
- Bone cyst formation: due to proliferation of tissue within the medullary canal
- Bowing of long bones
- Pseudoarthrosis of long bones

Scoliosis

The spine is the most common site of skeletal involvement. There are two types: dystrophic and non-dystrophic.
- Features of **non-dystrophic** scoliosis are similar to those of idiopathic scoliosis
- Feature of **dystrophic scoliosis** include:
  - Posterior vertebral body scalloping (saccular dilation of the dura)
  - Enlarged neural foramina (dumb bell tumour)
  - Rib or transverse process pencilling
  - Short, tight, sharply angulated curves that involve only a few vertebrae with severe apical rotation and wedging
  - Soft-tissue masses
  - Defective pedicles

Management

Non-dystrophic scoliosis is managed as idiopathic scoliosis.

A dystrophic curve is relentlessly progressive even when growth has finished, cannot be controlled by bracing and requires early fusion.

There can be associated kyphosis and correction deformity carries a high risk of paraplegia, pseudoarthrosis and loss of correction after anterior and posterior fusion.

Neurological involvement is common and may be caused by the deformity itself, soft-tissue mass, intraspinal tumour or dural ectasia (saccular dilation of the dura). MRI is therefore mandatory preoperatively.

It is not the condition itself that is the problem, but the amount of expression of the disease.

Examination corner

Paeds oral 1

Clinical photographs

- Severe scoliosis with café-au-lait spots (distinguishing feature)
- Thoracolumbar radiograph demonstrating short dystrophic curve

Paeds oral 2

- Neurofibromatosis diagnostic criteria
- Inheritance and chromosome defect

Pes cavus

Definition

A high arched foot deformity where the longitudinal arch fails to flatten with weight bearing. There is fixed plantar flexion of the forefoot relative to the hindfoot. Clawing toes are almost always present.

Classification

Congenital

- Idiopathic
- Arthrogryposis
- Residual congenital talipes equinovarus

Acquired

- Neuromuscular disorders:
  - Muscular: muscular dystrophies
  - Peripheral nerves: HMSN, polyneuritis
  - Spinal cord: spinal dysraphism, polio, spinal tumours, tethered cord, spina bifida
  - Central: cerebral palsy, Friedreich's ataxia, Charcot–Marie–Tooth disease
- Trauma: compartment syndrome, crush injuries

There are four basic types (Table 22.1).

Most idiopathic cases are simple cavus, whereas neurological cases are usually cavovarus. The cause of pes cavus is neurological until proven otherwise. Therefore, a thorough neurological examination is mandatory.

Coleman's lateral block test assesses hindfoot flexibility in the cavovarus foot. A flexible hindfoot corrects to neutral when a lift is placed under the lateral aspect of the foot.

Idiopathic pes cavus

- Presents in adolescence/adult life
- Pressure effects on the deformed foot
- Painful calluses are present under prominent metatarsal heads
- ±Associated claw toes – callosities over the dorsum of IP joints

Table 22.1 Classification of pes cavus

	Forefoot	Hindfoot
Simple	Balanced	Neutral
Cavovarus	Plantar flexed	Varus
Calcaneus	Fixed equinus	Calcaneus
Equinovarus	Equinus	Equinus

Neuromuscular pes cavus

- Presents earlier with concern about the appearance of the foot, difficulty with shoe fitting, excessive uneven shoe wear (lateral aspect of the forefoot) and recurrent giving way into inversion of the ankle
- Loss of sensation can lead to neuropathic ulcers over prominent bones (5th metatarsal)

Management

Non-operative management is rarely successful, and includes arch supports and special shoes.

Operative options for supple deformities

Plantar release with or without tendon transfers:
- Indicated in children <10 years old
- Fascia is cut while applying tension by dorsiflexion to the metatarsal joints
- Release the abductor hallucis fascia if it is tight
- Medial plantar release is indicated in fixed varus angulations
- Medial release involves releasing the medial structures such as the talonavicular joint capsule, the superficial deltoid ligament, and possibly the long toe flexors
- Consider transfer of tibialis anterior into the midtarsal region for flexible inversion deformity

Jones procedure
- Performed for clawing of the hallux with associated weakness of tibialis anterior muscle
- This procedure involves transferring the extensor hallucis longus to the neck of the first metatarsal with arthrodesis of the IP joint
- Improves dorsiflexion and removes deforming forces at MTPJ
- The most common complication is non-union of the IP joint

Operative options for rigid deformities

Calcaneal osteotomy
- Dwyer type of medial opening wedge osteotomy
- Performed for hindfoot involvement

- Usually combined with plantar fascia release
- Translate the distal and posterior calcaneal fragment laterally

Beak triple arthrodesis
- Indicated in rigid deformity once growth has ceased
- The technique involves mortising the navicular into the head of the talus and depressing the navicular, cuboid and cuneiforms to improve the forefoot cavus deformity
- Lengthening of tendo Achilles may be required
- This procedure is complex and technically demanding

Examination corner

Paeds oral

- Clinical photograph of pes cavus deformity
- Discussion of the Jones procedure

Congenital talipes equinovarus (CTEV)

Definition

A deformity in which the forefoot is in adduction and supination, and the hindfoot is in equinus and varus.

Epidemiology

- 1 per 1000 Caucasians, 3 per 1000 Polynesians
- ♀:♂ 2:1, bilateral 50%

Aetiology

Despite much research, the exact pathogenesis and aetiology remain obscure. Most infants who have clubfoot have no identifiable cause. Histological anomalies have been reported in every tissue in the clubfoot (muscle, nerve, tendon insertions, ligaments, vessels). Numerous theories include:
- Primary germ plasm defect
- Mechanical moulding theory: fallen out of favour in recent years

- Neurogenic theory: histochemical abnormalities secondary to denervation changes in various muscle groups of the foot
- Myogenic theory: primary muscle defect. Predominance in type I muscle fibres, fibre type IIB deficiency and abnormal fibre grouping
- Arrest of normal development of the growing limb bud
- Congenital constriction annular bands
- Retracting fibrosis: increased fibrous tissue and localised soft tissue contractures found in the muscles and ligaments of the clubfoot
- Familial incidence but precise genetics are unknown (25% of patients with CTEV have a positive family history)
- Viral causes

Pathology

- Malalignment of the talocalcaneal, talonavicular and calcaneocuboid joints fixed by contracted joint capsules, ligaments and foot/ankle tendons
- **Tendon contractures** include tibialis anterior, extensor hallucis longus, Achilles tendon, tibialis posterior, plantar aponeurosis, abductor hallucis, flexor digitorum brevis, extensor digitorum longus
- **Ligament contractures** include spring, bifurcate, deltoid, calcaneofibular, talofibular and calcaneonavicular (spring) ligaments
- **Joints**
- Ankle and subtalar joints: are in fixed equinus
- Hindfoot:
  - Heel inverted (varus)
  - Talus lies in equinus with its head palpable at the sinus tarsi and marked medial angulation of the head and neck of talus
  - Calcaneus is in equinus, varus and internal rotation
- Midfoot: navicular and cuboid are medially displaced
- Forefoot: inverted, adducted with forefoot supination relative to the hindfoot (forefoot varus)

Clinical assessment

- Examine the whole child to exclude associated abnormalities: myelomeningocele, intra-spinal tumour, diastematomyelia, polio, CP
- Also look for any associated developmental syndrome: arthrogryposis, diastrophic dysplasia
- Look for other moulding conditions
- Examine the spine (neurological cause)
- Pulses: usually present but vascular dysgenesis is possible. Dorsalis pedis artery may be absent
- Creases: medial, plantar, posterior
- Affected limb may be shortened, calf muscle is atrophic, and foot is short compared to opposite side

Investigations

- Radiographs
- MRI scan of the spine (if a neurological cause is suspected)

Scoring systems

There are various scoring systems described. The Pirani scoring system is a simple scoring system based on three midfoot and three hindfoot features. Each is considered as normal, moderately abnormal or severe abnormal. Maximum score is 6 points:

- Hindfoot contracture score (maximum score = 3 points)
  - Posterior crease
  - Equinus rigidity
  - Heel configuration
- Midfoot contracture score (maximum score = 3 points)
  - Medial crease
  - Talar head coverage
  - Curvature of the lateral border

The Clubfoot Assessment Protocol (CAP) is a more complicated system based on the degree of joint mobility.

Dimeglio classification (1995)

Based on the mobility of the clubfoot deformity.

Stiff: Irreducible
Severe: Slightly reducible
Mild: Partially reducible
Postural: Totally reducible

Harrold and Walker classification

Based on the reducibility of the equinovarus deformity by manipulation:

Grade I: Foot that can be manipulated to or beyond neutral

Grade II: Varus and/or equinus manipulable to within 20°

Grade III: Varus and/or equinus not manipulable to within 20°

Radiographic assessment

Weight-bearing AP view (Kite's)

- On AP view the talocalcaneal (Kite's) angle is normally 20°–40° (<20° is seen in clubfoot; Figure 22.6)
- The first metatarsal talus angle is between the longitudinal axis of the 1st metatarsal and that of the talus and is normally 0°–20° (a negative angle is seen in CTEV)

Forced dorsiflexion lateral view (Turco's)

- Turco's talocalcaneal angle is normally >35°. In CTEV, the angle is decreased and parallelism of calcaneus and talus is often seen

Management

Initially management is conservative regardless of the severity of the deformity. Serial casting and splinting are advised.

Ponseti casting technique

Serial casts or splints weekly for a month and biweekly for 3 months. Sequence of correction is:
- Correction of cavus
- Correction of adduction and heel varus
- Correction of equinus
- Achilles tenotomy in 90% of cases (under local or general anaesthetic)

Advocates assert nearly every case of idiopathic CTEV can be successfully treated this way. Critics note that this procedure is not a non-surgical technique.

Surgery

The aim is to achieve a plantigrade, pliable, cosmetically acceptable, pain-free foot (Ponseti).

Posteromedial release

- Cincinnati incisions: transverse incision around hindfoot
- Identify and preserve the neurovascular bundle and the sural nerve
- Z-lengthening of tendo Achilles
- Divide and lengthen TP, FHL and FDL
- Capsulotomies: ankle posteriorly, subtalar joint, calcaneocuboid joint
- Release plantar ligament, abductor hallucis, FDB
- Repair tendons and insert K-wires into the talus and calcaneus to hold reduction

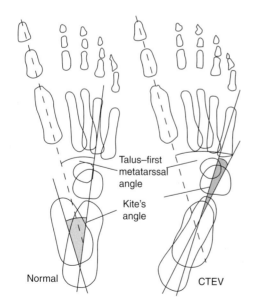

Talus–first metatarsal angle

Kite's angle

Normal   CTEV

Figure 22.6 Radiographic evaluation of club foot

Residue deformity

Consider spinal cord MRI to rule out spinal lesion. Must exclude a neurological cause. Residue deformity may be either:

- Dynamic
- Fixed

If it is dynamic consider SPLATT (split ant. tibialis transfer) tendon transfer if the patient is unable to actively evert their foot.

When the deformity is fixed consider a repeat release if there is not too much scarring and the patient is less than 5 years old. This is difficult, and in general poor results are reported. If patients are older than 5 years they need bony procedures to straighten the lateral border of the foot.

Adduction deformity

- Calcaneocuboid fusion (Dillwyn Evans procedure)
- Metatarsal osteotomy

These two procedures allow for lateral border shortening. Lengthening the medial border of the foot is rarely performed.

Hindfoot deformity

- Varus heel
- Opening medial wedge or laterally based closing wedge osteotomy of the calcaneum
- Residue cavus and adductus
- Wedge tarsectomy
- Salvage
- Triple arthrodesis salvage procedure for stiff, painful foot in patients >12 years old

Ilizarov multiplanar external fixator

- Can be used as a primary procedure but is generally reserved for recurrent CTEV

Complications of surgery

- Acute hypertension (unknown cause)
- Overcorrection
- Infection, wound breakdown
- Stiffness/restricted range of movement
- AVN of the talus
- Scarring

- Rocker bottom deformity
- Residue deformity (under-correction)

Examination corner

Paeds oral

Clinical photograph of bilateral clubfeet
Discussion about causes: arthrogryposis, dysraphism
Association with DDH

Curly toes

- Common disorder in children
- Frequently runs in families
- Often bilateral, look for symmetrical deformity in the opposite foot
- There is malrotation of one or more toes along with a digit flexion deformity (contracture of FDL and FDB)
- Noticed when child walks
- Usually asymptomatic
- Child may occasionally complain of discomfort, their toe may catch when putting their socks on, callosity of the dorsum of the toe with footwear

Management

- Conservative approach is mainstay of management
- Surgical management involves FDL tenotomy at age 4 years
- Girdlestone procedure is a flexor to extensor tenotomy that has gone out of favour. It is technically difficult and often produces stiff toes in extension with a rotational element

---

Examination corner

Paeds oral

Clinical picture of child with curly toes

- Management is conservative and operative

Tarsal coalition

Definition

A disorder of primitive mesenchymal segmentation and differentiation leading to fusion of tarsal bones and rigid flat foot. The coalitions can be fibrous (syndesmosis), cartilaginous (synchondrosis), or osseous (synostosis).

Calcaneonavicular (C-N) coalition

- Most common tarsal coalition, occurs in two-thirds of cases
- Rigid flat foot with contracture of the peroneal tendons, lateral foot pain and limited subtalar movement
- Radiographs: blunting of the subtalar process, narrowing of the posterior subtalar joint, elongated anterior calcaneal process, talar beaking
- Calcaneonavicular bony bridges are seen on lateral radiographs with the classic anteater nose sign arising from the calcaneus
- Presents between 8 and 12 years of age when ossification coalition occurs

Talocalcaneal (T-C) coalition

- Coalition between the calcaneus and talus may occur in any of the three facets. Usually involves the middle facet of the subtalar joint
- T-C coalitions account for approximately one-third of tarsal coalitions
- Pain in the medial side of the subtalar joint, repeated ankle sprains, patient is not able to take part in sports
- Contraction and spasm of the peroneal tendons with forced inversion, reduced subtalar movements
- T-C coalitions tends to ossify at 12–15 years of age
- T-C coalitions may be difficult to see on radiographs, which can often be normal. May see irregularity of the talus and calcaneus joint surfaces and occasionally the C sign of Lateur may be present
- Harris view – axial radiograph to visualize posterior and middle facet

Coalitions between calcaneum and cuboid, navicular and cuboid are rare.

Clinical features

- Visible peroneal spasm and flat foot
- Tenderness at the location of the coalition
- Antalgic gait
- Valgus hindfoot which on attempted correction induces peroneal spasm (peroneal spastic flat foot) and discomfort
- Calf pain
- Limited subtalar motion and peroneal tendon shortening
- In talocalcaneal coalition patients may have limited subtalar movement
- Increased laxity of the ankle joint

Investigations

- AP, lateral and oblique at 45° hindfoot radiographs. Harris views
- CT or MRI scan to rule out subtalar coalition. Coronal cuts are helpful in evaluating talocalcaneal bony bridges while transverse cuts are used for calcaneonavicular bars

Management

Conservative

- In children with mild symptoms
- Natural history unclear
- Supportive insoles or below-knee POP cast can be used

However, many children who present with pain have evidence of degenerative changes in the hindfoot joint. The vast majority of painful cases need surgical intervention.

Surgery options

Calcaneonavicular coalition

Ollier's approach. Wide bar excision such that one should be able to see across to soft tissues on the medial side of the foot through the excised bar. To prevent recurrence, all cartilage must be removed from both the calcaneus and navicular. Interposition of EDB into the defect reduces the risk of re-fusion.

Talocalcaneum coalition

Medial limb Cincinnati incision. FHL lies just plantar to the sustentaculum tali and the tendon can be used for orientation to the coalition anomaly. The FHL tendon sheath is incised, and the tendon is retracted inferiorly. The sustentaculum tali and its associated coalition are identified. Once the coalition is resected, interposition of one half of the FHL tendon will decrease the chance of recurrence.

Subtalar arthrodesis is performed when >50% of the middle facet is involved, with recurrence (failed resection), or if significant degenerative changes in the tarsal joints exist (talar beaking is not considered a degenerative change).

Triple arthrodesis may be indicated for severe symptoms with significant degenerative changes.

Arthrogrypotic syndromes

Definition

Congenital non-progressive limitation of joint movement due to soft-tissue contractures affecting two or more joints.

Many different subgroups exist but it is easier to group them into three major categories:
- Arthrogryposis multiplex congenita (classic form)
- In association with major neurogenic or myopathic dysfunction
- In association with other major anomalies and specific syndromes

Aetiology

- Exact cause is unknown; multifactorial as it is such a heterogeneous group, but factors likely to limit fetal movement in utero appear important

Arthrogryposis multiplex congenita (amyoplasia)

- Non-progressive congenital disorder with multiple congenitally rigid joints
- It is a sporadic disorder with no known hereditary pattern

- Incidence is variably quoted to be from 1 per 3000 to 1 per 50 000
- Aetiology is unknown, with possibly intrauterine viral infection, teratogenic or metabolic causes
- Joints develop normally in arthrogryposis multiplex congenita, but peri-articular soft-tissue structures become fibrotic, leading to development of an incomplete fibrous ankylosis and muscle atrophy
- The disorder can be myopathic, neuropathic, or mixed
- Associated with a decrease in anterior horn cells and other neural elements of the spinal cord
- Sensory function is maintained whilst motor function is lost

Clinical features

- Normal facies and normal intelligence. Head and neck movements are normal
- Skin creases are absent and there is tense, glossy, shiny skin. Muscle wasting
- Shapeless featureless cylindrical limbs
- Upper limbs: adduction and internal rotation of the shoulder, extension of the elbow, flexion and ulnar deviation of the wrist, fingers flexed at the MCP joints and IP joints, thumb adducted (similar to Erb's palsy deformity)
- Lower limbs: flexion, abduction and external rotation of the hip, teratological hip dislocations, knee contractures (flexion), equinovarus (club feet), vertical talus
- Spine: C-shaped neuromuscular scoliosis (33%)

Investigations

To establish the underlying diagnosis. Consider paediatrician, neurologist and clinical geneticist input.
- Nerve conduction studies, enzyme studies, muscle biopsy, chromosome analysis, collagen biochemistry, head scan (CT/MRI) and radiographs of the whole spine, anteroposterior pelvis and the involved limb

Management

Physiotherapy is an absolutely essential part of the management plan. The aim of management is to obtain maximum function, independent mobility and self-care.

- **Elbow**. Passive manipulation, serial casts, tendon transfer, posterior elbow capsulotomy, possibly osteotomies after the age of 4 years. One elbow should be left in extension for use of crutches when walking and the other in flexion for feeding
- **Wrist**. Flexion deformity common. FCU to extensor carpi radialis transfer and volar capsulotomy may be beneficial
- **Hand**. Release of thumb and palmar deformity by adductor pollicis lengthening, MCP joint fusion can be considered
- **Hips**. Surgery is nearly always associated with stiffness, which can be more disabling than a dislocated, but mobile, hip. In general unilateral dislocation is managed surgically because of concerns over LLD and asymmetry. Management of bilateral hip dislocation is controversial and there are two schools of thought: either medial open reduction without risking disabling stiffness or leave it alone. For a stiff, located hip following surgery, excision of the upper end of the femur, creating a Girdlestone-type arthroplasty, is required
- **Knees**. Both fixed flexion and fixed extension are common. Fixed extension responds well to stretching and serial casting, although occasionally quadricepsplasty is required. Fixed flexion is difficult to manage and often requires extensive posterior soft-tissue release with prolonged splintage. Reoccurrence can occur and repeat surgery is difficult. Femoral osteotomy with or without shortening (avoids stretching neurovascular bundle) is used towards the end of maturity
- **Foot**. The most common deformity is equinovarus; more rarely, vertical talus is seen. Severe equinovarus is initially managed with extended soft-tissue release; reoccurrences may need talectomy. Congenital vertical talus does not prevent the patient from standing and walking but it may cause problems with shoe wear. Surgical correction is only carried out if absolutely necessary
- **Scoliosis**. Early surgical intervention is recommended – either posterior spinal fusion alone or combined with anterior spinal fusion

The aim is to have finished surgery by the time the patient is 7 years old, if possible. The surgical principle in arthrogryposis is to do no harm.

Examination corner

Paeds oral

Clinical photograph of a child with congenital arthrogryposis multiplex

- Spot diagnosis
- Discussion about hip dislocation and other associated syndromes

Short case 1

A 9-year-old boy with mild arthrogryposis

Spot diagnosis, bilateral operated club feet and featureless limbs.

Asked to assess the upper limb. Typical features are internal rotation of shoulders, posterior release of the elbow and triceps lengthening, flexion of the wrist and stiff fingers.

Brodie's abscess

This is a chronic localized bone abscess. The lesion is typically single and located near the metaphysis of the bone. Preferred sites are proximal femur, proximal and distal tibia.

Clinical features

Subacute cases present with fever, pain and periosteal elevation. Chronic cases often present with apyrexia with long-standing, dull pain. There may be a limp, often slight swelling, muscle wasting and localized tenderness. The patient is usually apyrexic and has few signs or symptoms to suggest an infection. The white cell count is often normal but the ESR may be raised.

Pathology

Typically a well-defined cavity in cancellous bone lined by granulation tissue containing seropurulent fluid (occasionally pus). The cavity is lined by granulation tissue containing a mixture of acute and chronic inflammatory cells. Typically no organisms are found but if one is present it is usually *Staphylococcus aureus* (60%).

Radiology

Well circumscribed, round or oval cavity 1–2 cm diameter, most often in the tibia or femoral metaphysis. Sometimes the cavity is surrounded by a halo of sclerosis (classic Brodie's abscess). Metaphyseal lesions do not cause a periosteal reaction, whereas diaphyseal lesions may be associated with cortical thickening and periosteal new bone formation. A bone scan reveals markedly increased activity.

Differential diagnosis

- Osteoid osteoma
- Ewing's sarcoma
- Langerhans cell histiocytosis
- Aneurysmal bone cyst
- Pigmented villonodular synovitis (PVNS)
- Giant cell tumour
- Non-ossifying fibroma

Management

Brodie's abscesses are usually managed with biopsy and surgical debridement followed by intravenous antibiotics.

Examination corner

Paeds oral 1

Brodie's abscess

- Diagnosis
- Differential diagnosis
- Further tests
- Management
- Options

- Surgical management including types of incision and techniques
- The examiner wanted to know what kind of material is seen at curettage

Paeds oral 2

Radiograph of classic Brodie's abscess in the distal metaphysis of the radius

Examiner: These are radiographs of a young boy who presents with a several week history of localized pain and swelling in his wrist. What do you think of his X-rays?

Candidate: There is a well-defined cavity in the distal metaphysis of the radius. There is no periosteal reaction but a halo of sclerosis surrounding the lesion. The radiograph is suspicious of a Brodie's abscess.

Examiner: These are his MRI scans, which did confirm the impression of a Brodie's abscess. How are you going to treat him?

Candidate: I would treat him conservatively initially with IV antibiotics and see if it settles down. The condition may resolve in time.[1] If necessary, with recurrent flare-ups, the abscess should be curetted out.

Examiner: What you find is that the wall of the cavity becomes sclerotic and lined by a thick membrane and cannot be easily penetrated by antibiotics. The patient is then prone to recurrent flare-ups of pain. You need to go in and scrape the cavity out.

---

[1] Incorrect answer. Some older textbooks suggest that the lesion in certain circumstances may be managed with oral antibiotics alone. Most orthopaedic surgeons would disagree with this and fail you if you mention it as primary management of the condition.

Genu valgum

Definition

Genu valgum is the Latin-derived term used to describe knock-knee deformity.

Aetiology

Physiological genu varum (bowed legs) gradually improves as the child starts to stand and walk. By the age of 18–24 months the legs are straight.

By 2–3 years of age lower limbs have evolved naturally to genu valgum (knock-knees). There is a gradual transition to physiological valgus by 7 years of age by which time the leg has assumed a normal adult value of 7°–8° valgus. Pathological causes of genu valgum include:

- Skeletal dysplasias: multiple epiphyseal dysplasia, Morquio's syndrome, Ollier's disease
- Primary tibial valga
- Previous trauma: asymmetrical growth arrest following fracture
- Metabolic bone disease, particularly renal osteodystrophy
- Iliotibial band neuromuscular contracture: polio
- Infection: causing asymmetrical growth arrest
- Tumours: osteochondromas
- Congenital: congenital absence of the fibula

Unilateral genu valgum is suggestive of pathological genu valgum.

Clinical examination

- Is it unilateral or bilateral? If bilateral, is it symmetrical or asymmetrical?
- Measure standing and sitting height to rule out skeletal dysplasia
- Measure the distance between the medial malleoli with knees touching. Measure the mechanical axis projecting down from the ASIS. In genu valgum it passes medial to the first metatarsal
- Determine the site of valgus angulation, the degree of tibial torsion (tibia valga is associated with excessive lateral tibiofibular torsion) and carry out Ober's test to rule out iliotibial band contracture

If genu valgum is marked, the symptoms include:

- Intoeing to shift weight over the second metatarsal so the centre of gravity falls in the centre foot
- Lateral subluxation of the patella
- Fatigue

Management

- 95% resolve spontaneously
- Consider surgery if the intermalleolar distance (between medial malleoli when the child is standing with knees touching) is >10 cm or >15°–20° valgus at age 10 years
- Hemiepiphysiodesis of the distal femur and/or proximal tibial growth plate by either stapling or fusing the medial-side physis
- If skeletally mature carry out a tibial or femoral osteotomy

Valgus deformity in adults is usually due to:

- Sequel childhood deformity
- Secondary osteoarthritis or rheumatoid arthritis
- Ligament injury
- Mal-united fracture
- Paget's disease

Examination corner

Paeds oral 1

Clinical picture of a child with genu valgum within the physiological limit

- Discussion of whether this is normal or abnormal
- How will you assess this child in the outpatient clinic?
- Management

Genu varum

Aetiology

Normal in children under 2 years old. Pathological causes include:

- Metabolic bone disease
- Vitamin-D-resistant rickets
- Vitamin D deficiency
- Hypophosphatasia
- Asymmetrical growth arrest or retardation
- Trauma
- Infection
- Blount's disease
- Skeletal dysplasia: metaphyseal chondrodysplasia, achondroplasia, osteogenesis imperfecta
- Neuromuscular: polio, spina bifida
- Congenital: deficient tibia with relatively long fibula

Clinical features

- Chief complaint is that the foot turns in
- Parents notice bowlegs
- Frequent cause of parental concern

Clinical examination

- Document height, weight and percentiles for age
- Examine pelvis, knees and feet
- Shortened limb relative to trunk may suggest dwarfing condition
- Document general appearance during standing and gait
- Notice deformity: is there gradual bowing or abrupt angulation?
- Gait is characterized by painless varus thrust in stance phase
- Measure the inter-condylar distance: the distance between the knees when the ankles are held together
- Internal tibial torsion: this is measured by the angular difference between the transmalleolar axis and the bicondylar axis of the knee
- Thigh foot angle: this is measured with the child in the prone position and knee flexed 90°, by observing the angle of the foot and the thigh

Indications for radiographs

- Deformity outside the normal range
- Deformity – unilateral or asymmetrical
- Child over 3 years
- Positive family history (bone dysplasia, syndromes or renal rickets)
- Short stature or disproportion (bone dysplasia or endocrine disturbance)

Radiographic evaluation

- **Tibiofemoral angle**: measures varus severity
- **Metaphyseal-diaphyseal angle**: formed by intersection of a line through the transverse plane of the proximal tibial epiphysis with a line through the transverse plane of the metaphysis. Normal is <11°

Tibia vara (Blount's disease)

Tibia vara is a growth disorder of the proximal tibial physis caused by repetitive trauma to the postero-medial proximal tibial physis from early walking on a knee with physiological varus alignment. The aetiology of late-onset tibia vara is unknown.

The infantile form is commonly bilateral and associated with internal tibial torsion. The late-onset or adolescent form presents as a painful, unilateral, slowly progressive varus deformity of the knee:

- Unilateral or bilateral, asymmetrical
- Often a varus thrust
- The metaphyseal-diaphyseal angle (Drennan's) >11°
- Upper tibial metaphysis is fragmented
- Upper tibial epiphysis slopes medially
- Upper tibial physis is widened laterally

Langenskiold's classification of tibia vara[1]

Type I: Medial metaphyseal beaking
Type II: Cartilage-filled depression
Type III: Ossification at the inferomedial corner epiphysis
Type IV: Epiphyseal ossification filling the metaphyseal depression
Type V: Double epiphyseal plate
Type VI: Medial physeal closure

Management

- Bracing for Langenskiold's stage I and II disease in patients <3 years old
- Surgery for failed orthotic management and Langenskiold's stages III–IV
- Initial operation is proximal tibial valgus osteotomy distal to the tibial tubercle to avoid damaging the tibial apophysis

---

[1] I think you need to be aware of this classification for the exam but without necessarily knowing specifics. You would however be expected to spot the diagnosis on a clinical photograph (an overweight child with severe genu varum) or radiograph. Recognition of the radiographic features of the disease is important.

- If growth arrest has occurred a physeal procedure also needs to be performed, either stapling or epiphysiodesis of the lateral tibial physis (selective closure of half of the growth plate to allow the contralateral portion of the physis to correct with growth) or rarely a partial physeal bridge resection with interposition of fat

For late-onset tibia vara, carry out a tibial osteotomy below the growth plate with correction of the tibio-femoral angle.

Examination corner

Paeds oral 1

- Spot diagnosis – unilateral Blount's disease
- Differential diagnosis
- Causes
- Management

Paeds oral 2

Clinical photograph of a young child with mild, bilateral genu varum

Candidate: This is a clinical photograph, which demonstrates mild bilateral genu varum. The most common cause of this is a benign normal variant in which the knee will evolve into genu valgum and then a normal adult valgus angle will develop in time.

Examiner: This child comes to clinic with her mother. The mother is worried about the appearance of the knees. How will you reassure her?

Candidate: I would say that it is a very common condition, which is seen often in the clinic. In the vast majority of cases, it is just a feature of normal growth and development of the leg, and corrects as the child grows. I would take a full history and examination so as to reassure the mother. I would want to exclude any pathological cause for the genu varum.

Examiner: (Interrupts with) What pathological causes are you thinking about?

Candidate: Conditions such as Blount's disease.

Examiner: (Interrupting) Come on, is the child black? How common is Blount's disease in a young white girl with normal build?

Candidate: Not common. (Regains composure.) I would want to exclude rickets, a skeletal dysplasia or a syndrome. Other

causes could include infection, trauma, tumours but these are usually unilateral.

Next picture: Clinical photograph of an obese girl, approximately 15 years old, with severe unilateral genu varum with gigantism of the limb

Candidate: (Big influx of breath as answer is prepared.) This is a clinical photograph of a young girl, which demonstrates a severe genu varum of the left leg and gigantism of this leg. The situation is grossly abnormal and I would be worried about a pathological cause for the condition.

Examiner: Can you name any causes that can give the limb this appearance?

Candidate: The causes of gigantism are an AV malformation, nerve tumours, neurofibromatosis, lymphoedema of the leg, a neoplasm or idiopathic.

[Pass]

Candidate: I did not sound very convincing to the examiners in how I would have reassured the mother in the first picture or, more accurately, the examiners seemed unimpressed with my answer. This was a failure to deliver the facts rather than any glaring omission. The examiner was making life just a little bit too uncomfortable. In the second picture I had never seen anything like it before. Luckily I managed to say something sensible in my answer. The examiner was stony-faced and gave no feedback on my answer. Even a simple topic like genu varum can be made difficult by an examiner's line of questioning.

Congenital pseudoarthrosis of the tibia

Rare condition, incidence 1:250 000. Almost always unilateral. This is one of the most challenging conditions to manage in orthopaedics. The condition may not be obvious at birth. Present with a spectrum of disorders, ranging from anterolateral bowing to frank pseudoarthrosis or pathological fracture with an apex deformity.

Classifications

Boyd[14]

Boyd's is the best known and most complete classification of the disease and the most appropriate

---

[14] Boyd HB (1982) Pathology and natural history of congenital pseudoarthritis of the tibia. *Clin Orthop Relat Res* Jun (166): 5–13.

one for use in clinical practice. There is no specific disease entity, but there are several types, each with its own pathology, prognosis and natural history. Cystic lesions tend to do better whilst the dysplastic type is less favourable.

Type I: Born with anterior bowing and tibial defect

Type II: Born with anterior bowing and an **hourglass constriction. Spontaneous fractures occur before 2 years of age.** Often associated with neurofibromatosis

Type III: Those developing **bone cysts** often at the junction of upper and lower thirds. Anterior bowing may precede or follow a fracture

Type IV: Those originating in a sclerotic segment of tibia without narrowing or fracture. The medullary canal is obliterated

Type V: Those who also have **a dysplastic fibula** develop pseudoarthrosis later

Type VI: Those with **an interosseous neurofibroma** or schwannoma (very rare)

Management

- Non-operative management includes prophylactic total contact bracing to try to prevent fractures or control developing ones
- Surgical management options include:
  - Intramedullary rodding and bone grafting
  - Vascularized fibular graft
  - Ilizarov frame
  - Syme's amputation

Open reduction internal fixation includes excision of fibrous tissue at the pseudoarthrosis site, removal of sclerotic bone and correction of anterolateral angulation. Osteotomies to correct anterolateral bowing are contraindicated.

Complications

- Re-fracture or non-union
- Stiffness of ankle and subtalar joints
- Limb shortening
- Progressive anterior angulation of tibia
- Infection
- Repeated operations
- Soft-tissue scarring

Fibula hemimelia

Definition

Consists of a spectrum of anomalies from mild fibula shortening to total absence of the fibula. It is the most common long bone congenital deficiency.

Classifications

Achterman and Kalamchi[15]

Type I: Hypoplastic fibula

Type Ia: Proximal fibular epiphysis is more distal, and distal fibular epiphysis more proximal, than normal. There may be a ball and socket ankle joint

Type Ib: More severe deficiency with at least 30%–50% of the fibula missing and no distal support to the ankle

Type II: Complete absence of the fibula. Angular deformities of the tibia are common and are associated with severe foot and ankle problems (tarsal coalition, lateral ray deficiencies)

Coventry and Johnson[16] *(3 types)*

Based on the degree of fibular dysplasia and whether the deformity is unilateral or bilateral:

Type I: Shortened fibula – partial absence of upper portion

Type Ia: Normal foot

Type Ib: Equinovalgus foot

Type II: Complete absence of the fibula and foot deformities, etc.

Type III: Bilateral

Clinical features

- LLD always present
- Antero-medial bowing with a dimple over the apex of the tibia
- Absence of lateral rays of the foot

[15] Achterman C, Kalamchi A (1979) Congenital deficiency of the fibula. *J Bone Joint Surg Br* **61B**: 133–7.

[16] Coventry MB, Johnson EW (1952) Congenital absence of the fibula. *J Bone Joint Surg Am* **34**: 941–55.

- Equinovarus of the foot
- Stiff hindfoot with tarsal coalition particularly talus and calcaneus
- Ball and socket ankle joint
- Flexion contracture of the knee
- Ankle and knee instability
- Femoral shortening (if associated with PFFD)

Management

Management is difficult and complex. Generally the following principles apply in deciding on reconstruction versus amputation:
- **Mild deformity**: reconstruct
- **Severe**: amputate
- **Intermediate**: obtain a second opinion
Reconstruction options include:
- Posterolateral release to correct equinovalgus deformity of the foot
- Limb lengthening is indicated if the foot and ankle are relatively normal
Syme's amputation is ablation of the foot by ankle disarticulation, producing a sturdy end-bearing stump that can be walked on.

Tibia hemimelia

Definition

The condition represents a spectrum of deformities ranging from total absence of the tibia to mild hypoplasia. It is often associated with PFFD or a congenital short femur. This is the only skeletal deficiency with a Mendelian pattern of inheritance. Both autosomal-dominant and recessive patterns are described. Thirty percent of cases are bilateral.

Classifications

Kalamchi (3 types)

Based on radiographs, clinical appearance and functioning of the quadriceps mechanism:

Type I: Complete absence
Type II: Absence of the distal half of the tibia
Type III: Hypoplastic

Jones classification

Classified into four types on the early radiographic appearance:
Type I: Absent tibia
Type II: Proximal tibia present
Type III: Distal tibia present
Type IV: Tibia shortened, proximal migration of the fibula and diastasis. Distal tibiofibular syndesmosis

Clinical features

- The involved leg is short with a varus or calcaneo-varus foot
- There is often a skin dimple over the front of the leg
- Quadriceps muscle is often underdeveloped or absent; there are various degrees of fixed flexion at the knee

Management

Reconstruction options include:
- Distal fibulotalar arthrodesis or calcaneal-fibula fusion to stabilize hindfoot
- Tibiofibular synostosis (fusion)
- Tibial lengthening with epiphysiodesis of the ipsilateral distal fibula and contralateral limb

Amputation

Through-knee amputation indicated in:
- Severe deformity
- If there is marked fixed-flexion deformity of the knee
- Knee is unstable
- Tibia is completely absent
Avoid above- or below-diaphyseal amputations, because of associated problems with overgrowth of the residue diaphysis.

Popliteal cyst

The common site is medial, originating in the gastrocnemius-semimembranosus bursa just below the popliteal crease. The cyst arises from the synovial sheaths of the surrounding tendons and contains clear viscous fluid. In contrast to those in adults they do not communicate with the knee joint and are not associated with intra-articular pathology:

- Presents at 5–8 years of age as a painless, firm, rubbery swelling behind the knee
- Usually asymptomatic and of insidious onset; occasionally can cause vague mild local discomfort
- The mass is fluctuant and transilluminable. The rest of the knee examination is normal
- Ultrasound and CT scan demonstrate the lesion well although this is not usually necessary unless the diagnosis is in doubt

Management

Reassure the child's parents that the lesion is benign; the vast majority will resolve in time and the lesion should be left alone.

There are very few indications for surgery:
- When the diagnosis is in doubt
- Severe pain (check for other more obvious causes)

There can occasionally be great parental concern about this swelling. The desire for surgery from parents must be fiercely resisted because the majority (90%) resolve in time, surgery is not without its risks and the cyst can reoccur following excision.

Examination corner

Paeds oral

Clinical photograph of a child with obvious swelling at the back of the knee

Spot diagnosis with discussion afterwards of management, particularly how you deal with awkward parents demanding surgery for their child (second opinion!).

Candidate: This is a clinical picture of a child, which shows an obvious swelling in the popliteal fossa. The swelling appears to be about 3 cm by 2 cm, the skin overlying the swelling appears normal. The picture is very suggestive of a popliteal cyst.
Examiner: How will you manage this condition?
Candidate: Popliteal cysts are benign lesions, the vast majority resolve in time, surgery is not indicated and parents should be reassured about the condition.
Examiner: How long on average do they take to resolve?
Candidate: Ninety percent resolve over a 4-year period.

Assessment of rotational profile

Generally present as either intoeing or outtoeing (Table 22.2).

Foot progression angle (FPA)

Describes the direction in which the foot points during gait and can be altered by any abnormality at any level in the leg. The angle made by the feet with an imaginary straight midline on the floor. Normal –5° to +20°. Average +10°.

Range of hip rotation (Staheli)

Place the child in the prone position with their knee flexed at 90° and their ankle held in neutral position. The leg acts as a protractor indicating degrees of movement. Internal rotation (IR) is assessed by turning the legs away from the midline and external rotation (ER) by turning the legs one at a time towards the midline of the body. Normally IR is less than 70°. A value greater than 70° suggests anteversion of the femur. A normal value of ER is 20° and if it is less than 20° this suggests femoral anteversion.

Ryder method

For degree of femoral anteversion.

Place the child prone on the examination couch. Flex their knees to 90° and internally rotate their leg while palpating the greater trochanter. Rotate the leg

Table 22.2 Causes of intoeing and of outtoeing

	Causes of intoeing	Causes of outtoeing
• Most common causes	Persistent femoral anteversion	
	Metatarsus adductus	
	Internal (medial) tibial torsion	
• Femur and hip	Persistent femoral anteversion	Femoral retroversion
	Spasticity of internal rotators (CP)	Flaccid paralysis of internal rotators
• Leg and knee	Internal tibial torsion	External tibial torsion
	Genu valgum	
	Blount's disease	
• Foot and ankle	Pronated feet	Pes valgus
	Metatarsus varus	Talipes calcaneovalgus
	Talipes equinovarus	

until the greater trochanter is most prominent laterally. The degree of internal rotation at this point corresponds with the degree of femoral anteversion.

Normal value from approximately 40° at birth to between 10° and 15° in adults. Anteversion is likely to be present if internal rotation exceeds 70° and external rotation is less than 20°.

Foot thigh angle (FTA)

Tibial torsion is assessed by observing FTA. Flex the patient's knee to 90° and hold the ankle in neutral position by applying gentle downward pressure on the sole of the foot. Estimate the angle made by an imaginary straight line along the axis of the thigh and an imaginary line along the axis of the foot. Normally FTA is 10°–20° in external tibial torsion. If it is less than 10°, this indicates internal (medial) tibial torsion.

Transmalleolar-thigh angle

Tibial rotation is measured using the transmalleolar axis. This angle is derived from a line along the longitudinal axis of the thigh compared with a line perpendicular to the axis of the medial and lateral malleolus. Normal value is 0°–45°. If negative this suggests internal tibial torsion.

Examination corner

Paeds oral 1

Clinical measurement of anteversion of a femoral neck

- Description of Ryder's method
- Intoeing due to medial femoral torsion: assessment of severity (internal hip rotation, W position) and indications for surgery
- Torsional mal-alignment syndrome: features (increased Q angle, patellofemoral pain)

Paeds oral 2

Clinical photo of intoeing

How do you assess this child?

The trauma oral

23. Trauma oral topics 403
Abayomi Animashawun and
Paul A. Banaszkiewicz

Trauma oral topics

Abayomi Animashawun and Paul A. Banaszkiewicz

Introduction

The original plan was to write a concise account of orthopaedic trauma that would be all things to all candidates about to sit the FRCS (Tr & Orth) exam. The reality is that there are a lot of very good concise orthopaedic trauma textbooks available (to read and revise from). Therefore, what follows is an attempt to present an overview of the trauma oral section to give a candidate a flavour of what to expect. At the end of the chapter we discuss possible trauma long cases. Trauma long cases can be awkward as they usually involve complex management issues often secondary to complications from initial trauma care.

Differing oral styles

Many candidates regard the trauma oral as the easiest oral to pass. Perversely a fair number of candidates have come out of it saying it was the worst one of the lot. There seem to be broadly four styles of trauma oral that you may encounter in the examination:

1. The classic trauma oral

    A series of fast-moving slides where you describe the injury and your preferred method of management. There is barely enough time to catch your breath before the next slide is shown. This type of oral covers a lot of ground very quickly but the discussion is fairly superficial. It can be an enjoyable oral if you know your stuff well

2. The probing trauma oral

    The trauma oral where fewer slides are shown but the questions are more detailed and a more thorough answer is expected. Usually it contains one or more of the dreaded "describe the surgical approach you would use to fix this fracture" type of question

3. The complex trauma oral

    This is where complex trauma cases are shown and the discussion centres on the management of these difficult cases

4. The mixed trauma oral

    A combination of the above three styles: some straightforward questions, a couple of topics probed in detail and a couple of difficult fractures to discuss

A straw poll of candidates who recently sat the examination would seem to suggest most of the trauma orals were either style 1 or 4. Occasionally a candidate encountered oral style 2 or 3 but these were the exception. Essentially the style of trauma oral one gets depends on who examines you.

The classic trauma oral

With oral style 1 a large part of the exam can consist of straightforward bread and butter trauma cases that you come across on a daily basis in the fracture clinic. These should present no problem to the average candidate.

The oral usually consists of a series of fast-moving radiographs and clinical pictures. In the 30 min it is not uncommon to view upwards of over 15 slides.

Postgraduate Orthopaedics: The Candidate's Guide to the FRCS (Tr & Orth) Examination, Ed. Paul A. Banaszkiewicz, Deiary F. Kader, Nicola Maffulli. Published by Cambridge University Press. © Cambridge University Press 2009.

In general you are shown a radiograph, occasionally a clinical photograph or given a short history, etc.

Start off by describing the radiograph or clinical photograph in general terms. If possible classify the fracture (if appropriate). You are then most likely to be asked about the management of the condition, "what are you going to do next?".

It is not unreasonable to mention searching for other associated injuries (if the fracture is high velocity) and to discuss your initial resuscitation and management (of the injury). However, once you have alerted the examiner to this line of approach in the first couple of slides and set the tone, skip over it; do not keep repeating the same story line as it will slow you down, irritate examiners and not score you any points.

"Assuming that all things being equal and there are no other associated injuries or co-morbidity factors present and the patient is adequately resuscitated then I would manage this fracture with…"

You can either list various management options, discussing the pros and cons of each, or state your own management preference first and why you have chosen it over other possible methods of management.

When discussing management options the examiner may prefer that you answer how "you yourself" would manage the fracture rather than give the options available.

Candidate: This fracture is suitable for either conservative management initially in a long leg cast and then Sarmiento brace or closed reamed intra-medullary nailing.

Examiner: I didn't ask for the various treatment options I asked, "How are YOU going to manage this fracture?"

In many cases there will be several ways to manage a fracture and your own preferred method may be different to that of the examiners. If you suggest a particular management plan be able to defend your point of view if challenged by the examiners (assuming that it is a sensible option).

The probing trauma oral

Some examiners prefer to show fewer slides but expect a more thorough and detailed discussion of each one

shown. The style 2 orals are more likely to catch out the less prepared candidate. A candidate may only have a superficial working knowledge of trauma and be able to get through a rapid series of clinical slides without this being exposed. When grilled in detail about a trauma topic a lack of in-depth knowledge is easily uncovered by an examiner.

The complex trauma oral

The style 3 oral scenario probably arises because an examiner expects you to have a good working knowledge of the management of most trauma conditions. He or she therefore only shows you very difficult or complex clinical cases for you to discuss. This is the most difficult type of oral to deal with. Get the basics out first before jumping in with an elaborate management plan so at least you can score enough marks to scrape through. This is the nightmare type of oral, usually the last one of the day when everything seems to be going reasonably well and the end of the examination is in sight. The candidate is expecting to breeze through this final hurdle and then suddenly gets hit with an impossible oral, gets mixed up, starts to waffle and backtrack. Calm it down; get basic first principles out and hope you have done enough to pass.

The mixed trauma oral

There is not particularly much to say about a style 4 oral. It is neither one thing nor the other. Probably more difficult than style 1, it is probably easier to pass than either style 2 or 3.

There are certain key topics that tend to be asked in the trauma oral. Compartment syndrome is probably the most important topic to learn. You are almost certain to be asked about it and there are no excuses for not knowing this subject inside out and back to front. Ideally you should have gone through a couple of dry runs with a colleague so that you do not just answer the topic well, you go to town on it and murder it.

Other reasonably common topics are some sort of spinal fracture, a proximal humerus fracture or shoulder dislocation (usually posterior, spot diagnosis), a foot fracture, distal radius fracture and either a pelvic or acetabular fracture. There are usually two or three children's fractures shown as well.

As trauma surgeons we see a huge number of different fractures in the fracture clinic. It is therefore not uncommon to be shown two or three radiographs of some minor or obscure fracture that you will not have read about recently (mallet finger is a classic example and also a common question in the hands oral). With the experience gained from a reasonably busy trauma job you should be able to come up with some sort of half decent answer that satisfies the examiners, who will then hopefully move on to another topic, with which you are more familiar.

Scapula fractures

Scapula fractures account for fewer than 1% of all fractures and 3%–5% of shoulder girdle injuries. The mean patient age range is 35–45 years. RTAs account for 70% of all scapula fractures (50% motor car, 20% motor cycle). Major trauma is required to fracture the scapula so other injuries and complications are common (50%–90% of cases). In the majority of situations, closed management of these fractures is the norm.

Mechanism of injury

- Indirect – caused by axial loading on an outstretched arm
- Direct – usually high-energy trauma including falls from a height and RTA

The most common fracture site is the scapular body (35%) followed by scapular neck fractures (27%). Spine, glenoid and acromion fractures have similar occurrence rates.

Classification

Several classifications exist for scapula fractures. Ideberg's system[1] (1984) classifies intra-articular

fractures of the glenoid fossa. Mayo classification[2] (1998) is a modification of Ideberg's classification. The Zdravkovic[3] classification is based on anatomy.

Zdravkovic–Damholt classification of scapula fractures (1974)

Type I: scapular body fracture
Type II: coracoid or acromial fracture
Type III: scapular neck or glenoid fossa fracture

Clinical presentation

- Pain – with active/passive shoulder motion or deep inspiration
- Local tenderness
- Ecchymosis
- Local swelling
- Deformity – rare without associated clavicle fracture or ACJ separation

Imaging

- Often an incidental finding on a trauma skeletal survey
- AP/lateral scapular radiographs
- CT is useful for more complex fracture patterns, i.e. glenoid fossa

Management

- It is important to recognize the high incidence of associated life- and limb-threatening injuries
- Pulmonary injuries, including rib fractures, pulmonary contusions and haemo/pneumothorax (30% of cases)
- Significant closed head injury (33%)
- Ipsilateral clavicular fracture (25%)
- Brachial plexus and vascular injury

[1] Ideberg I (1984) Fractures of the scapula involving the glenoid fossa. In Bateman JE, Welsh RP (eds.) *Surgery of the Shoulder*. Philadelphia: Decker, pp. 63–6.

[2] Mayo KA, Benirschke SK, Mast JW (1998) Displaced fractures of the glenoid fossa: results of open reduction and internal fixation. *Clin Orthop* **347**: 122–30.
[3] Zdravkovic D, Damholt VV (1974) Comminuted and severely displaced fractures of the scapula. *Acta Orthop Scand* **45**: 60–5.

Simple fractures of the scapular body, even with significant displacement, may be managed by being closed in a sling followed by assisted mobilization. Displaced scapular neck fractures can result in a high incidence of residual disability. Greater than 40° displacement in the coronal/transverse plane or >1 cm medial displacement may require fixation. Displaced fractures of the glenoid, especially those associated with glenohumeral instability, need ORIF to prevent secondary osteoarthritic changes or shoulder instability. Malfunction of the rotator cuff may occur with spine fractures, and weakness on abduction and pain may follow. There is a risk of non-union with fractures at the base of the acromion with >5 mm displacement. The key factor that influences management of the scapula fracture is its effect on shoulder function including glenohumeral stability, rotator cuff function and glenohumeral movement. In recent years there has been a trend towards more thorough evaluation of these fractures as not all of them are benign, with a greater role of surgery for these fractures than previously was the case.

Surgical approach

- Anterior deltopectoral approach for anterior glenoid rim and coracoid fractures
- Posterior (Judet) approach for posterior glenoid rim, neck and glenoid fossa fractures
- Good/excellent results of surgical fixation as high as 79% have been reported in experienced hands

---

Examination corner

Radiograph of a glenoid fossa fracture

Classification system used
Indications for surgical fixation and surgical approach

Clavicle fractures

These account for 5% of all fractures and 35%–44% of fractures around the shoulder girdle. Caused by direct trauma in up to 91%–94% of cases and indirect trauma (fall on outstretched hand) in 6%–9% of cases.

The primary classification system divides fractures into medial third (5%), middle third (85%) and lateral third (10%) (Allman).

Neer's classification

Fractures of the lateral third are further divided based on the integrity of the coracoclavicular ligament (CCL) complex in relation to the injury:

Type I: Non-displaced

Type IIA: Fracture medial to conoid and trapezoid ligaments

Type IIB: Fracture between conoid and trapezoid ligaments

Type III: Fracture into the AC joint without CCL injury

Type IV: Epiphyseal separation (children)

Type V: Three-part fracture, with intact ligaments connected to middle fragment

Examination and investigation

- Neuromuscular examination – exclude brachial plexus injury
- Vascular injury – particularly the subclavian/axillary vessels
- Pneumothorax (3%)
- Open injuries or compromise of the skin
- Medial third fractures are usually associated with high-energy trauma and multiple injuries

Imaging

- AP radiographs
- 45° cephalic/caudal views
- Weight-bearing views of both shoulders are used to demonstrate ligament integrity in distal third fractures
- CT scan demonstrates intra-articular extension in medial/lateral third fractures

Management

Non-operative management

Broad arm sling or collar and cuff are the mainstay of non-operative management. Mobilize when clinical union occurs. Radiological union occurs after clinical union. Distal third fractures, types I and III, are usually managed conservatively.

Indications for operative management

- Open fractures
- Fractures with neurovascular injury
- Compromised overlying skin
- Floating shoulder
- Type II distal third fractures because of the high rate of non-union
- Polytrauma
- Symptomatic non-union or degenerate AC joint
- Greater than 1 cm of displacement or 2 cm of shortening

Contraindications for operative management

- Active infection in the operative area
- Prior soft-tissue irradiation of the operative area
- Burns over the clavicular area
- Significant co-morbidity medical factors
- A high risk of poor patient compliance, especially due to drugs and/or alcohol
- An elderly patient with a sedentary lifestyle

Methods of fixation

- Plate fixation (reconstruction plate, 3.5-mm dynamic compression plate (DCP), precontoured clavicle locking plate, hook plate). Semitubular plates should not be used. Reconstruction plates more easily contoured but greater risk of non-union
- Intramedullary fixation but traditionally a high complication rate including infection, non-union and implant migration. Newer designs and modifications in the technique used for fixation have recently led to renewed interest. Significant advantages over plate fixation including minimal soft-tissue and periosteal stripping, better cosmesis (smaller skin incision) and ease of removal. Ability to resist torsional forces is much less than with a conventional plate. Examples include the Rockwood clavicle pin, titanium elastic nail (TEN, Synthes) and Herbert cannulated bone screw

- External fixation is occasionally indicated in multiply injured patients
- Coracoclavicular screw fixation for distal third fractures with CCL disruption
- Resection of distal clavicle – following degenerative change with type III distal third fractures
- Arthroscopic fixation
- ORIF gives superior results in type II and type V fractures of the distal third as these have a higher rate of non-union if managed conservatively

Complications

Non-union

More commonly seen in middle third fractures due to their higher incidence, but lateral third fractures are more prone to develop non-unions. Lower rates following non-operative management (0.1%–4%) but more favourable fracture types are more likely to heal than those chosen for fixation. Predisposing factors in middle third fractures include:

- Severity of injury (high-velocity injuries)
- Primary operative management. Aggressive soft-tissue stripping, inability to reduce the fracture, and inadequate internal fixation
- Re-fracture
- Completely displaced fracture with shortening >2 cm
- Patient's age

Non-union rate is 30% for a non-operated type II distal third fracture. The management of a symptomatic non-union is open reduction, bone grafting and fixation.

Malunion

A distinct clinical entity with characteristic clinical and radiographic features. Defined as union of the fracture in a shortened, angulated, or displaced position with weakness, rapid fatigability, pain with overhead activity, neurologic symptoms (numbness and paresthesia of the hand and forearm with elevation of the limb), and shoulder asymmetry.

Neurovascular compromise

Acute compromise relates to fracture displacement while chronic compromise relates to excessive callus formation or a mobile non-union. Typically, the proximal part of the distal fragment in middle third fractures is pulled inferiorly/posteriorly against the neurovascular bundle.

Osteoarthritis

May follow SC joint and AC joint injury.

Floating shoulder

Double disruption of the superior shoulder complex (scapula, clavicle and soft tissue). This results from fracture of the clavicle and scapula and this combination of injuries should be stabilized. The clavicle should be plated. If the scapula fracture (usually of the glenoid neck) does not reduce spontaneously, ORIF is indicated.

Examination corner

Trauma oral 1

Adult middle third clavicular fracture

- Non-union rate
- Indications for ORIF
- Complications of fixation (non-union, delayed union, infection, skin breakdown over the plate, new fracture around the plate, etc.)

Trauma oral 2

Radiograph of a fractured lateral third of clavicle

- Classification
- Management

- Use of a clavicular hook plate
- Rehabilitation after hook plate fixation. Specifically the examiners wanted to discuss the possibility of causing rotator cuff damage with unrestricted range of shoulder movement
- Need for plate removal (yes, as part of planned treatment)

Acromioclavicular joint dislocation

Rockwood classification (1984)[4]

Type I: Sprain

Type II: Rupture of AC joint. Sprain of CCLs

Type III: Rupture of AC joint and CCLs with <100% displacement

Type IV: Rupture of AC joint and CCLs with posterior displacement (clavicle may be trapped in the trapezius muscle). Best viewed from the side or above

Type V: Rupture of AC joint and CCLs with >100% displacement

Type VI: Rupture of AC joint and CCLs with inferior displacement (clavicle may be trapped under the conjoint tendon)

Or more simply the "Six S's"

Type 1: Sprained

Type 2: Subluxed

Type 3: Superior dislocation

Type 4: Superior/posterior dislocation

Type 5: Severe superior dislocation

Type 6: Severe inferior dislocation

Types I–III account for 98% of these injuries. Controversies of surgical versus non-surgical management surround type III fractures, which make up 40% of all ACJ injuries.

---

[4] Rockwood CA Jr. (1984) Subluxations and dislocations about the shoulder. Injuries to the acromioclavicular joint. In: Rockwood CA Jr., Green DP (eds.) *Fractures*, edn. 2, vol. 1. Philadelphia: JB Lippincott, pp. 860–910.

Imaging

- AP with 10°–15° cephalic tilt – outlines joint/loose bodies
- Stress radiograph with 4-kg weight suspended from patient's wrist – helps differentiate between type II and III injuries

Management

Types I and II are managed non-operatively; types IV–VI, with surgery. Controversy surrounds the type III injury, as to whether to manage operatively or non-operatively. There is possibly a case for surgery in a heavy manual labourer or an athlete.

A wide variety of operative procedures have been described but none has been shown to be clearly superior to the others. Newer arthroscopic techniques to manage ACJ injuries are evolving, they cause less disruption to the soft tissue envelope but there is a steep learning curve.

Non-operative management

- Sling or brace for 6–8 weeks
- Loss of shoulder and elbow motion
- Soft-tissue calcification
- Interference with ADLs
- Late ACJ osteoarthritis

Operative management

- The use of K-wires to fix the ACJ is now contraindicated. It is dangerous as pin breakage and migration can occur, it gives relatively poor fixation and a second procedure for hardware removal is required
- Steinman pin across the ACJ. Given the wider range of better implants now available, this is not recommended
- Coracoclavicular lag screw (Bosworth screw) with repair of CCL and plication of the torn deltoid and trapezius. Gone out of favour as concerns with loss of screw fixation or screw breakage, etc.
- Dynamic muscle transfers. Transfer of the lateral half of the conjoined tendon to the distal clavicle augmented by EndoButton fixation of the ACJ. A

major procedure with more risks involved than are necessary such as musculocutaneous nerve injury and loss of fixation
- Coracoclavicular cerclage. A well-established technique, materials include tendons, wire loops and synthetic ligament substitutes such as Dacron or Mersilene tape
- Clavicular hook plate. Needs removing after healing of the soft tissues
- Arthroscopic techniques. The CCL is dissected from the undersurface of the acromion and is reinserted on the inferior clavicle by transosseous suture fixation. Other techniques involve the use of a semitendinosus allograft to reconstruct the CCL. The accuracy of reduction of the joint is more difficult to assess arthroscopically

Complications of conservative management

- Cosmetic "bump" on the distal clavicle
- Painful ACJ with degenerative changes. If severe, it is managed with excision of the distal clavicle and reconstruction of the CCL by using the coracoacromial ligament (Weaver–Dunn procedure)

Prognosis

- Up to 100% good/excellent results with type I/II injuries
- Patients with non-operative management of type III injuries may experience mild discomfort, but no reduction of strength or endurance compared to the non-injured side at 4 years
- Return to work and rehabilitation are quicker with non-operative management for type I–III injuries

---

Examination corner

Trauma oral 1

Radiograph of a grade V ACJ dislocation

Examiner: This is a 23-year-old male who sustained the above injury when playing football. It is a week later on and you see him in your fracture clinic. How are you going to manage him?

Candidate: This is either a Rockwood grade III or V injury to the AC joint. If this was a grade III injury I would manage the patient conservatively with a sling but if it was a grade V injury I would manage him surgically.

Examiner: How are you going to manage this gentleman "you yourself"?

Candidate: There is a large coracoid-clavicular interval so I would probably want to fix it.

Examiner: You would not really want to leave this injury alone would you?! (A very slight alarm in examiners voice – candidate has got to pick these types of clue up.)

Candidate: I would fix it with a Bosworth screw.

Examiner: Do you leave the screw in or take it out?

Candidate: I would take it out.

Examiner: When?

Candidate: At 8 weeks.

The candidate made it hard work for themselves. The injury was grade V, there was no real debate about this from the radiograph and it needed operative fixation. The candidate was too cautious (or unsure) with their answer; they should have been more definite and confident with their reply. Nowadays a Bosworth screw is a much less popular method used to fix these injuries and as such they would not be my first choice to mention to the examiners.

Trauma oral 2

Grade III ACJ dislocation

- Management: acute versus chronic
- Weaver–Dunn: "How do you do it?"

Trauma oral 3

Clinical photograph of a middle-aged man with a slightly prominent lateral end of clavicle. A grade II ACJ dislocation

- Describe what you see
- What is your management?
- Chronic symptoms
- Weaver–Dunn procedure

Sternoclavicular joint dislocation

Rare, typically follows RTAs and sporting injuries. Anterior dislocation is usually caused by forced backward and downward movement of the shoulder. A posterior dislocation is usually due to a blow over the posterolateral aspect of the shoulder or less commonly a direct blow over the clavicle. Diagnosis is made from the site of pain, swelling and deformity. Patients with hypermobility may exhibit voluntary joint subluxation. Anterior dislocation is more common (20:1) and less dangerous because of the mechanism of injury and potential complications from management.

Imaging

- Diagnosis can be difficult due to artefacts from neighbouring structures
- The serendipity view is a 40° cephalic tilt. In anterior SCJ dislocations the clavicle is high riding whilst in a posterior SCJ dislocation the clavicle is below the interclavicle line. Details of avulsion fractures and the relationship of the clavicle to the mediastinal structures are difficult to interpret
- CT is the investigation of choice
- Vascular studies should be considered in a posterior dislocation where there has been a significant risk of injury to the great vessels (superior vena cava, subclavian vascular system, laceration of the innominate vein and carotid artery compression) or severe thoracic outlet syndrome
- MRI may be useful in assessing the extent of soft tissue injury

Associated injuries

Posterior dislocation may impinge on closely related structures:

- Great vessels, trachea (lacerations), oesophagus (rupture – pneumomediastinum), heart and pleura (pneumothorax)
- Venous congestion in the neck or ipsilateral arm, hoarseness, cough, dysphagia or a feeling of choking suggest superior mediastinal obstruction from posterior dislocation, and are indications for urgent reduction

Anterior dislocation is relatively benign.

Management of anterior dislocations

Closed reduction under GA with a sandbag between the scapulae and shoulder abducted. Reduction is often unstable even with a figure-of-eight sling. The rate of recurrence following closed reduction varies from 20% to 60%. If recurrence is symptomatic stabilization with tendon grafting or resection of the medial end of the clavicle can be undertaken.

Management of posterior dislocations

One must first assess for any airway and vascular injuries. A closed reduction technique similar to that used for anterior dislocation should be initially attempted. A towel clip may be used to facilitate reduction. Reduction is usually stable and postoperatively, a sling is worn for 3 months. Fixation with K-wires, or similar devices, to stabilize the relocated joint has been described but is not recommended. There are concerns with the rotational and translational torques involved leading to breakage or migration. There are reports of fatalities following wire migration.

Shoulder joint dislocation

Thirty-eight percent of all traumatic dislocations involve the glenohumeral joint. Ninety-eight percent are anterior dislocations (usually subcoracoid). Less commonly, the humeral head sits in a subglenoid, subclavicular or an intra-thoracic position following anterior dislocation. The remaining 2% are posterior, with the exception of "luxatio erecta" and superior dislocations. The soft tissues including the rotator cuff, glenoid labrum and the glenohumeral capsular ligaments provide most of the stability of the shoulder.

Anterior dislocations occur when the shoulder is abducted and externally rotated. The dislocated arm is held in slight abduction and external rotation. It is characterized by emptiness felt beneath the acromion or squaring of the shoulder contour.

Fifty percent of posterior dislocations are missed on first presentation. Suspect a posterior dislocation with a flat anterior contour of the shoulder, a prominent coracoid and difficulty abducting the arm. The most striking feature is inability to externally rotate the shoulder.

Inferior dislocation presents with fixed abduction as the humeral head is locked underneath the glenoid.

Imaging

- AP shoulder (the plate is parallel to the scapula)
- Lateral scapular view
- Axillary view – single most important film to assess the presence and direction of glenohumeral dislocation
- "Light bulb" sign on AP view is classic of a posterior dislocation

Management

Closed reduction of anterior dislocation

- The principle is to apply *gentle* traction with muscle relaxation
- Kocher's method involves traction and abduction, followed by adduction and internal rotation. However, this has been linked with fractures of the humeral neck and higher rates of recurrent dislocation
- The Hippocratic method is still recommended using traction with or without rotation
- Counter traction is with the foot in the axilla or a sheet looped through the axilla

Closed reduction of posterior dislocation

- Traction is along the adducted arm
- Avoid forceful external rotation due to the risk of fracture

Closed reduction of inferior dislocation

- Traction alone is usually sufficient. Open reduction may be necessary if the head buttonholes through the capsule

Post-reduction care

Repeat radiographs to ensure adequate reduction. Immobilize for 3–6 weeks following anterior dislocation. Early mobilization is desirable in patients over 40 years old to avoid stiffness. Physiotherapy to strengthen the muscular stabilizers (rotator cuff muscles) is necessary. Avoid positions that provoke instability. Posterior dislocation is often unstable post-reduction. A shoulder spica in neutral rotation (handshake cast) is desirable.

Complications

Recurrent dislocation

Inversely related to age of first dislocation: 80% of those under 20 years of age have a recurrence within 2 years. The rate is 10%–15% over the age of 40 years. Recurrence is rare with a greater tuberosity fracture. A Bankart lesion is associated with younger patients (stripping of labrum and capsule from anterior glenoid). Older patients stretch the capsule or avulse the greater tuberosity. Early repair of Bankart lesion in the young reduces recurrence from 80% to 14%.

Rotator cuff tears

Common in older patients. Suspect with excessive bruising and slow rehabilitation. Repair is usually required.

Fractures

Intra-articular fractures of the head and extra-articular fractures are associated with dislocation. A Hill–Sachs lesion (impaction fracture of the posterolateral head seen in anterior dislocation) is seen in 35% of acute cases and 60% of chronic cases. Reverse Hill–Sachs is seen in posterior dislocations. Impaction exceeding 20% may need surgical correction. Glenoid fractures may need fixation if displaced or if associated with joint subluxation. Fractures of the greater tuberosity usually reduce after reduction. Persistent displacement of greater than 1 cm (0.5 cm in the young) requires ORIF and cuff repair.

Neurological injury

Incidence increases with age. Axillary, suprascapular and musculocutaneous nerves are the most commonly injured. Nerve injury is rare with posterior dislocation. Almost all luxatio erecta present with neurological compromise, which resolves with reduction.

Vascular injury

May occur at time of injury and manifest as vascular occlusion or haemorrhage. The second and third parts of the axillary artery are most commonly involved. Arterial occlusion may occur in the presence of palpable distal pulses.

Indications for acute operative management

- Associated vascular injury
- Open dislocation
- Failure of closed reduction (may be biceps tendon/rotator cuff interposition)
- Displaced greater tuberosity or glenoid fractures
- Significant impaction of humeral head
- Gross instability following posterior dislocation

Examination corner

Trauma oral 1

Posterior shoulder dislocation and reversed Hill–Sachs lesion

Trauma oral 2

Radiograph demonstrating inferior shoulder dislocation (luxatio erecta). Discussion and management of the condition. Incidence of rotator cuff injuries

Trauma oral 3

Radiograph shown of a young male patient with a fracture dislocation of the glenohumeral joint. You are called down to casualty because the A/E doctor has failed to reduce it.

- Your management
- What structures may be preventing reduction?
- The possibility of an associated occult humeral neck fracture and management if present

Trauma oral 4

Male aged 40 years. Radiograph shown of traumatic anterior shoulder dislocation

- Management
- Splint for how long? Evidence?
- Failure to recover: possible causes – rotator cuff tear, subclinical brachial plexus injury
- How would you investigate – ultra-sound scan or EMG (both!)

Proximal humeral fractures

Proximal humeral fractures account for 5% of all fractures and 75% of all humeral fractures in people >40 years. This fracture is associated with severe osteoporosis in the elderly. There are 70% as many proximal humeral fractures as there are femoral neck fractures. These fractures should be managed individually taking into account age, bone stock, fracture configuration and patient expectations.

Anatomy

The anatomical neck encircles the base of the articular surface. The surgical neck is more distal and closely related to the axillary nerve. The axillary nerve runs through the quadrangular space. The surgical neck is most frequently fractured. The anterior circumflex humeral artery primarily supplies the head although the posteromedial vessel alone can sustain it.

Codman divided the proximal humerus into four parts (head, greater/lesser tuberosity and the shaft).

- The rotator cuff muscles (teres minor, supraspinatus and infraspinatus) insert into the greater tuberosity and pull the fracture fragment posterosuperiorly
- Subscapularis inserts into the lesser tuberosity and pulls the fracture fragment anteromedially
- Pectoralis major inserts distal to the surgical neck, pulling the shaft medially with a surgical neck fracture

The humeral head lies under the acromial arch and the aim is to maintain adequate space under the arch to prevent impingement.

Neer's classification

- The classification system considers anatomy, biomechanical forces and displacement of fracture fragments, relating these to diagnosis and management. Defines the fracture according to the number of osseous segments (Codman's parts) that are displaced
- Displacement is defined as separation >1 cm or >45° angulation
- A further category is the fracture associated with dislocation
- Splitting or impaction of the articular surface, quantifying impaction according to the percentage of head involvement

Clinical examination

Neurovascular assessment is mandatory (neurological deficits are reported in up to 36% and vascular injury in 5% of patients).

Imaging

- AP, scapular lateral and axillary views (latter to determine displacement of the lesser tuberosity and humeral head injury)
- CT and/or MRI may be helpful in evaluating the fracture pattern, amount of articular involvement, the displacement of fracture fragments and soft-tissue involvement especially if surgical intervention is contemplated

Management

Non-operative management

- Suitable for up to 85% of cases that are impacted or non-displaced
- High arm collar and cuff
- Pendular exercises at 7–14 days followed by more vigorous mobilization and physiotherapy

Operative management

The aim is to restore the anatomy and function of the proximal humerus with an intact rotator cuff function, which does not impinge. Avoid devascularizing fracture fragments and leaving hardware that interferes with shoulder movements.

- ORIF of greater tuberosity fractures displaced by more than 10 mm (5 mm in the young patient). Rationale is to avoid prominence in order to prevent impingement. Usually associated rotator cuff tear which needs to be carefully repaired to relieve tension on the tuberosity repair
- Surgical neck fractures can usually be managed non-operatively. Displaced fractures can be managed with intramedullary nailing if the head is intact
- Three-part fractures have a better outcome if the bony anatomy is restored. Fixation with plates and screws is associated with AVN rates of 30%. Tension band wiring is also a popular method of fixation but technically difficult
- Four-part fractures have a poor result with non-operative management. The rate of AVN can approach 80%–90%. Reconstruction may be attempted with a fixed angle plate such as the PHILOS plate in young fit patients with good bone quality preferably by an experienced trauma upper limb/shoulder surgeon. Technical details include limited surgical exposure, careful soft-tissue dissection, use of small cancellous screws, and placement of the plate high on the head without impingement. Good results have been reported, therefore move towards ORIF as the initial management of four-part fractures, with primary prosthetic replacement hemiarthroplasty

for elderly patients with osteopenic bones and for any patient with poor bone quality
- Neer introduced the shoulder hemiarthroplasty in the 1950s. Primary hemiarthroplasty ideally provides a pain-free shoulder with active forward flexion to 90° or more. The rotator cuff should be re-attached and the natural humeral head retroversion of 35° maintained. Can be a challenging procedure with a number of technical issues. Complications include dislocation, infection, residue pain, stiffness, tuberosity malunion or non-union, nerve injury, loosening, heterotopic ossification and degenerative changes in the glenoid
- The results of early hemiarthroplasty are superior to those of delayed primary arthroplasty, or late arthroplasty to revise failed internal fixation

Fracture/dislocation

- Fracture of the greater tuberosity associated with dislocation of the shoulder often reduces spontaneously after reduction of the shoulder. If the fragment is still displaced, ORIF and cuff repair are necessary. Care must be taken not to displace the undisplaced fracture on manipulation. The tuberosity fragment displaces proximally and posteriorly to become incarcerated within the subacromial space
- Two- and three-part fracture dislocation may be treated with ORIF
- Four-part fracture dislocations generally have a poor outcome due to AVN. They should be managed with a hemiarthroplasty in an elderly patient. In younger patients an attempt at fixation is not an unreasonable option if there are large fragments and good bone quality
- Impaction or splitting of >45% of the articular surface is an indication for hemiarthroplasty

Complications

- **Neurological impairment** is seen in up to 36% of patients. Most commonly injured is the axillary nerve. Injuries to the suprascapular, musculocutaneous and radial nerves have also been reported

- **Axillary artery damage** occurs in up to 5% of these injuries with 27% of these still having palpable distal pulses
- **AVN** is related to the severity of the injury and occurs in 5%–15% of three-part fractures and 10%–34% of four-part fractures
- **Malunion** is not uncommon following proximal humeral fractures. Conservative management of surgical neck fractures often results in increased anterior angulation. Failed ORIF is due to excessive scar formation, muscle atrophy, tuberosity displacement, malrotation of the head, varus/valgus deformity of the shaft
- **Shoulder stiffness** may be a result of poor rehabilitation, myositis ossificans, malunion and AVN. Involvement of the soft tissues leads to adhesions and scar formation of the capsule and ligaments and rotator cuff atrophy

---

Examination corner

Trauma oral 1

Radiograph of a three-part fracture of the proximal humerus

- Classification
- Management options
- "What are you going to do?"
- Current literature and recommendations

Trauma oral 2

Anteroposterior radiograph of a four-part proximal humeral fracture

- Failed plate fixation with screw cut out and loosening
- Surgical exposure used: deltoid-pectoral approach to the shoulder
- Re-do surgery. Revision to a hemiarthroplasty is a technically difficult procedure. Problems encountered at surgery include soft-tissue contractures, scarring, malunion, etc.

Humeral shaft fractures

The humeral shaft extends from the upper border of pectoralis major insertion proximally to the supracondylar ridge distally. The proximal shaft is circular in cross-section and the cortex thin. By midshaft the cortex is very thick and the medullary cavity is narrow. Distally, the shaft cross-section changes to trapezoidal and there is a flat posterior surface between the medial and lateral cortical ridges.

Humeral shaft fractures are not common (3% of all fractures) and the majority are managed conservatively.

The majority are caused by direct trauma, either RTA or a fall. Rarer causes include gunshot or other penetrating missiles, arm wrestling, javelin throwing, using "bullworkers" and pathological fractures.

In high-energy mechanisms, soft-tissue disruption and extensive fracture comminution may be seen. This renders closed management less predictable. A thorough examination is required for associated injuries including the cervical spine and airway to exclude instability or intubation difficulties.

Clinical examination

As many as 18% of humeral shaft fractures have an associated radial nerve injury either a laceration or entrapment at the fracture site, so look for wrist and finger drop. The majority (90%) are neurapraxia and recover in 3–4 months. Examination of the shoulder and elbow is difficult in the presence of a shaft fracture, but they should be gently palpated to detect injury or stiffness as this may influence the decision of whether to IM nail.

In proximal fractures the rotator cuff abducts and internally rotates the proximal fragment, and the distal fragment is pulled medially by pectoralis major. Fractures that occur between the pectoralis major insertion and the deltoid insertion display adduction of the proximal fragment and lateral displacement of the distal fragment. In fractures distal to the deltoid insertion, the proximal fragment is abducted with proximal migration of the distal fragment.

Imaging

Full-length AP and lateral radiographs, which must include the shoulder and elbow joints.

Classification

The humerus is divided into thirds for descriptive purposes. The fracture pattern is described according to the configuration (transverse, spiral, oblique, segmental, etc.). The Holstein–Lewis fracture is a spiral fracture of the distal third of the humeral shaft that may be associated with a radial nerve injury.

Management

Non-operative management

This is associated with good/excellent results in 95% of patients. Acceptable displacement includes <3 cm of shortening, <20° of anteroposterior angulation and <30° of varus-valgus angulation. The reported mean time to clinical union is 8 weeks, with 95% of fractures radiographically united by 12 weeks and 90% of patients having normal function at 12 weeks.

Splinting may be by hanging cast. The length of the collar and cuff controls varus/valgus alignment. The position of the loop on the forearm controls AP alignment. Avoid a heavy cast distracting the fracture as this may lead to delayed or non-union, particularly in transverse fractures. A U-slab may be useful in the acute setting, but it is bulky and predisposes to axillary irritation. The slab should be applied beyond the fracture site to avoid the fractures levering around the end of the cast. The functional cast brace as described by Sarmiento (pre-fabricated anterior and posterior shells secured with Velcro strap) may be applied after 1–2 weeks when the swelling has decreased. This may be progressively tightened as the swelling further diminishes. Early mobilization of the elbow and shoulder is encouraged.

Attention to detail is required for conservative management. Problems associated with brace management include non-compliance and poor tolerance by elderly patients.

Indications for operative management

Surgery is the exception rather than the rule for humeral shaft fractures. For routine fractures the risks and problems of surgical intervention generally outweigh the benefits. Indications for surgical fixation include:

- Open fractures
- Pathological fractures
- Ipsilateral upper-limb fractures or dislocation (floating elbow)
- Fractures associated with a radial nerve palsy AFTER a closed reduction
- Bilateral humeral fractures
- Polytrauma/multiple injuries (lower extremity, pelvis)
- Associated vascular injury
- Intra-articular extension
- Inability to maintain reduction (failure of conservative management)
- Delayed/non-union

Methods of internal fixation

- **Compression plate and screws**. Using either a broad 4.5-mm plate or a 3.5-mm plate with a small humerus. Use either an anterolateral approach, extensile both proximally to the shoulder and distally to the elbow, or a posterior approach for distal shaft fractures. The radial nerve must be identified. A low threshold for bone grafting is advised. The complication rate averages 10%, including non-union (2%), radial nerve palsy and sepsis. Care with exposure and instrumentation is critical. Fixation may be difficult in osteoporotic bone.
- **Antegrade locked intramedullary nails**. Insertion may be antegrade, which is applicable to middle and distal fractures. Advantages of intramedullary nailing include limited surgical exposure with less soft-tissue stripping, the ability to perform indirect

reduction, rotational control of the fracture with cross screws and added stability in osteoporotic bone. Static locking (distal and proximal nail locking) is generally recommended to enhance both rotational and axial stability. Complications associated with antegrade intramedullary nailing include rotator cuff injury, shoulder pain, proximal prominence of the implant, non-union and fractures near the tip of the nail

- **Retrograde intramedullary locking nails**. They may result in decreased elbow extension, heterotopic ossification and distal implant migration. There is also a theoretical risk of supracondylar humeral fracture

- **A non-reamed, locked intramedullary nail**. Reasonable option for a pathological fracture to reduce operating time and avoid reaming the medullary canal (increased bleeding, embolization of marrow contents) in unfit patients. For proximal and distal fractures, a plate may be used with possible augmentation with methyl methacrylate

- **External fixation** with a conventional or ring fixator is only rarely utilized. Most common indication has been for severe open fracture (type III Gustilo open fracture). Pins must be inserted in a controlled fashion with some authors recommending an open technique under direct vision to guard against neurovascular injury. A safe portal for proximal pins is from lateral to medial. Distal pins can be placed from posterior to anterior. The radial nerve crosses the posterior aspect of the midshaft and so placing pins just proximal to the olecranon fossa is safe. Anterior distal pin placement is possible but requires an open technique

Complications

Radial nerve injury

Such injury occurs in 2%–20% of cases and whilst classically associated with the Holstein–Lewis fracture it is more common following middle third fractures. Neurapraxia or neurotemesis is most common, and 90% resolve without treatment. In cases of complete radial nerve dysfunction, EMG and nerve conduction studies should be performed 6 weeks after injury. If motor function is present (action potentials), continued observation is indicated. If studies show no evidence of innervation (denervation fibrillation), exploration of the nerve is usually indicated. Acute exploration is indicated in open injuries (64% involve nerve damage or nerve interposition). With post-manipulation palsy, many surgeons would advise exploration despite the fact that the majority will resolve spontaneously.

Vascular injury

Extremely rare but may follow direct trauma or compartment syndrome, most commonly in the proximal and middle third fractures. Requires urgent management with skeletal stabilization before arterial repair. Fasciotomies may be required. Ischaemic time should be kept below 6 hours. Note that distal pulses may be present in patients with brachial artery injury due to the collateral blood flow. The role of angiography is controversial as in many cases the clinical picture is clear and the delay in surgery needs to be justified.

Non-union

Defined as >4 months without healing. The incidence is 2%–5%. It is most common in the proximal and distal thirds. Predisposing factors include systemic factors (age, diabetes, nutritional status) and local factors (transverse fracture, distraction, soft-tissue interposition, segmental fractures, inadequate immobilization, poor fixation, high-energy trauma). Management is operative with plate and screw fixation with bone grafting at the fracture site (union rate 89%–96%) or with a reamed, locked intramedullary nail (union rate 87%). The complication rate with intramedullary nailing is lower (12% versus 21%). Osteoporotic bone and pathological fractures may be more amenable to intramedullary nail fixation to reduce the dependence on screw fixation.

Examination corner

Trauma oral 1

Management of radial nerve palsies occurring at the time of closed humeral shaft fractures

- Conservative initial management versus early surgical exploration. Advantages and disadvantages of each approach
- Definite indications for early exploration (open fractures, post-manipulation palsy)
- Literature on the subject
- Role of nerve conduction studies

Trauma oral 2

AP radiograph of a displaced midshaft humeral fracture in a 72-year-old female

- Discussion of the merits of conservative versus operative management
- This led to a more formal review of the indications for conservative and operative management. The examiners were pushing me towards operative fixation, implying it would be an extremely difficult fracture to manage conservatively
- Discussion of the advantages and disadvantages of compression plating versus intramedullary nailing fixation
- Rates of healing for each technique
- Any recent publications on the subject
- I was pushed by the examiners for what I would do myself; they wanted me to say plate fixation because of the risks of radial nerve injury from nailing with fracture location

Distal humeral fractures

Account for approximately 2% of all fractures and one-third of fractures around the elbow. Occur in three age groups: children, young adults usually following high-energy injuries and in the elderly (in whom there is typically an osteoporotic fracture pattern).

Distal humeral fractures may be intra or extra-articular. Supracondylar fractures are extra-articular. Intra-articular fractures include transcondylar, intercondylar, condylar (medial/lateral), epicondylar and isolated fractures of the articular surface. The principles of management are closed treatment whenever possible and ORIF for displaced, unstable or intra-articular fractures. Early mobilization should be encouraged to optimize outcome and prevent elbow stiffness.

Supracondylar fractures

The most common pattern is displacement into extension with the distal fragment posterior. Classified by Gartland into:
- Type I: undisplaced
- Type II: displaced with the posterior cortical hinge intact
- Type III: completely displaced

Undisplaced fractures are managed non-operatively in a long arm cast, with early mobilization after 3 weeks. Displaced fractures tend to be unstable and require MUA and percutaneous pinning or open reduction and K-wire fixation. Cross K-wires placed from the medial and lateral sides provide the greatest stability and rotational control. The risk of iatrogenic nerve injury is reduced by a small skin incision medially and dissection down to bone. With open reduction posterolateral displacement is exposed through an anteromedial approach and posteromedial displacement is exposed through an anterolateral approach. Neurovascular injury must be excluded. Displacement of a distal fragment into flexion is rare (<4%) but more difficult to reduce.

Very swollen limbs and cases where the radial pulse is compromised with flexion can be managed with Dunlop traction until the swelling subsides, followed by definitive plaster or K-wire fixation.

Transcondylar fractures

These are more distal to supracondylar fractures and are less common injuries. They are managed in the same manner as supracondylar fractures. They are more unstable, especially in rotation, and a lower threshold for fixation is necessary as there is a greater potential for non-union.

Intercondylar fractures

There may be T- or Y-shaped fracture patterns, passing between and separating the condyles.

Riseborough and Radin classification of intercondylar T or Y fractures

Type I: Undisplaced fracture between the capitellum and trochlea

Type II: Displaced, non-rotated fracture

Type III: Displaced, rotated fragments

Type IV: Severely comminuted with wide separation of the humeral condyles

Non-displaced fractures may be managed by immobilization in a plaster cast. Displaced fractures require ORIF through a posterior approach with olecranon osteotomy or triceps turn down. The principle is to reconstruct the two columns of the distal humerus and fix them back to the humeral shaft. Severely comminuted fractures may be managed with early elbow replacement.

Isolated condylar fractures

Isolated condylar fractures follow the Milch classification:

- Type I: fractures pass through the capitellum or medial condyle, leaving the trochlear ridge intact
- Type II: fractures pass close to the trochlear sulcus, and include the trochlear ridge in the fracture fragment
- Type III: fractures are associated with dislocation of the elbow and collateral ligament rupture. These fractures are usually childhood fractures.

Undisplaced fractures should be immobilized in pronation for medial fractures and in supination for lateral fractures. Displaced fractures need ORIF. A single lag screw is often sufficient.

Capitellum fractures

These fractures are rare. They follow a fall on to the outstretched hand. They often involve a shear fracture of the capitellum rather than the trochlea.

Bryan and Morrey classification of capitellum fractures

Type I: Complete fracture

Type II: Osteochondral (shear) fracture

Type III: Comminuted fracture

Non-displaced fractures may be managed with early mobilization. Unstable or displaced fractures need ORIF with a lag screw or a Herbert screw. Some comminuted fractures with minimal subchondral bone, or fractures in the elderly may not be amenable to stable internal fixation and are best managed by excising the fragment. Arthroscopic excision has resulted in improved motion compared to open excision.

Epicondylar fractures

May occur in younger adults and are usually managed non-operatively. They must be distinguished from delayed closure of the ossification centre. The medial epicondyle is more commonly affected. Persistent ulnar nerve symptoms require surgery, or an unsightly lump necessitates late excision of the bony fragment.

Management

Internal fixation of distal humeral fractures

Preoperative planning is essential as surgical reconstruction of the fracture can be very challenging. For complex fractures the posterior approach to the elbow is preferred. This gives optimal access to the distal humerus but requires an olecranon osteotomy. It is essential to identify and protect the ulnar nerve. A bright coloured rubber sling is used as a gentle retractor and protective marker. An olecranon chevron osteotomy is performed through a non-articular segment about 2 cm from the olecranon tip. It is advisable to pre-drill the olecranon fragment to enable TBW fixation with either a cancellous lag screw or K pins on closure. The tip of the olecranon, carrying triceps, is then retracted proximally to expose the distal humerus. Full exposure of the posterior aspect of the distal humerus by medial and lateral dissection is required. The distal intra-articular fragments are first reconstructed and then reattached to the humerus with a double-plate technique, without violating the articular surfaces or any of the three fossae around the elbow. DCP, malleable pelvic reconstruction plates or the newer low-profile pre-contoured plates may be used in planes at 90° to each other, one in the frontal plane and one in the sagittal. Provisional K-wire fixation is often required. A large defect of the articular surface should be filled with an iliac crest bone graft. Complications of surgery include neurovascular compromise, compartment syndrome, infection, mal-union, non-union, joint stiffness, heterotopic bone formation, myositis ossificans and post-traumatic osteoarthritis.

Timing of surgery should be within 24–36 h or after 7–10 days of the fracture, as the swelling begins to subside. By 10 days the risk of myositis ossificans greatly increases. With rigid fixation, mobilization may commence when wound healing is satisfactory. Good/excellent results are reported in 75% of cases (stable elbow, minimal pain, flexion from 15° to 130° and a return to pre-injury activity).

Examination corner

Trauma oral 1

- Radiograph of a distal extra-articular humeral fracture – surgical approach for fixation and structures at risk
- This was followed by a radiograph of an intra-articular distal humeral fracture – again what surgical approach would you take for fixation and what structures are at risk?

Trauma oral 2

- Radiograph of a comminuted intra-articular supra-condylar humeral fracture in a 40-year-old male
- Management
- Articular reconstruction and double plating discussed
- Shown post-fixation radiographs of such an ORIF and asked to critique – articular step present
- I was asked about what surgical approach I would use
- The examiner asked me to draw the Baumann's angle

Trauma oral 3

Paediatric Gartland III supracondylar fracture of the humerus

- Every possible scenario concerning the vascular status of this injury was covered including pulse, position fracture, capillary refill, loss of pulse post fixation and if/when to call the vascular surgeons

---

Trauma oral 4

Paediatric supracondylar fracture of the humerus

- Nerve injury patterns
- Methods of management including K-wire fixation (how many, where and when to remove)

Examiner: Do you really need to open up a Gartland III supra-condylar fracture? Can't you use just reduce it and fix it with K-wires?

Candidate: This question unnerved me and I stumbled a bit with it. I replied that it was worth attempting to percutaneously fix a Gartland III supracondylar fracture but that often closed reduction would be unsuccessful.

Trauma oral 5

Clinical picture of a child with a severely swollen, bruised, deformed elbow

- Diagnosis of supracondylar fracture with vascular compromise
- Initial management including the possibility of performing an angiogram and vascular reconstruction
- Possible complications

Trauma oral 6

Supracondylar fracture in a young boy approximately 8 years old

- Acute management
- Chronic (late) complications

- Supracondylar fracture presenting late at 1 day. Discussion of the role of Dunlop traction

Trauma oral 7

Radiograph of a supracondylar fracture of the humerus in a child

- Describe
- Do you know any classifications for this injury?
- What type is this?
- How will you manage this fracture?
- Detailed discussion about the management of various types of supracondylar fractures
- Complications and management of complications

Trauma oral 8

Radiograph of a Gartland type 3 supracondylar fracture of the humerus

Every possible scenario concerning management of this injury was discussed including how to reduce the fracture and vascular compromise:

Examiner:

- Would you wake your consultant in the middle of the night?
- Here, this is my arm; show me how you reduce a supracondylar fracture. How do you specifically correct the displacement and rotational deformity of the fracture?
- There is vascular compromise. What are you going to do?
- You cannot get into theatre because the general surgeons are doing an emergency laparotomy. What are you going to do?
- You fix the fracture with K-wires. There is good capillary refill of the fingertips but no radial pulse. What are you going to do?

Elbow dislocation

Dislocation at the elbow is second only to dislocation at the shoulder. A simple dislocation carries a good prognosis. The mechanism of injury is hyperextension of the arm causing the olecranon to impinge on the olecranon fossa, levering it out of the joint. Alternatively, axial loading of the slightly flexed joint is thought to cause dislocation.

Classification

According to the direction of forearm displacement:
- Anterior
- Posterior (most common)
- Medial
- Lateral
- Divergent dislocation
- Ulnar or radial dislocation in isolation

Divergent dislocation occurs when the radius and ulna dissociate to either side of the humerus. This may be anteroposterior with the radius anterior and the ulna posterior, or mediolateral. Ulnar and radial dislocation may also occur in isolation.

Clinical presentation

Presentation is usually acute. Delayed presentation of more than 7 days is classed as a "neglected" case and often needs open reduction. The equilateral triangle formed by the olecranon, medial and lateral epicondyles is disrupted, differentiating dislocation from supracondylar fracture. Neurovascular status must be thoroughly assessed and documented at presentation. It must be repeated following reduction.

Associated injuries

Vascular injury

The presence of distal pulses does not exclude vascular injury. An arteriogram may be necessary following reduction.

Nerve damage

The median, ulnar, anterior interosseous and radial nerves can all be injured. The ulnar nerve is most commonly injured, followed by the median nerve. The radial nerve is the least of all involved. An injury to the anterior interosseous nerve is difficult to diagnose due to lack of sensory involvement. The median and ulnar nerves can be trapped within the joint during reduction and the development of post-reduction palsy requires surgical exploration. Pre-reduction palsy is traditionally managed expectantly. After 3 months, if recovery has not occurred spontaneously and EMG studies indicate that the nerve is non-functioning, surgical exploration is indicated.

Fracture dislocation

The incidence of associated fractures ranges from 16% to 62%, reflecting the unreliable detection of osteochondral lesions. Fracture dislocation is associated with a poorer outcome than dislocation alone.

Medial condylar avulsion

• Needs to be recognized and managed, as retained fragments within the joint lead to articular surface damage. ORIF or removal is needed.

Management

Non-operative management

Posterior dislocations can often be reduced closed under sedation. Reduction may be by longitudinal forearm traction with digital pressure over the olecranon or extension of the elbow to "unlock" it (predisposes to nerve entrapment). The elbow is immobilized in 100° flexion in a plaster for 7–10 days before commencing mobilization. Forced passive mobilization should be avoided. If a significant fracture such as unfixed coronoid process fracture is present, immobilization may be increased to 3 weeks.

Indications for open surgery

• Open dislocation
• Significant fracture requiring fixation
• Entrapped soft tissue blocking reduction

• Vascular injury requiring surgery
• Ligamentous repair (seldom improving the result)
• Irreducible neglected dislocation

Management of persistent instability

• Ligamentous repair (usually lateral)
• Hinged external fixator or brace
• Pass a Steinman pin across the joint (stiffness, heterotopic ossification and pin breakage may follow)

Prognosis

Good in simple dislocation. Recovery takes 3–6 months. Many patients are left with 10°–15° fixed-flexion contractures.

Complications include heterotopic ossification and chronic instability.

Proximal radius and ulna fractures

Radial head fractures

Common injuries of the adult elbow.

Mason's classification

Type I: Undisplaced fracture
Type II: Marginal with displacement >2 mm or 30° articular surface
Type III: Comminuted
Type IV: Associated with elbow dislocation (added by Johnston)

Clinical examination

Swelling secondary to haemarthrosis. This may be aspirated and local anaesthetic infiltrated into the joint for pain relief. Pronation/supination can then be assessed.

Imaging

AP and lateral radiographs of the elbow. Note any "fat pad" sign.

Management

Type I injuries may be mobilized early. This approach may be followed with type II injuries if there is no mechanical block to pronation/supination. However, if a block exists, then ORIF should be performed. This provides pain relief, increased motion and grip strength. If reconstruction proves impossible, excision of the radial head may be performed. Where instability exists after radial head excision, radial head replacement using a Silastic® or metal head should be carried out.

ORIF is carried out, if possible, for type III injuries but it is often not achievable and radial head excision is the only viable option. Consider radial head replacement if there is valgus elbow instability or longitudinal forearm instability.

If the fracture is associated with dislocation (type IV), an attempt should be made to keep the radial head to prevent recurrent dislocation and valgus instability. If this proves impossible, then repair of the collateral ligaments is necessary. This may be augmented with a prosthetic radial head implant. In certain situations a hinged external fixator may be utilized to maintain mobility during recovery.

Coronoid process fractures

The coronoid process forms an anterior buttress to the elbow. The anterior capsule and the medial collateral ligament attach to the coronoid process and the brachialis inserts just distal to it. Two to ten percent of dislocations of the elbow are associated with fractures of the coronoid. One-third of fractures are secondary to elbow dislocation. Complications of a large coronoid fragment that has not united may include a mechanical block to motion and elbow instability.

Regan and Morrey classification

Type I: Simple avulsion fracture of the tip of the coronoid
Type II: Fracture involving half or less of the coronoid process
Type III: Fracture involving more than half of the coronoid process

Management

- All type I and most type II fractures are amenable to non-operative management. All type III and some type II injuries are unstable. This is caused by the disruption of the osseous integrity of the ulna-humeral articulation and disruption of the anterior capsule thereby rendering the MCL incompetent.
- These unstable injuries require ORIF. If instability persists, a collateral ligament repair should be undertaken. A hinged external fixator may be used for added stability.

Olecranon fractures

Olecranon fractures are classically caused by pull of the triceps mechanism, or a direct blow following a fall.

Colton's classification

Type I: Fractures are undisplaced/stable
Type II: Fractures are displaced. A: avulsion, B: oblique/transverse fracture, C: comminuted fracture, D: fracture dislocation

Management

- Undisplaced fractures are immobilized in a cast for 3 weeks followed by supervised mobilization
- Displaced fractures may be managed with ORIF (tension band wire, plating). Occasionally for unreconstructable fractures olecranon excision with reattachment of the triceps mechanism to the proximal ulna may be indicated, but this is usually associated with a poor functional outcome

---

Examination corner

Trauma oral 1

Radiograph of a Mason's type II radial head fracture in an adult

- Classification and management
- When to use radial head replacements

Trauma oral 2

Radiograph of radial head fracture fixed with mini fragment screws and plate

- Critique the fixation
- This led into a discussion about Essex–Lopresti injury

Trauma oral 3

Radiograph of a displaced comminuted oblique fracture of the olecranon

Examiner: Describe your surgical management of this patient.
Candidate: I would use an interfragmentary screw and then a contoured one-third tubular plate. The fracture is not amenable to management with a tension band wire as the compression achieved is axial along the ulna and will displace an oblique fracture.

Trauma oral 4

Radiograph of a displaced transverse fracture of the olecranon

A very long drawn out discussion of the principles of tension band wiring for this particular fracture. Biomechanics discussed in great detail. The candidate was invited to draw out a diagram of the elbow TBW to help them explain the biomechanical principles better. The examiner wasn't happy with the explanation and ended up drawing it out themselves.

Candidate: The examiner seemed to want punchy catch phrases which I wasn't able to deliver quickly enough for him. We therefore spent what seemed like forever labouring various biomechanical points.
Examiner: The candidate didn't come across as though they knew what they were talking about particularly well and as a result needed to be probed in greater detail than usual.

Fractures of the forearm

The most common mechanisms of injury are falls on the outstretched hand or a direct blow. Management of these injuries is dependent on the injury pattern,

associated injuries, bone quality and the patient's functional status and physical demands. The bowed radius rotates around the ulna allowing pronation and supination. The aim of treatment is to restore bony anatomy and preserve this movement.

Clinical examination

Examination must include evaluation of the elbow and wrist for tenderness. Also carry out a full neurovascular assessment, including a check of radial and ulnar pulses and an examination of median, ulnar and radial nerves. Check for early signs of compartment syndrome. Clinical signs include deformity, abnormal limb movement, prominent swelling, crepitus and severe pain.

Imaging

AP and true lateral radiographs of the forearm including careful assessment of the elbow and wrist to rule out associated joint instability, dislocation or intra-articular fracture. The radial head should pass through the capitellum in all planes in the normal elbow.

Signs of DRUJ injury include fracture of the base of the ulnar styloid, widening of the joint on AP radiograph, dislocation of the ulna on a true lateral projection and radial shortening of <5 mm. Assess fracture location, displacement, angulation, configuration, shortening and comminution.

Management

Non-displaced fractures are rare. Angulation of <10° and translation of <50% is acceptable. Closed reduction is difficult to achieve and maintain such that ORIF is the preferred method of management when both bones of the forearm have been fractured in an adult.

Non-operative management consists of an above-elbow cast that incorporates the hand to prevent pronation-supination with weekly radiographs for at least 4 weeks to monitor the fracture. Problems associated with conservative management include loss of fracture alignment, decreased forearm motion, delayed and non-union.

Surgical options include plates, intramedullary nails or external fixation.

Methods of fixation

- **Plate fixation** (DCP, locking plates). The advantages of plating include anatomical reduction, rigid fixation and early movement. Disadvantages include the extensive soft-tissue dissection that is required for application, the risks of neurovascular injury, infection and scarring. The use of supplemental bone graft is controversial. A useful guideline is to graft if cortical continuity is lost for more than one-third of the circumference. Union rates are >95% and good/excellent results are achieved in >90% of patients
- **Unlocked intramedullary nailing**. This does not provide rotational or longitudinal stability. It is difficult to re-establish the radial bow and non-union rates of 10%–20% have been reported. However, flexible nailing in paediatric fractures has proved very successful and is gaining increasing popularity in the management of forearm fractures in this age group
- **External fixation** is generally used for Gustilo type IIIB and IIIC severe open injuries with significant soft-tissue loss that are not suitable for plating or intramedullary nails. Ten percent require fixator adjustment and superficial infection is common. Otherwise, ORIF may be used for most other open injuries. Thorough debridement, irrigation and antibiotic prophylaxis are necessary. External fixation provides temporary stabilization of the fracture while permitting access to the soft tissues but long-term unilateral fixation is unable to maintain the radial bow or resist rotational loads

Henry's approach to the forearm

The muscle and neurological interval is between the brachioradialis (radial nerve) and the pronator teres/ flexor carpi radialis (median nerve). In exposing the proximal third, the supinator is stripped off the bone (to prevent damage to the posterior interosseous nerve). Distally flexor pollicis longus and pronator quadratus are stripped off the radius at their insertion.

Dorsal (Thompson) approach

The muscle and neurological interval is between the extensor carpi radialis brevis (radial nerve) and the extensor digitorum communis and extensor pollicis longus (posterior interosseous nerve). This approach allows the plate to be placed on the tension side of the bone, but is more technically demanding due to the risk posed to the posterior interosseous nerve.

Monteggia fracture

Middle to proximal ulna fracture with associated radial head dislocation. Comprises 1%–2% of all forearm fractures. Easily misdiagnosed because of the focus on the obvious ulna fracture.

Bado's classification

Based on the direction of radial head displacement:
Type I: Anterior (most common)
Type II: Posterior
Type III: Lateral
Type IV: Dislocation associated with both radius and ulna fracture
A stable reduction of the radial head is commonly achieved with ORIF of the ulna fracture. Open reduction is needed if reduction is blocked by an interposed capsule or annular ligament (10% of cases). Repair of the annular ligament is controversial. Some authors suggest repair is required for greater early elbow stability whilst others suggest that repair may contribute to scarring and loss of elbow motion.

Nightstick fracture

This is an isolated ulna fracture and is usually the result of a direct blow to the ulna. These fractures can be transverse with minimal displacement or comminuted and displaced. Angulation of 10° and translation of <50% may be accepted. ORIF is required for displaced fractures >50%, short oblique or comminuted fractures and for distal third ulna fractures.

Galeazzi fracture

Isolated fracture of the distal or middle third of the radius with DRUJ dislocation. Management is ORIF of the radius with plates and screws and reduction of the DRUJ. The injury is known as the "fracture of necessity" because closed conservative management is contraindicated. Careful assessment of the DRUJ is essential as the functional deficit associated with a missed ligamentous injury to the DRUJ can be severe. The DRUJ is often found to be stable following ORIF of the radius and DRUJ reduction. If reduction is unstable transarticular K-wire fixation is required for 4–6 weeks. In a small number of cases, the dislocation is irreducible due to interposition of the ECU tendon. This necessitates open reduction and pin fixation.

Early complications

- **Compartment syndrome** – seen with vascular injury, high-energy injuries and crush injuries
- **Nerve injury** – rare. Posterior interosseous nerve palsy is seen in 20% of Monteggia fractures. There is usually a neurapraxia and most resolve within 3 months
- **Vascular injuries** – more prevalent with open fractures, in particular high-energy or penetrating injuries

Late complications

- **Stiffness** – depends on the severity of injury and quality of reduction post ORIF
- **Failure of fixation** – caused by infection and poor fixation
- **Infection** – rates are low. Treat with debridement. Metalwork should be retained till loose

- **Non-union** – risk is increased by open fractures, severe comminution, segmental fractures, segmental bone loss and inadequate fixation. Treat with autogenous bone grafting
- **Radial ulnar synostosis** – reported in 2% of forearm fractures. Associated with:
  - High-energy complex fractures
  - Fractures with concomitant head injury
  - Open fractures
  - Fracture of both bones at the same level
  - Infection
  - A single surgical approach
  - Delay of surgery by >2 weeks
  - Mal-reduction with loss of the radial bow or screw fixation that crosses the interosseous membrane

---

Vince and Miller's classification of synostosis (1987)[1]

Type I: At the DRUJ. Responds poorly to resection
Type II: Middle two-thirds. Amenable to resection (relatively low recurrence rate)
Type III: Proximal third. Intermediate prognosis

[1] Vince KG, Miller JE (1987) Cross-union complicating fracture of the forearm. Part I: Adults. *J Bone Joint Surg Am* **69**(5): 640–53.

Resection of the synostosis is best performed between 1 and 2 years post injury. Bony resection after 2 years is less successful due to muscle atrophy and interosseous membrane fibrosis.

Forearm metalwork removal

- Late problems due to retained metalwork include symptomatic hardware, stress risers at the bone–implant interface and cortical bone atrophy
- Risks of metalwork removal include a re-fracture rate of 2.5%–20% and a neurological injury rate of 10%–20%
- Risk of re-fracture is increased by early plate removal, delayed or non-union, inadequate fixation techniques and removal of a 4.5-mm plate

- There is concern regarding the long-term effects of retained plates on bone mineral density and forearm grip strength
- Removal of symptomatic metalwork is associated with worsening of symptoms in 9%
- Bone density beneath a plate does not return to normal for a mean of 21 months

Distal radius fractures

Account for one-sixth of fractures. Young patients present following high-energy trauma. Elderly osteoporotic patients present following low-energy falls onto outstretched hands.

Classification

Several classifications for distal radius fractures exist such as Frykman,[5] Melone (1984)[6] and the AO system.

Frykman classification

Type I: Extra-articular
Type III: Intra-articular involving the radiocarpal joint
Type V: Intra-articular involving the radioulnar joint
Type VII: Intra-articular involving both the radiocarpal and radioulnar joints
(Even numbers denote an associated ulnar styloid fracture)

Imaging

- Volar tilt – 11° seen in the lateral radiographic view

[5] Frykman G (1967) Fracture of the distal radius including sequelae – shoulder-hand-finger syndrome, disturbance in the distal radio-ulnar joint and impairment of nerve function. A clinical and experimental study. *Acta Orthop Scand Suppl* **108**:3+.
[6] Melone CP Jr. (1984) Articular fractures of the distal radius. *Orthop Clin North Am* **15**: 217–236.

- Radial length – 11 mm between a transverse line across the radial styloid and across the distal ulna
- Radial inclination – 22°
- Step in articular surface – >2 mm

Management

- Below-elbow POP cast with three-point fixation
- MUA and percutaneous K-wire fixation. Poor at maintaining length in the presence of bi-cortical comminution or osteoporosis
- External fixation. Used in more complex comminuted fractures or open fractures of the distal radius
- ORIF with AO locking plate. Mandatory for most volar displaced fractures

Complications

- Loss of reduction – re-manipulation is possible at up to 3 weeks
- Neurological complication – occurs in 10%. Median nerve most common (carpal tunnel syndrome)
- Compartment syndrome – <1%
- Acute tendon injury – rare in closed reduction
- Late tendon rupture – 1% EPL classically following non-displaced or minimally displaced fractures (rupture at level of Lister's tubercle – a vascular watershed)
- Stiffness
- Reflex sympathetic syndrome – up to 25%
- Malunion – >2 mm residual displacement leads to symptomatic degeneration in 50% at 30 years. Reduced to 5%–10% with anatomical reduction

Prognosis

Ninety percent of patients regain 90% of function by 1 year. Grip strength is usually reduced. In extra-articular fractures, the main predictor of a good result is restoration of normal radiocarpal alignment.

Examination corner

Trauma oral 1

Lateral radiograph of Colles' fracture of the distal radius in an 81-year-old female

- Patient was previously self caring and the fracture is in her dominant hand. Dorsally angulated 30°.
- Discussion of management options, complications and outcome

Trauma oral 2

Radiograph of an extra-articular, displaced distal radius fracture in a 50-year-old female with carpal tunnel syndrome

- Management

Hand oral 3

Complication of a Colles' fracture

As soon as EPL rupture was mentioned there was a change of emphasis in the oral questions as how to manage an EPL rupture, which operative technique to use, principles of tendon transfers, etc.

Hand oral 4

- How will you manage this fracture?
- Principles of POP management (moulding, three-point fixation, etc.)
- When will you manipulate?

Hand oral 5

Radiograph of a closed fracture of the distal radius/ulna in a 12-year-old boy with the inferior radio-ulnar joint dislocated as well

- Management
- Missed DRUJ dislocation (loss of supination).
- How to correct and when

Pelvic ring fractures

Pelvic ring fractures follow high-energy trauma; they are usually due to motor vehicle accidents and are frequently seen in association with major skeletal, thoracic, abdominal and pelvic trauma. Stability of the fracture depends on the integrity of the pelvic ring. Approximately 25% of fatal accidents have associated pelvic fracture and the mortality rate following pelvic fractures is 10%–20%.

They may occur following a low-energy trauma in elderly osteoporotic patients, usually an accidental fall.

Anatomy

- Pelvic ring – two innominate bones and the sacrum
- Sacroiliac joint (SI joint) – stabilized by multiple ligaments
- Posterior SI ligaments – strongest ligaments in the body
- Also anterior SI ligaments, sacrotuberous, sacrospinous, iliolumbar and lumbosacral ligaments, which add stability to the pelvic ring
- Pubic symphysis stabilizes the pelvic ring anteriorly

Classification

Tile classification[7]

Combines mechanism of injury and stability and aids in prognosis and treatment:
Type A: stable
Type B: rotationally unstable. Vertically stable
Type C: rotationally and vertically unstable

Young and Burgess classification[8]

Considers mechanism of injury and alerts the surgeon to potential resuscitation requirement and associated injury patterns.

[7] Tile M (1988) Pelvic ring fractures:should they be fixed? *J Bone Joint Surg Br* **70**(1):1–20.
[8] Burgess AR, Eastridge BJ, Young JW (1990) Pelvic ring disruptions: effective classification system and treatment protocols. *J Trauma* **30**(7): 848–56.

Antero-posterior compression

Following direct anterior or posterior trauma. Divided into three subtypes: APC-I, APC-II and APC-III. Patients with APC-I have minimally displaced, usually vertical, pubic rami fractures or mild pubic symphysis diastasis. In type APC-II injuries the anterior sacroiliac, sacrospinous and sacrotuberous ligaments are torn and the pelvis is splayed open like a book. In type APC-III injuries all the sacroiliac structures are disrupted including the posterior ligaments and they have the highest incidence of life-threatening haemorrhage. This is the most common severe injury seen in pedestrians.

Lateral compression

Divided into three subtypes: LC-I, LC-II and LC-III, differentiated by disruption of the posterior sacroiliac structures. In LC-III injuries, the pelvis opens on the contralateral side as the deforming force is transmitted through the pelvis, resulting in a wind-swept pelvis.

Vertical shear

Usually occurs as a result of a fall from a height. There is a fracture pattern through the pubic rami and posterior pelvis with vertical displacement of the hemipelvis.

Combined mechanism

Combination of LC and VS or LC and APC.

Associated injuries

- **Haemorrhage** – from the sacral venous plexus and other great veins. Arterial bleeding, particularly divisions of the internal iliac artery (superior gluteal artery). Occasionally disruption of a major vessel such as the common (or internal/external) iliac artery and vein. Bleeding from exposed bone surfaces
- **Urethral injury** – 10%. More common in males. Bladder rupture in 5%. Check blood at the meatus, penile bruising, a high riding prostate on per rectum, and haematuria. Ureteric injury is rare

- **Nerve damage**. Sacral fractures through neural foramina – lumbosacral plexus damage. Sciatic/other nerve damage depending on injury

Imaging

- AP pelvis ✓
- Pelvic inlet/outlet views
- Judet views
  - Obturator oblique – view of anterior column and posterior rim
  - Iliac oblique – view of posterior column and anterior rim
- CT scans
- FAST scan to exclude intra-abdominal injury

Management

Mechanism of injury determines energy and the probability of associated injuries. Emergency care includes management of life-threatening injuries using ATLS protocols. Only one surgeon assesses the stability of the pelvis with bimanual compression/distraction at initial assessment. Anti-shock garment may be useful in the acute setting (risk of lower extremity compartment syndrome). Where there is uncontrolled haemorrhage despite an external fixator, the patient may need angiography and embolization. With an unstable pelvic injury, laparotomy presents great risk if an external fixator has not been applied.

External fixator

Applied in the haemodynamically unstable patient not responding to initial fluid resuscitation.
- Inverted A-frame external fixator (may be suitable for definitive treatment – retained for 8–12 weeks)
- Ganz pelvic C clamp (posterior closure of pelvis)

Definitive surgical management

- External fixator (open book – Tile type B1 – SI ligaments are intact)
- Internal fixation (dependent on the fracture configuration)
- Stabilize the pubic symphysis with two plates through a Pfannenstiel incision

- Displaced posterior injuries are fixed through a direct posterior approach (wound healing complications occur in 3%–25%) or an anterior (extended ilioinguinal) approach to the SI joint
- Reconstruction plates, iliosacral screws or inter-fragmentary lag screws (for crescent fractures if the intact portion of the ilium is large and firmly attached to the sacrum)
- Iliac wing fractures are fixed with plates and screws or lag screws
- Non-operative management includes protective weight bearing for stable injuries, skeletal traction for vertically unstable fractures where surgery is contraindicated or prolonged bed rest (this yields poor results)

Examination corner

Trauma oral 1

- Classification and management of open book fractures, haemodynamics, etc.
- External fixator – whether to put on in Accident and Emergency or in theatre. Discuss

Trauma oral 2

AP pelvic radiograph of a complex fracture

- ATLS protocol
- Urological problems
- Classification
- Surgical management options

Trauma oral 3

Radiograph of the pelvis with wide diastasis of the pubic symphysis

- Young female patient, RTA no other injuries
- Discuss the assessment and management of this patient
- Classification of pelvic fractures
- Management of pelvic fractures with shock
- Discussion about external fixation

Trauma oral 4

AP radiograph of pelvic fracture

- Management including indications for surgery and exposure
- Role of external fixators

Trauma oral 5

Clinical photograph of open supracondylar femoral fracture with pelvic fracture

History given of a young female patient involved in a high speed RTA with the above injuries and a pulseless leg.

Asked about management. ATLS, open fracture management, vascular injury, external fixation of the pelvis and LISS plate for the femoral fracture. This then led on to being asked about the principles of locking plates.

Trauma oral 6

Management of an open book pelvic fracture with life threatening haemorrhage.

Acetabular fractures

Acetabular fractures often occur in the younger population and are a significant skeletal injury. Seventy-five percent follow RTAs. Fifty percent are associated with another major fracture or injury.

Acetabular fractures may be associated with hip dislocation or impaired sciatic nerve function. Femoral head dislocations should be reduced as a surgical emergency and maintained with traction until definitive management is initiated.

Prognostic factors

- Velocity of injury
- Stability of the femoral head
- Restoration of congruency of the weight-bearing surface of the acetabular dome

Anatomy

The acetabulum is part of the innominate bone, formed from the ilium, ischium and pubis. Letournel described an inverted Y configuration with anterior and posterior columns:

- Anterior column – pelvic brim, anterior wall, superior pubic ramus and anterior border of iliac wing
- Posterior column – greater/lesser sciatic notch, posterior wall, ischial tuberosity and most of the quadrilateral surface

Letournel and Judet classification of acetabular fractures[9]

Simple fractures

- Posterior wall
- Posterior column
- Anterior wall
- Anterior column
- Transverse

Complex associated fractures (combination of two simple fractures)

- Associated posterior column and posterior wall
- Associated transverse and posterior wall
- T-shaped
- Associated anterior wall or column and posterior hemi-transverse
- Both columns

Imaging

Radiographs

- AP pelvis, pelvis inlet and outlet views
- Judet views: obturator oblique and iliac oblique views

CT

- Spiral CT with three-dimensional reconstruction. Useful for head fractures and intra-articular loose bodies. Improves understanding and surgical reconstruction of acetabular fractures

Management

Indications for conservative management

- Local/systemic infection
- Severe osteoporosis
- Non-displaced fracture (<2 mm of acetabular dome)
- Low column, low transverse and low T-shaped acetabular fractures
- Advanced age (considered with view to early total hip arthroplasty)
- Associated medical conditions
- Associated soft-tissue and visceral injuries

Conservative management

1. Non-displaced and minimally displaced fractures
   - Less than 4 mm displacement of the acetabular dome
2. Fractures with significant displacement but in an unimportant region of the joint
   - Low transverse fractures, low anterior column fractures
3. Secondary congruence in displaced fractures of both columns
   - Often comminuted, two-column fracture fragments assume a position of articular secondary congruency around the femoral head, even though the femoral head is displaced medially and there may be gaps between the fracture fragments

Manage with 8 weeks of traction and bed rest.

Indications for ORIF

- >4 mm articular step off
- Posterior wall fractures >40%

[9] Judet R, Judet J, Letournel E (1964) Fractures of the acetabulum:classification and surgical approaches for open reduction. *J Bone Joint Surg* **46** A:1615–1647.

- Marginal impaction fractures
- Loss of acetabular congruity
- Intra-articular debris
- Irreducible fracture/dislocation
- Roof arc measurement <45° suggests significant involvement of weight-bearing dome and need for ORIF
- All acetabular fractures resulting in hip joint instability

Reconstruction

The aim of reconstruction is to achieve anatomical reduction and fixation with a combination of screws and contoured pelvic reconstructive plates. Surgical approaches can be simple or extensile.

Anterior ilioinguinal approach
For anterior column fractures and possibly two-column fractures. Gives access to the interior ileum, anterior column and superior pubic ramus.

Extended Kocher–Langenbeck approach
This is indicated for a posterior injury and is the workhorse of acetabular surgery. Gives access to the posterior wall and posterior column below the greater sciatic notch.

Ipsilateral femoral shaft and acetabular fracture
Compression plate fixation or retrograde intramedullary nailing is indicated. Keep the wound away from the pelvis. Address acetabular fracture later following necessary investigations.

Complications of surgery

- **Sciatic nerve injury.** Occurs in up to 10%–15% of acetabular fractures
- **DVT/PE.** Occurs in one-third of patients (one-fifth of those <40 years old, half of patients >40 years old). PE occurs in 4%–7% of patients
- **Infection.** Reported to occur in 1%–5% of patients and may destroy the hip joint

- **Heterotopic ossification.** Incidence varies from 5% to 15% of surgically treated patients, but usually asymptomatic. Prophylaxis should be given
- **AVN.** Reported rate of 10% after posterior dislocation
- **Post-degenerative OA.** Where reduction is good 90% will have a favourable result; where reduction is poor 50%–70% will achieve a satisfactory result
- **Chondrolysis.** Following acetabular trauma it may occur with or without surgical intervention. It is usually a manifestation of early osteoarthritis without surgery. After ORIF, suspect infection or the presence of metal in the joint. On occasion, AVN of acetabular fragments causes early collapse and chondrolysis may ensue

Complications of non-operative management

- Severe osteoporosis
- Sepsis
- Systemic illness
- Age and functional demands

Examination corner

Trauma oral 1

- Classification of acetabular fractures
- Broad outline of management
- Approaches to the acetabulum: indications, complications of surgery
- Radiographs shown with both columns fixed and with trochanteric osteotomies

Trauma oral 2

Acetabular fractures

- Classification
- Principles of surgical treatment
- Heterotopic ossification
- Surgical approaches

Long case 1

Young man with AVN of his right hip and secondary osteoarthritis several years following acetabular fixation. Now presents with a painful and stiff hip requiring arthroplasty.

Discussion included:

• Acute management of acetabular fractures
• Surgical approaches to the acetabulum
• Complications and results of acetabular fixation
• What to do now with the hip
• MOM hip resurfacing
• Management of an infected MOM hip resurfacing presenting at 1 year

Traumatic hip dislocation

Background

The vast majority (80%) of traumatic hip dislocations are caused by RTAs, often secondary to severe violent injury. The remainder include falls from a height, industrial accidents and sports injuries. Hip dislocations can be either anterior, posterior or central. Dislocations with either acetabular or femoral fractures are almost always posterior (90%), whilst anterior dislocations often have an associated femoral head fracture and/or impaction injury. Reduction should be as a surgical emergency within 6 hours of injury to reduce the risk of AVN developing. Prognosis is proportional to the time interval between occurrence and reduction. One-half of patients have other fractures (patella, femoral or tibial condyles) and 30% have soft-tissue injury of the knee from hitting the dashboard (PCL injury and posterolateral rotational instability).

Classification

Classifications for hip dislocation include Epstein for anterior dislocation, Thompson and Epstein for posterior dislocation and central fracture dislocations within the AO comprehensive classification of fractures of the pelvis and acetabulum.

Thompson and Epstein classification for posterior hip dislocation (1951)[10]

Type I: Pure dislocation with or without minor fracture of the acetabulum

Type II: Dislocation with a large, single posterior rim fracture

Type III: Dislocation with a comminuted posterior wall fracture

Type IV: Dislocation with associated fracture of the posterior acetabular wall and floor

Type V: Dislocation with associated fracture of the femoral head (5%–10%)

Epstein classification for anterior dislocation[11]

Type I superior and type II inferior, with further sub-divisions as follows:

A: No associated fracture
B: Associated femoral head fracture
C: Associated acetabular rim fracture

Pipkin classification[12]

Thompson and Epstein type V fractures (posterior hip dislocation with associated fracture of the femoral head) have been subdivided by Pipkin into four types:

Type I: Caudal head fragment (below the fovea centralis)

Type II: Cephalad fracture (below the fovea centralis)

Type III: Type I or II injury with associated femoral head and neck fracture

Type IV: Type I or II injury with associated acetabular rim fracture

[10] Thompson VP, Epstein HC (1951) Traumatic dislocation of the hip; a survey of two hundred and four cases covering a period of twenty-one years. *J Bone Joint Surg Am* **33A**(3): 746–78.

[11] Epstein HC (1973) Traumatic dislocations of the hip. *Clin Orthop Relat Res* **92**: 116–42.

[12] Pipkin G (1957) Treatment for grade IV fracture dislocation of hip. *J Bone Joint Surg* **29**: 1027–42.

Imaging

- Anteroposterior radiograph of the pelvis. A careful search should be made for associated fractures of the acetabulum, femoral head and femoral shaft
- Pelvic inlet/outlet views
- Obturator/iliac oblique (Judet) views. Not always easy to obtain because of pain issues but they allow assessment of the anterior and posterior walls and columns of the acetabulum
- Repeat radiographs are obtained post reduction to determine adequacy of reduction, presence or absence of fracture fragments trapped within the joint and the presence of any associated fractures of the acetabulum or femoral head and neck possibly initially missed
- CT. Post reduction to assess congruity of the hip joint and to look for any free osteochondral fragments within the joint. The incidence of instability is high if the remaining posterior articular surface is <34%. Hips with >55% of the remaining posterior articular surface are stable
- MRI. Useful if post reduction radiographs suggest incongruency, to exclude soft-tissue interposition (labrum, muscle and capsule) in the articular space.

Initial management

- The injury follows major trauma so initial management must follow ATLS protocol
- Assessment and resuscitation of patient
- Neurological injuries must be assessed and documented before and after hip reduction. Sciatic nerve injuries occur in 10%–23% of posterior dislocations, the peroneal component more commonly involved and usually more severely affected than the tibial component
- Hip dislocation should be reduced as an emergency. Other fractures may be addressed later

Associated bony injuries

- Acetabular fractures – usually posterior wall (dashboard injury) but any fracture pattern is possible

- Femoral head fractures
  - Most femoral head fractures are seen with a posterior dislocation since posterior dislocations are more frequent (90%)
  - However, a higher percentage of anterior dislocations have an associated femoral head fracture (68% compared to 7%)
- Femoral neck fractures are uncommon with hip dislocation
- Femoral shaft fractures are uncommon but make reduction difficult
- Patella fractures and knee dislocations may lead to knee instability

Complications

AVN

The reported risk of AVN is between 2% and 17% following posterior dislocation. The medial femoral circumflex artery is the key vessel to the femoral head at the superolateral articular margin. A posterior dislocation puts this vessel at risk whereas an anterior dislocation will relax the vessel. Difficult problem to manage as these patients are usually young and active. THA may not be an appropriate option; consider trabecular metal AVN rod or vascularized fibular grafting.

Sciatic nerve palsy

Occurs almost exclusively with posterior dislocations, with a reported incidence of 10%–23%. At least partial nerve recovery can be expected in 60%–70% of patients. Sciatic nerve may be damaged by ischaemia secondary to sustained pressure from the femoral head or large fragments of bone or lacerated or impaled by bone fragments.

Acetabular labral injuries

May be source of symptoms (persistent pain) even after successful reduction. May cause intermittent clicking or catching. Clinically diagnosis is made with a positive impingement test. Hip arthroscopy is sometimes required for management.

Joint capsule injury

If the femoral head buttonholes through the capsule it can block reduction.

Muscle injury

Short external rotators are frequently torn during posterior dislocations.

Arterial injury

The femoral artery can be injured with anterior dislocations.

Chondrolysis

It is postulated that either an intra-articular haematoma results in enzymatic degradation of the articular cartilage, similar to the process of joint destruction seen in patients with hemophilia, or that ischaemia occurs secondary to increased capsular pressure.

Recurrent dislocation

May be associated with unrecognized or untreated acetabular fracture or impaction fractures of the femoral head. Very rare; most are posterior.

Post-traumatic osteoarthritis

Incidence varies from 11% to 16%. The incidence increases with age and significant acetabular fractures and is reduced with accurate ORIF.

Heterotopic bone formation

Incidence is approximately 2%. Increases with ORIF, delayed surgery, and associated head injury.

Methods of closed reduction for posterior dislocation

Allis and Bigelow technique

The patient is supine with counter traction applied to the ipsilateral anterior superior iliac crest. The leg is slowly flexed beyond 90°, internally rotated and adducted. Reduction of the hip is not subtle and is easily palpable.

Stimson technique

The patient is prone with the hip flexed 90° off the edge of the table. Force is applied to the back of the proximal calf. The reduction manoeuvres are the same as for anterior dislocation.

Anterior dislocation

Anterior dislocations are harder to reduce than posterior dislocations. Position of the leg is reversed. With the leg in external rotation, abduction and flexion, inline traction is applied.

Open reduction

Indications include hips that cannot be reduced closed, hips with associated fractures that are unstable after closed reduction and hips that are not congruent after closed reduction.

Significant rim fractures

Significant rim fractures usually require ORIF as the hip is generally unstable following reduction. Fragments are usually posterior and often comminuted. They should be stabilized with interfragmentary screws and a reconstruction plate.

Retained fragments

Retained fragments can be diagnosed on a post-reduction CT and are removed by arthrotomy or hip arthroscopy. There is a high risk of developing post-traumatic osteoarthritis when patients with intra-articular fragments are managed in traction. Widening of the hip joint on plain radiographs is not evident when fragments of 2 mm are present in the hip joint.

Large head fragments

Large head fragments require ORIF or removal if they are not involving the weight-bearing area.

Fractures of the femoral head associated with a posterior hip dislocation are usually managed with an anterior approach to the hip joint. Fragments are often cephalad and attached to the ligamentum teres and cannot be adequately visualized using the posterior approach. Fractures of the femoral head associated with anterior hip dislocation usually require a posterior approach to the hip joint.

The fragments are fixed using small fragment screws or Herbert screws.

Hip movements should be started early. Toe-touch weight bearing for 6 weeks is increased to full weight bearing over the next 6 weeks.

Examination corner

Trauma oral 1

Pipkin type III posterior dislocation of the hip with a fracture of the neck of femur in a 53-year-old patient

• Management of this patient. Least common Pipkin injury. Approach to use. Closed reduction contraindicated. The femoral neck fracture must be stabilized before reduction of the hip dislocation
• What is the management when there is concern regarding the vascular supply to the femoral head?
• Discussion regarding hemiarthroplasty against total hip arthroplasty and then unipolar hemiarthroplasty against bipolar hemiarthroplasty

Trauma oral 2

AP radiograph of the pelvis of a 45-year-old male driver in a car who has a front head-on collision with another vehicle

Presents to casualty with a shortened and externally rotated right leg and some paraesthesia in his right lower leg.
• Differential diagnosis, management of traumatic hip dislocation
• Pipkin femoral head fracture classification system, femoral neck fracture classification systems (Garden, Evans, Pauwels)

Trauma oral 3

• No prop used. Discussion of the clinical features of anterior versus posterior dislocation
• Posterior hip dislocations typically lie with the hip in a position of flexion, adduction and internal rotation. With an anterior dislocation the hip is externally rotated. Movement of the hip is painful and restricted. With ipsilateral fractures of the femoral neck or shaft the leg may assume a near-normal position and the dislocation may be missed
• Associated injuries
• Discussion of AVN of the hip
• Management of established AVN of the hip. Which type of hip replacement to use. Survival analysis tables

---

Extracapsular femoral neck fractures

Account for approximately 50% of all femoral neck fractures. The proportion is growing due to an increasingly elderly population and an increase in the age-specific incidence. Usually the fracture occurs in elderly osteoporotic patients. The majority are women (80%) with a mean age of presentation of 80 years, who often present following minimal trauma. Blood supply to the femoral head is preserved. Union rates are high (large surface area of cancellous bone at the fracture site). Fractures occur in young patients following high-velocity trauma.

Classification

Extracapsular fractures may be subdivided into trochanteric and subtrochanteric fractures. The term intertrochanteric refers to a fracture running transversely in between (but not through) the lesser and greater trochanters. The term pertrochanteric refers to a fracture running obliquely and through the greater to lesser trochanter.

Subtrochanteric fractures occur within 2.5 cm of the lesser trochanter and account for a minority of proximal femoral fractures (bimodal distribution in the young and those over 65 years old).

Evans' classification (1949)[13]

Based on the direction of the fracture and division of fractures into stable and unstable:

Type I: Undisplaced two-fragment fracture

Type II: Displaced two-fragment fracture

Type III: Three-fragment fracture without postero-lateral support, owing to displacement of greater trochanter fragment

Type IV: Three-fragment fracture without medial support, owing to displaced lesser trochanter or femoral arch fragment

Type V: Four-fragment fracture without posterolateral and medial support (combination of type III and type IV)

R: Reversed obliquity fracture

Seinsheimer's classification (subtrochanteric fractures)[14]

This classification is based on fracture fragments and the location and shape of the fracture lines:

Type I: Undisplaced fracture with less than 2 mm displacement of fracture fragments

Type II: Two-part fracture

Type IIA: Two-part transverse femoral fracture

Type IIB: Two-part spiral fracture with lesser trochanter attached to proximal fragment

Type IIC: Two-part spiral fracture with lesser trochanter attached to distal fragment

Type III: Three-part fracture

Type IIIA: Three-part spiral fracture in which lesser trochanter is part of third fragment, which has an inferior spike of cortex of varying length

Type IIIB: Three-part spiral fracture of the proximal third of the femur, with the third part being a butterfly fragment

Type IV: Comminuted fracture with four or more fragments

Type V: Subtrochanteric intertrochanteric fracture. This group includes any subtrochanteric fracture with extension through the greater trochanter

Imaging

- AP pelvis and lateral hip radiographs
- Only rarely is a CT or MRI scan required, if the diagnosis is disputed
- If no obvious fracture exists and pain persists, repeat X-rays after 3–4 days to check for fracture propagation

Management

Aim is for early mobilization of the patient. This prevents prolonged bed rest and its associated complications. Ideally, surgery should be within 24 h of hospital admission. Non-operative management is considered only in the very sick patient with a poor prognosis or where there is a definite contraindication to surgery, or the patient is completely immobile prior to surgery.

Non-operative treatment

Skilful neglect

Only appropriate for a patient who is completely immobile prior to the fracture. Fracture deformity with shortening and external rotation occurs. Nursing care is difficult.

Active conservative management

Consists of applying skin or skeletal traction for 6–8 weeks. Regular radiographs are required to check on fracture position. This is indicated if a patient is unfit for surgery, refuses surgery, where there is a lack of surgical implant, the absence of an experienced surgeon and a lack of surgical facilities.

Operative management

Extramedullary fixation (sliding hip screw-plate system)

Refers to applying a side plate to the proximal femur attached to a lag screw, which is passed proximally

[13] Evans EM (1949) The treatment of trochanteric fractures of the femur. *J Bone Joint Surg Br* **31B**: 190–203.

[14] Seinsheimer F (1978) Subtrochanteric fractures of the femur. *J Bone Joint Surg Am* **60**(3): 300–6.

across the fracture site up the femoral neck. These implants can be static or dynamic. Static implants have no capacity for sliding and cannot allow for any bone collapse that occurs around the fracture site. Examples of static implants include Jewett and McLaughlin nail plates. Dynamic implants do allow sliding at the plate–screw junction and allow for collapse at the fracture site. Examples include the dynamic hip screw (sliding hip screw) and the Pugh nail. Good anatomical reduction is required with alignment of the medial calcar. This hip screw should be in the centre of the head on both AP and lateral views and within 10 mm of the articular surface (in strong subchondral bone) to prevent cut out.

Cephalic-condylar intramedullary devices

This refers to an intramedullary implant that is passed distally within the femur from an insertion point in the greater trochanter. They are especially useful where the lesser trochanter is fractured. They provide better mechanical advantage as load sharing is improved and the bending moment is reduced. The hip screw position is the same as for the sliding hip screw.

Until recently results of all randomized trials found no major difference between intramedullary and extramedullary fixation. Latest research[15] with the newer intramedullary hip screw implants suggests a lower incidence of complications in the more difficult comminuted fractures (reverse fracture lines, subtrochanteric fractures).

Arthroplasty

A small number of cases have been reported using long-stem, cemented hemiarthroplasty for comminuted trochanteric fractures. This is probably a role best reserved for revision surgery after failure of internal fixation.

Basilar neck fractures

Basilar neck fractures are two-part fractures and are managed with a sliding hip screw. However, there is

a tendency for the head to rotate as the sliding hip screw is inserted. An anti-rotation screw or supplementary guidewire should be inserted superior to the sliding screw guidewire before insertion of the sliding screw.

Reverse oblique fractures

Reverse oblique fractures run in the inferolateral to superomedial direction, creating a tendency for the shaft to displace medially. The sliding axis of the sliding hip screw is therefore parallel to the fracture line as opposed to being perpendicular. The benefits of the sliding hip screw are therefore lost, leading to suboptimal fixation. This fracture pattern is best managed with an intramedullary device or a 90° fixed-angle plate system.

Subtrochanteric fractures

Subtrochanteric fractures can be managed with a sliding hip screw or a long intramedullary device.

Complications

A number of complications relating to the fracture can occur after an extracapsular fracture:

- Mortality: 33% at 6 months, 38% at 12 months (3% <60 years, 50% >90 years)
- In-hospital mortality: 15%
- Wound infection: 2%–15%
- Limb shortening
- Rotational deformity
- Re-fracture
- Detachment of the implant from the femur
- Breakage or disassembly of the implant
- Screw cut-out rate
- AVN: <0.5%

Examination corner

Trauma oral 1

Radiograph of the pelvis and both hips. One side of the trochanteric fracture fixed with a dynamic hip screw, the other side with a gamma nail.

Comment on the fixation methods used on both sides and the pros and cons of each.

---

[15] Parker MJ, Handoll HH (2005) Gamma and other cephalocondylic intramedullary nails versus extramedullary implants for extracapsular hip fractures. *Cochrane Database Syst Rev* **2005**(4): CD000093.

Intracapsular femoral neck fractures

They may be subcapital (junction of head and neck) or transcervical (passing through the neck). They account for just under half of all femoral neck fractures. Incidence is increasing. Mean age of presentation is around 80 years and 80% occur in women such that the fracture has been called widow's disease. It is uncommon in the presence of osteoarthritis.

Intracapsular fractures put the blood supply to the femoral head at risk. This is especially so with displaced fractures where there is a substantial risk of AVN or non-union.

Non-union

- Non-displaced and impacted <5%
- Displaced >20%–30%
- Patient's age
- Poor fracture reduction

Symptoms include progressive groin, thigh or buttock pain or a combination thereof.

AVN

- Non-displaced or impacted <8%
- Displaced 10%–20%

Classification

Garden classification (1961)[16]

Based on the degree of displacement of an intracapsular neck fracture on the AP radiograph of the pelvis:

Type I: Incomplete or impacted into valgus. Trabeculae are angulated

Type II: Complete fracture with minimal/no displacement. Trabeculae are interrupted but not broken

Type III: Displaced fracture with angulation of the trabecular lines

Type IV: Grossly displaced with trabecular lines of the head and acetabulum parallel

---

[16] Garden R (1961) Low-angle fixation in fractures of the femoral neck. *J Bone Joint Surg Br* **43**:647–61.

Pauwels' classification[17]

Based on the angle formed by the fracture line and the horizontal plane: the more vertical the fracture line, the higher the shear forces across the fracture and the poorer the prognosis:

- Type I: Fracture line 30° from the horizontal
- Type II: Fracture line 50° from the horizontal
- Type III: Fracture line 70° from the horizontal

Management

The pros and cons of ORIF versus hemiarthroplasty in intracapsular fractured neck of femur are given in Table 23.1, and the advantages and disadvantages of using cement are given in Table 23.2. These are favourite questions of examiners who, for an exit orthopaedic exam, would expect a snappy answer from a candidate

Impacted fractures

Early mobilization may be attempted if the head is tilted into valgus and weight bearing is tolerated. Stabilization with three parallel cannulated screws is generally advised.

Undisplaced fractures

Osteosynthesis with three parallel cannulated screws or a sliding hip screw with an additional anti-rotational screw is advised. Recommended for a patient with a physiological age of less than 75 years. Arthroplasty is generally indicated for patients older than 75 years. This usually equates with only one surgical procedure with no healing complications despite a higher complication rate.

Displaced fractures

There is a relatively low threshold for performing hemiarthroplasty in displaced fractures as the femoral head's blood supply is likely to be compromised.

---

[17] Pauwels F (1935) *Der Schenkelhalsbruch – ein mechanisches Problem: Grundlagen des Heilungsvorganges, Prognose und Therapie.* Stuttgart: Ferdinand Enke Verlag.

Table 23.1 Pros and cons of ORIF versus hemiarthroplasty in intracapsular fractured necks of femur

	Internal fixation	Arthroplasty
Non-union	20%–30%	Avoided
AVN	10%–20%	Avoided
Dislocation	Avoided	5% hemi 10% total
Acetabular erosion	Avoided	20% long-term survivors
Prosthetic loosening	Avoided	10%
Sepsis around implant		2%–5% (mortality >50%)
Re-operation rate 1 year	18.6% (Parker *et al.*)[1]	4.8%
Re-fracture around implant	Rare	2%–4%

[1]Parker MJ, Khan RJ, Crawford J, Pryor GA (2002) Hemiarthroplasty versus internal fixation for displaced intracapsular hip fractures in the elderly. A randomised trial of 455 patients. *J Bone Joint Surg Br* **84**(8): 1150–5.

Table 23.2 Use of cement

Advantages of cement	Disadvantages of cement
Less thigh pain	More demanding operation
Reduced revision rate	Revision more difficult
Increased mobility	Increased mortality
More secure fixation	Cement reaction

There are no healing complications of the fracture if the femoral head is replaced with a metal one. However, management depends on a patient's pre-fracture level of mobility and associated medical co-morbidity factors. Consider internal fixation in younger patients with displaced intracapsular fractures. If proceeding with arthroplasty a cemented bipolar prosthesis is recommended in younger, healthier patients. The theory is that the bipolar mechanism will decrease wear at the acetabulum. There are no reported benefits of bipolar prosthesis in patients over the age of 80 years.

Alternatively, a cemented mono-block hemiarthroplasty may be used in older patients. In very frail patients when a quick procedure may be required due to concurrent medical issues, then a non-cemented prosthesis such as the Austin–Moore hemiarthroplasty is used. However, this particular prosthesis is associated with anterior thigh pain due to the poor fit and "toggling" of the prosthesis.

Young patients

This constitutes patients under the age of 60. Preservation of the femoral head by reduction and internal fixation within 6 h of injury is the accepted management. The Leadbetter manoeuvre (traction along the line of the femur with the hip and knee flexed at 90°, followed by internal rotation and abduction) is used to reduce the fracture before internal fixation. A good result can be expected in up to 84% of cases. Alternatively, primary THA may be performed. Risks include a higher incidence of dislocation, infection, HO and earlier failure compared to elective THA.

Examination corner

Trauma oral 1

Radiograph of a displaced intracapsular fractured neck of femur

- Describe
- How will you manage this patient: details of history and preoperative assessment
- What is the mental test score?
- What operation would you advise and why?

Trauma oral 2

Radiograph of a displaced Garden type IV intracapsular fractured neck of femur

- Female aged 88 years
- Classification
- Management
- Differences between cemented, uncemented and bipolar hemiarthroplasty of the hip

Trauma oral 3

Radiograph of a displaced fractured neck of femur in a 70-year-old female

- Classification
- Management of Garden grade IV fracture and prognosis

Trauma oral 4

Radiographs of an undisplaced subcapital fractured neck of femur in a female aged 60 years with Parkinson's disease

- Describe the radiographs
- How do you manage this fracture?
- Closed reduction and fixation
- Aspiration of the joint to decrease the incidence of AVN – when is this indicated, what evidence is there for this procedure in the literature?

Distal femoral fractures

Background

Distal femoral fractures account for 4%–7% of all femoral fractures and are difficult fractures to manage. Fifty per cent are extra-articular supracondylar fractures. Fifty per cent have an intra-articular extension. Twenty-five per cent of all fractures are open. There is a bimodal age distribution: usually young males following high-energy trauma or elderly osteoporotic females following minimal trauma. Management may result in knee stiffness due to damage and scarring of the extensor mechanism and/or intra-articular pathology (cartilage contusion, osteochondral fractures and meniscal tears) and adhesions. Ligament injuries occur in 20% of fractures (collateral/cruciate ligament injuries).

Mechanism of injury

Several muscle groups insert or arise in the supracondylar region and cause deformity after fractures. The gastrocnemius rotates the distal fragment posteriorly while the strong adductors cause varus angulation. Intercondylar fractures are splayed open by discordant muscle action. The hamstrings muscles cause posterior fracture displacement and angulation with associated medial or lateral deformation. The quadriceps muscle shortens the fracture.

Management

Non-operative management

Undisplaced or minimally displaced fractures can be managed conservatively either with a long leg cast or with skeletal traction. Maintaining accurate reduction is difficult. The gastrocnemius muscle attachment causes a hyperextension deformity of the distal segment. Prolonged skeletal traction is associated with knee stiffness and medical risks of immobilization. Malunion and non-union are common.

Associated injuries

The associated injuries depend on the position of the patient's lower extremity at the time of the injury: simultaneous injuries can result in hip dislocation, femoral shaft fracture, tibial plateau fracture, tibial shaft fractures (floating knee) and patella fractures (10%). Popliteal vessel injury is rare.

Operative management

Several methods available, which are now discussed.

Cancellous lag screw fixation

For unicondylar fractures. Most commonly used as a supplement to other devices.

A 95° condylar blade plate

Technically demanding and requires precision in placement. Requires extensive soft-tissue exposure therefore compromising the blood supply to the bone. There may also be stress shielding of the bone.

Dynamic condylar screw (DCS)

The compression screw is cannulated to allow easy application over a guidewire. Bone grafting is often required. Requires an adequate distal fracture fragment to allow insertion of the compression screw.

Condylar buttress plate

Weaker construct than either a condylar screw or a blade plate. Errors in alignment, particularly valgus, are common.

LISS plate fixation

LISS stands for less invasive stabilization system. A LISS plate is similar to a buttress plate with several modifications. The screw holes in a LISS plate are round and threaded so that the screws are locked onto the plate. This allows adequate stabilization with only unicortical screws rather than the bicortical fixation required with standard compression

or buttress plates. The plate does not have to be close to the bone and therefore it does not need to be closely contoured to the periarticular surface as with a standard buttress plate. These modifications allow easier insertion and less damage to the bone and its blood supply. Specially shaped unicortical screws are used with the LISS plate.

Retrograde intramedullary nail

A retrograde intramedullary nail causes minimal soft-tissue damage and is associated with low infection rates. In the elderly fixation can be tenuous and a cast brace support is often necessary. Non-weight-bearing or cast bracing is encouraged for 3 months after the operation. However, due to the preservation of the soft tissue around the knee, early knee movement is often regained.

External fixation

External fixation is indicated for severe or open injuries. This may be with an anterior bridging fixator (when stabilization is needed for soft tissue and vascular reconstruction). A circular frame may be used to supplement minimal open reduction and percutaneous screw or wire fixation. This allows for early movement of the knee.

Complications

Early complications

- Vascular compromise
- Infection
- Mal-reduction
- Fixation failure

Late complications

- Malunion (rotational, flexion/extension, varus/valgus alignment)
- Non-union (especially fractures above a stiff knee)
- Knee stiffness
- Joint destruction (if intramedullary nail left prominent)

Examination corner

Knee stiffness following supracondylar fracture

Quite common as a potential trauma long case with other associated injuries. The discussion of management options can be difficult.

Results from injury to the quadriceps mechanism and/or articular surface either during the initial trauma or during surgery. The combination of muscle adhesions, arthrofibrosis and ligamentous contractures causes knee stiffness. Iatrogenic causes such as protruding hardware and articular mal-reduction can also contribute.

Difficult problem to manage; MUA with or without arthroscopic lysis of adhesions or quadricepsplasty are possible options.

Tibial plafond fractures

Also known as tibial pilon fractures, tibial plafond fractures account for fewer than 1% of all lower limb fractures and 5%–7% of tibial fractures. The fracture involves the weight-bearing articular surface of the distal tibia, the diaphysis and the distal fibula (75% of cases). Occasionally, there is diaphyseal extension into the tibial shaft.

Twenty percent of plafond fractures are associated with an open injury. The wound is often anteromedial. Swelling and skin contusions may be severe at an early stage, worsening with time.

Mechanism of injury

Rotational injuries cause low-energy fractures with relatively little associated soft-tissue injury or comminution. Axial compression causes high-energy fractures with extensive soft-tissue disruption and "explosive" comminution of the plafond.

- Axial loading with the ankle in plantar flexion (posterior articular comminution)
- Axial loading with the ankle in dorsiflexion (anterior articular comminution)
- Rotational (shear) forces (wide array of injury patterns are seen)

Imaging

- AP, mortise and lateral views
- CT scan demonstrates the fracture configuration and helps preoperative planning

Classification

Rüedi and Allgöwer (1979)[18] is the most widely used classification. It both helps planning and is of prognostic value. Other classifications include Kellam and Waddell (1979),[19] Ovadia and Beals (1986)[20] and the AO/ASIF (1996).

Rüedi and Allgöwer classification

Type I: Undisplacement T shaped intra-articular fracture of the distal tibia without comminution

Type II: Significant displacement of the intra-articular components without comminution

Type III: Displaced intra-articular multifragmentary fracture with impaction and comminution of the articular surface

Low-energy fractures tend to be type I or II. High-energy fractures are usually type III fractures.

Associated injuries

- **Skeletal** (calcaneum, long bone fractures, shear fractures of the pelvis and axial spine fractures)
- **Soft tissues**. There may be significant soft-tissue damage without an open fracture
- **Neurovascular injuries**. These must be excluded
- **Other injuries** secondary to high-energy injuries (head, thorax, abdomen)

[18] Rüedi TP, Allgöwer M (1979) The operative treatment of intra-articular fractures of the lower end of the tibia. *Clin Orthop Relat Res* **138**: 105–10.

[19] Kellam JF, Waddell JP (1979) Fractures of the distal tibial metaphysis with intra-articular extension – the distal tibial explosion fracture. *J Trauma* **19**(8): 593–601.

[20] Ovadia DN, Beals RK (1986) Fractures of the tibial plafond. *J Bone Joint Surg Am* **68**(4): 543–51.

Management

Objectives of surgical management

- Anatomical reduction of the articular surface
- Restoration of length
- Bone union
- Viable soft tissue, which is not infected
- Early movement and restoration of function

Timing of surgery

Timing is critical in the management of high-energy tibial plafond fractures. ORIF, if attempted early, should be within 6–12 h post injury. After 12 h post injury, profound swelling means there is a high risk of complications. Temporary stabilization with external fixation is preferable. Surgery should be delayed for 7–10 days while swelling resolves with elevation and cryo-cooling. Several centres advocate a two-stage procedure with high-energy injuries with extensively compromised soft tissues. In the first stage, primary reduction and internal fixation of the articular surface is performed using stab incisions, screws and K-wires. Temporary external fixation is applied across the ankle joint. After recovery of the soft tissues, the second stage entails internal fixation with a medial plate using a reduced invasive technique.

Surgical management

Type I fractures

Type I fractures are preferably managed non-operatively with cast immobilization and 6 weeks of non-weight-bearing, followed by a further 6 weeks of graduated weight-bearing. Surgical stabilization will allow earlier movement. Bourne *et al.*[21] reported >80% satisfactory results with type I and II fractures. Only 44% of type III fractures had a satisfactory result.

Type II and III fractures

Type II and III fractures are difficult to manage. Several methods of management are available:

[21] Bourne RB, Rorabeck CH, Macnab J (1983) Intra-articular fractures of the distal tibia: the pilon fracture. *Trauma* **23**(7): 591–16.

- **ORIF** with reconstruction of the fibular length with a plate, reconstruction of the articular surface with interfragmentary screws, cancellous bone grafting and stabilization of the medial tibia with a buttress plate (Rüedi and Allgöwer)
- **External fixation** with a unilateral external fixator spanning the ankle to provide ligamentotaxis and effect indirect reduction. The results are no better than ORIF for type III injuries. A circular external fixator such as the Ilizarov external fixator consists of fine wires (1.8 mm) for interfragmentary fixation. Ilizarov frames allow for early weight-bearing and ankle joint movement
- **Combined fixation** with a fibular plate to restore length and an external fixator placed medially, crossing the ankle joint. They are combined with minimal open reduction, bone grafting and interfragmentary screw fixation. The results are similar to ORIF in type II fractures. However, good results are achieved in >70% for type III fractures
- **Early arthrodesis** is a reasonable option in the severely comminuted fracture that is non-reconstructable. It facilitates earlier rehabilitation

Complications

Early complications

- Delayed wound healing or wound sloughing
- Infection of wound or pin tracks
- Osteomyelitis
- Neurovascular injury
- Loss of reduction

Late complications

- Mal/non-union
- Joint stiffness
- Ankle joint instability
- Post-traumatic arthritis (relates to cartilage damage at time of surgery despite optimal management)
- Late arthrodesis is 50% in some series for type III injuries
- Amputation

Trauma oral 1

Radiograph of a severe open pilon fracture

- ABC ATLS resuscitation in A&E: cut short by examiners, not wanted
- General management principles of open fractures: again cut short, not what the examiners want to talk about
- Classification
- Current thinking about management and recent literature

Candidate: Might have been better if I had cut to the chase and just described the radiograph and then moved onto classification rather trying the ABC ATLS waffle

---

Ankle fractures

High-energy injuries include RTAs, falls from height and sports injuries. Low-energy injuries include falls, twists and slips. Common in young sportsmen and in late-middle-aged obese women.

Classification

Lauge-Hansen classification[22]

The first description refers to the position of the foot at the time of injury (supinated or pronated). The second refers to the direction in which the talus moves within the ankle mortise (abduction, adduction or external rotation). The injuries occur in a step-wise fashion as the deforming force progresses.

Supination (inversion)/adduction injuries (SA)
1. Transverse distal fibula fracture or lateral ligament rupture
2. Vertical medial malleolar fracture

Supination (inversion)/external rotation injuries (SER)
1. Anterior talofibular ligament rupture ±avulsion of the anterolateral tibia (Tillaux fracture)

---

[22] Lauge-Hansen N (1949) Ligamentous ankle fractures; diagnosis and treatment. *Acta Chir Scand* **97**(6): 544–50.

2. Spiral/oblique fibular fracture (posterior at the proximal end to anterior distally) at the level of the syndesmosis
3. Posterior malleolar fracture or rupture of the posterior tibiofibular ligament
4. Medial ligament rupture of low medial malleolar fracture

Pronation (eversion)/abduction injuries (PA)

1. Deltoid ligament rupture (rare) or horizontal fracture of medial malleolus
2. Both the anterior and posterior tibiofibular ligaments rupture (syndesmosis rupture). In the case of the posterior ligament, the tibial attachment may be avulsed instead
3. Short transverse or oblique fibular fracture at the level of the joint. Comminution may occur with formation of a triangular fragment with its base directed laterally. The fibular fragment is tilted laterally

Pronation (eversion)/external rotation injuries (PER)
1. Deltoid rupture or oblique fracture of medial malleolus
2. Disruption of the anterior tibiofibular ligament causing avulsion of the tibial attachment (Tillaux fracture) or rupture
3. Spiral or oblique fibular fracture above the joint (obliquity fibular fracture is in the opposite direction found in supination-lateral rotation injuries). If the fracture is in the proximal fibula, this is a Maisonneuve fracture
4. Disruption of the posterior tibiofibular ligament or avulsion of the bony attachment (posterior malleolar fracture). If displacement of the talus continues, the interosseous membrane tears and gross diastasis occurs (Dupuytren's fracture dislocation)

Pronation-dorsiflexion (vertical compression fracture – pilon type fracture)

The anterior part of the talus is forced between the malleolus shearing off the medial malleolus.

Continued force fractures the anterior tibial margin and lateral malleolus. Finally the inferior articular surface of the tibia (pilon) fractures in an irregular fashion with severe communition.

Weber classification
This is based on the level of the fibular fracture relative to the syndesmosis:
A: Below
B: At the level
C: Above (more proximal type C fractures are unstable)

Imaging

- AP, lateral and mortise (15° internal rotation) radiographs
- CT scans for more complex patterns (pilon fractures)

Radiographic features to note

1. Medial and superior joint space. The joint space should be 4 mm throughout or <1 mm difference. Talar shift of 1 mm reduces the area of joint contact by 40%
2. Talar tilt is the angle between the tibial articular surface and the superior talus on the mortise view. This should be <5°
3. Talocrural angle is the angle between the tibial articular surface and the malleoli. This should be 8°–15°
4. A greater than 2-mm step in the articular surface
5. Tibiofibular overlap should be >1 mm on all views

Management

Conservative management

- Undisplaced fractures, including lateral malleolus alone without talar shift, are managed with below-knee cast for 6 weeks. Weight bearing may be allowed after 2–4 weeks if radiographs demonstrate no displacement

- Undisplaced fractures that are potentially unstable may be managed with below-knee cast as long as there is close radiographic monitoring for at least 3 weeks. If this is not possible, then fixation gives a better outcome. Note that 5%–10% of medial malleolar fractures go on to non-union and therefore should be followed-up closely
- Displaced bi- or tri-malleolar fractures may be managed non-operatively with reduction and POP cast only when surgery is contraindicated, i.e. poor skin, elderly, diabetics, alcoholics and the immunocompromised. Redisplacement is common when the swelling resolves

Operative management

Timing of surgery is essential to prevent soft-tissue problems. Surgery should be undertaken within 24 h of injury or after 7–10 days to avoid excess swelling of the tissues at the time of operation. It is essential that the limb be elevated as soon as possible. Cryo-cooling will help reduction of swelling.

- Displaced isolated malleolar fractures should be reduced and fixed with plates and screws, tension band wiring or screw fixation
- Displaced bi- and tri-malleolar fractures are generally unstable and require ORIF
- Accurate reduction of the lateral malleolus is the key to restoration of joint congruity. This fracture is addressed first. Oblique fractures are managed with a lag screw and a one-third tubular neutralization plate. A posterior anti-glide plate is recommended in porotic bone. Transverse fractures are stabilized with dynamic compression plates
- Medial malleolar fractures are fixed with lag screws or tension banding
- Posterior malleolar fractures need fixation only if >25% of the articular surface is involved. This is performed by lag screw fixation passed anteriorly to pick up the posterior fragment
- Stabilization of the syndesmosis is performed with one or two fully threaded 4.5-mm screw passed across at least three cortices just above the syndesmosis with the ankle in neutral (widest part of the talus is engaged in the mortise). Patient to

be non-weight-bearing for 6–10 weeks. The screw may be removed or left in situ after this time

Indication for fixation of Weber type C fractures

1. Associated medial ligament rupture (repair of ligament alone is not adequate). Medial fractures, if fixed, will prevent talar shift
2. Fractures 4.5 cm or more above the joint are likely to have residual diastasis despite fibular fixation. Those below 3 cm above the joint are generally stable. Fractures occurring within 3 and 4.5 cm may be assessed intra-operatively by hooking the fibula and pulling. This will identify significant dynamic diastasis
3. Proximal fibular fractures are rarely fixed. However, a diastasis screw should be inserted

Complications

Early complications

- Inadequate reduction
- Redisplacement (non-operative treatment)
- Delayed wound healing
- Wound infection
- Osteomyelitis
- Nerve injury (sural nerve)

Late complications

- Mal or non-union and diastasis
- Joint stiffness
- Ankle joint instability
- Post-traumatic arthritis (relates to cartilage damage at time of surgery despite optimal management)

Examination corner

Trauma oral 1

Radiograph of a trimalleolar fracture ankle

- Assessment and management

Trauma oral 2

Mechanism of ankle fractures

- Lauge-Hansen classification
- Fixation methods for Weber C fracture

Achilles tendon rupture

Classically occurs in middle-aged sedentary males performing unaccustomed sporting activity such as squash or tennis. The mean age of presentation is 35 years with 60% of ruptures occur during recreational sport.

Mechanism of injury

- Sudden ankle dorsiflexion
- Excessive strain during the heel-off phase of gait
- Following direct trauma

Diagnosis

- Hear or feel a pop
- Immediate weakness of push-off followed by pain and swelling, with difficulty walking
- Visible and palpable defect in the tendon
- Weakness of plantar flexion
- Inability to heel raise
- Simmond's test is positive for Achilles tendon rupture – with the patient prone or kneeling on a chair, squeezing the calf does not produce passive plantar flexion
- O'Brien's needle test

Where clinical findings are equivocal, the diagnosis can be confirmed by ultrasound or MRI scans.

Pathological process

The pathological process leading to rupture is poorly understood. A watershed area is present 3–6 cm above the calcaneal insertion. This is an area of relatively poor blood supply aggravated by decreased perfusion during stretching, contraction and advancing age. In addition there are changes to the cross-linking of collagen fibres and degenerative changes with age.

Two theories

- Chronic tendon degeneration
- Acute mechanical overload

Both factors usually involved.

Management

Non-operative management

- Basically avoids the risk of surgical complications
- Higher re-rupture rate approx 15% (4%–50%)
- Greater tendon elongation and weaker plantar flexion (20% versus 10% surgery)
- Cast for 8/52 initially in equinus
- Conflicting reports of whether the cast should be below or above the knee and when weight bearing is begun

Advantages of surgery

- Re-rupture rate is lower at 2% (0%–7%)
- Rehabilitation is more rapid
- Earlier return to work
- Quicker return to sport

Disadvantages of surgery

- Overall complication rate approximately 10%
- Deep infection
- Superficial infection
- Fistula
- Skin necrosis
- Suture granuloma
- Damage to the sural nerve

Surgical technique

- Posteromedial incision
- Lateral incision: risk of injury to sural nerve
- Midline: prone to adhesions and subsequent irritation by footwear

---

Examination corner

Examiner: What are the advantages and disadvantages of conservative versus operative management for acute tendon rupture?

Candidate: Non-operative management is favoured by a number of surgeons to avoid the complications of surgery, which are essentially wound healing problems. However, there may be situations in which operative treatment may be the preferred option. These would include, etc.

Examiner: What do you do? How do YOU treat an acute Achilles rupture tendon?

Candidate: I would sit down with the patient and explain the pros and cons of surgery versus non-operative treatment and let them decide. I would however be guided by age, level of sporting activity and any co-existing medical condition in recommending a choice.

Intramedullary fixation techniques

Implant design characteristics

- **Diameter**: stiffness is proportional to fourth power of the radius
- **Length**: working length is the distance over which the nail is unsupported by the bone. Bending stiffness is inversely proportional to the square of the working length. Torsional stiffness is inversely proportional to the working length
- **Shape:** unreamed nails have relatively small diameter, but are solid to give adequate stiffness. Cannulated nails may be rigid or slotted
- **Cross-sectional characteristics:** most are cylindrical (therefore lighter). Some are cloverleaf shaped in cross-section (increases stiffness)
- **Material:** infection may be higher with stainless steel implants
- **Locking screws:** reduce the need for close contact between the implant and the endosteal bone

Complications

- **Fat emboli:** excessive reaming is associated with increased fat and platelet aggregates. Identify patients at risk (polytrauma, ARDS, hypovolaemia). Unreamed nail can still cause fat emboli
- **Infection:** 1%–2% for closed fractures

- **Non- or delayed union:** non-union rates are low (2%). Dynamization occasionally needed. Bone grafting of large defects may be necessary. Exchange nailing can be performed for patients with delayed union or non-union
- **Malunion:** rare. This is best avoided by accurate reduction at the time of surgery. Two percent of femoral fractures will have >20° malunion
- **Neurovascular injury:** traction injuries. Caution in humeral shaft fractures

Principles of external fixation

Advantages of external fixation

- Rapid skeletal stabilization
- Versatile for different injuries and anatomy
- Adjustment of alignment and fixation during fracture healing (spatial frame, limb lengthening)
- Indirect reduction by ligamentotaxis
- Allows good access to the wound
- Soft tissues not disturbed
- Easy to remove
- Technically easy to perform

Indications for external fixation in trauma

- Fractures associated with significant soft-tissue trauma (grade III open fractures, closed degloving injuries)
- Polytrauma
- Peri-articular and metaphyseal fractures

Types of fixator

- **Simple fixators.** These may be uni- or multi-planar. They may use clamps or pins. Pin types allow little scope for adjustment once applied. Clamp type fixators allow reduction after application
- **Ring fixators.** These comprise rings or half-rings surrounding the limb with the use of pins and wires for stabilization. They allow considerable adjustment once applied. Examples are Ilizarov and Taylor Spatial frames
- **Hybrid fixators.** These are a combination of simple and ring fixators

The components and mechanics of external fixators

- Pins or wires for fixation to bone
- Frames (rods and/or rings) connect to the pins or wires
- Bone–pin interface important to frame stability
- Bending rigidity of the pin is proportional to the fourth power of the radius
- Diameter of pins is only limited by the size of the bone being fixed
- Pins greater than one-third of the bone diameter risk fatigue fracture of the bone
- Pins may be half pins (pass through one side of the limb only) or transfixion pins or wires (pass all the way through the limb)
- Most pins are stainless steel and have a threaded portion
- Transfixion wires of 1.5–1.8 mm are unthreaded
- These may be tensioned to 90–120 kg to enable deforming forces to be resisted
- Bone purchase is by tension and friction
- Some wires have enlargements (olives) at one end to prevent movement of bone during fixation, or to allow a deforming force to be applied

Factors affecting stability and rigidity

- Configuration of the frame
- Total number of Schanz screws used
- Degree of contact between bone ends
- Extent of the soft-tissue injury
- Degree to which the clamps are correctly tightened
- Quality of bone at Schanz screw interface

Factors affecting construct stiffness

- Clamp type
- Number and orientation of rods
- Clamp-to-bone distance
- Side bars/bone separation distance
- Type and number of pins and their orientation and size
- Pin separation across fracture site. Site the outer (peripheral) Schanz pins as far away from the fracture as possible. Inner (central) Schanz pins should be placed as near to the fracture site as possible

- Place the connecting rods (stainless steel or carbon fibre) as near to the skin as possible

Considerations for application

- Avoid neurovascular structures
- Avoid muscle tethering and the use of relieving skin incisions to reduce the risk of necrosis and infection
- Half pins are generally safe in the subcutaneous border of the tibia and ulna or around the lateral intermuscular septum of the humerus
- In the proximal tibia, transverse wires are safe in the anterior arc of 220°
- Avoid thermal injury at the pin–bone interface by cooled pre-drilling
- A strict pin-care regimen is important to reduce infection frequency and severity. The patient can be taught to self-care for their pin sites

Complications

- Pin tract infection (50% – from minor infection to osteomyelitis)
- Joint stiffness
- Non-union (5%–10% of all external fixations)
- Malunion (5%)
- Neurovascular damage
- Pin loosening
- Frame failure is rare

Compartment syndrome

Definition

Compartment syndrome is caused by increases in soft-tissue pressure within an enclosed fascial space of an extremity leading to tissue ischaemia, severe muscle necrosis and fibrosis, functional impairment and nerve damage.

Aetiology

- Fractures
- Soft tissue

- Crush injuries
- Burns
- Gunshot wounds
- Surgery
- Prolonged use of tourniquet or pneumatic anti-shock garment

Clinical features

The first sign is severe pain out of all character to the original injury. The earliest and most reliable feature is significant pain with passive stretching of an involved muscle group. Paraesthesia is another early sign (first web space of the foot for lower leg compartment syndrome). Pallor, pulselessness and paralysis are late features.

Compartment pressure monitoring is useful if the patient is paralysed or intoxicated. Clinical suspicion is enough to warrant surgical exploration without the need for fancy monitoring.

The normal fascial compartment pressure is around 0 mmHg. Pressures within 30 mmHg of the diastolic blood pressure or an absolute value >40 mmHg require urgent surgical decompression by fasciotomy. This should be done within 4 h of onset of symptoms.

Lower leg

Compartment syndrome of the lower leg follows closed or open fractures and intramedullary nailing. The four compartments in the lower leg are the anterior, lateral, posterior and deep posterior compartments. All four must be released. The anterior compartment is most commonly involved.

An anterolateral incision, 15–20 cm long, is made between the fibula and the tibial crest (anterior border tibia). This decompresses the anterior and lateral compartments. Use a gloved finger to palpate the intermuscular septum and beware of the superficial peroneal nerve.

Make a posteromedial incision, 15–20 cm long and 2 cm behind the posterior medial tibial margin (medial border tibia). Beware of the saphenous nerve and vein. This decompresses the superficial and deep posterior compartments. Muscle viability is determined by the 4Cs: colour, consistency, contractibility and capacity to bleed.

Forearm (volar ulnar decompression)

Incision begins above the elbow laterally. A curved incision is made across the flexor crease of the elbow. The incision is completed distally, staying on the ulnar side of the forearm and then into the carpal tunnel.

The dorsal incision is made in the line of the lateral epicondyle of the humerus and distal to the radioulnar joint.

Hand

There are four dorsal interosseous compartments, and three volar interosseous compartments: the abductor pollicis compartment, and thenar and hypothenar compartments.

Two dorsal longitudinal incisions over the second and fourth metacarpals are made. Longitudinal incisions parallel to the radial aspect of the first metacarpal and ulnar aspect of the fifth metacarpal are made.

Foot

There are five major compartments of the foot: medial, lateral, central, interosseous and calcaneal. Nine compartments in the foot have been recorded using injection studies. All can be reached through two dorsal incisions plus one medial incision. The dorsal incisions are placed over the second and fourth metatarsals (these allow access to all compartments). When no dorsal decompression is required or trauma is limited to the hindfoot, a plantar medial approach provides access to all compartments.

Full-thickness burns

Full-thickness burns cause contraction of the skin, which may be circumferential, and can cause elevated compartment pressures. The eschar should be released with a longitudinal incision. Full-thickness burns may be released in the emergency room if urgent, as the skin is rendered anaesthetic.

Fasciotomy wounds are inspected under GA at 48 h. At this stage part of the wound may be closed but usually a split-skin graft is needed for coverage.

Delayed or untreated compartment syndrome

Fibrosis of necrotic tissue leads to contracture and ineffective muscle function. Contracture may be mild (clawing of the toes), or florid (Volkmann's contracture). Tendon transfer may be indicated to improve function.

Examination corner

Basic science oral 1

Cross-section of calf: identify nerves and muscles
Compartment syndrome: diagnosis and management

Trauma oral 1

Compartment syndrome

• Definition
• Causes
• Diagnosis
• Use of compartment pressure measurements
• Incisions for lower leg fasciotomies

Trauma oral 2

Compartment syndrome: everything possible was asked. The examiner rolled up his trousers, waved his leg in my face and said "show me on my own leg exactly where you would perform your incisions". Then he asked about the superficial peroneal nerve and whether it travels posterior to anteriorly in the leg or vice versa. This was a tough and intimidating but fair grilling by the examiner.

Talar fracture

Talar fractures are uncommon but important due to the complex bony anatomy, articulations and vascularity. There are no muscle origins or insertions. Over 60% of the talus is covered by articular cartilage.

Talar neck fractures are classified by Hawkins[23] with type 4 later added by Canale and Kelly[24].

Examination corner

Hawkins type III fracture

Displaced fracture with dislocation of the body of the talus from both the subtalar and ankle joints. No other injury in the history.

Examiner:
- Describe what you see on the radiograph
- Classify the risk of AVN in each of the Hawkins subgroups
- How would you manage this fracture? This fracture requires urgent anatomical reduction and fixation. These fractures are open in 25% of cases. Document the neurovascular status of the foot
- What surgical approach will you use?

Candidate: Three surgical approaches are described: anteromedial, anterolateral and posterolateral. A medial malleolar osteotomy is sometimes used, which is said to preserve the blood supply through the deltoid ligament.

Examiner: A medial malleolar osteotomy is a recognized approach for a talar neck fracture. What is your postoperative management? When would you allow weight bearing? What is Hawkins sign?

Candidate: Hawkins sign is a radiographic appearance on AP radiograph with the foot out of plaster. After 6–8 weeks' disuse osteopenia is seen as subchondral atrophy in the dome of the talus. This would not occur if there was no blood supply. Subchondral atrophy generally excludes the diagnosis of avascular necrosis.

Examiner: If Hawkins sign is absent can you be sure there will be AVN?

Candidate: AVN may not necessarily occur with an absent Hawkins sign.

Examiner: If you suspect AVN what will you do?

Candidate: I would mange expectantly with non-weight-bearing but active ROM and wait for revascularization to occur, which may take up to a year.

Biomechanics of implants in trauma

Bone screws

A **screw** is a mechanism that produces linear motion as it is rotated. The main function of a screw is to fix together two or more objects by compressing them against each other.

The main components of a screw are the head, shaft, thread and tip.

The head

- Provides an attachment for the screwdriver (RECESS)
- Provides a buttress to stop the whole screw sinking into the bone
- The hexagonal head recess design most popular because:
  - It avoids slippage of the screwdriver
  - It allows better directional control during screw insertion
  - The torque is spread between six points of contact

Screw shaft

- Smooth link between the head and thread
- The run out is the transitional area between the shaft and thread. This is the area where screws break

Screw thread

- The standard orthopaedic screw has a single thread
  - Core/root diameter = the narrowest diameter
- Outer/thread diameter
  - The larger the outer diameter the greater the resistance to screw pullout

---

[23] Hawkins LG (1970) Fractures of the neck of the talus. *J Bone Joint Surg Am* **52**(5): 991–1002.

[24] Canale ST, Kelly FB Jr. (1978) Fractures of the neck of the talus. Long-term evaluation of seventy-one cases. *J Bone Joint Surg Am* **60**(2): 143–56.

- **Screw pitch** is the distance between adjacent threads
  - Cortical screws have a small pitch and cancellous screws a large pitch
- **Lead** is the linear distance through which a screw advances with one turn
  - The smaller the lead the greater the mechanical advantage of the screw

Tensile strength

- The resistance to breaking is proportional to the diameter of a screw (diameter of the core) squared

Pull-out strength

- This depends on the outside diameter of the threads and the area of thread in contact with the bone. To increase the pull-out strength of a screw, the outer diameter may be increased or the pitch reduced. Over the first 6 weeks following insertion, the pull-out strength increases to 150% of that at insertion

Shear strength

- Shear strength of a screw is proportional to the cube root of its diameter

Self-tapping versus non-self-tapping screws

A tap is designed in such a way that it is not only much sharper than the thread of the screw, but it also has a more efficient mechanism for clearing bone debris that therefore does not accumulate and clog its threads.

A non-self-tapping screw is generally superior at holding bone, except in extremely thin cortical bone, cancellous bone, and in flat bones such as those of the face, the skull, and the pelvis, where self-tapping screws have been shown to have better holding power.

Experimental evidence has shown that a self-tapping screw can be removed and reinserted without

weakening its hold in bone provided it is carefully inserted. If, however, the screw is inadvertently angled it will cut a new path and destroy the thread that has already been cut. Self-tapping screws should therefore not be used as a lag screw.

Cancellous screws do not have flutes, but gain a better hold when cancellous bone is not tapped.

Principle of the lag screw

This allows compression of two fracture fragments as the screw thread engages only the furthest fragment and slides through the proximal fragment. "Lagging" may be achieved in two ways:
- Use of a partially threaded screw
- "Lagging" the proximal fragment. By over-drilling the proximal fracture fragment to a diameter slightly larger than the thread diameter, this creates a gliding hole. The distal fracture fragment is drilled as normal to the core diameter and if needed tapped to the thread diameter. The screw thread only gains purchase in the distal fragment so when the head comes into contact with the proximal fragment it allows compression of the two objects.

Instruments for inserting screw

Drill bits: Usually have two to three cutting edges. Flutes allow bone cuttings (swarf) to escape. The direction of drilling is important, as drilling in the reverse direction means the drill bit will not clear the swarf.

Taps: Correspond to the thread diameter, shape and pitch of individual screws.

Depth gauge: Oblique holes may have two depth readings depending on which side the measurement is made. The longer measurement should be used. A screw hole will only be used optimally if completely filled with a screw.

Screw drivers: Ensure screwdrivers are not worn and that they are fully seated in the screw head to prevent stripping of the head. Stripping prevents purchase of the screwdriver in the screw head making screw removal difficult.

Examination corner

Basic science oral 1

- Various screws handed to candidate to describe

Basic science oral 2

- Handed a small fragment AO cortical screw to describe
- Asked to draw out the lag principle
- Asked about various drill and tap sizes

Basic science oral 3

- Given a pile of various screws (AO type screws, a wood screw) and asked to talk about them
- Discuss the size, pitch, type (cortical/cancellous, partial/fully threaded), core diameter, and the need to tap or not

Basic science oral 4

- Handed various types of screws
- Asked to describe them
- What do you think they are used for?
- Followed on by discussion of the biomechanics of implants

Trauma oral

- Screw design, etc.
- Basically discussed and pointed out the various features of a screw

Plates

Plate strength is defined by the formula BH^3 (B is width, H is height or thickness). Increasing the plate height increases plate rigidity to the power of three. Plate failure occurs as a result of metal fatigue. A gap between the bone ends following fracture fixation increases the risk of plate failure.

Functions of a plate include:

- **Neutralization.** To protect a lag screw from torsional, shear and bending forces
- **Compression**, achieved by:
  - A lag screw through the plate

- Use of eccentric hole in a dynamic compression plate (DCP). There is the potential of 1.8 mm of glide when two holes are compressed. This produces 600 N of compression
- An external tensioning device
- Pre-bending the plate by 1–2 mm
- Plating the tension side of the bone
- **Bridge plate.** In a multifragmentary fracture, the plate bridges fracture fragments
- **Buttress.** Usually periarticular, used to buttress up articular surfaces
- **Tension band.** Bones are not always loaded evenly along all axes. If the fracture is fixed on the side tending to open (tension side) then the tension forces on one side are converted to compression forces on the opposite cortex

Types of plate

- One-third tubular plates
- DCP
- Low-contact dynamic compression plates (LCDCP)
- Less invasive stabilization system (LISS) plates
- Locking compression plates (LCP)

Methods to avoid fracture following plate removal

Complications following removal of metalwork vary from 3% to >40%. The main problems include re-fracture and neurovascular damage. The removal of forearm plates is most frequently associated with problems. Causes of re-fracture are now discussed:

- Removed screws cause a stress riser in the bone. If the size of the screw is 20%–30% the diameter of the bone, the risk rises exponentially. Thus 3.5-mm screws are recommended for the forearm
- Demineralization of bone under a plate as a result of stress shielding or bone necrosis caused by the plate occluding periosteal blood supply
- Re-fracture may occur through an unhealed fracture site if the plate is removed prematurely
- Plates should be retained for at least 18–21 months to allow bone density to return to its pre-fracture level before removal of plates. This allows time for blood supply to be re-established. Fracture rates

drop with later plate removal. The forearm should be protected for 6 weeks following removal of a plate

- Fracture with initial comminution
- Plating with 4.5-mm DCP

Examination corner

Trauma oral 1

Plates: types of plate, uses, differences, strength, effect of making holes in the bone, stress risers, oval versus square hole, principle of tension band wiring.

Basic science oral 1

- What is biological plating?
- Causes of plate failure in a fracture
- What happens if you leave screw holes empty in a plate?
- Is there a difference if the empty holes are lying against the bone or lying against the fracture?

Basic science oral 2

LCDCP

- Material used and principles of the plate

Trauma oral 2

Radiograph of patella fracture

- Questions on the principles of tension band wiring

Biomechanics of intramedullary nails

A nail functions as a form of internal splint, which stabilizes long bone fractures with minimal damage to the surrounding soft tissues.

Working length

This is the length of a nail between the most distal point of fixation in the proximal fragment and the most proximal point of fixation in the distal fragment. More simply put, it is the unsupported portion of nail between the bone fragments.

- Torsional stiffness is inversely proportional to working length
- Bending stiffness is inversely proportional to the square of working length

Therefore, for a long working length the nail bone composite is less able to resist bending and torsional forces. The working length can vary 1–2 mm with transverse fractures at the isthmus to the distance between proximal and distal locking screws in very comminuted fractures.

Area moment of inertia

This is the resistance of a structure to **bending** during static loading. If an area is considered to be made up of infinitesimal sections, the moment of inertia measures the average of the square of the perpendicular distance that each of the infinitesimal sections is from the axis of bending.

Polar moment of inertia

This is the resistance of a structure to **torsion or twisting**. The polar moment of inertia measures the average of the square of the perpendicular distance of each infinitesimal section of material from the axis of torsion.

Torsional rigidity

Torsional rigidity is a measure of the resistance of a material of a particular size and shape to torsional forces.

- Proportional to 1/length – doubling the length decreases rigidity by a factor of 2
- Proportional to the fourth power of the radius – doubling the radius increases rigidity by a factor of 16
- The **rigidity or stiffness** of a cylindrical structure **in bending and torsion** is proportional to the fourth power of the radius (r^4; bending) (Young's E measure of stiffness)
- The **strength in bending** is proportional to the third power of the radius (r^3; breaking)

The relationship between stiffness and strength is not a simple one. Both factors are related to the diameter of the nail. As nails get a bit stronger they get considerably stiffer. Very stiff nails may damage bone if there is any discrepancy between the shape of the nail and that of the bone.

Nail diameter is the principle factor that alters bending stiffness. The cross-sectional shape also affects bending and torsional stiffness. A slot is the principle factor that alters torsional stiffness. A slot has little effect on nail bending stiffness but a non-slotted nail is 40× more stiff in torsion. A slot reduces torsional stiffness by 98%.

Examination corner

Trauma oral 1

Biomechanics of intramedullary nails

- Area moment and polar moment
- Working length of a nail
- Effect of reaming on the working length

Trauma oral 2

Radiograph of a patella fracture

Questions on the principles of tension band wiring

Examination corner

Trauma long case 1

Mr Jones is a 59-year-old retired joiner, married with 3 children.

The presenting complaint was of a left femoral mal-union with an external rotational deformity and shortening secondary to RTA and fracture 30 years previously.

The femur was treated with intramedullary nailing at the time, which became infected. There was subsequent removal of the nail and traction for 6 months.

Multiple sinuses. Recurrent osteomyelitis and abscesses.

Current problem now is of a degenerate arthritic knee with FFD 40°, hip and thigh pain.

Examination of the left knee included:
- Demonstration of FFD knee
- Lachman's test
- Varus/valgus instability

Discussion

- Current management of an infected femoral intramedullary nail at 2 weeks post surgery
- General discussion about osteomyelitis
- Cierny classification of osteomyelitis including condition of the host, functional impairment caused by the disease, site of involvement and extent of bony necrosis
- Draw different types of traction
- Principles of how traction works
- Management for the hip and knee
- Investigation of osteomyelitis

Trauma long case 2

The patient was male, about 28 years old. He had sustained a compound fracture of the right distal femur and a closed comminuted fracture of his right tibia 18 months previously.

These fractures had been treated with an Ilizarov frame fixation.

His main problems now were a leg length discrepancy of 4 cm in the right leg and a stiff but relatively painless right knee.

Difficult historian, not sure why he was in hospital and what else was going to be done with his leg.

Examination included:
- Gait
- Leg length measurements
- Assessment of rotation
- Examination of the knee including collateral and ACL ligaments

Trauma long case 3

History

Mr Brown is a 48-year-old married farmer with two children. He sustained a severe Lisfranc injury to his right foot 3 years ago, which was not anatomically reduced at the time of his injury. He now presents with a history, over several months, of progressively worsening pain and stiffness in this right foot. He has difficulty with shoe wear, particularly wearing his wellington boots. He is taking regular analgesia, up to eight paracetamol a day and ibuprofen 400 mg three times a day.
- His sleep is disturbed most nights
- He has an unremarkable past medical history
- He has had no other operations

- He denies any history of asthma, tuberculosis, angina, hypertension, myocardial infarction and epilepsy
- He is otherwise fit and healthy

Examination

- On examination he looks well for his age
- He is a tall, well-built individual
- There is a plantar deformity of the first ray and degeneration of the tarsometatarsal joints

Discussion

- Discussion concentrated on the classification of Lisfranc injuries and the associated patterns of injury
- Early management
- Early and late complications

Trauma long case 4

A 43-year-old lady previously fit and healthy, who had an RTA 6 months previously.

She sustained a posterior dislocation of the hip and extensive lacerations of the ipsilateral knee with an ACL rupture.

Examination of the knee included :
- Demonstration of an effusion
- Lachman and Pivot shift
- Apley's grinding test
- Explain the pathophysiology of the Pivot shift

Discussion included:
- Classification of hip dislocations
- Management of an acute hip dislocation
- Identification and classification of Pipkin's fracture/dislocation
- Complications of hip dislocation and their incidence
- Investigation and management of AVN
- Description of the surgical approach and fixation of an acetabular wall fracture
- Management of the ACL-deficient knee: the role of physiotherapy and bracing

Trauma long case 5

Middle-aged man. Infected tibial non-union with leg still in external fixator. Open comminuted tibial fracture managed initially with IM nailing and then severe infection occurred leading to nail removal and external fixator
- History: RTA, initial management

- On examination; describe scars, frame, sinus
- LLD: blocks, Galeazzi, test, tape measure, role of CT
- Discussion: management of the initial fracture; is it safe to nail a 3b tibial fracture and in the middle of the night?
- Exchange nailing for infected tibial non-union versus circular frame
- What to do now

Miscellaneous trauma oral questions

It is impossible to cover every possible trauma oral topic that could be asked in the FRCS Orth exam in detail. Below however are some less well known questions that candidates may be asked.

It is easy for these trauma questions to be read very superficially and then the whole process can become a pointless exercise consisting of a very long list of possible trauma topics that the examiners could ask. Imagine yourself in the trauma oral having to talk around each topic for 2–3 minutes. For example with the T12/L1 fracture subluxation a candidate will almost certainly be shown a radiograph demonstrating the condition. They would need to describe the radiographic abnormalities present. This will be a severe injury with disruption of all three columns of the spine with a high incidence of associated neurological deficits. The majority will probably require surgery.

- ATLS, assessment for associated injuries, mechanisms of injury, imaging
- Denis three column concept
- What are the indications for surgery?
- Do the indications for surgery differ if there is a complete neurological deficit?
- What type of surgery is required?
- What approach is to be used for the procedure? (You should be able to describe the anterior, posterior or thoracoabdominal approach to the lumbar spine fully to the examiners if asked)

Advantages and disadvantages to each approach The point being it is very easy to superficially glance over these questions without thinking about how it will run in the examination. Make sure you actively think through the following questions with due care and preparation rather than a passive read through of the list.

Examination corner

Trauma oral 1

- T12/L1 fracture subluxation
- Comminuted closed intercondylar fracture of the distal femur
- Os calcis fracture
- Fractured tibia: management options
- Fracture dislocation of the elbow
- Mid shaft clavicle fracture in a young adult >2 cm overlap. How do you manage it? Why do we operate on these fractures? Complications of surgery. What type of plate to use. Approach and surgical dissection. If it goes onto a non-union after surgery how do you manage it?

Trauma oral 2

- High-energy open fractured distal femur in a young female with vascular compromise: management
- Compartment syndrome: basic science and theory
- Severely comminuted, closed, distal radius fracture in the dominant hand of a young patient
- Management of a closed intercondylar fracture of the distal femur
- Haemarthrosis: radiographic findings in dislocation of the elbow
- Osteochondral fragment in a child's knee: management and surgical approach
- Monteggia fracture: Bado classification and management
- Stress fracture of the metatarsal

Trauma oral 3

- Clinical photograph of soft-tissue/degloving injury of the lower leg: management
- Compartment syndrome of the lower leg: everything, including incisions for fasciotomy
- Soft-tissue coverage – flaps, grafts, etc.
- Compound tibial fractures
- Gustillo classification of open fractures
- Distal radial fractures
- RSD
- DHS: modes of failure
- Four-part unstable intertrochanteric fracture of the femur. What are the management options for fixation and biomechanics of the fixation devices?

Trauma oral 4

- Bone screws: describe them, what do you think they are for? The biomechanics of implants
- Radiograph of a fixed-angle trefoil device for intertrochanteric fracture fixation put in badly, why did this fail and what would you do about it?
- Radiograph of the elbow of a radial head fixed with mini fragment screws and a plate. Discussion of Essex–Lopresti injury
- Radiograph of paediatric hip fracture: classification, management, AVN
- Fracture subluxation of knee: classification, management of knee dislocation, arteriography, ligament reconstruction
- Trans-scaphoid perilunate dislocation

Trauma oral 5

- Infected femoral nail
- Segmental femoral fracture including co-existing femoral neck fracture
- Calcaneal fracture: types, classification, surgical approaches, complications
- Removal of forearm plate: risks, literature, the Henry approach
- Humeral atrophic non-union with K nail protruding into cuff muscles of the shoulder: management
- Tibial hypertrophic non-union: management
- Displaced patellar fracture: principles of tension band wiring including drawing out a diagram to explain

Trauma oral 6

- Monteggia fracture
- Periprosthetic supracondylar fracture of the femur: pros and cons of conservative versus surgical management
- Hamilton Russell traction. "*Draw me Hamilton Russell traction for a femoral fracture*"
- Principles of cast bracing
- Crush injury of the foot
- Lisfranc fracture/dislocation: management and types, importance of the second metatarsal bone, assessment of reduction, prognosis
- Foot compartments and releases for compartment syndrome

The basic science oral

24. Basic science oral core topics   461
Simon Barker and Paul A. Banaszkiewicz

Basic science oral core topics

Simon Barker and Paul A. Banaszkiewicz

Introduction

The FRCS Orth examination will definitely test you on aspects of basic science – in the past there has commonly been a surgical approach question in the written paper, and although the format is changing it is highly likely that the emphasis and content of questions will not. Critical appraisal of a journal article will remain a part of the revised examination and will require a working knowledge of statistics.

The Basic Science Oral is often feared by candidates, but having established that there is no avoiding it, the key to understanding basic science in orthopaedics and to making it *stick in your head* is to keep it clinically relevant and to concentrate on understanding concepts rather than learning lists of esoteric facts.

The Basic Science section of the syllabus includes the following headings:

- Anatomy
- Tissues
- Physiology, biochemistry and genetics
- Biomechanics and bioengineering
- Bone and joint diseases
  - Osteoarthritis
  - Osteoporosis
  - Metabolic bone diseases
  - Rheumatoid arthritis and other arthropathies (inflammatory, crystal, etc.)
  - Haemophilia
  - Inherited musculoskeletal disorders
  - Neuromuscular disorders – inherited and acquired

- Osteonecrosis
- Osteochrondritides
- Heterotopic ossification
- Bone and soft-tissue sarcomas
- Metastases
- Orthopaedic oncology
- Investigations
- Operative topics
- Infection, thromboembolism and pain
- Prosthetics and orthotics
- Research and audit
- Medical ethics

This section of the guide will take you through areas that are commonly tested from the above list. The content cannot be comprehensive; you should check through the above list after reading this chapter and identify areas of weakness in *your* knowledge that remain.

Anatomy will not be covered here as it is a topic well dealt with in other revision texts. As you approach the exam you are strongly advised to develop a good working knowledge of surgical approaches, anatomical landmarks, methods for extending an approach and structures at risk. Do *not* ignore approaches that are out of day-to-day practice – the posterior approach to the knee and the anterior approach to the cervical spine have both been asked in the last few years!

What about a "top ten" for basic science? The following are *must-know* topics, but there are no guarantees! To do well you need to understand these subjects and their clinical relevance – it's not just a question of regurgitating them.

Postgraduate Orthopaedics: The Candidate's Guide to the FRCS (Tr & Orth) Examination, Ed. Paul A. Banaszkiewicz,
Deiary F. Kader, Nicola Maffulli. Published by Cambridge University Press. © Cambridge University Press 2009.

- Cartilage structure
- Growth plate structure
- Free body diagrams of hip
- Gait cycle
- The stress strain curve
- Calcium and vitamin D
- Osteonecrosis/AVN
- Radiological principles
- Paget's disease
- Infection

Remember – aim for a wide knowledge base so you can say something on almost any topic. The minutiae on one topic will be of no use if you are quizzed on the basics of another! You will not fail the exam for not knowing Young's modulus of stainless steel but you will if you cannot explain what Young's modulus is *and its relevance*.

Embryology

Limb embryology

At 3 weeks in utero (wiu)

Gastrulation occurs, i.e. the formation of ectodermal and endodermal plates. The primitive streak forms, and mesenchymal tissue gives rise to mesoderm. The notochord is formed of ectodermal tissue. Neurulation occurs, i.e. the ectodermal neural plate forms a neural crest and tube. Somatization occurs, i.e. mesoderm gives rise to 42–44 pairs of somites, each with a dermatome, myotome and sclerotome.

At 4 wiu

Folding of embryo into "C shape". The apical ectodermal ridge (AER) forms. Limb buds appear – mesoderm covered by a thin surface of ectoderm.

At 7 weeks onwards

Rays and then digits form under the control of the zone of polarizing activity (ZPA). Mesenchymal condensations form *cartilage anlage (models)*, which will become primary centres of ossification.

The limb buds develop between 4 and 6 weeks and quickly form the upper extremities with pronated forearms that then rotate externally. A few days later the lower extremities form and rotate internally. Vascular buds invade the cartilage model bringing in osteoprogenitor cells, which differentiate into osteoblasts and form primary centres of ossification at 8 weeks. Although finger rays are present at 7 weeks the hands continue to differentiate until 13 weeks.

Control of limb development

Apical ectodermal ridge (AER)
The AER is a thickening of the distal ectoderm covering the limb bud which influences the underlying mesoderm to promote and control growth. The AER directs the growth of the limb bud in a proximodistal (PD) direction. The AER releases chemical signals, particularly fibroblast growth factor (FGF). Experimental removal of the AER or loss of contact of the AER with limb bud mesoderm prevents limb development.

Zone of polarizing activity (ZPA)
The ZPA is a zone of tissue at the posterior aspect of the limb bud. It is important in specifying the number of digits along the AP axis. This activity is mediated by the gene SHH (*sonic hedgehog*). SHH activates a group of *homeobox genes*, which specify the number of digits.

Growth factors
Growth factors are important in signalling along the dorsoventral (DV) axis.

Spine embryology

- Vertebrae are each formed of two adjacent sclerotomes from the third week onwards
- There are two centres of ossification, one from each sclerotome, which fuse to form a single centrum
- Notochord persists as the nucleus pulposus of the intervertebral disc

- The neural arch also forms two centres, which do not fuse together until the postnatal period, and to the centrum at around 5 years of age

Pain

Physiology

- Aδ fibres. Myelinated. Sharp, acute pain
- C fibres. Unmyelinated (slow to conduct). Dull ache, prolonged pain

Pathways

- Via dorsal spinal roots
- C fibres to substantia gelatinosa (layers II and III of grey matter)
- A fibres to layers I and V of grey matter
- Second-order ascending fibres pass contralaterally via the dorsal/posterior column or spinothalamic tract
- Sympathetic – may increase blood flow (and therefore pain) in a limb

Gate theory

Afferent impulses to the substantia gelatinosa are modulated there. Descending neurones from the brain are thought to act as a "gatekeeper" to determine the extent of secondary neuronal activation.

Endorphins

Endorphins are endogenous opiates acting as inhibitors of the pain pathway. They act on δ, κ and μ receptors.

Acute pain management

Diagnosis

Ascertaining the cause of pain should take equal priority with efforts to reduce pain, since diagnosis may lead to a specific pain-reducing intervention (e.g. compartment syndrome will not be relieved by anything short of surgery, fractures require adequate splintage, etc.).

Management

Management broadly follows the pain ladder. An acute pain team service should be viewed as an adjunct to pain management and should be involved early where significant pain control issues are anticipated (e.g. amputees).

Pain ladder

Originally devised by the World Health Organization for cancer relief but more widely applied to pain of other aetiologies and chronicities. There are three main classes:

Non-opioid – paracetamol, aspirin (and other NSAIDs)

Weak opioid – codeine, dextropropoxyphene, co-codamol, etc.

Strong opioids – morphine, diamorphine

Where optimal use of a drug in one class does not give adequate analgesia, move up a level. Co-analgesics may be added to any step in the ladder.

Chronic pain management

A multidisciplinary team-based approach is favoured. Dedicated chronic pain clinics are appropriate for intractable pain:

Diagnosis – must be thorough to rule out causes where specific management may be curative (e.g. missed spinal stenosis).

Psychology – chronic pain of benign aetiology is frequently associated with clinical depression, whereas chronic pain of neoplastic aetiology is seldom associated with depression. Lifestyle change and antidepressants have a role.

Analgesia – the analgesic ladder should be applied (see above). Aim for regular medication with the option of extra doses for "breakthrough pain". Oral medication is favoured.

Co-analgesics – are drugs used in conjunction with traditional analgesic agents:

NSAIDs – good for bone pain (but have negative effect on bone and soft tissue healing!)

Tricyclic antidepressants – good for nerve damage pain.

Calcium channel blockers (nifedipine) – good for sympathetic mediated pain (e.g. Raynaud's).

Steroids – can relieve pain in inflammatory arthropathy.

Muscle relaxants – may have a role where spasticity is a problem (cord injury).

Stimulation – acupuncture, ice, heat, ultrasound, TENS are all thought to act via a gating effect on myelinated fibres.

Nerve blocks – temporary via local anaesthetic, permanent with phenol or radiofrequency ablation. Examples – epidural or peripheral plexus blocks.

Neurosurgery – has a limited role, e.g. rhizotomy, ablation of PIN at wrist.

Bone

Bone is a specialized form of dense connective tissue. For the oral examination you must have a grasp of the differences between cancellous, cortical and woven bone. Normal bone is lamellar and can be cortical or cancellous. Immature and pathological bone is made up of woven bone.

Functions

- Biochemical: calcium homeostasis and metabolism
- Biomechanical: support and protection of soft tissues, transmission of load and muscular force
- Haematological: haematopoietic marrow synthesizes erythrocytes, leucocytes and platelets

Matrix

Bone is a composite material consisting of cells (10%) within a matrix (90%) that has inorganic and organic components.

1. Inorganic (mineralized) matrix (60% dry weight of bone)

- Calcium hydroxyapatite – $Ca_{10}(PO_4)_6(OH)_2$, 80×5 nm crystals

- Calcium phosphate
- Responsible for the compressive strength of bone
- Inorganic matrix is the major calcium "reservoir" in the body (99%)

2. Organic matrix (40% dry weight of bone)

- Collagen
- Proteoglycans
- Non-collagenous matrix proteins
- Growth factors and cytokines

Collagen

- Approximately 90% of the organic matrix of bone is type I collagen (the word *bone* contains *one* as its last three letters so it is easy to remember *Type one collagen*)
- Responsible for the tensile strength of bone. Hole zones (gaps) exist within the collagen fibril between the ends of the molecule. Pores exist between the sides of parallel molecules. Mineral deposition (calcification) occurs within these hole zones and pores

Proteoglycans

- Proteoglycans are partially responsible for the compressive strength of bone. They have a half-life of 3 months. They are involved in mineralization, organization of collagen fibres and the binding of growth factors

Non-collagenous matrix proteins (bone-specific proteins)

- Promote mineralization and bone formation and include osteocalcin, osteonectin, osteopontin
  - Osteocalcin: levels measured in serum/urine as a marker of bone turnover; produced by osteoblasts; attracts osteoclasts to sites of bone resorption
  - Osteonectin: secreted by osteoblasts and platelets for regulation of mineralization
  - Osteopontin: cell binding protein anchoring osteoclasts to the mineralized matrix

Growth factors and cytokines

- Play a role/aid in bone cell differentiation, activation, and the growth and turnover of bone

Bone cells

Osteoblasts

- Bone-forming cells derived from undifferentiated mesenchymal stem cells. Osteoblasts have a well developed endoplasmic reticulum, Golgi apparatus and mitochondria to facilitate the synthesis and secretion of matrix. They deposit osteoid on pre-existing mineralized surfaces only (=the mineralization front). Produce type I collagen
- Osteoblasts have specific surface receptors for parathyroid hormone (PTH), vitamin D, glucocorticoids, prostaglandins, oestrogen
- Osteoblast differentiation is regulated by interleukins (ILs), TGF-β, insulin-like growth factor (IGF-1) and platelet-derived growth factor (PDGF)

Osteocytes

- Osteocytes maintain bone. They make up 90% of cells in the mature skeleton. Osteocytes are osteoblasts that become trapped within newly formed matrix. They are important in controlling extracellular concentrations of calcium and phosphorus
- Osteocytes are directly stimulated by calcitonin and inhibited by PTH

Osteoclasts

- Osteoclasts are large, multinucleated, irregularly shaped giant cells that resorb bone matrix
- Derived from pluripotent cells of the bone marrow, which are the haematopoietic precursors that also give rise to monocytes and macrophages
- Possess a ruffled (brush) border that increases surface area from plasma membrane enfolding. Bone resorption occurs in pits (depressions) known as Howship's lacunae on endosteal and periosteal surfaces of bone

- Osteoclastic bone resorption initially involves inorganic mineral dissolution, followed by degradation of components of the organic matrix by proteolytic digestion
- Osteoclasts bind to bone surfaces via cell attachment (anchoring) proteins called integrins (cell surface glycoprotein). The integrins seal the area below osteoclast attachment to bone. Osteoclasts produce hydrogen ions (via the carbonic anhydrase system) which lowers the pH and dissolves the hydroxyapatite crystals
- Osteoclasts actively synthesize acidic proteolytic lysosomal enzymes, in particular tartrate-resistant acid phosphatase and cysteine proteinases, which then hydrolyse the organic matrix components
- Regulators of osteoclast activity include IL-1 (stimulates osteoclast bone resorption), IL-10 (suppresses osteoclast formation) and calcitonin (inhibits osteoclasts)

Bone lining cells

- Bone lining cells are narrow, flattened cells that form an envelope around bone and possess cytoplasmic extensions that penetrate bone matrix and communicate with osteocytes
- Bone lining cells are considered inactive osteoblasts that may be reactivated back to osteoblasts

Osteoprogenitor cells

- Osteoprogenitor cells are mesenchymal cells that line Haversian canals, endosteum and periosteum awaiting the stimulus to differentiate into osteoblasts

Structure

Cortical bone (compact bone)

- Cortical bone has a slower turnover rate, a higher Young's modulus of elasticity (20 GPa) and a higher resistance to torsion and bending than cancellous bone
- Stress orientated. Comprises 80% of the adult skeleton, forming the cortex of long bones

- Osteoblasts deposit bone matrix in the form of thin sheets, which are called lamellae
- In the process of deposition of matrix, osteoblasts become trapped in small hollows within the matrix called lacunae and become osteocytes. Between adjacent lacunae and the Haversian canal are numerous minute interconnecting canals called canaliculi, which contain fine cytoplasmic extensions of the osteocytes
- In mature compact bone most of the individual lamellae form concentric rings or laminations known as concentric lamellae
- An osteon or Haversian system consists of a series of concentric layers (lamellae) surrounding a central neurovascular channel (Haversian canal). Nutrition is via the intraosseous circulation (canals and canaliculi)
- The remnants of lamellae no longer surrounding Haversian systems form interstitial lamellae and lie between the osteons
- Cement lines surround the outer border of an osteon – the demarcation between where bone resorption has stopped and new bone formation has begun. Collagen fibres and canaliculi do not cross cement lines
- A second system of canals called Volkmann's canals penetrates bone perpendicular to its surface and establishes connections between the inner and outer surfaces of the bone. Vessels in Volkmann's canals communicate with vessels in the Haversian canals

Cancellous bone (spongy or trabeculae bone)

- Cancellous bone is less dense than cortical bone and has a higher turnover rate and more remodelling
- Cancellous bone is more elastic and has a smaller Young's modulus of elasticity (1 GPa) than cortical bone
- Cancellous bone structure is a three-dimensional lattice of interconnecting trabeculae with each trabecula made up of parallel sheets of lamellae
- Honeycomb appearance

- Osteocytes, lacunae and canaliculi in cancellous bone resemble those in cortical bone
- The spaces between trabeculae contain marrow and sinusoidal vessels

Woven bone

- Immature or pathologic bone is woven and has a more random organization with collagen fibres and cells arranged haphazardly
- Weaker. More flexible. Increased turnover. Not stress orientated. More osteocytes
- Normally found in the embryo, in fracture callus and in the metaphyseal region of growing bone
- Often found in tumours, Paget's bone and in osteogenesis imperfecta

Periosteum

- Has an outer layer with fibroblasts and an inner layer of osteoblasts. Transmits vessels to bony canaliculi

Biomechanics

- Bone is a composite material consisting of collagen and hydroxyapatite. Bone strength is derived from this composite nature
- Collagen has a low Young's modulus, high tensile strength and poor compressive strength
- Calcium hydroxyapatite is stiff, brittle material with high compressive strength

This combination forms an "anisotropic material" that resists forces with respect to loading direction – bone is strongest in compression, weakest in shear, and intermediate in tension.

Bone metabolism

A complex interplay and interaction of various hormones, growth factors and cytokines regulates plasma calcium and phosphate levels:
- Parathyroid hormone (PTH)
- Vitamin D
- Calcitonin

Stimulators of bone formation (osteoblastic activation)

- Transforming growth factor β (TGF-β)
- Insulin-like growth factors
- Growth hormones
- Bone morphogenetic proteins (BMPs)
- Sex hormones: oestrogen, androgens

Inhibitors of bone formation (osteoblastic inhibition)

- Gamma interferon
- IL-4
- IL-10
- Bisphosphonates

Stimulators of bone resorption (osteoclastic activation)

- Thyroxine
- Leukotrienes
- Glucocorticoids
- Prostaglandins F_2, E_2
- IL-1, IL-3, IL-6
- Tumour necrosis factor α (TNFα)
- Epidermal growth factor (EGF)
- Platelet-derived growth factor (PDGF)
- Fibroblast growth factor (FGF)

Inhibitors of bone resorption (osteoclastic inhibition)

- Oestrogen
- Calcitonin

Osteoclastic formation and differentiation

- IL-1, IL-3, IL-6
- Prostaglandins F_2, E_2
- TNFα

Osteoblastic formation and differentiation

- IL-1
- Insulin-like growth factors

Examination corner

Basic science oral 1

Examiner: What factors inhibit osteoclast function?

Candidate: I was not sure if the examiner had said osteoclasts or osteoblasts. I decided not to ask them to repeat the question and set about trying to remember the inhibitors of osteoclast function. This was actually quite a tricky question and in hindsight I should have asked the examiner to clarify the above point.

I mentioned calcitonin and oestrogen but the examiner seemed unimpressed and was looking I presume for a big list of various hormones, growth factors and cytokines that could be reeled off verbatim. The only difficulty was that I was not aware of any more!

We changed direction and ended up discussing vitamin D metabolism and again the examiner seemed unimpressed by my answers. In this situation the best solution would have been to improvise and mention the various factors that have a beneficial effect on bone formation. This may have saved the day (even though strictly their action is primarily on osteoblasts and osteoblastic activation). The examiners would probably have been no wiser. Begin with mentioning that there is a complex interplay, interaction and overlap between various hormones, growth factors and cytokines on both the formation and resorption of bone and continue on from there hoping that your answer meets with the examiner's approval.

In truth I am not sure if my examiners really knew their basic sciences particularly well, for most of the oral they were using written cards for the cue to ask questions. I am sure they would have been completely lost without these cards and I couldn't help thinking that it was an odd question to ask.

I would again emphasize the need to clarify the examiner's question if you are not sure what they asked. Once or perhaps twice per oral is probably OK but don't do this too often, otherwise you will severely irritate the examiners.

They of course had the last laugh as they failed me!

On balance (I think) the topic the examines wanted me to discuss was "regulators of osteoclast activity", which include:

- **Parathyroid hormone (PTH) and 1,25-dihydroxycholecalciferol (active form of vitamin D)**: PTH and 1,25-dihydroxycholecalciferol are unable to stimulate osteoclastic bone resorption in vitro in the absence of osteoblastic cells. These agents stimulate osteoclasts to resorb bone via a "coupling" factor. Osteoclasts do not have receptors for 1,25-dihydroxycholecalciferol and until recently were not believed to have PTH receptors, although the functional significance of PTH receptors on osteoclasts remains to be established

- **Calcitonin**: osteoclasts do have calcitonin receptors and this inhibitor of bone resorption acts directly on the osteoclast to reduce cellular motility, retract cytoplasmic extensions and reduce ruffled border size
- **Glucocorticoids**
- **Prostaglandins**
- **IL-1, IL-6 and TNFα**: stimulate the proliferation of osteoclast precursors
- **TGFβ**: stimulates proliferation of osteoclast precursors in vitro. Also has osteoblastic activation potential
- **Oestrogens**: increased expression of TGFβ
- **Androgens**
- **Thyroid hormones**
- **Bisphosphonates**: act as inhibitors of osteoclast-mediated bone resorption

All this information may be a bit too complicated to throw at the examiners but is included for the sake of completeness. Maybe half of it would be enough.

Basic science oral 2

Describe the structure of collagen in bone

Composed primarily (90%) of type I collagen (b-one) which consists of a triple helix of two alpha$_1$ chains and one alpha$_2$ chain arranged in a quarter staggered structural array producing single fibrils. Collagen is responsible for the tensile strength of bone. Mineral deposition occurs in the hole zones that exist between the ends of fibrils and the pore zones that lie between the sides of fibrils of collagen. Crosslinking increases the tensile strength of collagen.

Basic science oral 3

- What cells are found in bone?
- What are their functions?
- What receptors are present on osteoblasts?

Basic science oral 4

- Explain how an osteon is formed
- How does remodelling of bone occur?

Bone circulation

Bone, as an organ, receives 5%–10% of the cardiac output.

Anatomy

Blood supply is from three sources:
- High-pressure nutrient artery system
- Metaphyseal–epiphyseal system
- Low-pressure periosteal circulation (capillaries)

High-pressure nutrient artery system

- The nutrient artery originates as a branch from the major artery of the systemic circulation
- Enters the mid-diaphysis cortex (outer and inner tables) through the nutrient foramen to enter the medullary canal. Foramen passes at an angle to the cortex with respect to epiphyseal growth centres in long bones, hence *"from the knee I flee, to the elbow I go"*
- Branches into ascending and descending arteries, which divide into arteriole branches supplying the inner two-thirds of the diaphyseal cortex from within (endosteal)

Metaphyseal–epiphyseal system

- The periarticular vascular complex penetrates the thin cortex and supplies the metaphysis, physis and epiphysis
- In epiphyses with large articular surfaces, such as the femoral and radial heads, the vessels enter in the region between the articular cartilage and physis and hence the blood supply is tenuous

Periosteal system

- The periosteal system forms an extensive network of capillaries covering the entire length of the bone shaft
- Supplies the outer one-third of the cortex
- Low-pressure system
- Very important in children, for circumferential bone growth (appositional)

Physiology: direction of flow

- Arterial flow in mature bone is centrifugal (inside to out) as a result of the net effect of the high-pressure nutrient artery system
- The direction is reversed in a displaced fracture (centripetal) with complete disruption of the endosteal (nutrient) system
- Arterial flow in immature developing bone is centripetal because the periosteum is highly vascular and is the predominant component of bone blood flow
- Venous flow in mature bone is centripetal, with cortical capillaries draining to venous sinusoids to the emissary venous system
- Remember *Batson's valveless venous plexus* – accounting for the spread of infection/tumour between the spine and the retroperitoneum

Regulation

- Bone blood flow is under the control of metabolic, humoral and autonomic inputs
- The arterial system of bone has greater potential for vasoconstriction than for dilatation
- The vessels within bone possess a variety of vasoactive receptors

Fracture healing[1]

- Bone blood flow is the major determinant of fracture healing
- Bone blood flow delivers nutrients to the site of bony injury
- The initial response is decreased bone blood flow after vascular disruption at the fracture site
- Within a few hours to days, bone blood flow increases (a regionally accelerated phenomenon) and peaks at 2 weeks, returning to normal at between 3 and 5 months

---

[1] A typical oral question might be "Describe the blood flow changes that occur with fracture healing". This may lead into a discussion on the stages of fracture healing.

Examination corner

Basic science oral 1

- Blood supply of a long bone
- Describe the blood flow changes that occur with fracture healing

This may lead into a discussion on the stages of fracture healing and then possibly into general management principles for a non-union

---

Bone formation and remodelling

Endochondral

Undifferentiated cells secrete a cartilaginous matrix and differentiate into chondrocytes. The cartilage matrix then calcifies and the chondrocytes die. Vascular invasion brings osteoblast precursors so that mineralized osteoid is laid on the surface of the calcified remnants of the cartilage matrix. Simultaneously the periosteal sleeve lays down a cortical shell. The junction of cartilage and bone is called the *physis* (see "The growth plate/physis" below).

Intramembranous

Intramembranous ossification occurs within membranes (layers) of condensed, primitive mesenchymal tissue. Mesenchymal cells differentiate into osteoblasts, which begin the synthesis and secretion of osteoid at centres of ossification. Mineralization of osteoid closely follows. Early woven bone is later replaced by lamellar bone. Examples of intramembranous ossification include embryonic flat bone formation (pelvis, clavicle, vault of skull).

Remodelling mechanism

Bone formation and resorption are closely coupled and result in no net change in bone mass. Bone remodelling occurs in small packets of cells known as basic multicellular units (BMUs). Each unit consists of a group of all the linked cells that participate in remodelling a certain area of bone.

Endosteal lining cells are stimulated and collagenase digests unmineralized type I collagen, exposing the mineral to osteoclasts.

Cortical bone remodels via osteoclastic cutting cones – "miners sinking a new shaft". The inorganic apatite crystals are dissolved by the acidic pH generated within Howship's lacunae at the ruffled borders of osteoclasts. Cutting cones or sheets of osteoclasts bore holes through the hard bone leaving tunnels that appear in cross-section as cavities. The head of the cutting cone consists of osteoclasts that resorb the bone. Closely following the osteoclast front is a capillary loop and a population of osteoblasts that actively lay down osteoid to refill the resorption cavity.

Matrix lamellar "seams" 10 µm thick are laid down, entombing osteoblasts. By 20 days mineralization of the seam occurs via a calcification front under the control of vitamin D_3.

Histologically reversal lines are seen where osteoclast activity has stopped and osteoblast activity has laid down new bone.

Control mechanisms

Control of this process is exercised by *Hox* and *Pax* genes via systemic hormones and local cytokines, growth factors, matrix metalloproteins and their inhibitors. These may in turn be controlled by mechanical load – bone responds to piezoelectric charges:

- Compression side is electronegative, stimulating bone formation by osteoblasts
- Tension side is electropositive, stimulating bone resorption by osteoclasts

Resorption–formation coupling

Osteoblasts produce:
- ODF (osteoclast differentiation factor) also known as RANK ligand
  - ODF/RANK-L binds with RANK on osteoclasts thereby stimulating osteoclasis
- OPG (osteoprotegerin)

- OPG acts as a decoy receptor for ODF/RANK-L and thereby reduces osteoclasis
- PTH, vitamin D_3, PGE_2 and IL-1/2 stimulate ODF/RANK-L and inhibit OPG

By this mechanism a homeostatic balance between resorption by osteoclasts and formation by osteoblasts is achieved. Uncoupling occurs in disease states.

Wolff's law

Bone remodels according to the stress applied to it: more stress, more bone formation.

Heuter–Volkmann law (of growth plate)

Increased pressure causes decreased growth and decreased pressure causes increased growth.

Limb lengthening – callotasis

- Involves low-energy fracture of a (long) bone, a short latent period for callus to form and then traction of the callus, which stimulates distraction osteogenesis
- Usually carried out at 1 mm per day in four increments, although it may be faster in the juvenile skeleton
- Reliant on a soft-tissue envelope (periosteum)
- Endochondral bone forms as columns in the gap
- Cortex formation is late
- Consolidation time is usually 1 month per centimetre of elongation

The growth plate/physis

Zones of the growth plate

- Reserve zone
- Proliferative zone
- Hypertrophic zone: maturation, degeneration, provisional calcification
- Primary spongiosa
- Secondary spongiosa

Reserve zone

The reserve zone is a resting zone that is involved in matrix production, the storage of lipids, glycogen and proteoglycan aggregates. It contains germinal cells (stem cell population) existing singly or in pairs, separated by an abundant extracellular matrix and not clearly ordered in columns. There is a low oxygen tension, as epiphyseal arteries pass through this region but do not form terminal capillaries.

Proliferative zone

In the proliferative zone chondrocytes are highly ordered in columns directed along the axis of growth of the long bone. Longitudinal growth occurs with stacking of chondrocytes (the top cell is the dividing mother cell). This zone is involved with cell division and matrix production. There is a high oxygen tension and high proteoglycan concentration (inhibits mineralization).

Hypertrophic zone

The hypertrophic zone is involved in the maturation of cells. Chondrocytes increase in size (×5–10), accumulate Ca^{2+} in their mitochondria and then undergo programmed cell death, releasing calcium from matrix vesicles and allowing calcification of the matrix to occur. There is a low oxygen tension. Physeal fractures are classically believed to occur through the zone of provisional calcification (within the hypertrophic zone). The rate of chondrocyte maturation is regulated by systemic hormones and local growth factors. Parathyroid-related peptide inhibits chondrocyte maturation. Indian hedgehog is produced by growth plate chondrocytes and regulates the expression of parathyroid-related peptide.

At times the hypertrophic zone is subdivided into three zones:
- Maturation zone – preparation of matrix for calcification
- Degeneration zone – cell deterioration and death

- Provisional calcification zone – chondroid matrix becomes impregnated with calcium salt from mitochondria from destroyed cartilage cells

Primary spongiosa

Vascular invasion and resorption of transverse septa. Calcified cartilage bars are resorbed by chondroclasts, formation of woven bone (primary trabeculae) by osteoblasts.

Secondary spongiosa

Remodelling in the metaphysis to trabeculae of lamellar bone.

Physeal–metaphyseal junction

The physeal–metaphyseal junction is the "weakest" link of the growth plate

Shearing forces are reduced by:
- Microscopic irregularities – mammillary processes
- Macroscopic contouring – undulations

Periphery of the physis

Groove of Ranvier. A wedge-shaped area of chondrocyte progenitor cells laterally that supplies reserve zone cells to the periphery of the growth plate for lateral growth

Perichondral ring of Lacroix. Dense fibrous band at the periphery of the growth plate, which anchors and supports the physis

Premature growth plate arrest (physeal injuries)

Physeal injuries can result in a bridge of bone forming across the physeal cartilage. The bars can be central, peripheral or linear. A central bridge may lead to a limb-length discrepancy while a more peripheral bar may produce an angular deformity.

Diseases affecting the growth plate

Reserve zone

- Diastrophic dwarfism
- Pseudo-achondroplasia
- Kniest syndrome
- Gaucher's disease

Proliferative zone

- Achondroplasia (deficiency in cell proliferation)
- Gigantism
- Malnutrition, irradiation, glycocorticoid excess

Hypertrophic zone (maturation, degeneration)

- Mucopolysaccharidosis

Hypertrophic zone (zone of provisional calcification)

- Rickets (insufficient calcium for normal calcification of the matrix)
- Osteomalacia
- SUFE

Primary spongiosa

- Metaphyseal chondroplasia
- Acute osteomyelitis

Secondary spongiosa

- Osteopetrosis (abnormality of osteoclasts, internal remodelling)
- Osteogenesis imperfecta
- Scurvy

Effect of hormones and growth factors

The growth plate is affected by:
- **Hormones** (GH, thyroxine, insulin, PTH, calcitonin)
- **Growth factors** (transforming growth factors, BDGF, EGF and FGF)
- **Vitamins** (vitamins A, C, and D)

These factors influence chondrocyte proliferation, maturation, synthesis and matrix mineralization. Some factors have a specific effect on a particular zone whilst others affect the entire growth plate.

Reserve zone

- Parathyroid hormone
- IL-1

Proliferative zone

- Thyroxine
- GH
- Insulin
- TGFβ

Hypertrophic zone

- TGFβ
- BDGF
- Vitamin D
- Calcitonin

Thyroxine

- Essential for cartilage growth
- Increases DNA synthesis in cells from the proliferative zone

Parathyroid hormone

- Direct mitogenic effect on epiphyseal chondrocytes and stimulates proteoglycan synthesis

Calcitonin

- Acts primarily in the hypertrophic zone
- Accelerates growth plate calcification and cellular maturation

Glucocorticoids

- Decrease in proliferation of chondroprogenitor cells in the zone of differentiation

Growth hormone

- Affects cellular proliferation

Insulin

- May affect the concentration of circulating growth plate factor

Vitamin D

- Vitamin D deficiency results in an elongation of the cell columns of the growth plate

---

Examination corner

Basic science oral 1

Draw and describe the growth plate

Just like "Sit down and draw articular cartilage", this is a top-ten topic for the basic science oral and is an absolutely classic question favoured by examiners. Practise drawing it out and explaining what you are drawing beforehand; it can be surprisingly easy to lose one's way when explaining out loud what you are drawing to someone.

Basic science oral 2

Draw the growth plate

- Discussion of cell maturation through the layers of the growth plate
- Effect of various hormones on the growth plate
- Location of various disease processors in the growth plate: SUFE, rickets, etc.

Basic science oral 3

Histology picture of the growth plate

Examiner: What is this? Can you name the various parts?
Examiner: What are the resting cells?
Candidate: Pluripotent stem cells.
Examiner: Where does the blood supply come from for this layer?

Examiner: What is the pinkish staining in this layer between the cells?
Examiner: Why are the cells hypertrophic in this layer (hypertrophic layer)?
Candidate: I wasn't sure. I said because they are rich in stored material probably glycogen granules.
Examiner: What happens to cells after hypertrophy?
Examiner: Where do fractures occur and why?

Basic science oral 4

Electron micrograph picture of the growth plate

Examiner: What is the structure the picture is demonstrating?
Candidate: The growth plate.
Examiner: Can you point out the various layers?
Candidate: A bit trickier than expected. Slightly different in appearance than the classic text book drawings.
Halfway through I got a bit lost but managed to recover with some prompting. Not asked anything else and we quickly moved on to another topic.

Basic science oral 5

Draw and explain the architecture of the physis and its relation to fractures

Basic science oral 6

Growth plate and its blood supply

Bone graft

Indications

- Augmentation of fracture repair
- Reconstruction and replacement of skeletal defects
- Stimulation of arthrodesis

Function

- Mechanical (support)
- Biological (bone healing)

Properties

Osteoconductive

The graft functions as a three-dimensional scaffold or matrix on which new bone growth occurs. The graft has the ability to support the ingrowth of capillaries, perivascular tissues and osteogenic precursor cells, e.g. coral scaffolds.

Osteoinductive

Mediated and regulated by graft-derived factors (which include TGF), bone morphogenetic proteins (BMP), insulin-like growth factors 1(IGF-1) and 2 (IGF-2), interleukins, etc. The graft provides a biological stimulus that has the capacity to activate and recruit from the surrounding bed of mesenchymal-type cells, which then differentiate into cartilage-forming and bone-forming cells, e.g. fresh frozen allograft.

Osteogenesis

The graft contains living cells that are capable of differentiation into bone. Inherent biological activity, e.g. autograft.

Genetics

- Autograft (same individual)
- Allograft (another individual, same species)
- Xenograft (different species)
- Isograft (genetically identical – twins or clones!)

Tissue composition

- Cortical
- Cancellous
- Corticocancellous
- Osteochondral
- Bone marrow aspirate

Preservation method

- **Fresh** (increased antigenicity): viable, living cell population and associated cytokines and growth factors; need and availability may not coincide
- **Fresh frozen**: less immunogenic than fresh, preserves BMP
- **Freeze dried**: loss of structural integrity, depletes BMP, least immunogenic
- In **bone matrix gelatin** (BMG)

Graft incorporation

The process by which invasion of the graft by host bone occurs, such that the graft is replaced partially or completely by host bone.

The key to the whole process of graft incorporation is the initial inflammatory response, which is similar for both cortical and cancellous grafts. Analogous to fracture healing.

Important differences exist in the latter stages (secondary phase) of osteoconduction and remodelling between cortical and cancellous bone.

The process of incorporation is also different for autografts and allografts. Allograft incorporation is slower than autograft incorporation and is accompanied by a variable amount of inflammation as a result of the host's immune response to the graft. Possible outcomes following allograft implantation include:

- Accepted as an autogenous graft
- Rejected because strong genetic differences exist (few)
- Reluctantly accepted due to some genetic disparity (majority of cases)

After bone grafting a haematoma rich in nutrients forms around the bone graft. Platelet-derived growth factor (PDGF) attracts lymphocytes, plasma cells, osteoblasts, and polynuclear cells to the bone graft. Necrosis of the bone graft occurs and an inflammatory response is established in which granulation tissue forms, with an ingrowth of capillary buds bringing macrophages and primitive mesenchymal cells with it. Fibrovascular stroma develops with an influx of osteogenic precursors and blood vessels. IL-1, IL-6, BMP and IDGF are secreted, stimulating osteoblast and osteoclast activity. The graft is penetrated by osteoclasts, which initiates the resorptive phase and incorporation.

Table 24.1 Autograft incorporation in cancellous and cortical bone

Autograft incorporation	Cancellous	Cortical
Revascularization rate	Rapid	Slow, used for structural defects
Mechanism and order of repair	Osteoid laid down on dead bone, donor bone later reabsorbed	Donor bone reabsorbed before laying down of appositional new bone
Radiographs	Radiodense	Loss of mechanical strength and reduced radiodensity
Completeness of repair	All donor bone eventually removed. Creeping substitution	Some necrotic bone remains. Cutting cones

Cancellous graft incorporation

Autogenous non-vascularized cancellous grafts undergo an inflammatory response. Analogous to fracture healing. There is subsequent remodelling, with all cancellous graft eventually replaced by creeping substitution. Creeping substitution is the process whereby osteoblasts lay down new bone on the scaffold of dead trabeculae with simultaneous osteoclastic resorption (Table 24.1).

Cortical graft incorporation

Autogenous non-vascularized cortical grafts undergo a similar but slower process of inflammation but then incorporate in a different manner to cancellous grafts. Osteoclastic resorption via cutting cones into the graft has to precede osteoblastic bone formation. Therefore, mechanical strength is lost in the first 3–6 months and returns over 1–2 years. The entire graft is not incorporated and there is no remodelling phase (Table 24.1).

Types of graft

Best considered in terms of the advantages and disadvantages of each.

Vascularized grafts

- Reduced necrosis (bulk graft remains viable), reduced reliance upon host bed, rapid host–graft union

- Systemic route of transportation of osteogenic cells
- Less articular chondral collapse
- Microsurgical transfer of rib, iliac crest, radius, fibula
- Early mechanical strength
- Best for large tissue defects and irradiated tissues

Versus
- Technically difficult to perform
- Limited donor sites
- Sacrifice of normal structures
- Significant donor site morbidity

Autografts

- No immunogenicity
- No disease transmission
- Cheap

Versus
- Limited availability
- Donor site morbidity (scar, haematoma, pain, infection)
- Increased operative and anaesthetic time

Allografts

- No donor site morbidity
- Large amounts available

Versus
- Disease transmission
- Immunogenic
- Slow incorporation

Stages of graft healing: five stages (Urist)

- Inflammation. Chemotaxis stimulated by necrotic debris
- Osteoblast differentiation. From precursors
- Osteoinduction. Osteoblast and osteoclast function
- Osteoconductive. New bone forms over scaffold
- Remodelling. Process continues for years

Processing

To remove superfluous proteins, cells and tissues in order to:
- Reduce disease transmission
- Reduce immune sensitization
- Allow better graft preservation

By:
- Physical debridement of unwanted tissue
- Ultrasonic processing with or without pulsatile washing to remove remaining cells and blood
- Ethanol to denature cell proteins and reduce bacterial and viral loads
- Antibiotic soak to kill bacteria
- Preservation (freezing, freeze-drying)
- Sterilization (aseptic versus irradiate if contaminated)

Bone banking

Bone allograft donor exclusions (contraindications to allograft bone donation):
- Any evidence of current symptomatic infection
- History or suspicion of past infections: TB, hepatitis B and C, and venereal diseases
- Malignancy
- HIV and high-risk activities for HIV
- Dementia
- Long-term steroid use
- Metabolic bone disease
- Any condition with uncertain aetiology where altered immune competence or viral involvement is suspected or implicated: rheumatoid arthritis, CJD, multiple sclerosis, etc.

Detailed past medical history and social history obtained.

Serological testing for the following is routinely carried out:
- Hepatitis B and C
- Syphilis
- HIV
- Rhesus status

Demineralized bone matrix

- Proteins are acid-extracted from bone
- Offers no structural support
- Moderately osteoinductive due to bone morphogenetic proteins
- Must be kept refrigerated to avoid protein denaturation
- Most effective when used as an adjunct to internal fixation

Bone marrow

- An autograft source of osteoprogenitor cells
- Harvested from ilium by aspiration
- Often used in a **composite** graft as the osteogenic component with an osteoconductive allograft or xenograft

Corraline xenograft

- Natural sea coral is calcium carbonate based, and can be used as a xenograft
- Replamineform corals involve hydroxyapatite substitution for the calcium carbonate by a hydrothermal mechanism
- *Goniopora* and *Porites* corals are used

Ceramics

- Osteoconductive
- Hydroxyapatite ($Ca_{10}(PO_4)_6(OH)_2$) or tricalcium phosphate ($Ca_3(PO_4)_2$)
- Brittle, of limited structural value
- Biologically inert

Table 24.2 The make up of cartilage

Cells (chondrocytes)			
Extracellular matrix	Fibres	Collagen	Type II, IX, XI Type V, VI, X
		Elastin	
	Ground substance	Water	
		Proteoglycans and glycosaminoglycans	
		Glycoproteins	
		Degradative enzymes (matrix metalloproteinases)	

Examination corner

Basic science oral 1

- Types of bone graft: autograft, allograft, vascular, etc.
- Storage
- Sterility
- Antigenicity
- What is bone graft used for?

Basic science oral 2

- Exclusion criteria for femoral head donation
- Method of collection
- Storage including temperature (–70°C ultracold freezer)
- Dose of gamma irradiation for re-implantation (2.5 megarad)

Basic science oral 3

- How are allografts processed?

Cartilage

A definite "A-list topic" for the basic science oral. You need to rehearse and practise drawing out the layers of cartilage, as invariably the examiner asks you to do this and explain the diagram as you go along.

Function

- Shock-absorbing structure
- Decreases friction in joints (low friction coefficient of 0.002). The best artificial joint is 30 times higher!

Contents

The contents of cartilage are given in Table 24.2.

Chondrocytes

- Form 5% of the wet weight
- Are important in the control of matrix turnover
- Produce collagen, proteoglycans and some enzymes for cartilage metabolism

Water

- Is a major constituent of the extracellular matrix
- Accounts for 65%–80% of the wet weight of articular cartilage
- Allows for deformation of the cartilage surface in response to stress by shifting in and out of cartilage
- Is responsible for nutrition and lubrication
- Increased water content leads to increased permeability, decreased strength and decreased Young's modulus of elasticity

Collagen

- Accounts for 10%–20% of wet weight or 40%–70% dry weight
- Responsible for the high tensile strength of cartilage
- Composed mainly of type II (90%–95%)
- Small amounts of types V, VI (content increases in early osteoarthritis), IX, X and XI collagen are present in the matrix of articular cartilage
- Collagen type X is only produced by hypertrophic chondrocytes during endochondral ossification
- Collagen type XI acts as a constrainer of the proteoglycan matrix

Proteoglycans

- These molecules are complex. They account for 10%–15% of the wet weight of cartilage
- Are produced by chondrocytes and are secreted into the extracellular matrix. Proteoglycans are strongly bound to collagen and are responsible for the **compressive** strength of cartilage
- Serve to trap and hold water to regulate matrix hydration. Half-life of 3 months
- Are responsible for the elasticity and resistance to compression of articular cartilage. Present in increased concentrations in the deeper layers of cartilage
- Look like a **test tube brush** with glycosaminoglycans bound to a protein core by sugar bonds to form a proteoglycan aggrecan molecule
- Link proteins stabilize these aggrecan molecules to hyaluronic acid to form a proteoglycan aggregate
- Glycosaminoglycans (GAGs) include the subtypes
  - Keratin sulphate (increases with age)
  - Chondroitin-4-sulphate (decreases with age)
  - Chondroitin-6-sulphate (increases with age)

The proteoglycan aggregates have a highly fixed negative charge, allowing them to hold enormous amounts of water, which contributes to the shock-absorbing properties of cartilage.

Decreased proteoglycan leads to decreased stiffness (chondromalacia) and collagen will tend to break and fray (fibrillate).

Structure

The structure, composition and mechanical properties of articular cartilage differ with depth from the surface and determine the zones or layers:

1. **Surface**
2. **Superficial tangential zone (10%–20%) (gliding zone)**

   High concentration of collagen fibres, arranged parallel to the articular surface like a mat, with the greatest ability to resist shear stresses. Water is at its highest level; proteoglycan content at its lowest level. Water is squeezed out by mechanical pressure and helps create a fluid lubrication layer. May function as a barrier to the passage of large molecules from the synovial fluid. In osteoarthritis, this layer is the first to show degenerative changes
3. **Middle zone** (40%–60%) (transitional zone)

   Collagen fibres are arranged obliquely, composed almost entirely of proteoglycans. This zone forms a transition between the shearing forces of the surface layer to compressive forces in the deeper layers
4. **Deep zone** (30%) (radial zone)

   Collagen fibres attached radially (vertical) to the tidemark. There is a high concentration of proteoglycans between the collagen fibres, which draws water in. This creates a hydrostatic pressure that assists in distributing load and resisting compression
5. **Tidemark**

   Straddles the boundary between calcified and uncalcified cartilage and is made visible by histological staining. It is cell free
6. **Calcified zone**

   The calcified zone forms a transitional region of intermediate stiffness between articular cartilage and subchondral bone. Hydroxyapatite crystals anchor the cartilage to the subchondral bone. The calcified zone forms a barrier to diffusion from blood vessels supplying the subchondral bone
7. **Subchondral bone**

Nutrients and metabolic mediators are provided by synovial fluid via diffusion through the matrix cartilage and help to maintain the metabolic state of the cartilage. Intermittent load and motion are essential for cartilage nutrition; immobilization leads to atrophy of cartilage. Water flux occurs under load allowing for cartilage nutrition.

The compressive stiffness of cartilage is directly proportional to the aggregate (proteoglycan) content.

Classification of cartilage degeneration (Jackson):

1: Softening of articular cartilage
2: Fibrillation and fissuring of articular cartilage
3: Partial-thickness cartilage loss, clefts and chondral flaps
4: Full-thickness cartilage loss with bone exposed

Causes of cartilage breakdown
(see also Table 24.3)

- Chondral and osteochondral fractures
- Ligamentous injuries

- Idiopathic AVN
- Osteochondritis dissecans

Characteristics of cartilage

- Type II collagen
- No nerve supply (aneural)
- No blood supply (avascular)
- No lymphatics (alymphatic)
- Almost non-immunogenic
- Few cells, which are locked into matrix
- Repair capacity poor

Injury and healing

Superficial laceration (does not cross the tidemark)

- Chondrocytes at the site of injury die and matrix becomes disrupted
- Attempt at chondrocyte division, forming clusters or clones and increased matrix synthesis
- However, chondrocytes do not migrate to the site of the injury and the matrix they synthesize does not fill the defect

Table 24.3 Biochemical changes of articular cartilage. Ageing versus osteoarthritis. PG, Proteoglycan; MMPs, metalloproteinase.

	Ageing	Osteoarthritis
Water content	Decreases	Increases then decreases
Synthetic activity	Decreases	Increases
Collagen	Unchanged	Breakdown of cartilage collagen network
PG content	Decreases	Decreases
PG synthesis	Decreases	Increases
PG degradation	Decreases	Increases
Keratin sulphate	Increases	Decreases
Chondroitin sulphate	Decreases	Increases
Hydroxyapatite	Increases	Decreases
Enzymes		Increased activity MMPs
Matrix subunit molecules		Increased
Chondrocyte size	Increases	
Chondrocyte number	Decreases	
Modulus of elasticity	Increases	Decreases

- A haematoma does not form and therefore inflammatory cells, undifferentiated cells and fibroblasts do not migrate to the site of cartilage damage
- Inability of chondrocytes to respond effectively to the injury
- Inability of undifferentiated mesenchymal cells to invade the tissue defect
- Short-lived inadequate response that fails to provide sufficient numbers of new cells or matrix to repair even a small defect

Deep laceration (extending below the tidemark)

- Penetration of the underlying subchondral bone causes haemorrhage, fibrin clot formation and inflammation
- Injury to bone and fibrous clot formation causes the release of growth factors, which attracts inflammatory cells, fibroblasts
- Serves as a scaffold for some repair, forming a fibrocartilaginous scar
- Tissue is unsuitable for repetitive load bearing without any layered zonal organization
- The size, shape and location (high- or low-load-bearing areas) of the defect are important in terms of the likelihood of healing and the progression to degeneration
- V-shaped defects are more likely to heal with hyaline-like cartilage than U-shaped defects
- These defects may progress to focal OA

Response to blunt trauma

- Chondrocyte death, matrix damage, fissuring of the surface, injury to the underlying bone
- Loss of proteoglycans and chondrocyte clumping
- Increase in subchondral bone stiffness
- Cartilage fibrillation, which causes an increased water content and softening

Management of defects

No one method for managing cartilage defects has been shown to be superior over the others.

Abrasion arthroplasty

An arthroscopic technique that combines lavage and removal of unstable cartilage at the defect rim with abrasion of the subchondral bone at the base of the defect with a burr. This exposes vascularized subchondral bone which contains pluripotential stem cells which are thought to infiltrate the clot formed in the cartilage defect. This differentiates into fibrocartilage rather than hyaline cartilage but provides relief of pain in approximately 70% patients with a full thickness defect at 1 year. A crude type of repair, essentially a cartilage repair from subchondral bone by turning the defect into a deep injury.

Microfracture

Marrow-stimulating procedure directed at the recruitment of mesenchymal stem cells in the bone marrow. The subchondral bone is penetrated to allow fibrin clot formation within the defect and then the creation of repair tissue. The procedure consists of accurate debridement of all unstable and damaged cartilage in the lesion including the calcified layer down to the subchondral bone plate. All loose or marginally attached cartilage is also debrided from the surrounding rim of the defect to form a stable perpendicular edge of healthy cartilage. An arthroscopic awl is then used to make multiple holes in the defect, 3–4 mm apart.

Mosaicplasty (osteochondral plugs)

Cylindrical plugs of exposed bone are removed from the defect. Plugs of normal non-weight-bearing cartilage and bone are harvested and placed into the defect.

Autologous chondrocyte implantation

The management of articular cartilage defects using cells that have been taken from a patient and grown in a laboratory and re-implanted into an articular cartilage defect in the same patient. Chondrocytes are implanted over the damaged area under a layer of periosteum stitched or glued into position.

Cartilage is harvested arthroscopically from a low-load-bearing area on the proximal part of the medial femoral condyle of the affected knee.

After cell culturing, approximately 4 weeks later, the cells are re-implanted. An arthrotomy is performed and the defect debrided to healthy surrounding cartilage. Periosteum is taken from the proximal part of the tibia or distal part of the femur and sutured to the rim of the debrided defect. The cultured chondrocytes are then injected beneath the patch.

Examination corner

Basic science oral 1

Sit down and draw articular cartilage

An absolute classic top 10 "must-learn" topic. One of the examiner's favourite questions. Numerous candidates have been asked this one in the basic science oral. Don't forget to practise your drawing skills beforehand rather than in the examination itself.

Basic science oral 2

Discuss the mechanism of repair of cartilage lacerations

An extremely common question, which tends to crop up in both the basic science and general orthopaedic and pathology orals. Previously the topic was not particularly well covered in the various orthopaedic textbooks available. The *AAOS Orthopaedic Basic Science*, 3rd edition now provides an excellent overview of the topic.

For some reason in one particular diet of exams this was the basic science flavour-of-the-month topic. Every candidate seemed to be asked this particular question (and no – not all candidates had been examined at the same examination table!).

Candidate: The examiners were not satisfied with the usual basic two or three sentences from my favourite textbook of orthopaedics and wanted a much more detailed answer.

The examiners kept looking at me expecting me to say something more but there wasn't anything else that I could think of.

In retrospect I wasn't expecting to be asked this question and with just a bit more preparation I could have dealt with it that much more easily and passed this oral, whereas in fact I failed.

Examiners: The candidate was unsure of the mechanisms of repair of articular cartilage.

Basic science oral 3

- Cartilage changes with age

Basic science oral 4

- Articular cartilage – draw the layers
- Discussion on the different types of cartilage
- Asked about different types of collagen and the basic structure of collagen

Basic science oral 5

Articular cartilage

- Draw the structure
- Types of collagen in cartilage
- Role of type IX collagen
- Pathogenesis of osteoarthritis

Basic science oral 6

- What pathological processes are involved in the development of osteoarthritis?

Tendon

Tendons are dense, regularly arranged collagenous structures that transmit loads generated by muscle to bone.

Composition and structure

- Cellular material (20% of total tissue volume)
- Extracellular matrix (80% of total tissue volume)
  - 70% of matrix is water
  - 30% of matrix is solid
    - Collagen type I (75% dry weight)
    - Ground substance: (2% dry weight) proteogly-cans, glycoproteins, phospholipids (acting as a cement-like structure between collagen microfibrils)
    - Elastin

Collagen

Type I collagen fibres are arranged in a parallel fashion to withstand unidirectional tensile loads. Parallel fibres undergo elastic deformation at low load and then exhibit a largely linear stress/strain curve (actually it is viscoelastic and therefore exhibits creep and stress relaxation so the stress/strain curve exhibits hysteresis). Crimping (wavy fascicles) occurs at low tension due to cross-linking of proteoglycans, but there is straightening out when a load is applied. Primary, secondary and tertiary fascicles are embedded in proteoglycans within the tendon. Each fascicle contains collagen fibres within an endotenon. Tenocytes are collagen-forming and repair cells. In tendons, the collagen content is higher and the elastin content lower than in ligaments.

Architecture

Collagen molecules combine in a quarter-staggered array to form ordered units of microfibrils (five collagen molecules). Further aggregation of collagen microfibrils results in the formation of subfibrils and fibrils. Fibril units are arranged in closely packed, highly ordered, parallel bundles with proteoglycans, glycoproteins and water incorporated in a matrix, binding the fibrils together to form fascicles.

Insertion into bone

There are four transitional tissues/zones to the insertion of tendons and ligaments into bones:
- **Zone 1**: parallel collagen fibres at the end of the tendon or ligament
- **Zone 2:** collagen fibres intermeshed with unmineralized fibrocartilage
- **Zone 3:** mineralized fibrocartilage
- **Zone 4:** cortical bone

This allows a gradual increase in the stiffness of the tissue, so there is less of a stress-concentrating effect at the insertion of tendon/ligament into the bone, minimizing injuries at the insertion site.

Surrounding connective tissue

The fascicles within a tendon are surrounded by loose areolar tissue – the **endotenon**, which permits longitudinal movement of collagen fascicles and carries blood vessels, lymphatics and nerves. Surrounding the endotenon is a white glistening synovial-like membrane – the **epitenon**. In some tendons the epitenon is then circumscribed by a loose areolar tissue called the **paratenon**. This paratenon functions as an elastic sheath allowing free gliding of the tendon against the surrounding tissue. Together the epitenon and paratenon comprise the **peritenon**.

In some tendons, the paratenon is replaced by a true synovial sheath consisting of two layers lined by synovial cells. This double-layered sheath is referred to as a **tenosynovium**.

Therefore, two types of tendon exist:
1. Tendons surrounded by **paratenon** are referred to as vascular tendons because vessels enter from many points on the periphery and anastomose with a longitudinal system of capillaries
2. Tendons surrounded by a **tendon sheath** are referred to as avascular tendons. The avascular tendons contained within synovial sheaths have mesotenons within these sheaths that function as vascularized conduits called vincula, which carry a vessel that supplies only

one segment of the tendon. Avascular areas receive nutrition via diffusion pathways from the synovial fluid

Due to these differences in vascular supply paratenon-covered tendons heal better than sheathed tendons. Healing is initiated by fibroblasts that originate in the epitenon and macrophages.

Tendon healing

There is longstanding controversy over the relative contributions of the extrinsic processes and intrinsic capabilities of the tendon to heal.

- **Intrinsic** healing results in the formation of longitudinally aligned collagen fibres within the tendon substance with minimal adhesions
- **Extrinsic** healing provides scar tissue that envelops the injured tendon; it also has the deleterious effect of producing undesirable adhesions between the tendon and its surrounding soft tissues
- It is now generally agreed that relative contributions of intrinsic and extrinsic mechanisms vary with the type and site of tendon injury and the postoperative regime selected

The healing phase is divided into three sequential phases:

1. Haemorrhagic/inflammatory phase
2. Proliferative/collagen-producing phase
3. Remodelling phase

Haemorrhagic/inflammatory phase

- Formation of haematoma within the damaged region
- Invasion by polymorphonuclear cells and monocytes/macrophages with the release of a complex cascade of cytokines and growth factors
- The monocytes remove debris and the fibroblastic cells appear
- Three days after injury the inflammatory stage of healing predominates, with both intrinsic and extrinsic cellular sources for healing

- Extrinsic cells arise by the proliferation and migration of inflammatory cells from the synovial sheath and surrounding soft tissues
- Intrinsic cells arise from tendon cellular elements, mainly the outer layer of the epitenon
- The function of these cells is primarily phagocytic and involves the removal of cellular debris and collagen remnants
- The migration of fibroblasts is facilitated by the chemotactic effects of fibronectin

Proliferative/collagen-producing phase

- By day 5 proliferating fibroblasts lay abundant collagen (type III is predominant initially) in a haphazard way
- The collagen content continues to rise to reach its maximum level at approximately 4 weeks

Remodelling phase

- By the end of the 4th week the collagen fibres begin to align themselves along the long axis of the tendon in line with the tensile forces
- There is progressive maturation and conversion of collagen fibres (to type I)
- Complete maturation of the repair site and reversal of the active fibroblasts into quiescent tenocytes takes place by 3 months

---

Examination corner

Basic science oral 1

Mechanisms of tendon repair

Theories of intrinsic and extrinsic tendon repair

Basic science oral 2

How do tendons and ligaments heal after injury?

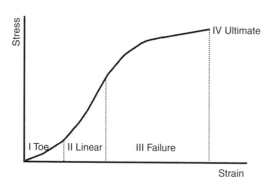

Figure 24.1 Stress/strain curve for a tendon

Stress/strain curve

The stress/strain curve for tendons is similar to that for ligaments and other tissues predominantly composed of collagen (Figure 24.1).

I Primary/non-linear toe region

This region of the stress/strain (load-elongation) curve is concave. Elongation here is believed to be the result of straightening of the wavy pattern of relaxed collagen fibres (crimped fibres begin to straighten). A small increase in stress/load causes a large increase in strain/length.

II Secondary or linear region (elastic region)

The fibres have straightened out and the stiffness of the ligament has increased and become constant. The deformation of tissue has a more or less linear relationship with load.

III Early sequential failure

Small force reductions (dips) can sometimes be observed at the end of the linear region. These dips are caused by failure of a few very stretched collagen fibres.

IV Ultimate stress/strength

The maximum load/stress before the ligament completely fails. May get a series of small drops as ultimate failure occurs due to the sequential failures of fibre bundles. Alternatively there is low resistance to elongation after ultimate failure has occurred. The ligament is intact but very lax.

Examination corner

Basic science oral 1

Examiner: Please draw me the stress/strain curve of a ligament.

The candidate performed poorly, drawing the curve incorrectly, and with this the examiners drew it themselves to demonstrate to the candidate the correct diagram. They then began to explain the significance of each particular area on the graph.

Basic science oral 2

Draw the stress/strain curve of a ligament/tendon and explain its various parts

---

Muscles

Structure

- Fundamental units are actin and myosin molecules. These are arranged linearly and myosin "ratchets" along the actin to achieve shortening using energy from ATP
- Troponin blocks the binding sites on the actin to limit contraction; calcium unblocks these sites
- **Myofibrils** are the grouped functional units of actin and myosin
- Myofibrils are segmented into functional contractile repeating units known as **sarcomeres:**
  - I band = actin filaments (lightest band on electron microscopy) where there is no overlap with myosin filaments

- A band = myosin filaments
- H band = myosin filament segment where there are no interdigitating actin filaments
- M line in the middle of the A band – where myosin filaments are joined together
- Z line in the middle of the I band – where actin filaments are joined together
- The arrangement of actin and myosin filaments is that of a hexagonal lattice in the centre of a sarcomere, i.e. each myosin filament is bounded by six actin filaments
- **Myofibres** are the cells containing fibrils; they are multinucleate in skeletal muscle, surrounded by endomysium
- Myofibres are grouped into **fascicles** surrounded by a perimysium
- Fascicles are grouped into a muscle surrounded by an epimysium

Muscle spindle

- Sensory structure within a muscle that regulates tension and acts as a proprioceptive organ:
  - Primary afferent endings (annulospiral fibres), which respond mainly to the rate of change of stretch
  - Secondary afferent endings (flower spray fibres), sensitive to steady level tension

Physiology

- Type 1 – slow oxidative, slow to fatigue, require oxygen for sustained activity, large concentration of myoglobin (red in colour) many mitochondria – for *endurance*
- Type 2a – fast fibres, oxidative and glycolytic, resist fatigue (white in colour), rich in mitochondria
- Type 2b – fast glycolytic, high levels of ATPase, few mitochondria, anaerobic and quick to fatigue – for *sprinting*

Hill model – biomechanically we can consider muscle to have a force due to its elasticity and its contractility (Figure 24.2).

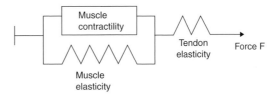

Figure 24.2 Hill model

Types of muscle contraction

Isotonic (dynamic) (t in isotonic, same as in tension)

- Muscle tension is constant through the range of motion
- Muscle length changes through the range of motion, e.g. the biceps curls with weights

Isometric (static)

- Muscle tension is generated but the length of the muscle remains unchanged, e.g. pushing against a wall

Isokinetic

- Muscle tension is generated as the muscle maximally contracts at a constant velocity over a full range of motion

Concentric contraction

- Muscle shortens during the contraction

Eccentric contraction

- Muscle lengthens during the contraction
- Eccentric contractions have the greatest potential for high muscle tension and muscle injury

Muscle–tendon junction

- Muscle and tendon fibres are almost parallel, which generates high shear forces

- This area has a specific morphology, which is adapted to its function
- Specific features include shorter sarcomere lengths, greater synthetic ability, greater number of organelles per cell, interdigitation of the cell membrane and intracellular connective tissue
- A high degree of membrane folding generates a large surface area, reduces stress at the junction and reduces the angle of the force vector applied. The net result is that the junction is very strong

Transfer principles

The "S"s
- Sensible patient
- Sufficient age (>4 years)
- Sacrificable donor, which is a synergist of strength ≥MRC 4 with sufficient excursion
- Sensate hand with supple joints
- Scar-free tissue with single action and straight line of pull

In reality these principles are always compromised to some extent.

Ligaments

- Shorter and wider tissue than tendon; connect bone to bone
- Major role in stability of joints
- Type I collagen 75%
- Higher elastin content compared to tendon, of 15%

Ligament–bone junction

- Similar in principle to tendon–bone junction
- With indirect insertions into bone the superficial fibres insert at acute angles into periosteum while the deep layers anchor to bone via Sharpey's fibres
- Direct insertions into bone contain transition of bone to ligament in four phases: ligament, fibrocartilage, mineralized fibrocartilage and bone. This facilitates transmission of forces

- Early ligament healing is composed of type III collagen that is later converted to type I
- Ligaments do not plastically deform

Nerves

Anatomy

- **Cell body** – site of metabolic activity, must be in continuity for regeneration
- **Axon** – *a*lways carries impulse *a*way from cell body; **dendrite** carries impulse towards it. Thus sensory fibres are always dendrites and motor fibres are always axons!
- **Myelinated nerve fibre** – axon/dendrite with its **Schwann cell** and surrounding **endoneurium** (basement membrane)
- **Unmyelinated nerve fibre** – single Schwann cell has several axons/dendrites embedded in it, called a **Remak bundle**
- **Perineurium** – cellular layer round groups of fibres, creating **fascicles**
- **Epineurium** – everything outside the perineurium that is not blood vessel or nerve. Mostly collagen

Physiology

- Myelinated conduction velocity is proportional to diameter
- Unmyelinated conduction velocity is proportional to the square root of the diameter
- Type A fibres – >2 μm in diameter, fast, motor, touch, pain
- Type B fibres – 3–15 μm in diameter, autonomic preganglion
- Type C fibres – 0.5–2 μm in diameter, chemonociceptors

Clinical tests

Objective sensory

- Ninhydrin colour change test for perspiration (sympathetic)
- Denervation test (failure of skin to wrinkle in water)

Subjective sensory

- Weber's two-point discrimination test
- Hoffman–Tinel sign, due to hyperexcitability of regenerating nerve end
- Pain (pin prick)
- Temperature – recovers at same rate as pain
- Vibration – 256 Hz fork
- Tactile/light touch – Semmes–Weinstein hairs
- Proprioception – variable recovery

Motor – MRC

- No contraction
- Perceptible contraction proximally
- Perceptible contraction proximally and distally
- Contraction against gravity
- Contraction against resistance
- Complete recovery

Nerve conduction studies

Stimulation of a peripheral nerve generates:
- A compound sensory nerve action potential (SNAP) of 5–30 μV
- A compound muscle action potential (CMAP) of 5–10 μV (in response to a supra-maximal stimulus)
- A preserved SNAP implies that the dorsal root ganglion is in continuity; if motor function is reduced, pathology at the root or more proximally is implied
- If both SNAP and CMAP are reduced then a peripheral lesion is more likely

The following properties can be investigated:
- **Latency** – time between onset of stimulus and response
- **Amplitude** – size of response or "evoked potential", usually an average recording to reduce background "noise"
- **Nerve conduction velocity** – distance between stimulating and recording electrodes divided by time; may be slowed by demyelination or focal entrapment

Entrapment sites include:
- **Median nerve** – carpal tunnel, pronator teres, ligament of Struthers, upper brachial plexus, C5–C8 roots, cord
- **Radial nerve** – forearm, lateral elbow, spiral groove, posterior plexus, C6–C7 roots, cord
- **Ulnar nerve** – Guyon's canal, cubital tunnel, ligament of Struthers, lower plexus, C8–T1 roots, cord

Electromyography (EMG)

Two needle electrodes are placed in the muscle to be studied:
- Electrical activity in response to voluntary movement
- Characteristic recruitment of motor units with increased force in a muscle
- Normal: no muscle activity at rest
- Immediately after section: EMG normal
- Between 5 and 14 days: positive sharp waves consistent with denervation
- Between 15 and 30 days: spontaneous denervation, fibrillation potentials present
- Evidence of re-innervation: highly polyphasic motor unit potentials

Somatosensory-evoked potentials

- Stimulation of a peripheral nerve (median or posterior tibial is standard)
- Electrical recordings at scalp electrodes are very small, therefore averaged over 100 or 200 stimulations
- Used for intra-operative monitoring of cord function
- Not absolute

Nerve injury (Seddon)

Neurapraxia (note spelling!)

- Nerve contusion involving reversible conduction block without Wallerian degeneration
- Selective demyelination of the axon sheath

Axonotmesis

- Conduction block with axonal degeneration
- Axon and myelin sheath degenerate but endoneurial tubes remain intact

Neurotmesis

- All layers of nerve are disrupted and there is Wallerian degeneration
- No recovery without repair; 1 mm/day in adults
- 3–5 mm/day in children

Sunderland

- First degree – same as neurapraxia
- Second degree – same as axonotmesis
- Third degree – axonal injury associated with endoneurial scarring (perineum is intact); most variable degree of ultimate recovery
- Fourth degree – in continuity but, at the level of injury, is complete, scarring across the nerve preventing regeneration. Perineurium and endoneurium are disrupted, and the continuity of the nerve is maintained by the epineurium
- Fifth degree – same as neurotmesis

Wallerian degeneration

- Axon and myelin degraded and removed by phagocytosis
- Existing Schwann cells proliferate
- Nerve cell body swells up and enlarges
- Rate of structural protein production increases

Factors affecting nerve recovery

- Age – there is a noticeable change often after the age of 30
- Level of injury – distal repairs have a better prognosis than proximal ones
- Nature of injury – sharp lacerations do better than crush or avulsion injuries
- Delayed repair – 1% of neural function is lost for each week of delay beyond the 3rd week from injury

Repair

Epineurial

- Epineurium repaired in a tension-free fashion

Fascicular

- Repairs the perineural sheaths. Individual fascicles are re-approximated

Group fascicular

- Ulnar and median nerves: distal third of the forearm
- Sciatic nerve: thigh

Neuropathy

- Exclude malignant or traumatic aetiology
- May be axonal or demyelinating

Classification

- **Chronic**
  - Genetic
  - Metabolic (including B_{12} deficiency)
  - Amyloidosis
  - Nutrition (alcoholism)
  - Iatrogenic (phenytoin, bleomycin)
  - Neoplastic
- **Acute**
  - Autoimmune – Guillain–Barré

Genetics

You need to have an understanding of inheritance patterns – both as a general principle and for specific conditions. It's a good idea to learn one or two conditions that obey each particular inheritance pattern to impress the examiners. Remember there are two approaches to this topic – the "top-down" population genetics that looks at patterns in large groups (closely allied to epidemiology) and the "bottom-up" approach of molecular genetics.

Chromosomes are made up of DNA. They carry the genes that specify amino acids as triplets of bases. The human has 46 chromosomes of which two are sex chromosomes, XX or XY.

Problems with chromosomes can include duplication, e.g. trisomy 21.

Gene/locus – the DNA sequence responsible for production of a protein. Has intron and exon regions, the latter being responsible for protein coding via transcription to RNA then translation to amino acids.

Mutation – irreversible alteration in the DNA of a gene; may be a deletion, insertion or substitution.

Phenotype – the expression of the underlying **genotype**.

Mendelian inheritance – single-gene traits are predictably inherited in fixed proportions. A gene can be autosomal or X-linked, dominant or recessive.

- **Autosomal dominant** – commonest mechanism, children of affected individuals have a 50% likelihood of being affected
- **Autosomal recessive** – both copies of a gene must be abnormal to manifest the condition; where a single copy is affected that person is a carrier. The risk of affected sibling is 1 in 4 if parents both heterozygotes
- **X-linked recessive** – males are more commonly affected since they only have one copy of the gene, which will be expressed even if it is recessive
- **Mosaicism** – occurs in females due to lyonization (switching off) of one copy of the X-chromosome in each cell at 1 week of development. Therefore the phenotype may vary
- **X-linked dominant** – all daughters of affected males will be affected. Females are more commonly affected than males

Penetrance – where the phenotype may or may not be clinically manifest in spite of a common genotype. A statistical concept.

Expressivity – often confused with penetrance, but describes the differing extent of clinical manifestation between individuals, e.g. in polydactyly 1, 2 or more digits can be affected.

Non-Mendelian inheritance – polygenic inheritance involving more than one gene; multifactorial conditions where environmental factors may precipitate the phenotype to manifest itself.

Risk factors – a variable that influences the occurrence of a disease. Include demographic, physical, biological and behavioural agents.

Genetic testing

- Karyotype test – demonstrates chromosomal abnormalities
- Hybridized DNA probes – for specific DNA sequences
- Northern blot – RNA quantification
- Western blot – protein quantification
- Southern blot – DNA quantification

Biomechanics

- The physical properties of materials used in medicine

Bending

- Depends on cross-sectional area and the distribution of a material in a structure
- A cylinder resists bend more than a solid rod because material is distributed further from the axis of the bend in a cylinder than in a rod
- Structural integrity resists bending by increased rigidity. For example, an intramedullary nail that is a complete tube will resist bending more than one with a slit in the circumference
- Screw holes in a plate may decrease the bending resistance ten-fold
- Beam length (also known as lever arm) is the distance at which load is applied from a fixed point. A doubling of beam length generates an eight-fold deflection for a given load
- Bending resistance is proportional to the thickness raised to the power 3

Torque

- The turning force applied about the long axis of a material
- = Force × perpendicular distance from axis of rotation
- Torsional stiffness = angular deformation due to torque and beam length
- Torque generates maximal shear stresses at 45° to the axis, hence spiral failure of tubular structures such as long bones

Material properties – definitions

- **Tensile force** – a pulling force applied to a stationary object
- **Compression force** – a pushing force
- **Fatigue failure** – occurs with repetitive loading cycles at stresses below the ultimate tensile strength. Usually does not occur if loads are kept below 0.5 of the yield stress
- **Endurance limit** – maximum stress under which material will not fail regardless of how many loading cycles are applied
- **Brittle** – little or no capacity to undergo permanent (plastic) deformation prior to failure. Exhibits a linear stress/strain curve up to the point of failure. The yield stress is almost equivalent to the fracture stress
- **Ductile** – undergoes a large amount of permanent (plastic) deformation prior to catastrophic failure
- **Ductility** – the amount of permanent deformation required to cause failure as a percentage of elongation
- **Anisotropic** – exhibits different intrinsic mechanical properties when loaded along different axes
- **Isotropic** – intrinsic mechanical properties do not depend upon the direction of loading
- **Hardness** – the surface property of a material; the ability of a material to resist scratching and indentation on the surface
- **Toughness** – the amount of energy per unit volume absorbed by a material before breakage (represented by the area under the stress/strain curve)
- **Stress raiser** – a change in cross-sectional area (e.g. screw hole, scratch or notch) of a material acts as a *stress raiser*, which increases fatigue failure

Deformation

- **Plastic** – a permanent change in length after a load has been removed
- **Elastic** – a temporary change in length that completely resolves after the load is removed

Viscoelastic – a property of biological and some plastic materials sensitive to the speed at which the load is applied. In general the faster the stress rate (rate of loading), the higher the stiffness. Bone is stiffer and more brittle and can sustain a higher load to failure when loads are applied at higher rates.

Viscoelastic materials have the following properties:

- **Creep** – deformation of a material over time to a constant load
- **Stress relaxation** – with a constantly applied strain the stress in the material decreases
- **Hysteresis** – under cyclical loading there is loss of energy in the material during each cycle (the stress/strain relationship during the loading process is different from that in the unloading process)

Stress/strain curve

An important "A" list subject in the basic science oral. You *must* understand the diagram in Figure 24.3a, b and be able to draw it out.

The curve is derived by axially loading a body and plotting stress (y axis) versus strain (x axis). The resulting curve consists of two lines: an almost vertical and an almost horizontal component. The vertical element is the elastic portion, where deformation is temporary and if the deforming force is removed the structure returns to its original length (like an elastic band). In this elastic region stress is proportional to strain and the stress/strain ratio is known as the Young's modulus of elasticity. The horizontal element is the plastic portion where increasing the stress on the material leads to permanent deformity. The point of change from plastic to permanent deformity is known as the yield point of proportional limit. Once the yield point has been exceeded there will always be some residual deformation that will be locked into the material specimen. Unloading from any part of the curve (even after the yield point has been reached) will always result in a straight-line relationship, which will follow a path that is parallel to the section that determines the elastic modulus. If loading continues every point represents a new yield point for the material. If the material is then unloaded and reloaded it will exhibit linear elastic behaviour

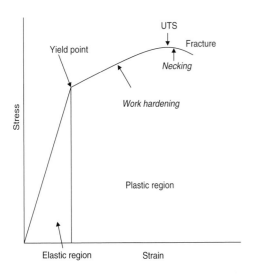
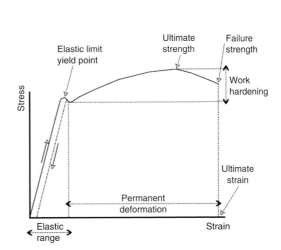

Figure 24.3a, b Ideal stress/strain curves

up to the last yield point from which additional loading will follow the path of the remainder of the curve with additional permanent deformation induced. Each subsequent yield point is higher than the previous one. This phenomenon is known as *work hardening*. The **ultimate tensile strength** (UTS) is the highest stress observed on the stress versus strain diagram while the failure strength is the stress value at which the material eventually fails. The reason for the drop off in magnitude is due to a phenomenon known as "necking".

Yield point (proportional limit): transition point from the elastic to the plastic range. This is reduced in plastics as temperature rises.

Strength: the stress at the failure point for a single cycle.

Ultimate strength: maximum strength obtained by material.

Breaking point: point where material fractures.

Plastic deformation: change in length after removing load (before breaking point) in the plastic range.

Strain: change in length divided by the original length is called strain. Strain is a proportion; it has no units.

Stress: force divided by the cross-sectional area perpendicular to its direction of action. Expressed as force per unit area ($N \cdot m^{-2}$).

Strain energy: when the material is loaded in the elastic region, the area under the stress/strain curve is known as the "strain energy".

Load/deformation: this graph is similar to the stress/strain concept, where the area under the graph represents the *work done*.

Stiffness: stress/strain (Young's modulus). The stiffness of most tissues is not constant but increases with increasing strain.

Compliance: the reverse of stiffness.

Young's modulus of elasticity

A measure of the stiffness of a material or its ability to resist deformation.

E = stress/strain = slope in the elastic range stress/strain curve

Shear stress

Occurs when two forces are directed parallel to each other but not along the same line or in the same direction. A couple is created by two equal, non-collinear, parallel but oppositely directed forces. Vector quantities are added according to the parallelogram law of vector addition.

Newton's laws

Newton's first law: For a body in equilibrium, the sum of forces and moments = 0.

Newton's second law: Force = mass × acceleration.

Newton's third law: To every force there is an equal and opposite one.

Moment

The moment of a force is the effect of a force at a perpendicular distance from an axis, which results in rotational movement and angular acceleration:

   Moment = Force × Distance (of lever arm perpendicular to fulcrum).

Free body diagrams

- Used to solve questions regarding forces acting at a joint
- Consider a body at rest or at constant velocity such that Newton's first law applies
- Sum of forces in any given direction equals the sum of forces in the opposite direction
- Anticlockwise moment = clockwise moment

Ground reaction force

- The force acting on the body whilst standing/walking/running, etc.
- Equal to the weight of the subject if static
- Measured on a force plate, having x, y, z components to the force and the moment about each axis

Joint reaction force (JRF)

- A concept to describe the equal and opposite forces between two bones due to weight and inertia
- Has a direction and magnitude that can be calculated by free body diagram analysis
- These diagrams *must be known and understood* for the exam

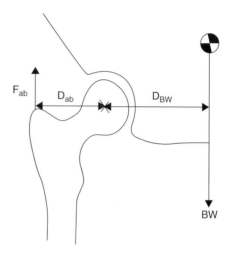

Figure 24.4 Hip free body diagram. BW, Body weight; D_{ab}, perpendicular force of F_{ab} from the fulcrum; D_{BW}, perpendicular distance of body weight from fulcrum; F_{ab}, abductor force

Hip

- Pauwels (1976)[2] gave a basic model of a two-dimensional hip with a single abductor acting upon it. His model predicts a JRF at the hip in single stance of 2.5 times body weight (Figure 24.4)

$$F_{ab} \times D_{ab} = 5BW/6 \times D_{BW}$$

So,

$$F_{ab} = 5BW/6 \times D_{BW}/D_{ab}$$

- The parallelogram of forces using F_{ab} and BW therefore allows the JRF direction and magnitude to be predicted
- F_{ab} = abductor force, D_{ab} = perpendicular distance of F_{ab} from the fulcrum, BW = body weight, reduced by one-sixth to account for leg weight, and D_{BW} = perpendicular distance of body weight from the fulcrum

Hip with walking stick

- When a walking stick is employed in the opposite hand, a force F_{ws} opposes body weight at

---

[2] Pauwels E (1976) *Biomechanics in the Normal and Diseased Hip*. Berlin: Springer-Verlag, p. 26.

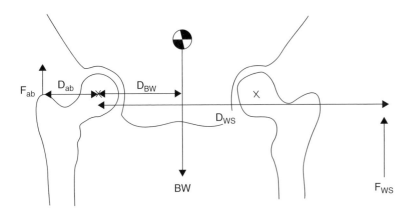

Figure 24.5 Hip with walking stick free body diagram. D_{ws}, distance of walking stick from fulcrum; F_{ws}, force walking stick

D_{ws} perpendicular distance from the fulcrum (Figure 24.5)

Now

$$F_{ab} \times D_{ab} = 5dw/6 - F_{ws} \times D_{ws}$$

- The transmission of 15% of body weight via the walking stick may reduce the JRF by up to 60%
- Berme and Paul (1979)[3] utilized a three-dimensional mathematical model and force plates to estimate that hip JRF in single stance is 2.25 times body weight, with components of 1.8 times body weight in anteroposterior, and 0.8 times body weight in medial–lateral, directions
- Bergmann (1993)[4] measured the forces directly using implanted transducers in hip prostheses and confirmed a hip JRF of 3 times body weight for walking, 5 times body weight for jogging and 7 times body weight at a stumble
- Proximal femoral angulation affects the hip joint reaction forces:
  - In a varus hip, the abductor moment arm (D_{ab}) is increased. The abductor pull is weaker. This results in increased shear forces but decreased JRF at the hip. The result is a broad, medially based sourcil in the acetabulum
  - In a valgus hip, the abductor moment arm (D_{ab}) is decreased. The abductor pull is strong. This results in reduced shear but increased JRF at the hip. There is a narrow lateral sourcil in the acetabulum
- These principles can be used in proximal femoral osteotomy and may also affect the performance of an implant in hip arthroplasty

Knee

- Any joint can have a free body diagram constructed. The knee is the other common exam question (Figure 24.6)

To calculate force in patellar tendon,

$$PT = (BW/2) \times d/e$$

If

BW=700 N, d=200 mm and e=35 mm

then PT=2000 N or 2.9 times the body weight

Mechanical axis of lower limb = centre of head of femur to centre of ankle (usually 3° with respect to vertical)

Vertical axis = centre of gravity to ground

[3] Berme N, Paul JP (1979) Load actions transmitted by implants. *J Biomed Eng* **1**(4): 268–72.
[4] Bergmann G, Graichen F, Rohlmann A (1993) Hip joint loading during walking and running, measured in two patients. *J Biomech* **26**(8): 969–90.

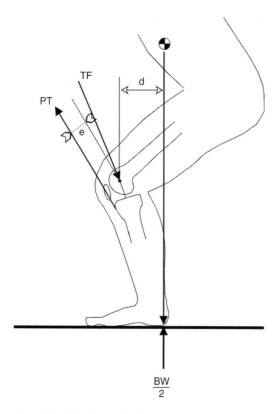

Figure 24.6 Knee free body diagram

Anatomical axes of long bones = along shafts of tibia and femur (usually 6° for femur and 3° for tibia with respect to vertical)

Mechanical axis of femur = centre of head of femur to centre of knee

Q angle = angle of quadriceps with respect to patellar tendon

Dynamics

- Use Newton's second law for motion analysis
- Derive motion from known forces (whereas *inverse dynamics* derives forces from known motion)
- When analysing human muscles or limbs, dynamics suffers from the problem of "indeterminacy" –

where there are more unknown quantities than equations to solve them

- Work done = force × distance moved
- Efficiency = work done divided by the energy expended in doing it

---

Examination corner

Basic science oral 1

Candidates were asked to draw the stress/strain curve for a typical material and explain the diagram as they were drawing.
They were then asked:

- To identify features on the curve such as yield point, ultimate tensile strength and breaking strength
- The differences in the shape of the stress/strain curve between a ductile and brittle material
- What the area under the stress/strain curve represents

If the examiners want to make life difficult for you they will ask you to draw out the stress/strain curve of either a ligament or tendon.

Basic science oral 2

Stress/strain curve

Several questions asked about various parts of the curve – breaking point, yield point, etc.

Basic science oral 3

Draw the stress/strain curve for ceramic and silicone and explain as you go along

Basic science oral 4

Stress/strain curve – discuss each part of the curve

Gait analysis

Gait analysis on its own is fairly useless and a thorough clinical history and examination are also required to put the condition into a clinical context.

If the child is a non-walker it is stupid to refer them for gait analysis.

A bipedal gait allows energy conservation "carry over" between steps.

History

- Birth, motor milestones (especially ability to sit unaided, crawled at x months, walked at x months), progression/deterioration, current/previous intervention

Examination

- Standing posture and spine
- Walking gait
- Recumbent lower limb – tone, power, co-ordination, fixed deformity, scars, wasting
- Look for walking aids including prosthetics, shoe wear patterns

Types of analysis

- Observational – what you do in the clinic!
- Video
- Specialized – pressure platforms, video, force plate studies, EMG, energy consumption, computer assisted

Gait analysis can be divided into two approaches:
1. Kinematics – the study of motion and the breakdown of this into its component parts
2. Kinetics – the study of forces that produce motion using force plates and computer modelling of the lower limb joints

The gait cycle

The gait cycle begins when the foot strikes the ground and ends when the same foot strikes the ground again. It is divided into two major phases: **stance** and **swing.** The stance phase starts when the foot strikes the ground (initial contact) and ends when the foot leaves the ground, at which point the swing phase commences. In normal walking, stance makes up 60% of the cycle, with swing making up 40%.

Perry[5] divided the gait cycle into eight descriptive stages for the purpose of assessment. These are an artificial division but provide reference points – you must be able to describe these!

Stance

Initial contact
- Usually of the heel (but note "heel strike" is no longer acceptable nomenclature)
- Flexed hip, extended knee, dorsiflexion at ankle
- Known as first/heel rocker

Loading response 13%
- First double limb support
- Plantar flexion occurring at the ankle to get the foot to the ground
- Eccentric contracture of the gastrocnemius-soleus, slows plantar flexion
- Flexed hip, flexed knee

Mid-stance 37%
- Weight of body passes forward over stable foot
- Momentarily there is no muscle action
- Ankle dorsiflexes (gastrocnemius-soleus contracts eccentrically)
- Known as second/ankle rocker

Terminal stance
- Heel leaving ground, foot plantar flexion
- Concentric contracture of gastrocnemius to plantar flex the foot
- Coincides with initial contact of other limb
- Known as third/toe rocker

Pre-swing 13%
- Second double limb support

---

[5] Perry J (1992) *Gait Analysis: Normal and Pathological Function*. Thorofare, NJ: Slack Incorporated.

Swing phase

Initial swing
- Knee flexed, hip flexed, foot dorsiflexed

Mid swing 40%
- Tibia swings forward under thigh

Terminal swing
- Prepositioning of the dorsiflexed foot ready for initial contact

Three foot and ankle rockers
- First: heel strike
- Second: ankle trunk forward over the shank
- Third: toe heel rise, push ourselves forwards

Cadence (steps/minute) – number of steps taken per unit time.

Stride length – the horizontal distance covered from initial foot contact to the next ipsilateral foot contact during one stride.

Step length – the horizontal distance covered from foot contact to the next contralateral foot contact.

Uses of the gait cycle
- Cerebral palsy, evaluating the effectiveness of prosthetic limbs, assessing orthotic devices, assessing the progression of neuromuscular disease, assessing the function of total hip or knee arthroplasty, documenting rehabilitation after sports injury
- Specialized techniques are not universally accepted – inter-laboratory variation, intra-laboratory variation and questionable clinical application have cast doubt on the validity of gait analysis in the past. Avoid singing the praises of gait analysis until you can determine whether your examiner is an enthusiast or sceptic. It is safest to discuss gait analysis as a "diagnostic tool" with limitations – like MRI

Ground reactive force
- Related to Newton's third law
- In normal gait the ground reactive force passes anterior to the hip and knee until just before

toe-off – reduces the force needed by the quadriceps for extension
- During the terminal stance and pre-swing ground reactive force passes behind the hip and knee and acts as a flexor – so reducing the work required by the hip and knee flexors
- If anything prevents this normal progression, it also increases energy expenditure

Gage's five prerequisites for normal gait
1. Prepositioning of the foot
2. Clearance of foot in swing
3. Stability in stance
4. Adequate step length
5. Energy conservation

Examination corner

Basic science oral

- What are Gage's five prerequisites for gait?
- What do you understand by gait analysis – how does it work (infra-red cameras, reflective markers)?
- What are the components of the gait cycle?

Ballistics

St Petersburg Declaration (1868) and Hague Declaration (1899)

- These basically set out terms to minimize unnecessary suffering

Velocity

- Measured at the muzzle
- Low – 300–600 m·s^{-1}
- High – >923 m·s^{-1}. Generally result in *cavitation*, where a wider area than the track is damaged by acceleration of the surrounding tissues
- Determines kinetic energy (KE) = $\frac{1}{2}mv^2$, where m is the mass and v is velocity

Assessment

- Primary – track of projectile

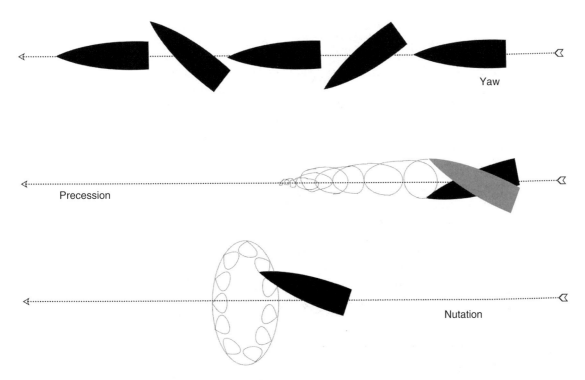

Figure 24.7 Ballistics

- Secondary – zone of contusion
- Tertiary – zone of concussion

Impact – "terminal ballistics"

- May be "nose on" (i.e. straight, ±spin) or may have yaw, tumble, precession or nutation (Figure 24.7), which all alter the surface area presented to the tissues

Expandable bullets deform on impact and cause maximal damage, and may fragment in different directions. Hence "full metal jackets" to prevent this. High-density, low-elasticity tissues such as bone absorb kinetic energy readily and fragment. Lower-density, higher-elasticity tissues allow the projectile to pass with less damage.

Shotgun pellets act as single mass at close range, and cause less damage the greater the distance. Wadding may enter tissue and require retrieval.

Management principles

- Antibiotics ("cauterization" of tissue by bullet is a myth)
- Debridement of entry and exit wounds (this has superseded traditional advice to "flay open the track" except where a joint or a viscus has been transgressed)
- Open reduction and internal fixation of fractures
- Remove foreign bodies and wash out joints

Non-operative fracture management

Suggested reading is *The Closed Treatment of Common Fractures*, John Charnley.[6]

[6] Charnley J (2003) *The Closed Treatment of Common Fractures*, 4th edn. Cambridge: Cambridge University Press.

Casting

Materials

- Plaster of Paris ($CaSO_4 \cdot H_2O + H_2O \leftrightarrow CaSO_4 \cdot 2H_2O$ + heat)
- Synthetic polymer

Technique

- Non-padded (Bohler)
- Padded (Bologna)

Principles

- Choice of analgesia/anaesthesia
- Planning
- Reduction
- Splintage – three-point fixation
- Ongoing assessment

Mechanics (after Charnley)

Soft tissue (specifically periosteum) acts as a hinge in most fractures. This can hinder reduction when fractures overlap and fragments interlock, but it also forms the basis for three-point fixation.

Traction aligns fragments by the (relative) splintage of soft tissues held in tension around the fragments (like a chain). Elongation may occur and is resisted by muscle tone, the continuity of soft tissues, and hydraulic forces (since a sphere has the greatest volume:surface area relationship and traction acts against the tendency of the swollen soft tissues to form a sphere, hydraulic forces are generated).

Transverse fractures are stable to shortening and require splintage to avoid angular and rotational deformity.

Short oblique fractures (<45° from transverse) are relatively stable in response to shortening if periosteal hinge is put in tension (i.e. three-point fixation).

A single plaster slab is not capable of delivering three-point fixation.

Charnley (in contrast to Sarmiento) believed that three-point fixation with padding is superior to a tube-like plaster.

Late deformity is commonly:
- Varus in the proximal femur
- Valgus in the lateral femur
- Varus in the humerus

Most joints eventually recover full range of movement after immobilization – as defined in Charnley's "Law of Closed Treatment": "After fracture of the shaft of a long bone, the associated joints will tolerate fixation for the duration of *normal* union without either permanent or significant loss of motion".

Functional bracing (Sarmiento)

- Concept of "fluid tube" to maintain position
- Use of soft tissues to maintain reduction

Traction

- Axis determined by the deforming forces acting on the proximal segment
- Opposing force can be **fixed** (e.g. Thomas splint in isolation) or **balanced/dynamic** (e.g. Hamilton Russell)
- Skeletal traction is achieved via a Denham pin (threaded centrally) or a Steinman pin (not threaded) for forces >4 kg
- Suspension avoids pressure points

Types

- Skin (Bucks) traction limited to <4 kg
- See Figure 24.8

Biomaterials

Stainless steel 316L

- The number 316 refers to 3% molybdenum and 16% nickel added to the normal alloy of iron, chromium (major corrosion protection) and carbon

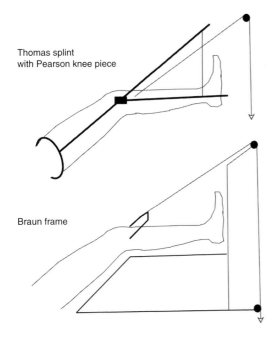

Thomas splint with Pearson knee piece

Braun frame

Hamilton Russell traction

Sling

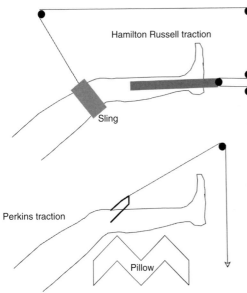

Perkins traction

Pillow

Figure 24.8 Traction

- The letter "L" denotes low carbon (less than 0.03%)
- Strong, cheap
- Relatively ductile and therefore it is easy to alter its shape. Useful in contouring of plates and wires during operative procedures
- Relatively biocompatible
- High Young's modulus of elasticity; can lead to stress shielding of lower modulus bone
- Usually cold worked by 30% to improve its yield and ultimate stress
- A small number of people are hyper-sensitive to nickel or chromium
- Good fatigue resistance
- Reasonably resistant to corrosion although it is susceptible to pitting, stress and crevice corrosion

Titanium alloys

The most commonly used alloy is titanium 64, referring to the proportions of the alloying elements aluminium (6%) and vanadium (4%) used to enhance tensile properties.

Advantages

- Outstanding biocompatibility and corrosion resistance
- Excellent resistance to pitting, intergranular and crevice corrosion
- Titanium forms an oxide layer by passivation, which protects the material from corrosion
- Relatively low Young's modulus, roughly half that of stainless steel and cobalt chrome, therefore less stress shielding of bone
- Less interference with CT/MRI

Disadvantages

- Poor resistance to wear compared to stainless steel or cobalt chrome and so it cannot be used as a bearing surface. Can produce large amounts of wear debris; these wear particles appearing black within the body. Particles can promote a histiocytic response

- Sensitive to surface flaws and scratching. Very notch sensitive and when notched this predisposes to fatigue failure
- Uncertain association with neoplasm
- Low tensile strength
- High coefficient of friction
- Relatively expensive

Cobalt chromium

- Vitallium® = chromium, cobalt and trace amounts of molybdenum, carbon and nickel
- Has a similar Young's modulus to stainless steel
- Ultimate strength and fatigue strength are very high, which means that it is extremely strong
- Good biocompatibility
- Its major advantage over stainless steel or titanium is its substantially better wear properties when used as an articulating surface in joint replacement surgery
- Excellent resistance to corrosion especially crevice corrosion

Metal processing

Casting

The liquid metal is poured into a pre-shaped mould. It is prone to trapping impurities, and shrinkage voids and internal cracks may develop as the material hardens during cooling.

Wrought

The cast metal is modified by rolling or extending.

Forging

The metal is heated and then subjected to force. This involves heating the material until it is red hot and then reshaping it using a series of hammer blows.

Cold working

The metal is repeatedly loaded. This confers strength on the material by increasing its yield strength.

Annealing

This involves beating the material at relatively low temperatures for extended periods of time to allow the grains or molecules of the material to realign themselves to a lower stress state.

Passivation

An oxide covering is applied over the surface of the metal. A chemical treatment is applied to a metallic implant surface to develop a very thin oxide layer to improve the biocompatibility of the surface.

Sintering

Sintering generates a porous layer on a bulk substrate. It generally involves very high temperatures (>1000°C) and high pressures. In the particular case of titanium (and its alloys) these temperatures are near the melting point and cause the microstructure to become so altered that what results is a much weaker material.

Hot pressing

A heat treatment that has been used to improve the surface finish of tibial plateau components. It involves "ironing" the surface, which removes machine tool marks and any minor imperfections.

Fatigue failure: crack propagation

Defined as the growth of cracks in a structure subjected to repetitive loading below the failure load of that structure. A crack usually starts at a stress concentration or stress riser, which may be a scratch, a hole, a corner or a change in cross-section. At these places the stress is greater than the average stress in the material. Once a crack occurs then, because of the reducing cross-sectional area, it propagates and accelerates towards ultimate failure of the material.

Metal allergy

- Of uncertain significance in metal prosthetic implantation including joint replacement

- It is unknown whether metal sensitization causes loosening or vice versa
- Joint replacements:
  - For metal-on-plastic it is not thought to be an issue. There is some evidence for a beneficial effect on immunological tolerance of metal!
  - Metal-on-metal (original 1960s versions) is associated with cobalt>nickel>chromate sensitivities and with loosening
  - Modern metal-on-metal – single series[7] suggests nickel sensitization and loosening but there have been no controlled trials to investigate this
- Low-sulphur stainless steel reduces nickel release and reduces sensitization
- A prospective study[8] of patch testing pre- and post-implantation of extremity stainless steel fracture plates showed no evidence of sensitization, even in nickel-allergic patients. Case reports of problematic eczematous reactions exist[9]

Ceramics

Ceramics are compounds of metallic elements bound ionically and/or covalently with non-metallic elements; they are bioinert or bioactive:

- Bioinert – alumina, zirconia
- Bioactive – hydroxyapatite, glass ceramic

Properties

- Extremely hard materials that are very resistant to wear
- Excellent abrasive resistance
- Low coefficient of friction
- Excellent wettability
- High impact strength
- Low moisture absorption

- Chemical resistance
- No observed toxic effects
- High Young's modulus of elasticity (high stiffness)
- High compressive strength
- Their big drawback is brittleness, they display almost no plastic deformation before failure. Occasionally they can fail catastrophically in THA, a so-called brittle femoral head fracture. This is much less common with newer ceramic designs
- Susceptible to abrasive wear and edge loading in THA especially if the acetabular cup is placed too open
- Zirconia has fallen out of favour as a ceramic used in THA. Although it has high fracture toughness it can undergo phase transformation at high temperatures which substantially weakens the material and roughens the surface, reducing its wear properties. The uncontrollable transformation of **zirconia** from its stronger to weaker phase led to the 2002 recall of ceramic heads manufactured by Saint Gobain Advanced Ceramics Demarquest (Monreuil, France). Its use as a bearing surface with polyethylene is controversial as high failure rates have been reported but this has been attributed to the poor quality of the polyethylene cup.[10]

Examination corner

Basic science oral 1

Exhibit – A metal hammer was shown which had broken off at the junction between the head and shaft

Examiner: This hammer broke while I was using it in theatre a couple of days ago and I brought it along so that we can discuss why it broke where it has. If you look carefully it is broken at the junction between its head and shaft. Can you explain why this is so?

Candidate: A difficult question, which was also found tricky by most of the other candidates I discussed it with after the oral. I managed to scrape some sort of answer together in a roundabout way, albeit with much prompting by the examiner.

---

[7] Thomas P, Gollwitzer H, Maier S, Rueff F (2006) Osteosynthesis associated contact dermatitis with unusual perpetuation of hyperreactivity in a nickel allergic patient. *Contact Dermatitis* **54**(4): 222–5.

[8] Hindsén M, Carlsson AS, Möller H (1993) Orthopaedic metallic implants in extremity fractures and contact allergy. *J Eur Acad Dermatol Venereol* **2**(1): 22–6.

[9] Rostoker G, Robin J, Binet O *et al.* (1987) Dermatitis due to orthopaedic implants. A review of the literature and report of three cases. *J Bone Joint Surg Am* **69**: 1408–12.

[10] Clarke IC, Manaka M, Green DD *et al.* (2003) Current status of zirconia used in total hip implants. *J Bone Joint Surg Am* **85** Suppl 4: 73–84.

The question concerns crack propagation and appears reasonably straightforward in a non-exam situation but trying to work it out from first principles in the stress of the examination is an entirely different matter.

Basic science oral 2

Structural properties of titanium

What is the head made of in a titanium-on-plastic THA implant?

Basic science oral 3

Fatigue fractures and endurance limit

Ultra high molecular weight polyethylene (UHMWPE)

- Polyethylene (PE) is a long-chain polymer formed of ethylene monomer molecules in which all of the carbon atoms are linked
- PE is made by low-pressure, oxygen-catalysed addition polymerization of ethylene (C_2H_4)
- UHMWPE has been the preferred acetabular-bearing material for more than 30 years
- UHMWPE has a molecular weight of 2×10^6–5×10^6 MW and a powder particle size of 63–250 μm
- Linear wear rates of up to 0.27 mm per annum have been reported (decreases with increasing head size)
- Volumetric wear rates are 40–80 mm^3 per year (rate increases with increasing head size)
- Wear particles are usually 1–100 μm; 10 000 particles per step are created by THA
- Manufacturing techniques are aimed at reducing this wear

Positive features

- High impact strength
- Low coefficient of friction
- Low moisture absorption

- Extremely tough
- Chemical resistance
- No observed toxic effects

Negative features

- Difficult to machine
- Wear debris (highly prone to abrasive wear)
- Creep

Production methods

Ram extrusion
Powdered resin is forced through a die with external heat to form a block from which components are cut. The high-temperature/high-pressure treatment is chosen to reduce product inconsistency and to increase Young's modulus, and produces "Hylamer™".

The disadvantage of this method is the product's susceptibility to non-uniformity.

Sheet compression moulding
The resin is heated and then cooled under pressure between two metal sheets.

The disadvantage of this method is that pressure differences in moulding may alter product consistency.

Direct compression moulding
To address the problem with compression moulding, a small volume is directly moulded onto a metal backing or into a shaped mould with a shaped plunger.

Isostatic moulding
The resin is packed cold into a mould under vacuum. Heat and isostatic compression are applied. This generates a uniform polymer with reduced oxidative degradation.

- **Calcium stearate** – used as moulding lubricant. May deposit crystals within PE and be a source of crack propagation
- **Fusion defects** – incomplete consolidation, fusion defects and the formation of non-consolidated

particles are associated with pitting and delamination. These defects act as stress concentrators, which can lead to the initiation of subsurface fatigue cracks

Sterilization of polyethylene

The sterilization process of PE has been implicated as a factor causing high wear rates and rapid PE wear. Irradiation of PE generates unstable free radical formation.

There are four outcomes from this:
- **Recombination** (to form the original polymer molecule)
- **Unsaturation**
- **Chain scission**
- **Cross-linking**

The two important pathways concerning PE wear are chain scission and cross-linking.

Chain scission

In the presence of oxygen chain scission (fragmentation and shortening of the large polymer chains) is favoured.

Cross-linking

Cross-linking of PE strengthens the polymer and improves the resistance to adhesive and abrasive wear, but the mechanical properties are altered. It is believed that cross-linking of the PE molecules resists intermolecular mobility making the PE more resistant to deformation and wear in the plane perpendicular to the primary molecular axis. Cross-linking has a detrimental effect on yield strength, ultimate tensile strength and elongation to break. The decrease in these properties is proportional to the degree of cross-linking. This fact has generated debates on the optimum degree of cross-linking since cross-linked PE may fail catastrophically if excessive stresses are applied.

Gamma sterilization
- Generates short-chain free radicals that cross-link to form a stronger polymer

- If oxygen is available, short chains unite with it (scission) to weaken the polymer and oxidative degradation will occur
- Oxidized PE should be avoided, as the polymer is weakened and vulnerable to fatigue wear, which can cause pitting, cracking and subsurface delamination
- Gamma sterilization in air was the industrial standard in the 1980s but has now largely been replaced by alternative methods
- Gamma irradiation in an oxygen-free environment favours the formation of cross-linked PE, so strengthening the polymer with improved resistance to adhesive and abrasive wear, however it does diminish its mechanical properties

Ethylene oxide
- Using ethylene oxide to sterilize PE decreases the production of free radicals so that oxidative degradation of PE does not occur
- This method of sterilization does not cause cross-linking of PE, reducing the PE resistance to wear by around 30%
- There is some concern regarding harmful residues left by gas on surrounding human tissue
- Some feel this method of sterilization does not achieve the level of cup sterility required for hip arthroplasty surgery

Post-irradiation oxidation of UHMWPE
- Sterilization within inert atmospheres reduces the level of oxidation by allowing a greater degree of cross-linking and/or recombination. However, some free radicals may remain which would allow oxidation at a later date. However, provided that the component is implanted soon after the sterilization process then the risks are thought to be reduced as the synovial joint has a low oxygen content
- When PE components are sterilized by gamma radiation and stored in an oxygen environment, this generates oxidized PE that, under repetitive loading, may lead to delamination, cracking and catastrophic failure

- Shelf ageing may cause oxidation and free radical formation thus vacuum packing is frequently used now. Maximum oxidation occurs 1–2 mm below the surface, the so-called subsurface white band, whose thickness increases with time
- Methods have been developed to entirely remove residual free radicals in PE so that there is no potential for oxidation on the shelf or in vivo
- Free radicals created in PE by ionizing radiation can be driven to a cross-linking reaction by re-melting the polymer and subsequent final sterilization with ethylene oxide or gas plasma[11]
- Re-melting the PE does induce changes in the crystalline structure of the material that may be associated with a decrease in some mechanical properties. Controversy persists regarding the relative detriment of re-melting compared with that of the retention of some residual free radicals

Tribology

- *NOT "tribiology"*
- *The science of interacting surfaces in relative motion*
- *Derivation: Tribos (Gk) meaning rubbing*

Friction

- Defined as the resistance to sliding motion between two bodies in contact
- The frictional force (F) is directly proportional to the applied load (W) across a bearing surface
- This is represented mathematically as $F = \mu W$
- Where, to clarify, F is frictional force, μ is the coefficient of friction, which depends on the combination of surface materials, and W is the normal load on the interface on each surface (in newtons)
- The force needed to initiate movement is greater than that needed to continue movement [μ_d

(dynamic coefficient) is approximately 70% of μ_s (static coefficient)]
- The frictional force is independent of the apparent contact area

Contact area

- The true contact area is between asperities (bumps) on the surfaces and is usually 1% of the apparent contact area. The asperities deform in proportion to load and inversely with respect to surface hardness
- Bonds form at contact points and must be broken to initiate movement (hence $\mu_s > \mu_d$)

Lubrication

Synovial fluid

- Synovial fluid is produced by the type B fibroblast-like cells of the synovium
- Type A fibroblast-like cells are involved in phagocytosis, the clearing away of debris created by joint movement
- Synovial fluid is made up of proteinase, collagenase, hyaluronic acid, lubricin and prostaglandins
- Synovial fluid is a clear, sometimes yellowish, viscous liquid
- Synovial fluid is a dialysate of blood plasma without clotting factors or erythrocytes
- It has unique fluid properties conferred by hyaluronic acid
- It exhibits non-newtonian flow properties, i.e. when the shear rate is varied, the shear stress does not vary in the same proportion (or even necessarily in the same direction)
- Pseudoplasticity = fall in viscosity as shear rate increases
- Thixotropy = time-dependent decrease in viscosity under constant shearing

Main functions

- Lubrication
- Cartilage nutrition through diffusion

[11] Key Reference: Hopper RH Jr, Young AM, Orishimo KF, Engh CA Jr (2003) Effect of terminal sterilization with gas plasma or gamma radiation on wear of polyethylene liners. *J Bone Joint Surg Am* **85-A** (3): 464–8.

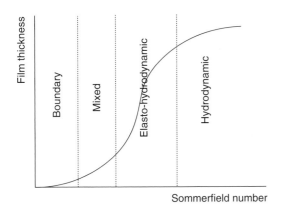

Figure 24.9 Lubrication

Sommerfield number
- This is a property of a given lubricant = viscosity × velocity/stress (Figure 24.9)
- This affects frictional properties in systems where boundary lubrication is exceeded
- Lambda value λ = fluid thickness/surface roughness
- Hence a rougher surface with higher asperities will require a thicker fluid film to achieve hydrodynamic lubrication
- The critical lambda value for reduced friction is ≈3
- Most artificial joints have a lambda value of <3, although metal-on-metal and ceramic-on-ceramic may approach this value
- As the lambda value exceeds 3 the friction starts to increase again due to viscosity within the fluid film layer itself

Basic types of lubrication

1. Boundary lubrication

- Occurs when the fluid film has been depleted and the contact-bearing surfaces are separated only by a boundary lubricant of molecular thickness, which prevents excessive bearing friction and wear
- This involves adsorption of a single monolayer of lubricant on each surface of the joint
- In synovial joints the glycoprotein lubricin, which is found in synovial fluid, is believed to be the adsorbed molecule

- Friction here is independent of the Sommerfield number

2. Fluid film lubrication

- Separation of surfaces by a fluid film whose minimum thickness exceeds the surface roughness of the bearing surface, which prevents asperity contact

Types of fluid film lubrication in synovial joints

Hydrodynamic

- Rigid bearing surfaces, which are not parallel and are separated by a fluid film, slide tangentially in relation to each other
- A converging wedge of fluid forms and the viscosity within this wedge of fluid produces a lifting pressure between the two surfaces
- Two surfaces are shearing relative to each other. The sliding speed and viscosity of lubricating fluid are sufficient to create a thin film capable of supporting the applied load. There is no contact between surfaces and hence no wear
- A poor model for synovial joints, however this may occur during the high-speed non-accelerating rotatory motion of the femur during the swing phase of gait

This model assumes that:
- Surfaces are rigid and non-porous when in fact they are elastic and deformable
- The lubricant velocity is constant (newtonian)
- The relative sliding speed is high
- Loads are light

Elastohydrodynamic lubrication

This type of lubrication occurs in bearing surfaces that are not rigid.

Macroscopic deformation of the bearing surface serves to trap pressurized fluid and increase the surface area. An increased surface area decreases the shear rate between the two surfaces, thereby increasing the viscosity of the synovial fluid. These factors increase the capacity of the fluid film to carry load and decrease stress within the cartilage.

Microelastohydrodynamic lubrication

- Assumes that asperities of articular cartilage are deformed under high loads to smooth out the bearing surface and create a film thickness of 0.5–1 μm, which is sufficient for fluid film lubrication

Squeeze film

- This occurs when two bearing surfaces approach each other without a relative sliding motion
- Because a viscous lubricant cannot instantaneously be squeezed out from the gap between two surfaces that are approaching each other, pressure is built up as a result of the viscous resistance offered by the lubricant as it is being squeezed from the gap
- As the fluid is forced out, so the layer of fluid lubricant becomes thinner and the joint surfaces come into contact
- This mechanism is capable of carrying high loads for short lengths of time

Weeping lubrication

- Articular cartilage is fluid filled, porous, permeable and capable of exuding and imbibing lubrication fluid
- Tears of lubricant fluid are generated from the cartilage by compression of the bearing surface upon relative motion
- The exudation and imbibition of lubrication fluid are also thought to contribute to nutrition of the chondrocytes

Boosted lubrication

- Assumes that under squeeze film conditions water and synovial fluid are pressurized into cartilage leaving behind a concentrated pool of hyaluronic acid protein complexes to lubricate the surface

Wettability

Describes the relative affinity of lubricant for another material. It can be measured by the angle of contact at the edge of a drop of lubricant applied to the surface of the material.

Hydrostatic

This is an unnatural system where fluid is pumped in and pressure is maintained to reduce surface contact.

Lubrication mechanisms in synovial joints

Despite extensive investigations, no one knows exactly when each type of lubrication comes into play in a synovial joint under particular conditions. The fact that intact synovial joints have a very low coefficient of friction, about 0.02, suggests that synovial joints in the human are likely to be at least partly lubricated by fluid film lubrication.

The articular cartilage surface is not flat and has numerous asperities on it.

The kind of lubrication occurring at any one time in a synovial joint varies according to the loading conditions encountered:

- In a situation where the fluid film thickness is in the same order of thickness as the asperities on the articular surfaces boundary lubrication occurs
- In areas where no surface contact occurs load is thought to be sustained by fluid film lubrication. Cyclical loading of joints may permit squeeze films to develop

---

Examination corner

Basic science oral 1

Examiner: What types of lubrication exist?
Candidate: There are two basic types of lubrication: boundary and fluid film lubrication.

Fluid film lubrication includes hydrodynamic lubrication, elastohydrodynamic lubrication, and microelastohydrodynamic lubrication, weeping lubrication, squeeze film and boosted lubrication.

Hydrodynamic lubrication is the most basic form of lubrication. Rigid bearing surfaces that not parallel and are separated by a fluid film slide tangentially in relation to each other.

Examiner: That's fine you don't need to go into any more detail. What type of lubrication exists in artificial joints?
Candidate: It is thought that boundary lubrication predominates. In this regime, the synovial fluid (lubricant) is not thick enough to prevent contact between the asperities of the

two opposing surfaces. However, the boundary lubricant can separate the two surfaces enough to prevent severe wear.

[Pass]

Basic science oral 2

What are the various types of lubrication in synovial and artificial joints?

Wear

- The progressive loss of material from the surface of a body due to relative motion at that surface
- Generates further "third body" wear particles
- Softest material is worn

Wear mechanisms

Wear is either chemical (usually corrosive) or mechanical.

Types of mechanical wear include:
- Adhesive
- Abrasive
- Fatigue

Adhesive wear

- Adhesive wear occurs when a junction (bond) is formed between the two opposing surfaces as they come into contact
- This junction is held by inter-molecular bonds between the solids and this force is responsible for friction
- If this junction is stronger than the cohesive strength of the individual bearing material surface and if the bond does not break at the original interface, fragments of the weaker material may be torn off and adhere to the stronger material (spot welding/transfer)
- Steady low wear rate

Abrasive wear (ploughing)

- Abrasive wear occurs when a softer material comes into contact with a significantly harder material

- Under these circumstances the microscopic counterface aspirates on the harder material surface cut and plough through the softer material, producing grooves and detaching material to form wear debris
- This is the main mechanism in metal/polymer prostheses
- Third body abrasive wear occurs when extraneous material enters the interfacial region. Trapped wear debris produces a very high local stress, which quickly leads to localized fatigue failure and a rapid, varying wear rate. Third body particles generate further debris through an abrasive process at articulating surfaces. This is also thought to be responsible in part for "backside wear" at "rigid" metal/polymer couplings and other modular interfaces

Fatigue wear

- Caused by accumulation of microscopic damage within the bearing material due to repetitive/cyclical stressing
- Depends on the frequency and magnitude of the applied loads and on the intrinsic properties of the bulk material
- Also dependent on contact stress
  - Decreased by:
    - Conformity of surfaces
    - Thicker bearing surface
  - Increased by:
    - Higher stiffness of material
    - Misaligned or unbalanced implants
- Mainly a problem in TKA as the joint is less conforming and the PE more highly stressed
- Delamination: repeated loading causes subsurface fatigue failure

Corrosive wear

Mechanical wear may remove the passivation layer of the metal surface allowing chemical corrosion to occur.

Fretting wear

Localized wear from relative motion over a very small range. Can produce a large amount of debris.

Wear sources in joint replacement

- Primary articulation surface
- Secondary articulation surface
  - Surfaces not involved in the primary articulation but still subject to wear (backside of modular poly insert with metal, screw fretting with the metal shell of acetabular liners)
- Cement/prosthesis micromotion
- Cement/bone or prosthesis/bone micromotion
- Third body wear

Linear wear

Linear wear is the loss of height of the bearing surface and is expressed in mm/year.

Volumetric wear

The total volume of material that has been worn away. Expressed in mm^3/year.

Wear rate

- Debris volume; highest in the first year – "wearing in"
- A steady state is then achieved where debris volume is not related to the contact area but to the load and sliding distance
- Accelerated wear occurs at the end of a prosthesis' life when its integrity may be jeopardized
- In the knee joint, rectilinear sliding generates alignment of the linear polymeric molecules, which reduces wear
- Cross-links increase the strength but also increase the brittleness of the polymer

Head size

- The larger the femoral head the greater the sliding distance and volumetric wear
- On the assumption that the femoral head produces a cylindrical bore, the volume of wear debris $= \pi P r^2$ where P is the penetration and r is the radius of the femoral head
- A smaller head size decreases the sliding distance (travelling distance) and reduces volumetric

wear, but there are increased stresses at the joint surface (increased penetrative wear). $P \propto 1/r^2$ and therefore the smaller the femoral head the greater the penetration

Laws of wear

The volume of material (V) removed by wear increases with load (L) and sliding distance (X) but decreases as the hardness of the softer material (H) increases:

$V \propto LX/H$

$V = kLX$

$k =$ a wear factor for a given combination of materials that incorporates the hardness of the softer material, material properties (stiffness, wear resistance), local environment (lubrication) and surface roughness.

Factors that determine wear

Patient factors

- Weight (applied load)
- Age and activity level (rate of applied rate load)

Implant factors

- Coefficient of friction (lubrication)
- Roughness (surface finish)
- Toughness (abrasive wear)
- Hardness (scratch resistance, adhesive wear)
- Surface damage
- Presence of third bodies (abrasive wear)

Wear in prosthetic hips

Penetration of the femoral head into the acetabular PE is due to a combination of wear and creep. Creep usually dominates the initial penetration rate but as creep decreases exponentially with time the majority of the linear penetration that occurs after the first year is due to wear. The direction of creep is superomedial as this is the direction of the compressive joint-contact force in the hip, whereas the direction of wear is superolateral, as this is perpendicular to the instantaneous axis of rotation.

Cup penetration can be measured in the following ways:
- By comparison between initial and follow-up radiographs, corrected for magnification
- Shadowgraph technique
- Computer software scan imaging

Biological effects of wear particles

Large (micron sized) particles have localized effects at the bone/implant/cement interfaces. Small (nanometre sized) particles are thought to have the potential for systemic effects.

Local

Particles of diameter 0.1–10 μm are phagocytosed by macrophages and stimulate the release of soluble pro-inflammatory mediators such as tumour necrosis factor (TNF), interleukin (IL)-1, IL-6, PGE2, matrix metaloproteinases and other factors.

Mediators released near bone cause osteolysis by stimulating bone resorption by osteoclasts and impairing the function of osteoblasts.

Macrophages themselves may also be able to resorb bone directly by the release of oxide radicals and hydrogen peroxide.

The major factors that affect the extent of macrophage activity induced by the wear particles, and therefore the extent of osteolysis, are:
- Volume of wear debris – >150 mm³ per annum is thought to be the "critical" level
- Total number of wear particles
- Morphology of particles (irregularly shaped and elongated particles are more active than spherical, globular-shaped particles)
- Size of particles
- Immune response to the particles

Systemic

Metal ion release is increased five-fold by metal-on-metal instead of metal-on-polymer bearing surfaces.

Metal ions are not phagocytosed. Controversy surrounds the long-term effects, which remain unknown.

Immune sensitization and neoplastic transformation are concerns. Recent worries with MOM hip articulations include ALVAR/pseudotumours and metal hypersensitivity leading to early hip revision.

Examination corner

Basic science oral 1

- Handed a femoral prosthesis
- Discussion about the mechanisms of component wear

Basic science oral 2

- Aseptic loosening of hips
- Wear particles
- Sources
- Third body wear
- Measurement of linear and volumetric wear

Basic science oral 3

- Airport metal detectors and various prostheses
- Metals/alloys in prostheses
- Statistics on new THA and mechanisms of testing wear
- Fatigue failure

Basic science oral 4

I was shown a failed knee prosthesis that had been removed from a patient and asked to describe it.
- General discussion on wear
- PE tibial insert – how can you improve its properties?
- Cross-linking of polymer in PE.
- Discussion on strength, stiffness, etc.

Basic science oral 5

Prosthetic wear mechanisms.
I discussed the mechanisms, modes and effects of wear, as well as suggestions for its reduction. I discussed the various

types of wear and followed on with a brief description of each type of wear mentioned. I then went on to discuss the four modes of prosthetic wear.

Basic science oral 6

Exhibit – a stainless steel femoral component was presented and the candidate was asked to comment.

Candidate: It's worth taking a second or two to look carefully at the prosthesis before launching in. The trick here was to recognize that it had been used and retrieved, but avoid using the word "failed" in your assessment unless pressed as the examiner might feel piqued by your judgement, and it could be that it was retrieved from a cadaver and did not fail!

Apart from noting the general features of a hip femoral prosthetic component, look for wear on the shaft and comment on it. The wear pattern may well give away the side of the patient on which it was used (think about rotational forces at the femur/cement interface with the prosthesis) and you will get "gold stars" for this. Avoid saying the specific type of prosthesis unless you are certain – you are safe saying collarless/collared, etc.

If it's going well you might be led off into a discussion about offset, cement technique, and the place of cementless stems.

Corrosion

Corrosion is the reaction of a metal with its environment resulting in its continuous degradation to oxides, hydroxides or other compounds.

Passivation

- Oxide layer forms on the alloy surface; strongly adherent; acts as a barrier to prevent corrosion. Can be jeopardized by mechanical wear

Types of corrosion

- Uniform attack
- Galvanic
- Crevice
- Pitting
- Fretting (combination of wear and crevice corrosion)
- Intergranular
- Inclusion corrosion
- Leaching corrosion
- Stress corrosion

Uniform attack

- Most common type of corrosion
- Occurs with all metals in electrolyte solution uniformly affecting the entire surface of the implant

Galvanic

- Two dissimilar metals are electrically coupled together
- An anode and cathode form – in essence a small battery develops as ions are exchanged

Crevice

- Occurs in a crevice or crack and is characterized by O_2 depletion
- Tip of the crack cannot passivate due to lack of O_2 accelerated by high concentrations of H^+ and Cl^-

Pitting

- Similar to crevice but the corrosive attacks are more isolated and insidious; a localized form of corrosion in which small pits or holes form
- Dissolution occurs within the pit

Fretting corrosion

- Synergistic combination of wear and crevice corrosion of two materials in contact
- Relative micro movement between the two so that the passivity layer is removed
- Can cause permanent damage to the oxide layer, and particles of metal and oxide can be released from fretting

Intergranular

- Metals have a granular structure, with grain being the name for areas of continuous structure and the grain boundaries being the disordered areas between grains
- Intergranular corrosion occurs at grain boundaries due to impurities

Inclusion corrosion

- Occurs due to impurities left on the surface of materials, e.g. metal fragments from a screwdriver
- Similar to galvanic

Leaching corrosion

- Similar to intergranular corrosion but the result of electrochemical differences within the grains themselves

Stress corrosion (fatigue)

- Metals that are repeatedly deformed and stressed in a corrosive environment show accelerated corrosion and fatigue damage

Ideal implant

- Biocompatibility: inert, non-immunogenic, non-toxic, non-carcinogenic
- Strength: sufficient tensile, compressive and torsional strength, stiffness and fatigue resistance
- Workability: easy to manufacture and implant
- Inexpensive
- No effect on radiological imaging
- Corrosion free

Examination corner

Basic science oral 1

- What is corrosion?
- What are the different types of corrosion?

Arthroplasty

When considering biomaterial issues of any prosthesis *think about the following*:
- Material
- Geometry
- Fixation

You must be able to discuss these features of hip replacements coherently.

Hip

- The femur normally transmits forces via trabeculae in a gradual fashion to a cortex that thickens distally towards the isthmus. A prosthetic stem inevitably alters load transmission
- Variables that may affect load transmission include:
  - Collar – presence/absence
  - Stem shape
  - Stem surface and interface with cement/bone
  - Stem material

Stem material (see "Biomaterials" above)

- Material stiffness is related to cross-sectional area, the shape and modulus of elasticity of a given material
- A reduced modulus of elasticity (for example, titanium) increases the transfer of load to the proximal femur and aims to reduce stress shielding

Stem geometry

- Two broad categories, straight and curved, the latter aiming to more closely mirror femoral anatomy
- May cause issues with stress risers (in both the metal of the stem and the surrounding cement mantle) where shapes alter abruptly
- Neck-shaft angle determines the:
  - Medial offset – describes the medial–lateral distance from the head axis of rotation to the stem long axis. Important in abductor muscle tension, minimizing the risk of dislocation

- Vertical offset – describes the height of the head axis of rotation from the shaft. Important for leg length and abductor muscle tension, minimizing the risk of dislocation
- Longer stems make for increased stress distribution but make revision difficult
- Thicker stems are stronger but of necessity reduce the potential thickness of the cement mantle. This is not significant if the cement is to form a "grout" but a mantle >2 mm is desirable for load transmission in a tapered, polished stem

Collar

- Devised to load the calcar and thereby reduce the stress at the cement interface
- Collars have been shown to restore load proximally to 70% of physiological levels
- Resorption of the calcar may occur due to "stress shielding"
- Ling (1992)[12] demonstrated that it is possible to load the calcar proximally without a collar

Stem fixation

- *Surface smoothness* is defined by the mean of the deviations from a mean plane
  - <0.04 μm – known as "smooth"
  - >0.30 μm – known as "rough"
- There is a fundamental difference in the ethos between a rough-finished and a polished stem
  - Cementless and fixed cemented are rough – they generate high shear forces, low compression forces and medium tensile forces. The aim is for a strong interlock with the bone or cement
  - Tapered polished stem (e.g. Exeter) cemented – generates low shear forces, high compression forces and almost no tensile forces. The ability of bone cement to undergo creep and stress relaxation is primarily responsible for the conversion of tensile forces to compressive forces at the bone–cement interface

- Hydroxyapatite coating of the stem encourages bone on-growth. Long-term dissociation of coating from stem has led some experts (Lee[13]) to conclude that the ultimate effect of hydroxyapatite coating is to generate an effect similar to a cemented polished stem

Head material

- Stainless steel, ceramics and their wear characteristics (see "Friction" and "Wear" above)
- Brittle first-generation ceramic heads (alumina) have failed catastrophically (fractured) in high-energy transfer situations. However third-generation alumina ceramic is less prone to this problem. Their mechanical properties have vastly improved with reduction in grain size and number and size of inclusions. This has been achieved with the use of hot isotatic pressing process, which has led to a denser, finer grain size in the alumina

Head geometry

- Diameter – 26 or 28 mm is the usual size used to achieve a compromise between conflicting biomechanical principles (wear volume increases with diameter but impingement risk decreases with diameter)
- Increased head diameter
  - Reduced dislocation risk
  - Increased range of movement (before impingement)
  - Reduced friction
  - Increased sliding distances (therefore *increased* wear particles)

Head fixation

- Monoblock stems remove the problem of the head–neck interface, however they also prevent adjustment of neck length after stem implantation

[12] Ling RS (1992) The use of a collar and precoating is unnecessary and detrimental. *Clin Orthop Relat Res* 285: 73–83.

[13] Jeffrey R, McLaughlin K, Lee R (2008) Total hip arthroplasty with an uncemented tapered femoral component. *J Bone Joint Surg Am* **90**: 1290–6.

- A "cold weld" is achieved at the machined interface between the components
- Tapered fit head–neck interfaces of different metal alloys may be subject to corrosion (galvanic coupling) and fretting
- Taper stiffness is related to the radius raised to the power 4

Acetabulum material

- UHMWPE has been the standard [see "Ultra high molecular weight polyethylene (UHMWPE)" above]
- Ceramic and metal cups are also in use
- Modular cups may combine two materials

Acetabulum geometry

- Half-spherical cups are in general use
- Modifications include:
  - A flange for cement pressurization and better centring of the cup in the cement mantle
  - Supplementary screw fixation (metal-backed polyethylene or ceramic)
  - Semi-constrained and constrained cups (where the cup is deeper than the radius of the head; this aims to reduce dislocation but can reduce the range of movement before impingement and levering forces are applied to the cup)
  - Posterior lip augmentation device ("PLAD") is used to constrain the cup along one axis of movement. May cause early impingement

Acetabulum fixation

- Can be monoblock or modular
- Modularity offers advantage of additional screw fixation, better load transmission from polyethylene and the possibility of liner exchange; however, disadvantages include potential for dissociation, thinner polyethylene (with poor wear characteristics) and backside wear
- Swedish National Hip Registry supports the use of cemented cups. Non-cemented cups are also in wide use (especially in the USA)

- For a good discussion on modularity in hip prostheses see McCarthy et al.[14]

Resurfacing arthroplasty

- A larger head diameter is associated with a much reduced dislocation rate and a return to higher levels of pre-morbid activity
- Reduced wear characteristics are associated with:
  - High carbide content
  - Wrought manufacturing
  - Large diameter
  - Low mismatch (clearance) clearance (head-cup geometry match)
  - Ability to self heal. The ability to polish out isolated surface scratches caused by third body particles
- Failure rates of <1% at 6 years reported[15] (Birmingham hip resurfacing arthroplasty)
- Reported series often include several different versions of a given prosthesis – this has drawn criticism
- There is some evidence[16] (Sulza) that offset is less in the resurfacing group due to prosthesis positioning, and therefore that these patients are more prone to shortening of the limb than those with a traditional, stemmed prosthesis
- Associated with lymphocyte aneuploidy and gene translocations. Metal ion release remains an issue of uncertain long-term significance to the patient

For a good discussion (but with a North American slant) see Huo and Gilbert.[17]

[14] McCarthy JC, Bono JV, O'Donnell PJ (1997) Custom and modular components in primary total hip replacement. *Clin Orthop Relat Res* **344**: 162–71.

[15] Treacy RB, McBryde CW, Pynsent PB (2005) Birmingham hip resurfacing arthroplasty: a minimum follow-up of five years. *J Bone Joint Surg Br* **87-B**: 167–70.

[16] Girard J, Lavigne M, Vendittoli P-A, Roy AG (2006) Biomechanical reconstruction of the hip: a randomised study comparing total hip resurfacing and total hip arthroplasty. *J Bone Joint Surg Br* **88-B**(6): 721–6.

[17] Huo MH, Gilbert NF (2005) What's new in hip arthroplasty? *J Bone Joint Surg Am* **87-A**(9): 2133–46.

Bone cement

How it works in arthroplasty

- Allows secure fixation of the implant to bone
- It is a space-filling, load-transferring material or "grout"
- It is not a glue; it has no adhesive properties
- It does not bond chemically to bone or to the implant surface
- The mechanical interlock between cancellous bone and cement is achieved by forcing cement into the bone interstices

Mechanical properties

- Poor tensile strength of 25 MPa
- Moderate shear strength of 40 MPa
- Strongest in compression of 90 MPa
- Brittle, notch sensitive
- Low Young's modulus of elasticity (E) =2400 MPa (this is one-hundredth the value of E for metal and one-tenth the value for cortical bone)
- Viscoelastic

Function in joint arthroplasty

- Fixation of implant component in bone
- Transmission of load from the component into bone
- Maintenance/restoration of bone stock

Composition

Liquid is added to the powder or vice versa depending on the brand of cement.
- **Liquid monomer** – supplied as a glass vial containing methyl methacrylate monomer; in the cold curing process an **inhibitor/stabilizer** (usually hydroquinone) is added to prevent spontaneous premature polymerization during storage and an **activator** (*N,N*-dimethyl-*p*-toluidine) is also added, which promotes the cold curing process and offsets the effect of hydroquinone once the reaction has begun
- **Powder polymer** – contains polymer granules of polymethyl methacrylate (PMMA), a polymerization **initiator** (1% benzoyl peroxide) and a radio-opaque material (zirconium oxide or barium sulphate)

Polymerization process (curing)

Carbon-to-carbon double bonds are broken down and new carbon single bonds form long-chain polymers that are essentially linear and relatively free of cross-linking. This is an exothermic reaction.

The curing process is characterized by the following time periods:

Dough time: starts from the beginning of mixing and ends when the cement will not stick to an unpowdered surgical glove

Setting time: the time from the beginning of mixing until the surface temperature is half maximum

Working time: the difference between dough time and setting time

Factors affecting the curing of cement

- Humidity. Increased humidity increases the setting time
- Temperature. Increases in room temperature shorten both the dough and setting times by 5%/degree centigrade
- Rate of mixing

Factors affecting bone cement strength

Uncontrollable factors
- Ageing of the cement after implantation, storage temperature, moisture content

Partially controllable factors
- Cement thickness, inclusion of blood or tissue, stress risers (sharp edges in implant), constraint

Fully controllable factors
- Antibiotics (reduce mechanical properties by 4%), pressured insertion, mixing speed, vacuum, radio-opaque material

Note: any admixture of antibiotic must be in powder form and of a drug that remains stable at 80°C.

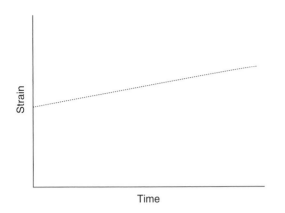

Figure 24.10 Creep: time-dependent deformation under constant load

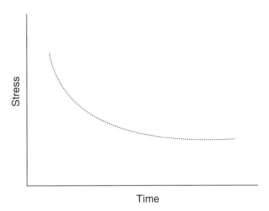

Figure 24.11 Stress relaxation: the change in stress with time under constant strain (deformation)

Three long-term properties of cement are of interest:

1. Creep
   - Time-dependent deformation under constant load (Figure 24.10)
   - All conventional bone cement creeps
   - The creep rate reduces with time after polymerization
   - Increases with increased temperature (37°C ×3.5 rate at 20°C) and increased stress level
   - Conceptually the load of daytime activities causes creep and increased stress level
2. Fatigue
   - The effect of repeated load cycles below the level needed to induce failure of a material in a single-application load
   - Usually 10^6 cycles at half-ultimate stress will produce fatigue failure
3. Stress relaxation
   - The change in stress with time under constant strain caused by a change in the structure of the cement polymer (Figure 24.11)
   - Conceptually, the rest at night of reduced load allows stress relaxation to occur, reducing the tensile stress level in the cement

Cement pressurization

- Improves cement strength by reducing voids in the cement, giving a more consistent material; improves the bone–cement interface and counters the effect of bone bleeding
- Insertion of components should be via a smooth and fully controlled push
- Reduction in the number of voids (porosity) with insertion (vacuum mixing, centrifugation, good technique)
- Increases cement strength and decreases cracking

Cementing techniques

Improvements in cementing techniques are typically referred to in terms of generations. These modifications are aimed at improving the initial interlock between cancellous bone and cement.

First generation

Original technique of Charnley:

- Hand mixing of the cement
- Finger packing of cement in an unplugged and uncleaned femoral canal and acetabulum
- No cement restrictor, no cement gun and no reduction in porosity

Second generation

- Femoral canal plug
- Cement gun to allow retrograde filling
- Pulsatile lavage

Third generation

- Pressurization of cement after insertion
- Some form of cement porosity reduction (vacuum or centrifugation)
- Spacers to ensure uniformity of cement mantle
- Surface changes to the implant

The mechanical properties of cement are weakened by the presence of blood at the bone–cement interface. Inclusions such as air, blood or tissue debris result in poor cement penetration into trabecular bone. Shear and tensile strength are reduced by the formation of debris laminations in the cement. Plugging of the femoral canal allows for increased pressurization and the guarantee of a uniform cement mantle distal to the prosthetic tip. Pressurization of cement helps to decrease the back flow of blood, which occurs from the host bone. Maintaining pressurization until the cement has increased in viscosity improves its penetration into the bone and the interlock at this interface. Cement should be a constrained, complete cement mantle; cement thickness should be 2–3 mm.

Concerns with PMMA

1. Cement reaction

Hypotension can occur on pressurization of the cement, possibly due to vasodilatation and direct myocardial depression secondary to monomer leakage and/or fat, air and marrow emboli have been reported as passing into the systemic circulation.

The transient hypotension does not correlate with the level of monomer in the circulation but with deficits in circulating blood volume. Can lead to cardiovascular collapse, cardiac arrest and death. Risk factors include older age and a patent foramen ovale (paradoxical embolization).

2. Local tissue effects of PMMA

Thermal necrosis of bone.

Data from the Swedish Hip Registry have shown that the type of cement used has an effect on the risk of revision for aseptic loosening. Palacos with gentamicin has the lowest risk followed by Palacos without gentamicin. The highest revision rates were associated with Sulfix.

Examination corner

Basic science oral 1

Tell me about your post-operative plan for a patient following THA

In some ways this question is a gift, inviting you to discuss your day-to-day practice. Beware, however, and lead with your strongest suit; if you start with your anti-thrombotic plan be prepared to be interrupted and to have to discuss it and the controversies that surround it. Pain control is a good starter as it's not very controversial and will get you beyond the awkward silence that follows the question.

Basic science oral 2

You may be asked a straight question such as "what is bone cement?" or shown a clinical photograph/video clip of a scrub nurse mixing cement.

The examiners started by asking me what the scrub nurse was doing.

Candidate: I began by saying that the scrub nurse was mixing cement and I then just kept on talking about cement. I mentioned everything possible that I knew. My answer just seemed to come together very well and the examiners were very happy with my discussion.

I started by saying that cement functioned as a "grout", a space-filling load-transferring material, that it was not a glue, and that it had no adhesive properties. I then continued to discuss dough times, setting times and working times. It was a very detailed discussion and we covered just about everything possible you could talk about.

Examiner: This candidate was always a little self-depreciating about their oral performance but had prepared well for the topic and had obviously rehearsed the answer beforehand.

Osteoarthritis/osteoarthrosis

Arthrosis is the preferred term over *arthritis* (Kellgren 1961), since there is no inflammation at the onset of disease.

Classification

- Primary – where no cause is identifiable
- Secondary – haemochromatosis, gout, acromegaly, trauma, etc.

Aetiology

- Age – early; 45 years is the peak for IP joint and CMC joint of the thumb, later for the hip/knee
- Occupation
- Obesity
- Mechanical factors – micro and macro trauma
- Metabolic – raised uric acid associated, diabetes mellitus
- Genetic – Heberden's nodes are strongly heritable
- May coexist with rheumatoid arthritis
- Developmental – especially CDH, Perthes and SUFE
- Polyarthritis is more common in females
- *Not* socioeconomic (except in the male trauma group)

Pathology

- Degenerative process of hyaline cartilage results in exposure of bone, becoming eburnated (polished)
- Classically: subchondral sclerosis, cysts, joint space narrowing and osteophytes
- Controversy regarding the primary event; theories include altered proteoglycans within cartilage, subchondral impaired venous drainage, altered synovial biochemistry
- Osteoarthritis is thought to be a failed attempt by chondrocytes to repair damaged cartilage; an imbalance of wear and repair
- Chondrocytes attempt to compensate by increasing their rate of synthesis

Molecular changes in osteoarthritic cartilage

- Increased water content (90% compared with normally 65%–80%)
- Alterations in proteoglycans (shorter chains and increased chondroitin/keratin sulphate ratio)
- Proteoglycan synthesis increases

Table 24.4 Radiographic features of osteoarthritis versus rheumatoid arthritis

Osteoarthritis	Rheumatoid
Loss of joint space	*Loss of joint space*
Osteophytes	*No osteophytes*
Subchondral cysts	*Marginal erosions*
Bony sclerosis	*Osteoporosis*
Deformity and mal-alignment	*Deformity and mal-alignment*
Loose bodies	*Loose bodies uncommon*
Asymmetrical	*Symmetrical*
Normal soft tissue	*Soft-tissue swelling*

- Proteoglycan degradation significantly increases
- Proteoglycan content decreases
- Collagen abnormalities (weakening of the type II collagen network)
- Disruption of binding of proteoglycans to hyaluronic acid
- Decreased numbers of link proteins
- Increased numbers of cathepsins B and D
- Increased levels of metalloproteinases (MMPs) (collagenase, gelatinase, stromelysin)
- Increased levels of IL-1 and IL-6
- Modulus of elasticity is decreased due to the increased water content; the increased water content also causes increased permeability and decreased strength (Table 24.3)

Differential diagnosis

- Seldom at issue
- RA, gout and infective *arthritis* may mimic or coexist with *arthrosis* (Table 24.4)

Management options – use an "intervention ladder":

- Offload joint – weight loss, active non-weight-bearing exercises, walking stick
- Topical analgesia – ibuprofen gel
- Systemic analgesia – paracetamol, NSAIDs, opiates
- Debridement – very limited indications
- Osteotomy – aimed at force realignment across joint

- Arthrodesis – still an option in young hips
- Arthroplasty – excision, hemi and total replacement
- Other options to be aware of include allograft (very limited indications) and autograft

This is a pass-fail topic. If you do not excel at this you will not pass the exam.

Arthrofibrosis

Characterized by:
- Exaggerated scar response
- Limited range of movement at joint (classically of knee)

Note: ≠ complex regional pain syndrome (CRPS), which is defined by its features of neuropathic pain and trophic changes. CRPS can however occur in an arthrofibrotic joint.

Aetiology

- Trauma
- Surgery
- Sepsis
- HLA predisposition (?)

Incidence

- 2%–11% of ACL reconstructions[18] (Karistinos 2005)
- 1%–18% of TKAs (Nelson 2004, Reuben 2004)[19]
- Generalized versus localized (e.g. cyclops lesion)

Differential diagnosis of stiff knee

- Patellofemoral joint is overstuffed
- Tight flexion gap

[18] Prodromos C, Brown C, Fu FH, Georgoulis AD *et al.* (2008) *The Anterior Cruciate Ligament: Reconstruction and Basic Science.* Philadelphia: Saunders.
[19] Reuben SS (2004) Preventing the development of complex regional pain syndrome after surgery. *Anesthesiology* **101**: 1063–5.

- Tight extension gap
- Tight PCL
- Mal-rotated components
- Arthrofibrosis
- "Jammed" mobile bearings
- Bony impingement

Pathology

Granulation tissue with cartilage islands leading to disorganized fibroconnective tissue

Management

Avoid it!
- Fat pad as a source of inflammatory cytokines – query resection
- Timing of surgery post ACL rupture – generally accepted to wait 3 weeks but some still advocate immediate surgery
- Accurate tunnel placement in ACL rupture
- Adequate postoperative analgesia to permit early mobilization
- Avoid prolonged immobilization
- Early rehabilitation

When it's too late …
- Minimize the inflammatory response – NSAIDs
- Physiotherapy
- Seek cause
  - Weight-bearing AP, lateral and skyline radiographs
  - Limited extension – ACL rupture – intercondylar notch
  - Limited flexion – TKA – suprapatellar pouch and gutters
- Antibiotics if there is infection
- Abnormal pain – consider CRPS!
- The role for surgery is limited:
  - MUA
  - Arthroscopic lavage *and* debridement
  - Open debridement – quadriceplasty
  - Formal revision surgery of mal-placed components, etc.
  - Surgery *worsens* prognosis if CRPS is present

Outcomes

- ACL
  - <5% prevalence
  - MUA and debridement
  - 60% satisfactory outcome cf. 80%+ of controls
  - 90% degenerative changes to joint (PFJ)
- TKA
  - <1% prevalence
  - Benefit of MUA diminishes the longer the time from TKA
  - Expect limited improvement of 20°–30° from MUA/revision

Complex regional pain syndrome

I Sudeck's atrophy, RSD – no overt nerve injury
II Causalgia – causative nerve injury

Incidence

Depends on your definition but up to 40% of TKAs in some series; 33% mild/"self-limiting",[20] 1% "catastrophic/late", 2F:1M.

Implicated factors

Trauma, pain, inflammation, psychology, sympathetic nervous system, immobilization, HLA predisposition.

Aetiological theories

I Localized inflammation, delayed free radical clearance, changed nerve sensitivity
II Enlarged field of undamaged nerve fibres

Clinical features

- Pain: neuropathic, unendurable and spontaneous
  - Hyperalgesia – increased sensitivity
  - Allodynia – pain from non-noxious stimulus
  - Hyperpathia – summative effect of allodynia

- Bone scan: early increase, late decrease
- Swelling and contracture
- Vasomotor instability: early only → temperature sensitivity, thin skin, spindle fingers, tendon adhesions, brittle nails, muscle wasting
- Biphasic: early pain and swelling – treatable; late atrophy and contracture – untreatable

Investigation

- A clinical diagnosis, high index of suspicion
- Excluded by normal bone scan and radiographs
- MRI – early bone and soft-tissue oedema = non-diagnostic
- Exclude other causes – DVT, infection and inflammatory arthropathy

Management

- Prevent – split tight casts applied early
- Early recognition
- Optimize analgesia (opioids, topical, local anaesthetic)
- Maintain movement – reassure, NSAID, physiotherapy
- Avoid splintage
- *Intensive* physiotherapy
- Early pain clinic referral
- Special analgesia – amitriptyline, gabapentin, regional blocks
- *Rarely* surgery – makes it worse, consider late for contracture, amputation seldom required
- Experimental – calcitonin, vitamin C (single randomized controlled trial[21] showing benefit)

CRPS myths

- Does *not* cause arthritis
- Is *not* caused by sympathetic nervous system
- Is *not* "rare"

---

[20] Atkins RN (2003) Complex regional pain syndrome. *J Bone Joint Surg Br* **85-B**: 1100–6.

[21] Zollinger PE, Tuinebreijer WE, Breederveld RS, Kreis RW (2007) Can vitamin C prevent complex regional pain syndrome in patients with wrist fractures. A randomized, controlled, multicenter dose-response study. *J Bone Joint Surg Am* **89(7)**: 1424–31.

- Is *not* helped by surgery
- Is *not* (necessarily) a disease of the barking mad
- Is *not* the same as arthrofibrosis

Osteoporosis

Definition

- The WHO consensus definition states that osteoporosis is a systemic skeletal disease characterized by low bone mass, micro-architectural deterioration of bone tissue leading to enhanced bone fragility and a consequent increase in fracture risk
- A simpler definition is decreased bone mass per unit volume of bone
- Quantitative not qualitative defect in bone (not strictly true, see WHO definition). Bone mass decreased, normal mineralization. Biochemistry normal

Risk factors

Primary osteoporosis

- Genetic: female, positive family history, white or Asian, thin
- Hormonal: loss of oestrogen protection
- Environmental/lifestyle: smoking, excessive alcohol, inactivity
- Diet: increased Ca^{2+} or vitamin D deficiency

Secondary osteoporosis

- Chronic medical conditions: endocrine, GI, chronic liver disease, chronic renal disease
- Drugs

Riggs and Melton

Type I: Affects mainly cancellous bone at the time of menopause so vertebrae and distal radius fractures are common; related to loss of oestrogen at the menopause; high-turnover osteoporosis.

Type II: Age-related and affects cortical and cancellous bone; poor calcium absorption; low-turnover osteoporosis, occurs 10–15 years later than type I.

Assessment

Pitfall: avoid commenting on osteoporosis on a single plain radiograph; the most you can say is that the bones appear osteopenic.

Radiographic absorptiometry

This measures density from a digital radiograph of the hand in comparison with an aluminium reference wedge.

DEXA

Dual energy X-ray absorptiometry. Regarded as the current standard measurement for bone mineral density. Simultaneous measurement of the passage through the body of X-rays with two different energies. The machine computes the relative amount of bone, fat and lean tissue mass together with an image of the bones under investigation from which an area measurement is made. Associated with a low radiation dose, it is accurate, quick and simple to perform.

Quantitative CT

The vertebra is scanned alongside an artificial phantom, and the two are compared. Associated with a large radiation dose, it is expensive but very accurate for vertebral cancellous bone.

Quantitative ultrasound

This is inexpensive and requires just a small, portable machine. There is renewed interest in the technique, there is no associated ionizing radiation and it yields information about the architecture and elasticity of bone.

- *T*-score is the number of standard deviations below the mean peak bone mass. Osteoporosis is based on 2.5 standard deviations below this
- *Z*-score is the number of standard deviations away from the mean for an age-, sex- and race-matched population. The *Z*-score is not used to define osteoporosis

Evaluation of vertebral fractures in the osteoporotic patient (acronym TOMEO)

- T – Tumour screening
- O – Osteopenia screening
- M – Marrow screening
- E – Endocrine screening
- O – Osteomalacia screening
- Tumour screening: radiographs, bone scan, MRI and CT
- Osteopenia screening: DEXA scan
- Marrow screening: full blood count and serum electrophoresis for myeloma
- Endocrine screening for parathyroid, Cushing's disease, thyroid function, diabetes
- Osteomalacia screening for vitamin D deficiency: perform this before making a diagnosis of osteoporosis

Steroids: an adverse effect is definite at 5 mg/day, prophylactic bisphosphonates should be considered.

Management

Simple measures

- Stop smoking, cut down excessive alcohol intake, exercise, healthy diet, hip protectors

Calcium and vitamin D

- Decreases bone resorption but does not increase bone mass or density
- There is evidence to suggest a modest protective effect, more effective for type II osteoporosis

Bisphosphonates

- Inhibit osteoclasts

Oestrogen therapy (HRT)

- Increases the risk of breast cancer and uterine cancer (if progesterone is not included)
- Helps to decrease bone resorption and slows the progression of osteoporosis but does not increase bone mass

- Best within 6 years of menopause
- Doubles the risk of DVT/PE

Selective oestrogen receptor modulators, e.g. raloxifene

- Works like oestrogen to prevent bone loss but may enhance menopausal symptoms
- Good evidence for protection again vertebral but not hip fractures

Calcitonin

- Inhibits osteoclastic resorption
- Hypersensitivity reactions, expensive

Teriparatide (recombinant PTH)

- Increases bone formation and improves micro-architecture
- Activates bone lining cells and osteoblasts
- Reduces the likelihood of both vertebral and non-vertebral fractures

Laboratory

- Blood tests normal
- Serum Ca^{2+}, PO_4, and alkaline phosphatase all normal

Examination corner

Basic science oral 1

- Discuss osteoporosis and osteomalacia
- Presenting symptoms
- Difference in pathology and blood tests in each

Basic science oral 2

DEXA scan results – comment on the findings of whether the patient is osteoporotic or osteopenic

Definition of osteoporosis (try to remember WHO definition)

Metabolic bone diseases

Calcium homeostasis

Calcium metabolism is a very reasonable question that you may be asked about in the basic science oral. Some candidates consider it a definite pass/fail question. It may be combined with questions on vitamin D action.

- Over 99% of body calcium is sequestered in bone
- The extraosseous fraction, although only amounting to 1%, has important effects on neuromuscular excitability, cardiac muscle and in the clotting cascade
- The normal plasma concentration of calcium is between 2.2 and 2.6 mmol/l. Calcium circulates in the plasma in two main forms:
  - That bound to albumin accounts for a little less than half the total calcium and is physiologically inactive
  - The free ionized calcium is physiologically important
- Whenever a plasma total calcium concentration is interpreted, an assessment of the level of the free ionized fraction should be made by noting the albumin concentration in the same specimen

Phosphate

Physiologically important in:
- Enzymic systems
- Molecular interactions (metabolite and buffer)

In renal failure serum phosphate rises and precipitates with calcium to cause a fall in serum calcium. High PO_4 and low calcium cause secondary hyperparathyroidism (see "Renal osteodystrophy" below).

Hypercalcaemia

"Bones, stones, groans and moans"

Clinical features

- May be asymptomatic

- Bones: excessive bone resorption
- Stones: renal calculi, polyuria, polydipsia
- Groans (gastrointestinal): nausea, vomiting, constipation, abdominal pain, anorexia
- Moans (CNS): lethargy, disorientation, hyperreflexia
- Other effects: SUDDEN cardiac arrest, hypotension

Causes

- Malignancy (most common, usually bone metastases)
- Hyperparathyroidism (raised PTH confirms diagnosis)

Other rare causes include:
- Vitamin D intoxication
- Excess steroids
- Addison's disease
- Milk-alkali syndrome
- Sarcoidosis
- Familial syndromes
  - MEN type 1
  - Parathyroid adenoma
  - Pancreatic tumours
  - Pituitary tumours
  - MEN type 2
  - Parathyroid hyperplasia
  - Medullary thyroid carcinoma
  - Phaeochromocytoma

Hypocalcaemia

Clinical features

Acute
- Neuromuscular irritability (tetany, seizures, Chvostek's sign, Trousseau's sign)
- Depression
- Perioral paraesthesia
- ECG shows prolonged QT interval

Chronic
- Cataracts
- Fungal nail infections

Causes

- Thyroid surgery or hypothyroidism
- Hypoparathyroidism

Control of calcium metabolism

- PTH
- Vitamin D
- Calcitonin
- (Thyroxine)

Vitamin D

- These naturally occurring steroids are either ingested in the diet from fish oils, such as cod liver oil, and plants or are activated in the skin by ultra-violet light
- UV radiation on the skin transforms 7-dehy-drocholesterol (precursor in skin) to vitamin D_3 (cholecalciferol)
- Hydroxylated to 25-hydroxycholecalciferol [25(OH)-vitamin D_3] in the liver (inactive form)
- Further hydroxylation to 1,25-dihydroxychole-calciferol [1,25(OH)$_2$-vitamin D_3] in the kidney (active form of vitamin D)
- In the presence of hypercalcaemia, 25-hydroxy-cholecalciferol is converted into the inactive metabolite 24,25-dihydroxycholecalciferol

Factors stimulating production

- Elevated PTH

Factors inhibiting production

- Decreased PTH
- Elevated serum Ca^{2+}
- Elevated serum phosphate

Effect

Intestine

- Increases gut calcium and phosphate absorption

Kidney

- Increases calcium absorption and phosphate excretion

Bone
- Dual action on bone
- Direct: Osteoclastic resorption of bone
- Indirect: Increases osteoid mineralization

PTH

PTH is an 84-amino-acid peptide secreted by the chief cells of the four parathyroid glands.

Factors stimulating production

- Decreased serum Ca^{2+}
- Decreased serum phosphate

Factors inhibiting production

- Elevated serum Ca^{2+}
- Elevated serum 1,25 (OH)$_2$-vitamin D_3

Effect

Intestine

- No direct effect
- Increases gut calcium absorption via effect on vitamin D_3

Kidney

- Increases reabsorption of filtered calcium in the kidney and increases phosphate urinary excretion
- Stimulates hydroxylation of 25-hydroxycholecal-ciferol in the proximal tubular cells

Bone

- Stimulates osteoclastic resorption of bone
- Mobilizes calcium and phosphate from bone

Calcitonin

A 32-amino-acid peptide secreted by the parafol-licular C cells of the thyroid gland.

Factors stimulating production

- Elevated serum Ca^{2+}

Factors inhibiting production

- Decreased serum Ca^{2+}

Effect

Kidney

- Decreases calcium resorption in the kidney and absorption from the gut

Bone

- Decreases osteoclastic resorption of bone

Examination corner

One candidate was not very sure about calcium homeostasis and vitamin D action. He struggled to come up with a decent answer during the basic science oral and believes this was the single reason why he failed the oral. This is probably not entirely correct but does serve to highlight the importance of this topic. One ex-examiner is unofficially quoted as saying that any candidate not knowing such a basic thing as vitamin D and calcium metabolism deserves to fail the oral.

Examiner: I still can't believe how many candidates fail to learn about calcium metabolism and also do not know the biochemical changes that occur with various bone diseases such as osteoporosis or Paget's disease. This is basic 2nd MB stuff that you should know inside out for your exit examination.

Hyperparathyroidism

Primary

Clinical features

- Of hypercalcaemia
- Gout (decreased uric acid excretion)
- Pseudogout (due to hypercalcaemia)

Radiographs

- Diffuse demineralization (osteopenia)
- Subperiosteal resorption (radial borders of proximal phalanges and tufts of distal phalanges, skull, medial end of the clavicle)

- Osteitis fibrosa et cystica or brown tumours (increased giant cells, extravasation of RBCs, haemosiderin staining, fibrous marrow replacement)
- Chondrocalcinosis and metastatic calcification of soft tissues
- Shaggy trabeculae
- Deformed osteopenic bones
- Rugger jersey spine
- Bilateral sacroiliac joint widening and erosion

Increased osteoclastic resorption of bone. Attempts to repair bone fail (poor mineralization due to low phosphate). Diagnosis based on signs and symptoms and hypercalcaemia.

Laboratory findings

- Excessive PTH production
- Increased plasma calcium
- Decreased plasma phosphate

Secondary

Parathyroid overactivity to compensate for a low serum calcium concentration. Excess PTH is an appropriate response to attempt to maintain a normal calcium concentration. The serum calcium concentration is low or normal, but never raised.

Causes

- Reduced intake of calcium, vitamin D
- Impaired absorption of calcium
- Hypercalciuria (renal tubular acidosis)
- Hyperphosphataemia (chronic renal failure)

Examination corner

Adult elective orthopaedics oral 1

Radiograph of brown tumour in the hand

Cystic lesion at the metacarpal, often expansile and aggressive looking.

Only rarely seen without other evidence of HPT (see above)

Candidate: This is a plain radiograph of the right hand demonstrating multiple well margined lytic lesions within the ring

---

and middle finger metacarpal. In addition there is diffuse subperiosteal bone resorption involving the radial aspect of the ring and index finger.

Adult elective orthopaedics oral 2

Radiograph of a skull demonstrating classic salt and pepper appearance.

Difficult one, a spot diagnosis. Differential diagnosis which included myeloma, GI malignancy with bony metastases. Symptoms of hypercalcaemia. Due to granular demineralization.

Renal osteodystrophy

Describes a group of disorders of bone mineral metabolism seen in chronic renal disease.
- Renal disease leads to:
  - Insufficient renal synthesis of vitamin D
  - Acidosis
  - Phosphate retention secondary to uraemia
  - Hypocalcaemia leading to secondary hyperparathyroidism
  - Aluminium toxicity of dialysis, which leads to osteomalacia
- This compromises mineral homeostasis which leads to abnormalities:
  - Osteitis fibrosa cystica – lytic lesions
  - Osteomalacia
  - Osteoporosis
  - Osteosclerosis – increased number of trabeculae, *not* increased mineral content
  - Ectopic calcification
- Two types:
  - High-turnover disease (chronically elevated serum PTH)
  - Low-turnover disease (normal or reduced serum PTH, excess deposition of aluminium into bone)

High-turnover disease

- Uraemia and phosphate retention from glomerular dysfunction

- High plasma phosphate promotes the secretion of PTH by three mechanisms
  - It directly lowers serum calcium, which stimulates PTH secretion
  - It impairs the synthesis of 1,25-dihydroxycholecalciferol by inhibiting renal 1-alpha-hydroxylase
  - Direct stimulation of PTH secretion
- Hypocalcaemia produces secondary HPT and ultimately tertiary HPT
- Impaired action of vitamin D
- Symptoms of hypercalcaemia
- Skeletal resistance to the actions of PTH
- As renal function deteriorates, acidosis exacerbates the negative calcium balance

Low-turnover disease

- These patients do not have secondary hyperparathyroidism
- PTH levels are normal or mildly elevated
- Bone formation and turnover are reduced (adynamic lesion of bone)
- Slowed mineralization (osteomalacia)
- Aluminium toxicity negatively affects bone metabolism
  - Impairs the differentiation of precursor cell osteoblasts
  - Impairs the proliferation of osteoblasts
  - Impairs the release of PTH from the parathyroid gland
  - Disrupts the mineralization process

Most patients have bone pain and tenderness and may have pathological fractures. Children are clinically more affected than adults.

Effects

- Hypocalcaemia
  - Osteomalacia or rickets
  - Osteoporosis
- SUFE
- Secondary HPT
  - Brown tumours – lytic lesions in the pelvis and long bones
  - Osteosclerosis

- From secondary HPT and increased osteoblast activity
- Rugger jersey spine due to alternating lucent and dense bands
- Metastatic calcification: soft-tissue calcification of periarticular tissues and blood vessels, calcium and phosphate solubility affected
- Amyloidosis

Laboratory

- Raised urea and creatinine
- Normal or low serum calcium
- Raised serum phosphate
- Raised alkaline phosphatase
- Raised PTH

Osteomalacia (adult equivalent of rickets)

Defect of skeletal mineralization caused by inadequate activity of vitamin D. Results in the accumulation of increased amounts of unmineralized matrix (osteoid) and a decreased rate of bone formation.

Osteomalacia is a qualitative defect in bone.

Aetiology

- Dietary deficiency
- Gastrointestinal malabsorption
- Renal tubular defects (renal phosphate leak)
  - Vitamin-D-dependent rickets type I and type II
  - X-linked familial hypophosphataemic osteomalacia (or rickets). Also known as vitamin-D-resistant osteomalacia or phosphate diabetes
  - Multiple renal tubular defects, leading to aminoaciduria (Fanconi's syndrome)
  - Renal tubular acidosis
- Renal osteodystrophy
- Hypophosphatasia – due to low levels of alkaline phosphatase
- Miscellaneous
  - Drugs – anticonvulsant medication, phenytoin (enhances 25-hydroxy-vitamin D_3 breakdown in the liver)

- Chronic alcoholism
- Chronic liver disease

Clinical features

- Much more insidious onset than rickets
- Bone pain is initially vague and non-specific but gradually becomes more severe and sometimes localized
- Proximal muscle weakness

Radiology

- Looser's zones (microscopic stress fractures on the concave border of long bones)
- Milkman pseudofracture on the compression side of the long bone (fractures that have healed but not mineralized)
- Biconcave "cod fish" vertebrae – can lead to kyphosis
- Thin cortices; indistinct fuzzy trabeculae
- Generalized osteopenia

Bone biopsy

Biopsy is required for the diagnosis (transiliac) of widened osteoid seams. Tetracyclines are deposited as a band at the mineralization front. After two courses of antibiotics, separated by several days, the growth of the skeleton is estimated in iliac crest biopsies by measurement of the distance between the bands of deposited tetracycline

Laboratory

- Low or normal Ca^{2+}
- Low phosphate
- High alkaline phosphatase
- High PTH

Rickets

Definition

Rickets is the juvenile form of osteomalacia with impaired mineralization of cartilage matrix (chondroid) affecting the physis in the zone of provisional calcification.

Clinical features

The clinical features depend on the severity of the deficiency and the age of onset.

General
- Retarded bone growth and short stature
- Symptoms of hypocalcaemia
- Under the age of 18 months an infant may present with failure to thrive, restlessness, muscular hypotonia, convulsions or tetany but only minimal bone changes

Skull-toe
- Delayed fontanelle closure and frontal and parietal bossing
- Dental disease
- Rachitic rosary (enlargement/hypertrophy of costochondral junction)
- Harrison's sulcus (groove/sulcus/depression develops in the sternum where the diaphragmatic attachments pull on the softened ribs)
- Pigeon chest
- Protuberant abdomen, hepatomegaly
- Scoliosis
- Genu valgum or varum, anterolateral bowing of the distal tibia and secondary adaptive changes in the foot
- Coxa vara, anterolateral bowing of the femur
- Waddling gait

Radiographs

- Pathological fractures (Looser's zones, Milkman pseudofractures on the compression side of bone[22])

[22] A Looser's zone is a thin transverse band of rarefaction in an otherwise normal looking bone. These zones are due to incomplete stress fractures, which heal with callus that is lacking in calcium (milkman pseudofracture). They are often symmetrical and tend to occur on the concave surfaces of long bones.

- Stunting of bone growth (defect in the hypertrophic zone with widened osteoid seams, physeal cupping)
- Centrally depressed cod fish vertebrae, dorsal kyphosis (cat back)
- Metaphysis is cupped, flared and jagged
- Trefoil pelvis
- Growth plate is enlarged, thickened and widened, disorientated

Causes

There are several different clinical variations of rickets.

Nutritional rickets
- Vitamin-D-deficiency rickets – dietary, malabsorption, leads to secondary hyperparathyroidism. Laboratory results: low/normal calcium, low phosphate, increased PTH, low vitamin D
- Calcium-deficiency rickets
- Phosphate-deficiency rickets

Hereditary vitamin-D-dependent rickets
Type 1 – the defect is in renal 1-alpha-hydroxylation
There is inhibition of conversion of the inactive form of vitamin D to the active form. Autosomal recessive, chromosome 12q14. Low levels of vitamin D.
Type 2 – end-organ resistance due to mutated vitamin D receptor. Normal levels of vitamin D.
Both present with features similar to nutritional rickets but may be more severe. Baldness (alopecia totalis) is a distinctive feature of type 2 disease.

X-linked familial hypophosphataemic rickets
- Vitamin-D-resistant rickets, also known as phosphate diabetes
- X-linked dominant disorder
- Impaired renal tubular resorption of phosphate, which results in a low plasma phosphate concentration
- Probably the commonest cause of rickets in Western societies

- Clinical features include symmetrical anterolateral femoral and tibial bowing
- Radiographs resemble those of ankylosing spondylitis, with ligamentous calcification and ossification
- Unresponsive to physiological doses of vitamin D
- Management requires the addition of phosphate to correct the low serum phosphate as well as large doses of vitamin D

Hypophosphatasia
- Autosomal recessive disorder
- Low levels of alkaline phosphatase, which is required for bone matrix formation
- Inborn error in the tissue of the non-specific isoenzyme of alkaline phosphatase
- 1-alpha-hydroxylase enzymic activity in the kidney is affected by PTH, Ca^{2+}, phosphate, oestrogen and prolactin

---

Examination corner

Adult elective orthopaedics oral 1

Classical radiographic changes of rickets at the wrist

- Spot diagnosis
- Describe the radiographic features
- Osteopenia of the bones and widening of the growth plates of the distal radius and ulna with flaring of the metaphysis
- What is rickets?
- What types of rickets exist?
- How do you manage it?

Adult elective orthopaedics oral 2

Classical radiographic changes of rickets of the lower limbs

- Spot diagnosis
- Distal tibial bowing
- Widening and cupping of growth plates
- Flaying and splaying of the epiphysis

Paget's disease

Paget's disease is a favourite topic of the examiners and generally comes up at some stage during the exam whether it is in the clinicals or orals.

Epidemiology

- 3%–4% prevalence in those >40 years old (10% >90 years)
- Most common in North America, England, Australia and Northern Europe
- Very rare in Scandinavia, Asia and Africa
- Family history in 15%–25% of cases
- Monostotic 17%, polyostotic 83%

Pathology

- Increased osteoclast size and number leading to increased bone resorption. This is followed by a compensatory increase in disorganized osteoblastic bone formation
- Accelerated but disorganized bone remodelling. A chaotic overactivity of bone
- Bone is rapidly laid down and is also rapidly resorbed
- Bone is both enlarged and biomechanically weak

Bone
- Very vascular
- Poor quality
- Thickened and bent
- Weak (delay between osteoid production and mineralization)
- Tendency to bend and break
- Marrow tends to become fibrous
- Erratic cement lines
- Mosaic pattern with irregular areas of lamellar bone

Aetiology

- Precise cause is unknown
- Thought that the osteoclast cell is responsible (increased size and number)

- Probably a viral origin as Pagetic osteoclasts have been shown to contain mRNA from paramyxoviruses and canine distemper virus

Clinical features

- A: Arthritis
- B: Blood flow complications (high-output cardiac failure)
- C: Cranial nerve compression
- D: Deformities (long bones, spine)
- P^3: Pain, pathological fracture, pseudoarthrosis
- M^2: Metabolic abnormalities (hypercalcaemia), malignant change

Asymptomatic in the majority of patients. Lesions detected on bone scan are usually painful whereas many seen on radiographs are not. Bone pain is unrelated to activity and is worse at night. Acute pain is related to fractures. Severe pain in a previous asymptomatic joint should arouse suspicion of sarcomatous change.

Radiographic features

Long bone

- Trabeculae of cancellous bone are thickened, coarse, irregular and wide
- Cortex is thickened, irregular and sclerotic
- Bones are thick, bent, widened and bowed
- Candle-flame-shaped lesions (arrow or flame sign) and V-shaped lytic defects in the diaphysis of long bones
- Loss of corticomedullary differentiation
- Disease involvement from one end of bone (proximal) along the shaft
- Stress fractures (convex side of long bones)
- Lateral bowing of the femur, anterior bowing of the tibia

Skull

- Osteoporosis circumscription: discrete areas of osteolysis (well-defined lytic lesions) (destructive active state)

- Cotton wool appearance: mixed lytic and blastic pattern of thickened calvarium
- Diploic widening with inner and outer table involvement

Pelvis

- Acetabular protrusion

Spine

- Picture frame vertebral body: enlarged, square vertebral body with thickened peripheral trabeculae and radiolucent inner portion
- Ivory vertebra (increased density)

Differential diagnosis

Differential diagnosis includes other causes of increased and disorganized bone turnover with fibrosis, such as:
- Osteitis fibrosa cystica (hyperparathyroidism)
- Fibrous dysplasia
- Osteoblastic secondaries
- Osteopetrosis
- Lymphoma
- Multiple myeloma

Pathological phases (acronym: LAB)

- L: Lytic (osteolytic): a front of osteoclastic resorption is seen, usually near the metaphyseal region of a long bone or osteoporosis circumscription in the skull
- A: Active (mixed): both osteoclastic resorption and osteoblastic bone formation occur in the same area of bone
- B: Burnt-out phase (sclerotic): a dense mosaic pattern of bone is seen

Laboratory

- Serum calcium usually normal
- Raised alkaline phosphatase

- Raised serum acid phosphatase
- Raised urinary hydroxyproline and collagen-derived cross-linked peptides (marker of collagen turnover)

Management

- Most patients require no active treatment

Calcitonin

Must be given parenterally. When stopped, bone activity levels quickly return to pretreatment levels but relief of pain may persist for months. Lowers bone turnover by decreasing the activity and number of osteoclasts.

Bisphosphonates

Slow down the formation and also dissolution of calcium hydroxyapatite. The main concern is that bisphosphonates have a narrow therapeutic window between resorption inhibition and mineralization defect, which may be associated with increased bone pain and fractures.

Mithramycin

A cytotoxic antibiotic with side-effects on the bone marrow, liver and kidney. It is not currently used because of its side-effects. It is useful in patients with severe disease who are unresponsive to other drugs.

Total hip arthroplasty

- Hypercalcaemia
- Metabolic acidosis
- Increased intraoperative bleeding
- Bisphosphonates are used for 3 months prior to surgery
- Increased incidence of heterotopic calcification after THA

- Protrusion
- Proximal femoral deformity

Oral question

Examiner: What are stress fractures?

Candidate: Stress fractures, which resemble Looser's zones, occur on the "tension/convex side bone" These are small horizontal stress/fissure fractures sometimes called banana fractures. They tend to be painful and locally tender and persist despite anti-Pagetic treatment.

This is a favourite basic science spot question of examiners with or without comparison with osteomalacia.

Examination corner

Basic science oral 1

Classic radiograph of Paget's disease affecting the proximal femur shown

A candidate would be expected to pick up the spot diagnosis and it is the follow-on discussion that will determine a pass or fail mark.

Examiner: What is Paget's disease?

Candidate: Paget's disease is a bone disease that results from rapid turnover of bone. There is increased bone formation and bone resorption.

Examiner: Are you sure about this?

(The examiner was not convinced or happy with the answer and attempted to prompt the candidate. Possibly a more detailed initial answer was wanted by the examiner.)

Candidate: (Hesitating as they were unsure whether their answer was wrong, what exactly the examiner wanted to hear and what they could say next to redeem the situation. The examiner wants to hear something!) The osteoclasts and osteoblasts are both overactive in Paget's disease.

The examiner mumbles something incoherent and then goes onto the next topic.

I think the candidate did not hit the ground running with this question and seemed to struggle initially with it. The candidate never got going with an answer and the examiner quickly lost patience with them. The examiner moved on to another topic with another nail in the candidate's coffin. [Fail]

Osteopetrosis – marble bone disease

A skeletal dysplasia. A group of rare congenital disorders characterized by a marked increase in bony sclerosis.

- Impaired osteoclast function. Osteoclasts lack the normal ruffled border and clear zone required for effective resorption
- Increased sclerosis and obliteration of the medullary canal
- Marrow spaces are filled with necrotic, calcified cartilage
- Empty lacunae and plugging of Haversian canals

Aetiology

Autosomal recessive

- Infantile, "malignant" form
- Bone encroachment on marrow results in pancytopenia, anaemia, haemolysis and hepatosplenomegaly
- Causes severe disability
- Repeated infection or haemorrhage usually leads to death

Autosomal dominant

- Tarda, "benign" form
- Patients live into adult life
- Seldom causes symptoms
- May present as an incidental radiographic finding

Clinical features

- Pathological fractures
- Bone infection
- Cranial nerve compression

Radiology

- Increased bone density
- Cortices widened
- Narrow medullary canals

- Sandwich vertebrae. The end plates are densely sclerotic giving the appearance of a sandwich. This is virtually pathognomonic for osteopetrosis when present and should *not* be confused with the ill-defined bands of sclerosis seen in the rugger jersey spine of HPT
- Skull thickened and the base is densely sclerotic
- The demarcation between cancellous and cortical bone is lost

---

Examination corner

Basic science oral

Radiograph of the pelvis, spine or legs

Spot diagnosis. An exercise in radiographic pattern recognition. There are several rare but commonly shown radiographs of various bone diseases that you have to pattern recognize, i.e. Paget's, osteogenesis imperfecta, melorheostosis (candle bones)

This may lead on to a discussion of pathogenesis of the disorder.

In less severely affected individuals it is not unusual to find areas of affected bone alternating with apparently normal bone, particularly in the pelvis. Lack of metaphyseal remodelling in the femur gives a characteristic Erlenmeyer flask deformity of the distal end of the femur.

Osteochondroses

- The above term is preferable to "osteochondritis" since there is no inflammation
- Occurs in the juvenile skeleton; a similar process to AVN in adults
- Think of three subgroups with respect to mechanical loading:
  - **Compression** – presents as necrosis of the centre of ossification. Initial radiodensity followed by later collapse (e.g. Kienböck's disease of the lunate)
  - **Shearing** – articular cartilage with adjacent subchondral bone split off from the joint surface. Classically "osteochondritis dissecans"

affecting knee with swelling, pain ±locking of loose body

- **Distraction** – the pull of a tendon can cause "traction apophysitis", classically at the tibial tuberosity

Eponyms abound here, you need to know them:

Femoral head – Legg–Calvé–Perthes disease

Tibial tuberosity – Osgood–Schlatter disease

Inferior patella – Sinding–Larsen and Johansson disease

Proximal tibial epiphysis – Blount's disease

Calcaneus – Sever's disease

Navicular – Kohler's disease

MT head – Freiberg's disease

Vertebral end plate – Scheuermann's disease

Lunate – Kienböck's disease

Capitellum – Panner's disease

Hand phalanges – Thiemann's disease

- Management is generally non-operative in these time-limited conditions. Rest and unloading have been traditionally favoured in the hope that anatomical structure can be maintained whilst biological recovery of bone takes place
- Where intervention is considered, it often attracts controversy [see "Perthes disease (coxa plana)" in Chapter 22]

Heterotopic ossification

aka myositis ossificans = extraskeletal ossification, usually in striated muscle.

Distinguished from soft-tissue calcification by histological structure:

- Peripheral woven bone
- Central trabecular bone
- May mimic the appearance of osteosarcoma

Myositis ossificans progressiva

This is a rare, atraumatic, autosomal-dominant condition. It is associated with fibrodysplasia, short thumbs and may cause respiratory compromise.

Traumatic local myositis ossificans

Associated with early vigorous movement after trauma/surgery:

- Elbow commonly affected
- Occurs symptomatically in up to 7% of total hip replacements
- May occur in soft-tissue trauma without fracture

Atraumatic myositis ossificans

- Occurs in thighs of young athletes. Unknown cause

Management

- Avoid further surgery (especially in proximity to the original insult to tissues) as this may provoke more heterotopic ossification
- Good surgical technique – tissue planes, haemostasis, tissue handling
- Prescribe indomethacin 75 mg daily for 6 weeks
- Low-dose radiotherapy 800–1000 CGy postoperatively[23]

Osteonecrosis/AVN

This is a favourite of examiners. You *must* be familiar with AVN as you are unlikely to emerge from the test without coming across it at least once.

Aetiology

Primary/idiopathic

- Responsible for one-third of AVN
- Young adults
- Usually bilateral
- Males>females

[23] Sell S, Willms R, Jany R *et al.* (1998) The suppression of heterotopic ossifications: radiation versus NSAID therapy – a prospective study. *J Arthroplasty* **13**(8): 854–9.

Secondary

- Sickle cell disease – causes rapidly progressing femoral head necrosis
- HIV – ?due to reduced anticardiolipin and increased triglyceride
- Gaucher's – accumulation of glucocerebroside in the reticuloendothelial system
- Haemophilia
- Trauma
- Alcohol
- Steroids
- Renal transplant
- SLE
- Caisson's disease (NB *Caisson* = chamber used to build bridge piles on a river bed. Generalized to all who experience symptoms of nitrogen dissolution in the blood when rapidly decompressing upon surfacing from a dive)
- Chronic liver disease, liver storage diseases
- Burns
- Gout
- Pregnancy
- Radiotherapy/radiation
- Chemotherapy
- Hyperlipidaemia

Pathology

Hypothesis (corresponding Ficat grade):
- Vascular obstruction – ischaemic event – bone marrow oedema (0)
- Anoxia – pain (1)
- Bony necrosis – microfracture (2)
- Segmental collapse (3)
- Secondary osteoarthritis (4)

Osteocyte cell death occurs at 48 hours of ischaemia. Infarcted area is thought to be in the territory of the end-artery, with prognosis relating to the relationship with load bearing. Attempted repair results in granulation of tissue and creeping bone substitution, which is responsible for the **junctional band** seen on MRI. The **crescent sign** occurs at the transition from Ficat grade 2 to grade 3 and is associated with a worse prognosis.

Diagnosis

History

- Risk factors, secondary causes, pain (especially nocturnal) is out of proportion to radiographic appearances, usually affects the hip(s)

Examination

- Examine for associated features of secondary causes

Investigation

- Radiographs, bone scan, MRI

Radiographs

Changes (e.g. crescent sign, collapse) are "too late" since the prognosis at this stage is already poor

MRI

Contrast with normal contralateral side (where unaffected) is 100% sensitive. The **double line sign** is diagnostic at Ficat grade 0 (a low signal on a T_1-weighted scan at the reactive interface, a high signal on a T_2-weighted scan due to hypervascularity).

Bone scan

- Initially "cold", becoming "hot" at 2 months

Differential diagnosis

- Neoplasia, transient osteoporosis (bone marrow oedema syndrome)

Management

- Avoid risk factors
- Analgesia
- Address the cause where possible (e.g. clotting factor levels for haemophilia)
- With respect to Ficat grade:

0: Offload (aim to reduce microfractures) by reduced activity, crutches, cushion sole shoes, etc.

1: + Core decompression ±vascular bone graft

2: ± Osteotomy

3: As above

4: ± Proceed to arthroplasty

Core decompression

Variable technique to introduce hole(s) into the neck/head of femur to "decompress" and/or permit revascularization of affected bone.

Bone graft

May be intra-articular via an osteochondral "trap-door" or via neck corticotomy. May be a vascularized strut (e.g. fibula).

Hip arthroplasty

Early loosening is common (especially in haemophilia, sickle cell and Gaucher's).

Extent of involvement may include the acetabulum therefore total arthroplasty is usually indicated, though surface replacement has been used in limited disease.

Haemophilia A

- 1 per 10 000 male births
- Due to lack of factor VIII
- X-linked recessive
- One-third are new mutations

Haemophilia B

- = Christmas disease
- Lack of factor IX
- X-linked inheritance

von Willebrand's disease

- Lack of factor VIII and cofactor
- Affects mucosae more than joints

Pathology

- Atraumatic joint haemorrhages cause synovial hypertrophy, synovitis and more bleeding
- Haemosiderin deposition in synovial villi
- Release of enzymes causes cartilage destruction
- Disuse osteoporosis
- Asymmetric physeal arrest in juvenile skeleton

Clinical

- Family history
- Haemarthroses in walking children
- Joint pathology during childhood, especially in weight-bearing joints
- Investigate with clotting screen then specific factor tests

Radiology

- Synovitis, distended capsule
- Thin cartilage
- Widened intercondylar notch on knee AP
- Enlarged ossification centres and widened epiphyses
- Flat femoral condyles
- Osteopenia

Management

- Haematologist leads multidisciplinary effort
- Prophylactic or "on demand" factor replacement
- Avoid NSAIDs
- Orthoses to prevent contractures and stabilize joints

Surgery

- Aseptic aspiration
- Arthroscopic synovectomy (if joint preserved)
- Arthroplasty
- Arthrodesis
- Pseudotumour excision (MRI/angiography first)
- Fractures – heal as per normal
- Factor replacement should be 100% of normal for bony surgery

Sickle cell disease

Inherited substitution of normal HbA with HbS (mutated chromosome 11). Homozygotes have disease, heterozygotes have trait. Common in malarial endemic areas due to protective quality.

Pathology

Low O_2 tension causes polymerization of HbS into longitudinal fibres, hence sickling of erythrocytes. Only manifests when HbF is lost, after 1 year old. Reduced RBC lifespan to 20 days (normal 120 days).

Clinical

Remember HBSS PAIN CRISIS
H Haemolysis
B Bone marrow hyperplasia
S Stroke
S Skin ulcers
P Pain
A Anaemia
I Infections
N Nocturia
C Congestive heart failure
R Renal failure
I Infarction of bone
S Sequestration in spleen
I Increased spontaneous abortion
S Sepsis
- Osteomyelitis – *Staphylococcus aureus* commonly
- AVN of the femoral head – occurs in up to 10%

Management

- Mostly by haematologist
- Surgical drainage of osteomyelitis/septic arthritis
- AVN – see "Osteonecrosis/AVN" above

Vitamin C deficiency – scurvy

- The disease is characterized clinically by haemorrhage secondary to capillary fragility

- Haemorrhages occur in the skin, gums, muscle attachments and, in children, subperiosteally in the bone
- Vitamin C deficiency leads to a failure of collagen synthesis and osteoid formation
- Decreased chondroitin sulphate synthesis and defective collagen growth and repair

Clinical features

- Fatigue
- Anaemia
- Bleeding gums
- Ecchymosis
- Intra-articular haemorrhages
- Poor wound healing

Radiology

- Generalized bone rarefaction most marked in long bone metaphysis
- Thin cortices and trabeculae
- Metaphyses may be deformed or fractured
- Subperiosteal haematomas

Oral question

Unlikely oral question; probably a difficult spot radiograph, which would be most likely shown as part of a series of radiographs demonstrating various metabolic bone diseases (e.g. Paget's, osteoporosis, etc.). You either pattern recognize the radiograph or not.

Rheumatoid arthritis

You are very likely to come across this in the short cases – rheumatoid arthritis is a chronic disease and lends itself to exams.

Definition

Symmetrical, erosive, deforming, inflammatory polyarthropathy involving both small and large joints.

Incidence

• Approximately 1% of the population

Diagnostic criteria

Rheumatoid arthritis is defined by the presence of four of the seven diagnostic criteria established by the American College of Rheumatology:
• Morning stiffness >1 h for >6 weeks
• Swelling of at least three joints for >6 weeks
• Involvement/swelling of the wrist or hands for >6 weeks
• Bilateral symmetrical polyarthritis for >6 weeks
• Rheumatoid nodules
• Positive serum rheumatoid factor
• Radiographic changes typical of rheumatoid arthritis (periarticular erosions, osteoporosis, etc.). Table 24.4 demonstrates the key differences between osteoarthritis and rheumatoid arthritis.

Rheumatoid factor

Rheumatoid factor has significant false-positive and false-negative results and it is not diagnostic for the disease. Being rheumatoid factor positive tends to indicate a more severe disease course.

Aetiology

The aetiology is still unclear; it is thought to be an autoimmune disease with a disordered immune response that causes an inflammatory response against soft tissues, cartilage and bone, involving antigen-presenting cells, T-helper cells, natural killer cells and plasma cells.

Autoimmune mediator of tissue destruction: macrophages, lymphocytes and plasma cells.

Environmental trigger is superimposed on a genetic predisposition (HLA DW4, HLA DR4).

Staging of rheumatoid disease

Early

Acute or subacute synovitis without destruction of soft tissues or articular cartilage. Management is largely medical although occasionally synovectomy or nerve decompression is required.

Intermediate

Involvement of synovial-lined tendon sheaths impairs tendon excursion and may lead to rupture. Erosions appear in articular surfaces. Synovectomy with or without soft-tissue reconstruction or re-alignment, tenosynovectomy and nerve decompression are typical of the procedures performed during this stage.

Late

Reconstructive procedures such as arthroplasty or arthrodesis are required to relieve pain, improve function and correct deformity of joints.

General characteristics

Insidious-onset of morning stiffness, joint pain (polyarthritis), symmetrical swelling of the peripheral joints, hands and feet are involved early.

Systemic manifestations (rheumatoid extra-articular manifestations)

• Rheumatoid nodules
• Vasculitis
• Ocular inflammation
• Amyloidosis
• Nephropathy and renal failure
• Cardiac (pericarditis, myocarditis, conduction defects, aortitis)
• Respiratory (pneumonitis, pleuritis, interstitial fibrosis)
• Myositis and muscle atrophy
• Neuropathy
• Anaemia (normochromic and microcytic)
• GIT (salivary problems and peptic ulceration)
• Cerebral complication
• Felty's syndrome (splenomegaly, leucopenia, lymphadenopathy, anaemia, skin pigmentation, weight loss)
• Sjögren's syndrome (conjunctival dryness or sicca syndrome)

Blood tests

- Rheumatoid factor (+ve 80%), ESR, CRP, FBC (anaemia), urea and electrolytes

Principles of management

- Control synovitis and pain
  - Stop synovitis: rest, splintage, non-specific drugs, specific drugs (alter disease process) and synovectomy
- Maintain joint function
  - A multidisciplinary approach is required: drugs, physiotherapy and sometimes surgery
- Prevent deformity
  - Prevent deformity: physiotherapy and splintage, tendon reconstruction and joint surgery (soft-tissue stabilization)
- Reconstruction: arthrodesis, excision arthroplasty and joint replacement

Atypical presentations

- Explosive arthritis
- Monoarticular arthropathy (chronic pain and swelling)
- Isolated second MTP joint swelling

Differential diagnosis

- Seronegative arthropathy: psoriatic arthritis, ankylosing spondylitis, Reiter's disease
- SLE
- Polyarticular gout
- Calcium pyrophosphate deposition disease
- Sarcoidosis
- Polymyalgia rheumatica

Radiological classification (grades)

I Osteoporosis and soft-tissue swelling
II Marginal erosions and very slight narrowing of joint space
III Joint space narrowing becomes marked
IV Punched-out erosions through subchondral plate
V Normal anatomical contours of the articular surface are destroyed

---

Examination corner

Adult elective orthopaedics oral 1

General discussion on the preoperative evaluation of the rheumatoid patient, which led into a discussion about cervical spinal involvement of rheumatoid arthritis.

Adult elective orthopaedics oral 2

AP radiography of either the pelvis or knee

Long-standing rheumatoid arthritis developing secondary degenerative joint disease.

Tricky one, especially in the heat of the exam, with several candidates assuming the diagnosis was osteoarthritis. The examiners gently led these candidates down the wrong path into a discussion of the radiographic features of osteoarthritis only to tell them at the end of the oral that the diagnosis was rheumatoid arthritis. When rheumatoid arthritis is long-standing it is not unusual for secondary degenerative joint disease to superimpose itself on the findings one would expect with rheumatoid arthritis. The key point is that sclerosis and osteophytes indicate secondary degenerative joint disease but are fairly mild compared to the amount of severe joint space narrowing.

Short case 1

Patient with obvious rheumatoid hands. Be certain to expose the patient's forearms above the elbow and check for rheumatoid nodules. Be systematic – start proximal and work distal describing the features as you go.

Gout

Definition

A disorder of nucleic acid metabolism causing hyperuricaemia, which leads to monosodium urate (MSU) crystal deposition in joints and recurrent attacks of synovitis.

Pathology

- Humans lack the enzyme uricase, which is involved in the elimination of excess nucleic acid purines and nitrogenous waste products through the production and excretion of allantoic acid, hence in humans uric acid is the end-product of purine degradation

- Characterized by the presence of crystals in and around joints, tendons and bursae
- Crystals activate macrophages, platelets, phagocytosis and the complement system
- Release of inflammatory mediators into the joint
- Cartilage erosion and periarticular cyst formation secondary to deposition of MSU
- Recurrent attacks of arthritis, usually in men aged 40–60 years, especially the great toe (podagara)
- Crystals are deposited as tophi (ear, eyelid, olecranon, Achilles tendon)

Clinical

Two types are recognized:
1. Primary (95%) (inherited)
   - Overproduction or underexcretion of uric acid
2. Secondary (5%)
   - Resulting from acquired conditions, which cause either overproduction, or underexcretion of uric acid (renal disease, multiple myeloma and polycythemia)

This division is somewhat arbitrary as people with a susceptibility to gout may only develop the condition when secondary (precipitating) factors are introduced, such as diuretic treatment, excessive alcohol, aspirin or localized trauma. Only a small number of people with hyperuricaemia develop gout.

Radiographs

Radiographic changes occur late in the disease, usually associated with the chronic tophaceous stage. These changes are of two main types:
1. Well-circumscribed, punched-out periarticular cystic erosions with sclerotic overhanging borders. The size of the cysts is the differentiating feature from other arthritides. Cysts larger than 5 mm are suggestive of gout

2. Degenerate arthritis with joint-space narrowing, osteophyte formation and sclerosis

Diagnosis

Elevated serum uric acid levels are not diagnostic of gout; one needs to demonstrate MSU crystals under polarized light microscopy.

Crystals

Thin, tapered intracellular and extracellular needle-like crystals that are strongly negatively birefringent under polarized light microscopy.

Acute attack

Sudden onset of severe joint pain, which lasts for a week or two before resolving. Commonest sites are the first MTP joint of the big toe, the elbow, finger joints and ankle. The skin is shiny, red and swollen. The joint is hot and tender. Large joints are infrequently involved. The spine is very rarely affected.

Chronic gout

Recurrent attacks merge into polyarticular gout. Joint erosion causes chronic pain, stiffness and deformity.

Differential diagnosis

- Infection
- Reiter's disease
- Pseudogout
- Rheumatoid arthritis

Management

- Rest
- Elevation
- Indomethacin
- Allopurinol (xanthine oxidase inhibitor) for long-term prophylaxis

- Colchicine for an acute attack
- Aspiration and intra-articular steroid injection

Laboratory

- Hyperuricaemia, leukocytosis
- Synovial fluid: leukocyte count similar to that in septic arthritis

---

Examination corner

Basic science oral 1

Examiner: This man presented with acute onset of pain in his foot (photograph shown).

Candidate: This is a picture of a left foot. It shows an inflamed and swollen big toe, and the surrounding skin is erythematous and shiny. There are no other obvious features of note. The diagnosis would be suggestive of gout. My differential diagnosis would include cellulitis, infected bunion and septic arthritis.

This was a classic picture of gout affecting the big toe.

The candidate would be expected to describe the photograph, say that the picture is suggestive of gout and give a differential diagnosis.

This type of question is fairly straightforward but there is little margin for error in your answer.

Your answer needs to be smooth and polished quickly describing what you see in the picture, the probable diagnosis and differential diagnosis. The examiners may then ask you one or two peripheral questions about the condition but more likely will move you on to another topic. If you do not recognize the condition, have to be prompted or are slow off the mark, you will fail the question no matter how well thereafter you talk on the subject (not recognizing a common condition demonstrates a lack of basic, core knowledge).

Other clinical pictures that you may be shown might include:
- Tophi deposited in an olecranon fossa or pinna of ear
- Ulcerated tophi through the skin with surrounding chalky material
- Radiograph of gouty arthropathy in a big toe: the periarticular erosions or cysts are larger and slightly more peripheral than those in rheumatoid arthritis and are filled with uric acid deposits

- Arthroscopic picture of a knee with small whitish crystal deposition on the menisci

Again these pictures are spot diagnoses, the condition needs to be recognized immediately or the question can very easily be lost. A useful tip would be to spend time pattern-recognizing pictures of the condition from two or three larger orthopaedic textbooks.

Basic science oral 2

Gout and pseudogout

- Difference between the microscopic appearances of the crystals
- Metabolism of uric acid, DNA, purines and pyrimidines

An unexpected question to catch you off guard, certainly not one I would have expected to be asked.

Basic science oral 3

AP radiograph of the hand

Look for oval periarticular erosions. Multiple punched-out erosions distributed throughout the carpi and phalanges. Erosions have sclerotic borders and often overhanging edges (unlike classic rheumatoid arthritis). In early gout, the hand and wrist joints have well-preserved joint spaces and normal mineralization. Later on there is often overlying soft-tissue swelling which may contain small calcified fragments – subcortical explosion. In the most advanced stages total joint destruction suggestive of a Charcot joint may be seen.

Examiner: When do you start long-term treatment for gout?

Candidate: Less than one attack per year – no indication for prophylaxis. More than five attacks per year – prophylaxis indicated.

Adult elective orthopaedics oral 1

Gout

- Causes
- Diagnosis
- Management

Psoriatic arthritis

Definition

Seronegative polysynovitis with an erosive, destructive arthritis and a significant incidence of sacroiliitis and spondylitis.

Clinical features

Mild asymmetrical polyarthritis affecting some of the IP joints of the fingers or toes. Sacroiliitis and spondylitis are seen in about one-third of patients and are similar to those in ankylosing spondylitis. Affects up to 10% of patients with psoriasis. HLA B27-positive in 50% of cases (other loci also involved).

Diagnosis

The main difficulty is to distinguish psoriatic arthritis from psoriasis with seronegative rheumatoid arthritis.

Important characteristic features of psoriatic arthropathy include:
- Asymmetrical joint distribution
- Involvement of distal finger joints
- Presence of sacroiliitis and spondylitis
- Absence of rheumatoid nodules
- Nail pitting, fragmentation
- Sausage digits
- "Pencil-in-cup" deformity (where the distal end of the middle phalanx is the pencil in the cup of the distal phalanx)
- Finally, rheumatoid factor is usually negative in psoriatic arthropathy

Ankylosing spondylitis

Background

One of the seronegative spondyloarthropathies. A generalized chronic inflammatory condition with a predilection for the sacroiliac joints and spine. Strong familial tendency. Cause is unknown but 90% of patients are HLA B27-positive, as are half of their first-degree relatives (but HLA B27 is *not* diagnostic and there is a high false-positive rate). It is more common in males than females, with estimates ranging from 2:1 to 10:1.

Clinical features

- Insidious-onset low-back pain and stiffness in an adolescent or young adult reoccurring at intervals
- Progressive spinal flexion deformities
- Early – little to find on clinical examination apart from slight loss of lumbar lordosis, limitation of spinal extension, sacroiliac joint tenderness
- Late – characteristic posture with loss of the normal lumbar lordosis, thoracic kyphosis, chin-on-chest deformity, flexed hips and knees
- Inability to perform the wall test
- Entire spine is ankylosed
- Limited chest expansion
- Peripheral joint involvement, usually the hips (flexion deformities and pain)
- Pronounced morning stiffness
- Protrusio acetabuli
- Heterotopic bone formation
- Whiskering enthesis

Differs from rheumatoid arthritis in that the disease is asymmetrical and affects large joints more than small joints.

Extraskeletal manifestations (eyes, heart, lungs, gastrointestinal, etc.)

- Heart disease (carditis, aortic valve disease)
- Pulmonary fibrosis, osteoporosis, uveitis, colitis, arachnoiditis, amyloidosis, sarcoidosis
- Poor outcome if there is pulmonary involvement, hip involvement, or a young age at onset of the disease

Spinal deformities

- Chin-on-chest deformity (corrective osteotomy at the cervicothoracic junction)
- Severe kyphotic deformity (posterior closing wedge osteotomy)

- Difficult spinal fractures (associated with epidural haemorrhage), high mortality rate, best diagnosed with CT scan, 75% neurological involvement
- May result in fixed cervical, thoracic or lumbar hyperkyphosis and inability of the patient to face forwards

Radiographic changes in the spine

- Earliest vertebral change is flattening of the normal anterior concavity of the vertebral body (squaring due to ossification of ALL)
- Ankylosis of the sacroiliac joints is followed by ossification of the interspinous and interlaminar ligaments, ankylosis of the facet joints, ossification of the annulus fibrosus and syndesmophyte formation. This proceeds in a cranial direction and may produce a characteristic radiographic appearance (bamboo spine)
- Erosion and fuzziness of the sacroiliac joints occur and then later sclerosis, especially on the iliac side of the joint, and finally bony ankylosis and obliteration of the sacroiliac joint

Pathology

Preferential involvement of tendon and ligament insertions has been coined the term **enthesopathy**. Inflammatory and erosive destruction of:
1. Diarthrodial joints
    - Sacroiliac joints, vertebral facet joints, costovertebral joints
    - Chest pains aggravated by breathing indicate involvement of the costovertebral joints
2. Fibro-osseous junctions, syndesmotic joints and tendons
    - This affects the invertebral discs, symphysis pubis, sacroiliac ligaments, manubriosternal joint and the bony insertions of large tendons

Pathological changes proceed in three stages:
1. Inflammatory reaction with round cell infiltration, granulation tissue and destruction of bone
2. Replacement of the granulation tissue with fibrous tissue

3. Ossification of the fibrous tissue leading to ankylosis of joints

Management

The majority of patients, despite the disease, can lead an active life.

Physiotherapy, NSAIDs, etc. are advised. Surgery is indicated to correct deformity or improve pain. Corrective osteotomies of the lumbar and cervical spine can be performed if the deformity is severe enough, but are difficult and potentially hazardous. Total joint arthroplasty especially THA, may be needed but these patients have a higher than normal infection rate and require prolonged rehabilitation.

Differential diagnosis

- Mechanical disorders
- Ankylosing hyperostosis (Forestier's disease). Common disorder in older men with widespread ossification of ligaments and tendons. Superficial resemblance to AS but not an inflammatory condition, the spinal pain and stiffness are rarely severe and bloods are normal
- Other seronegative spondarthritides

Atypical onset of AS occurs in 10% of cases. The disease starts with an asymmetrical inflammatory arthritis usually of the hip, knee or ankle.

Radiographic differential diagnosis of the sacroiliac joint lesions

- Reiter's disease
- Psoriatic arthritis
- Ulcerative colitis
- Crohn's disease

Examination corner

Basic science oral 1

Usually the adult and pathology oral. Watch out for the "trap!" – a radiograph of the pelvis demonstrating bilateral sacroiliac fusion is shown that the candidate fails to spot as they have been told that the patient has a hip problem.

Examiner: This is an X-ray of the pelvis of a 20-year-old male with bilaterally painful hips. What do you see?

Candidate: There is a slight loss of joint space of both hips and possibly some mild sub-articular sclerosis of the femoral head. There are no osteophytes present. The overall bony texture suggests an element of osteopenia. The radiograph is suggestive of an inflammatory arthritis, possibly rheumatoid arthritis.

Examiner: What about the sacroiliac joints? You have failed to mention them.

Candidate: There is bilateral sacroiliac fusion suggestive of ankylosing spondylitis.

If you initially fail to mention that the sacroiliac joints are fused you are in trouble. No matter what you say about ankylosing spondylitis afterwards, how many clinical features you mention, the latest theories regarding aetiology or the newest treatments you have read, you have still failed this question. You are unsafe in your practice as you have missed an obvious diagnosis and you have possibly failed the oral as well.

Other radiographic features to mention on a pelvic radiograph would be:
- Owl's eyes of the obturator foramen due to flexion spine
- Sacroiliac joint: bony ankylosis
- Pubic symphysis: erosions
- Traction spur of the lesser trochanter
- Fuzziness of the ischial tuberosity

With every radiograph of the pelvis look at:
- Hips
- Spine
- Iliac wings
- Sacroiliac joints
- Pubic symphysis
- Bones
- Soft tissues

Basic science oral 2

Shown radiograph of bamboo spine of ankylosing spondylitis. What is the pathology, what are the clinical symptoms they get? How do you manage a patient with painful bilateral hips with 30° fixed flexion deformity?

Systemic lupus erythematosus (SLE)

Defined as a chronic inflammatory disease of unknown aetiology associated with multisystem involvement.

Pathogenesis

Distension of soft tissues rather than direct destruction and fibrosis of supporting elements.

Clinical features

SLE arthritis affects >75% patients with SLE although this is often overshadowed by systemic symptoms. Typically the arthritis is not as destructive as rheumatoid arthritis. Disease occurs mainly in young females:
- Fever
- Butterfly malar rash across cheeks and bridge of the nose
- Pancytopenia
- Pericarditis
- Nephritis
- Raynaud's phenomenon
- Peripheral vasculitis
- Splenomegaly
- Polyarthritis

Laboratory

- Anaemia, leucopenia, elevated ESR, autoantibodies positive

Management

Corticosteroids are indicated for severe disease. Progressive joint deformity is unusual and the arthritis is usually controlled by anti-inflammatory drugs, physiotherapy and intermittent splintage. An unusual complication of SLE is AVN of the femoral head. This may be related to corticosteroid use but the disease itself seems to predispose to bone ischaemia.

> Examination corner
>
> ## Basic science oral 1
>
> ### Clinical picture of SLE hands
>
> - Rheumatoid pattern of arthropathy
> - Ulnar drift in the hands (due to ligament laxity)
>
> ## Basic science oral 2
>
> ### Radiograph of SLE hands
>
> Radiograph with ulnar deviation of the phalanges. Joint erosions are not typically seen. Joint narrowing and juxta-articular demineralization. Joint effusion. Joint destruction, even in severe long-standing disease, is unusual.
>
> ## Basic science oral 3
>
> - Clinical picture of typical butterfly rash

Radiology

Science dealing with diagnostic imaging, originally limited to ionizing radiation (X-rays, bone scans and PET) but now incorporating ultrasound, magnetic resonance and interventional radiology.

X-rays

- X-rays lie at the upper end (high frequency, short wavelength) of the electromagnetic spectrum
- X-rays are produced by electrons striking the tungsten target. Only 1% efficient: 99% of energy is liberated as heat, hence the rotating target to avoid meltdown!
- Parameters:
  - kV – unit of measurement of penetration of X-rays (i.e. how much energy they carry). Increased kV increases forward scatter
  - mA – unit of measurement of the number of X-rays (i.e. the exposure, which can also be increased by a longer time interval)

- Two types of X-rays result from an interaction with the patient:
  - *Primary* – direct from tube to plate, producing the desired image
  - *Scatter* – reflected from and within the patient/other objects and can blur the image. Reduced by *grids* of lead/aluminium
- *Resolution* is the minimum separation between objects for their identification as separate objects
- *Contrast* is the ability to identify objects of differing density
- *Contrast media* – use of high-atomic-number elements to enhance contrast between structures
- *Analogue images* have an infinite range of density between black and white
- *Digital images* have a discrete greyscale (levels of grey) between black and white
- *Orthogonal images* are captured at 90° mutual planes to convey three-dimensional images in two dimensions
- *Dose*
  - Total dose is measured in *gray*
  - Effective dose is measured in *sieverts*, enabling comparison of risk between procedures
  - Chest X-ray = 0.05 mSv
  - Flight to USA = 0.10 mSv
  - CT spine = 3.6 mSv
  - Bone scan = 5.0 mSv
  - *Remember X-rays are a form of radiation, radiographs are the recorded images*

Computerized tomography

- X-rays from an axially rotating source are received by a circle of stationary detectors
- Data are digitized such that every point within the patient is a labelled *pixel*, although because each "slice" has depth it is termed a *voxel*
- Slices are imaged sequentially, or on faster and newer machines in a helical or spiral fashion. Fastest machines now use multiple slices in a spiral fashion
- Transverse anatomical sections can be produced with high resolution. Data can be reformatted to

any chosen plane, but coronal and sagittal planes are the traditional ones
- CT is better at looking at bone than at soft tissue
- Windows:
  - Hounsfield units (HU) are a measure of attenuation
  - Image is centred on a particular attenuation value and greyscale compressed within a window
  - This gives a contrast range appropriate to the desired tissues; "bony windows" are usually centred on 300 HU with a width of 1200
- Resolution – is less on CT than plain radiographs due to the averaging within a voxel that occurs at the edges of objects

Bone scan

Involves intravenous injection of a bone-seeking radionuclide, which localizes at sites of increased bone blood flow with increasing osteoblastic activity.

A radionuclide is an unstable form of an element that decays spontaneously to a more stable form with emission of ionizing radiation.

An "ideal" radiopharmaceutical is one that has:
1. Low cost
2. Low toxicity
3. Localization to bone/pathology
4. Rapid elimination

Technetium 99m

- *Technetium*-99-labelled MDP (methylene diphosphonate) localizes in bone by absorption onto, or chemical interaction with, the surface of the hydroxyapatite crystal of bone
- The phosphorus component interacts with the endogenous calcium to produce insoluble technetium calcium phosphate complexes
- Uptake occurs in areas of:
  - **Increased blood flow**, e.g. hypervascular tumours, fractures, inflammatory processes
  - **Increased cellular activity and mineral turnover**. Osteoblastic activity produces immature osteoid with numerous binding sites for

developing apatite crystals, e.g. callus of healing fractures, reparative processes around inflammatory foci, growth zones of epiphyseal plates, remodelling of trabeculae in response to stress
  - **Metabolic bone disease**, where there may be abundant immature unmineralized collagen
- Emits gamma rays detected by gamma cameras
- The gamma camera is passed over the patient or the affected part 4 h after the injection when soft-tissue activity has cleared, giving better delineation of the skeleton

Three-phase scan

First phase: flow or dynamic images (vascular phase)
- Angiogram of blood flow through the arterial system, 1–2 min

Second phase: blood pool or equilibrium images
- Displays the equilibrium of tracer throughout the extracellular space at 5 min
- Increased uptake in the blood pool phase reflects increased vascularity in the soft tissues, the commonest cause of which is inflammation

Third phase: static or delayed images (bone phase)
- 4 h later
- Displays sites where tracer accumulates in skeletal structures

(Fourth phase)
- Delayed bone scan at 24 h

Indications
- Assessment of **occult bone** or **joint pain**
- Assessment of **metastatic disease** (95% sensitivity)
- **Infection**: flow and blood pool phases are hot in cellulitis; all three phases are hot in osteomyelitis
- **Trauma**: occult, stress fractures
- **Tumour**: e.g. osteoid osteoma and osteoblastoma, especially the spine
- **Postoperative**: painful joint arthroplasty
- **AVN**
- Assessment of **Paget's disease**

Gallium scan (67-citrate)

- Binds to plasma proteins and localizes to sites of inflammation and neoplasia due to exudation of labelled serum proteins
- Entry via leaking capillaries into inflamed tissues
- Delayed imaging (24–48 h required)
- Frequently used in combination with a technetium bone scan: a double tracer technique
- Less dependent than technetium on vascular flow
- Difficulty in distinguishing between cellulitis and osteomyelitis

Indium scan (indium-111-labelled white cells)

- Labelled white cells accumulate in areas of inflammation but not in areas of neoplasm
- Useful in diagnosing osteomyelitis or infection around joint replacement

Radiolabelled monoclonal antibodies

- Labelling specific to particular cell lines, e.g. granulocytes, thus localizes to infection

SPECT

- Tomographic images obtained by rotating a camera around the patient 360°, which are then reconstructed in sagittal, coronal and axial planes
- Enhances sensitivity
- Improves anatomical location

PET

- An emerging modality
- Specific radionuclides (^{11}C, ^{15}O and ^{18}F) are manufactured in a cyclotron
- Radionuclides are used to label biologically active molecules that are introduced into the subject. They are short half-life radionuclides
- When a positron (e^+) emitted by the radionuclide interacts with an electron (e^-), two γ rays result at 180° to one another and can be received by an array of detectors

- Useful for physiological investigations, e.g. blood flow in bone

---

Examination corner

Basic science oral 1

- What is a bone scan?
- How does it work?
- What are the indications for its use?
- What are the various phases of a bone scan?

Basic science oral 2

Examiner: How do bone scans work?

Candidate: A bone scan involves the intravenous injection of a bone-seeking radionuclide, which localizes at sites of increased bone blood flow with increasing osteoblastic activity. The tracer uptake has three phases: vascular phase, static blood pool and bone phase.

Examiner: How long after the injection are the bone images available?

Candidate: Four hours.

Examiner: What is the half-life of technetium-99 phosphate?

Candidate: Six hours (mask-like and expressionless face of the examiner relaxed for a brief second to register mild surprise that the answer was known).

Examiner: Why use an isotope with a half-life of six hours?

Candidate: You want to get rid of the radioactive material from the body as soon as possible.

Examiner: Yes you don't want to glow in the dark any longer than necessary.

Basic science oral 3

Bone scan

- Principles of technetium and indium scanning

Basic science oral 4

Bone scan

- Half-life, advice re avoiding pregnant women and urinating!

Basic science oral 5

- Principles of the isotope bone scan
- Value of the triple phase component
- Other types of isotope scans
- Indium-labelled white cells
- SPECT scanning

MRI

- Uses nuclei of hydrogen atoms (protons) in compounds of hydrogen (water, fat, etc.) to produce an image
- The key feature is sensitivity to abnormal water distribution
- When a body is placed in a uniform magnetic field protons align with the field
- Radiofrequency pulses are applied for a few milliseconds
- **Excitation** – protons pick up energy from the radio wave (resonance) lifting some protons into a higher energy level and decreasing their longitudinal magnetization
- **Precession** – protons spin about an axis (like a gyroscope) moving in turn or in phase together and induce a transverse magnetization
- Protons possess both a longitudinal and a transverse magnetization in relation to the main magnetic field
- **Relaxation** – occurs when the radiofrequency pulse is switched off
  - T_1 – longitudinal relaxation, the time constant within which longitudinal magnetization is regained
  - T_2 – transverse relaxation, the time constant for loss of phase when the transverse magnetization decreases
  - $T_1 = 300$–2000 ms and $T_2 = 30$–150 ms
- The changes in magnetic field induce currents in the antennae that can be digitized into an image

- Further enhancement is obtained by a **pulsed sequence**, where a succession of radiofrequency pulses is employed to demonstrate particular tissues:

- T_1: short repetition time (TR) and short echo time (TE)
- T_2: long TR and short TE
- STIR: **s**hort T_1, **i**nversion **r**ecovery; sequence is very sensitive to water (very sensitive to marrow pathology), suppresses the normal fat signal
- Contrast medium is a chelated compound of gadolinium (works due to its unpaired proton), whose use is controversial
- Contraindications – unfixed ferromagnetic material (cerebral aneurysm clips) and electronic implanted devices (pacemakers, implanted defibrillators)

Image interpretation

- T_1 images weighted towards fat – good for anatomical structures
- T_2 weighted towards water – contrasting normal and abnormal tissues, good for pathology
- Water, CSF, acute haemorrhage, soft-tissue tumours appear dark in T_1 studies and bright in T_2 studies
- Cortical bone, rapidly flowing blood and fibrous tissue all appear dark

Ultrasound

Based on the transmission of sound waves through tissue and the time it takes for the waves to be reflected back to the transducing probe.

Since different tissues transmit sound waves at different velocities and the waves are reflected at tissue interfaces, sound waves that originate from the transducer at the same time will return to the transducer at different times. This information is used to create an image. The acoustic impedance for different materials is proportional to the density of that material and the speed of sound through that particular medium. An ultrasound transducer is a device that is capable of both converting an electrical signal into ultrasound waves and converting ultrasound back into electrical signals.

- Fluid-filled cysts are echo free
- Fat is highly echogenic

- Semisolid organs vary in echogenicity
- Advantages:
  - Non-invasive
  - No radiation
  - Gives real-time dynamic images cheaply
  - Easily accessible in most hospitals
- Disadvantages:
  - Operator dependent
  - Difficult to interpret
  - Limited views
- Uses:
  - Trauma (degree and quality of fracture healing)
  - Sports injuries (Achilles tendon rupture)
  - Infection (differentiating between cellulitis, abscess, osteomyelitis)
  - Congenital paediatric disorders (DDH)
    - Extent and nature of soft-tissue masses
    - Muscle pathologies (rupture, inflammation, haematoma)
    - Tendon pathologies (tendonitis, tears, tumours)

Tourniquets

Tourniquets are used to provide a bloodless field in limb operations, which:
- Aids recognition of tissue
- Reduces operative time
- Reduces operative blood loss

No absolute value can be given for pressure of inflation; the surgeon should consider:
- Age of patient
- Soft-tissue condition and extent under the tourniquet
- Intercurrent medical conditions (especially vascular pathology)
- In the upper limb the inflation pressure should be 50 mmHg higher than the systolic blood pressure
- In the lower limb it should be double the systolic blood pressure

There are two main types of tourniquet:
- **Non-pneumatic**

- **Pneumatic**

Pneumatic may be:
- Non-automatic
- Automatic

Non-pneumatic

- Appropriate only for short operations on a finger or toe
- A rubber catheter is tightened around the base of a digit and held by an artery forceps

Non-automatic pneumatic tourniquet

- Consists of a cuff with a hand-operated pump and pressure gauge
- This is a closed system with no automatic compensation for leaks in the system

Automatic pneumatic tourniquets

- Use a continuous supply of pressurized gas from a compressed air line or electric pump in theatre

Contraindications

- Peripheral vascular disease (relative)
- Severe crushing injuries
- Sickle cell disease

Exsanguination

- Either by elevation or expression
- Contraindications to expression include venous thrombosis, malignancy or infection, all of which may be spread by embolism
- In frail patients cardiac arrest may occur from circulatory overload if both lower limbs are exsanguinated at the same time

Tourniquet paralysis syndrome

- Caused by cuff pressure rather than ischaemia
- Flaccid motor paralysis with sensory dissociation

- Pain sensation is often altered although temperature appreciation is usually preserved
- Colour, skin temperature and peripheral pulses are usually normal
- EMG – nerve conduction block at the level of the tourniquet
- May take up to 3 months to recover
- Nerves in patients with diabetes, alcoholism and rheumatoid arthritis have increased susceptibility to pressure

Post-tourniquet syndrome (tourniquet-induced skeletal muscle ischaemia)

This is a reperfusion injury and is due to ischaemia. After release of the tourniquet, the following occur:

- Oedema
- Stiffness
- Pallor
- Weakness
- Subjective numbness

Myonephropathic metabolic syndrome

- Metabolic acidosis
- Hyperkalaemia
- Myoglobinuria
- Renal failure

Complications

Local

- Compression neurapraxia
- Bone and soft-tissue necrosis
- Direct vascular injury
- Post-operative swelling and stiffness
- Delayed recovery of muscle power
- Wound haematoma
- Wound infection

Systemic

- Cardiorespiratory decompensation
- Increased CVP

- Deep vein thrombosis
- Cerebral infarction
- Alterations in acid–base balance

Examination corner

Basic science oral 1

General discussion about tourniquets

- Responsibility for maintenance of tourniquets
- Tourniquet pressures used in the upper and lower limb
- Complications of tourniquet application
- Safe tourniquet time

Candidate: A bit of a vague, awkward and waffly start to the basic science oral. The examiner seemed to go on for what seemed like forever about who was responsible for tourniquet maintenance without asking me any specific question. The examiner asked me if I knew any papers published on the subject. I remembered a paper published from Liverpool[1] a few years previously that had shown they were poorly maintained and looked after. The examiner agreed and continued to waffle on for another minute or so before asking me about tourniquet pressures.

Examiner: It was just a general discussion about tourniquets. I wasn't after anything too complicated.

The Rhys-Davies exsanguinators in our local hospitals were poorly maintained (inflation pressure, storage conditions, replacement age) when compared to the manufacturers' recommendations.

Basic science oral 2

Use of tourniquet in orthopaedic surgery

- Complications

[1] Harris PC, Cheong HL (2002) Rhys-Davies exsanguinator: effect of age and inflation on performance. *Ann R Coll Surg Engl* **84(4)**: 234–8.

Compartment syndrome

This is a "pass/fail" topic. You *must* be able to explain the mechanism clearly.

Compartment syndrome is defined as increased pressure in an enclosed osteofascial space resulting in decreased capillary perfusion below that necessary for sustained tissue viability.

Normal compartment pressures are on the order of 5 mmHg.

There are two possible mechanisms:
1. Increased content – haemorrhage, ischaemic swelling, reperfusion injury, AV fistulae
2. Decreased space – tight cast, premature closure of fascia

The final common pathway involves:
1. Compartment pressure exceeds the venous pressure
2. The venous outflow from the compartment is impaired and tissue ischaemia follows
3. Pressure within the compartment increases whilst arterial inflow is not impaired
4. As compartment pressure approaches systolic pressure the flow into the compartment will cease

Clinical presentation

- Pain out of proportion to the injury
- Pain on passive movement (pain on stretch of the involved compartment)
- Pallor of the extremity
- Paralysis
- Paresthesiae
- Pulseless
- "Perishing cold"

Of the above, pain out of proportion and pain on passive movement are the diagnostic features of most clinical relevance since the others are all *too late* and imply muscle death.
- At 1 h of ischaemia, a reversible neurapraxia develops
- At 8 h irreversible axonotmesis occurs

Measurement

Compartment syndrome is a clinical diagnosis except where pain cannot be assessed (polytrauma, ventilated/unconscious patients, head injury or other mental incapacity or regional anaesthesia), when pressure monitoring is indicated.
- A catheter/needle and pressure transducer are used with simultaneous blood pressure measurement
- In trauma the measurement is taken within the zone of injury and should be undertaken in all compartments
- The threshold can be an absolute value of 30 mmHg or pressure within 20–30 mmHg of diastolic blood pressure – Edinburgh group[24])

Fasciotomies

- A diagnosis of acute compartment syndrome is a surgical emergency
- Tibia – anterolateral and medial incisions are made to access all four compartments
- Forearm – volar decompression to include carpal tunnel, then check the dorsum and decompress if necessary
- Foot – two dorsal incisions are made over the medial aspect of the second metatarsal and the lateral aspect of the fourth metatarsal; one 6-cm medial incision is made, releasing the medial, calcaneal and lateral compartments
- Closure not before 48 h; there is a low threshold for skin grafts rather than delayed primary closure
- Late presentation – once muscle necrosis is established there is no indication for fasciotomy and it may provoke rhabdomyolysis and infection. Timing of "late" is controversial

Electrosurgery

- An electric circuit is made involving the patient, where the patient is the point of current resistance, generating heat
- Frequency chosen is above 100 kHz in order to avoid nerve and/or muscle stimulation

[24] McQueen MM, Court-Brown CM (1996) Compartment monitoring in tibial fractures. *J Bone Joint Surg Br* **78(1)**: 99–104.

- Bipolar electrosurgery involves active and return point electrodes at the surgical site. The forceps points (electrodes) must be separated for current to pass through tissue. This has the advantage of avoiding the risks of monopolar systems, and is especially indicated in the extremities
- Monopolar electrosurgery involves an active electrode (high current density) at the surgical site and a return electrode elsewhere on the patient. The return electrode must be of large surface area (therefore low current density) to avoid burns
- Waveforms:
  - "Cut" involves continuous current to generate heat and vaporize tissue
  - "Coag" involves intermittent current (on for <10% of the time) with less heat and permits coagulum to form. If this waveform is used to cut, higher voltages are involved with more surrounding tissue damage
  - "Blend" involves a longer "on time" than coag
  - "Fulguration" means the coagulation/charring of tissue over a wider area and employs a coag waveform with the diathermy point held slightly away from the tissue
- Safety:
  - "Grounded system" – original technology; the risk of a return electrode being formed by patient contact with metal on the operating table resulting in iatrogenic skin burns
  - "Isolated system" – the return electrode becomes the only route back to the generator, so "grounding" is no longer a risk
  - Return electrode – placement over well-vascularized muscle mass. Most systems now monitor the impedance at the return electrode to reduce burn risk here
- Note that, in electrocautery, direct current is applied as a heated instrument in contrast to electrosurgery, which involves alternating current

Infection control

Two approaches are taken to address this issue:
- Reducing the size of the inoculum
- Enhancing the host defences

Reducing inoculum

- Ward hygiene
- Screening/separation of infected cases
- Skin cleanliness (*not* antisepsis – as this encourages resistance)
- Theatre design and practice (see below)
- Limiting dressing changes

Enhancing host defences

- Good nutrition
- Antibiotic prophylaxis where appropriate
- Tetanus prophylaxis
- Optimize the skin preoperatively (e.g. psoriasis treatment, avoid blisters)
- Avoid unnecessary antibiotics (resistance)

Antibacterials

Resistance of two types:
- Genetic – resistance transferred via DNA (plasmids, integrons and transposons)
- Proteomic – altered target site on bacterium or altered enzyme that is the target of drug action

Skin flora includes coagulase-negative *Staphylococcus epidermidis*, *Staphylococcus aureus* and Gram-positive diphtheroid bacilli. These are accessed by lipophilic antibiotics secreted in perspiration.

Biofilms (associated with inert, e.g. stainless steel, implants) reduce access to bacteria for antibiotics and host defences. Rifampicin has good penetration of biofilms.

Therapeutic index = effective concentration at site/minimum inhibitory concentration.

Antibiotic mechanisms

Penicillin/cephalosporin – Cell wall enzyme
Glycopeptides (vancomycin, teicoplanin) – Cell wall enzyme
Rifampicin – DNA-dependent RNA polymerase
Fucidin and clarithromycin – Block ribosomal peptides

Panton-Valentine leukocidin (PVL)

This is a hot topic in the USA, where it is more common than in the UK.

PVL is a toxin produced by *Staphylococcus aureus* resulting in invasive infections including necrotizing pneumonia. It occurs in both methicillin-sensitive and methicillin-resistant forms of *Staphylococcus aureus*.

Operating theatre design and practice

Source of pathogens

- 98% floor-borne pathogens are from skin scales (12 μm in diameter)
- The floor is only a minor source (15%) of air-borne pathogens
- Theatre air counts (Lidwell 1988[25]) of <10 colony forming units (cfu) per cubic metre significantly reduced wound sepsis

Theatre clothing should be changed regularly to:
- Avoid transmission of ward-based pathogens to the theatre environment
- Reduce skin-scale load on clothing

Stryker hoods protect the operator from body fluids, but may increase patient risk due to contamination outside the reduced field of view.

Charnley suits void exhaust fumes out of the theatre, and have been shown to reduce air counts.

Instrument sterilization methods

- Dry heat (ineffective, used for glass, liquid and powders)
- Moist heat (under pressure, requires less heat for less time)
- UV light (surface sterilization only)
- Radiation (used commercially)
- Filtration (for sterilization of liquids)
- Gas (ethylene oxide used and is slow)
- Liquid bath (4%–8% glutaraldehyde, for heat-sensitive instruments, staff sensitization risk)

Drapes

- Efficacy of different types remains unproven
- A pore size in cotton fabric of 80–100 μm will admit skin scales

Clean air

- Classic paper – 1982 MRC Hip arthroplasty study[26]
  - Multicentre, $n \geq 8000$, *not* a randomized controlled trial
  - Showed 3.4% infection rate in conventional theatre without antibiotic prophylaxis
  - Ultraclean air reduced infection rates to 1.7%
  - Ultraclean air and prophylactic antibiotics reduced infection rates to 0.4%
  - When using exhaust suits in addition to above precautions, rates as low as 0.2% were achieved
- Options include
  - Continuous positive pressure ventilation – the standard for modern theatres (air counts <35 cfu/m^3, 20 air changes per hour)
  - Clean air theatres – use "HEPA" filters to deliver air counts (<10 cfu/m^3 and 400 air changes per hour are the orthopaedic arthroplasty standards)
  - Laminar flow – is a theoretical ideal that cannot be achieved in practice as it is spoilt once objects (patient, surgeon, etc.) get in the way

Theatre design principles

- Separated preparation and disposal areas
- Air flow is dictated by pressure, therefore highest to lowest pressure:
  - Preparation room
  - Theatre
  - Scrub room
  - Anaesthetic room
  - Disposal room

---

[25] Lidwell OM (1988) Air, antibiotics and sepsis in replacement joints. *J Hosp Infect Suppl C* **11**: 18–40.

[26] Lidwell OM, Lowbury EJ, Whyte W, Blowers R, Stanley SJ, Lowe D (1982) Effect of ultraclean air in operating rooms on deep sepsis in the joint after total hip or knee replacement: a randomised study. *Br Med J* **285(6334)**: 10–14.

- Minimal cross-traffic through theatre
- No entry/exit during arthroplasty
- No blockage of air vents and pressure flaps by equipment

Hand washing

- Bacterial counts are reduced by 99% with chlorhexidine, 97% with povidone-iodine
- Residual effect after time is maintained best by chlorhexidine (97% at 3 h compared with 90% for iodine)

"Universal precautions"

- A ubiquitous term governing any steps to reduce the potential exposure to body fluids and tissues during an intervention
- Described by local "infection control" policies in place within each NHS organization
- Include:
  - Surgical shoes and theatre clothing
  - Gown (±apron)
  - (Double) glove
  - Mask
  - Eye protection
  - (Sharp) instruments passed via tray
  - Safe disposal of sharps
  - Safe disposal of tissues

Prosthetics and orthotics: wheelchair design

- Depends on daily use, fixed deformities, head/trunk control, environment
- Frame weight, rigid/portable
- Wheel/tyres
- Back – height, reclining or fixed
- Foot rests
- Seat cushion, trochanteric pads, scoliosis pads
- Strapping – seat belt, pelvic belts
- Ambulation – hand operated (requires good upper limb function), electric

Assistive devices

- Crutches
- Walking sticks
- Zimmer frames

Orthoses

Orthoses are external appliances that are used to:
- correct flexible deformity
- accommodate fixed deformity
- control motion
- augment weakness
- redistribute forces

The same biomechanical principles as described for bones and joints apply to orthoses. Usually three-point pressure is required to achieve immobilization.

Naming orthoses is straightforward – they are described by the structures that they cross:
- TLSO – thoracolumbar spinal orthosis
- KAFO – knee-ankle-foot orthosis

The commonest one is an *ankle-foot orthosis (AFO)*:
- Usually made from polypropylene
- Has a posterior leaf spring – to augment the weakness of ankle dorsiflexion, a 5° preloading in dorsiflexion can be used
- Solid – controls medial/lateral ankle movement and prevents dorsal/plantar flexion of the ankle. Ambulation will be helped by a rocker bottom sole
- Clamshell – an anterior polyethylene gaiter increases control over movement
- Floor reaction – an AFO that extends anteriorly in front of the knee and encourages stretching of the gastrocnemius
- Patellar tendon bearing – off-loads the foot and ankle in diabetic or Charcot feet

Orthoses in paralysis

L1   TLHKAFO "ParaWalker" – requires upper limb function

L5   AFO to address inverted/supinated foot

Prosthetics

- Functional versus cosmetic
- Suspension – belt or socket
- Endoskeletal (modular) versus exoskeletal (formed plastic or wood)
- Limb fitting for infants from 8 months (who are starting to stand and can manage two-handed play)
- Levels:
  - Hip disarticulation
  - Transfemoral – silicone Iceross® sockets
  - Through-knee – problematic for artificial knee mechanism
  - Transtibial – patellar tendon bearing, supracondylar suspension
  - Ankle disarticulation "Syme's" – silicone feet
  - Prosthetic feet – SACH (solid ankle cushion heel), multi-axis, dynamic response (carbon fibre springs)
- Upper limb – body powered (shoulder) or external power (myoelectric or switch)

Statistics

Statistics is an important part of the examination. What you should aim for is a good basic grasp of the subject rather than encyclopaedic knowledge. It is important to try to avoid spending too much time reading up on the subject in large textbooks. Time is tight in preparation for the examination. Use summarized handouts from various courses to maximize your gain of information. Our aim is to cover some important basic principles and definitions so that you can quickly go over them two or three days before the exam to refresh your memory.

Statistics is involved in the collection, presentation and interpretation of data. Data are recorded as *variables* (measurable properties), and each recording is a *variate*.

Types of data

Qualitative

- Nominal = not ranked (e.g. cast, traction, surgery)
- Ordinal = ranked (e.g. 1st, 2nd, 3rd)

Quantitative

- Discrete integers (e.g. 1, 2, 3, 4)
- Continuous (e.g. 0–100 and all decimals between)

Parametric tests: data are normally distributed on a Gaussian curve. By definition they must be continuous quantitative data. Can be subjected to t-test.

- More powerful than non-parametric tests
- Assumes that data are sampled from a normal distribution
- Observations must be independent
- Populations must have the same variance
- Rarely exist in orthopaedics

Non-parametric tests: data are not normally distributed, e.g. skew curve with a tail. Can only be subjected to less powerful tests (Wilcoxon signed rank, Mann–Whitney U, etc.).

- No assumptions are made about the origins of the data
- Less likely to give type II errors
- Less likely to be significant
- Rank order of values
- Cannot relate back to any parametric properties of the data

Transformation: the process by which non-parametric data are converted to the parametric form to permit more powerful analysis, e.g. logarithmic scale.

NOTE: Scoring systems (e.g. Harris Hip) include ordinal data. Even if final values appear to be continuous, they remain non-parametric data and appropriate tests must be used.

Outcome measures

Outcome measures need to be valid, reproducible, responsive to change, clinically relevant and easily measured. Other factors to consider are blinding and quality control. Outcome measures may be primary or secondary, objective or subjective.

Measures of central tendency

- **Mean:** the average of the data
- **Median:** central value of the data
- **Mode:** value with the greatest frequency

Measures of spread/variability

- **Range**: extreme values of the data set. The lowest and highest values of the data. The range does not give much information about the spread of data about the mean
- **Variance:** the measure of the spread, where the mean is the measure of the central tendency. Variance is the corrected sum of squares about the mean of the data
- **Standard deviation:** the square root of the variance; abbreviated to SD
- **Standard error of the mean:** defined as the SD divided by the square root of the sample size. It measures how closely a sample mean approximates the population mean. Can be used to calculate confidence intervals
- **Confidence intervals**: ranges on either side of a sample mean giving a rapid visual impression of significance
  - Only applicable to normal distributions (parametric data)
  - Confidence intervals are equal to the values between the confidence limits and are a set number of standard errors of estimate of the mean (SEM) from the mean on either side
  - For a large sample 95% confidence intervals are approximately two SEM from the mean on either side
  - It allows for comparison of statistical and clinical significance

Data interpretation

Null hypothesis: that no difference exists between two groups (hence any difference seen has occurred purely by chance). Tests including outcome measures are then employed to disprove null hypothesis.

The p value: the probability that the difference seen occurred by chance. The usual level is set at a 5% probability ($p = 0.05$) that the difference was due to chance, although any level can be set.

Type I (α) error: a false-positive result, incorrectly rejecting the null hypothesis, i.e. deciding there is

a difference when there isn't. Reduced by setting the p value smaller but then bigger study samples are needed in order to protect against a type II error.

Type II (β) error: a false-negative result, incorrectly accepting the null hypothesis, i.e. finding no difference when there is one. Increased by sample size being too small or by the p value being too small.

Type II (γ) error: occurs when the researcher correctly rejects the null hypothesis but incorrectly attributes the cause. In other words, the researcher misinterprets cause and effect.

Power analysis

Power $=1-\beta$: the probability of demonstrating a true effect and correctly rejecting the null hypothesis. The method of determining the number of subjects you need in order to have a reasonable chance of showing a difference, if one exists. Usually set at 80%.

Factors affecting power analysis:

- Size of the difference between the means
- Spread of the data
- Significance level (the p value that is set)
- Sample size (power increases with increasing sample size)
- Variability in observations (the larger the variability, the lower the power)
- Experimental design
- Type of data (parametric versus non-parametric)

Screening

Testing of asymptomatic people to look for disease/carrier status.

   Criteria
- Valid
- Test acceptable – no harm
- Specific, sensitive
- Natural history of the condition is known
- Early pick up – leads to intervention
- Intervention – leads to improved outcomes

- Potential yields, cost-effective
- Incidence known

Surveillance: the study of trends in a population

Accuracy: how often is the test correct

Precision: repeatability of measurement

Validation: evidence that a test measures what it is intended to measure

Incidence: the rate of occurrence of new disease in a population previously free of disease. It is found by dividing the number of *new* cases per year by the number in the population at risk

Prevalence: the frequency of a disease at a given time. Found by dividing the number of *existing* cases per year by the number in the population at risk

Sensitivity: true positive (test positive)/all true positive (all with the condition). The ability of a test to exclude false negatives: $a/(a+c)$

Specificity: true negative (test negative)/disease negative (all without the condition). The ability of a test to exclude false positives: $d/(d+b)$

Positive predictive value: true positives/all who test positive, i.e. the probability that a subject who tests positive is truly positive: $a/(a+b)$

Negative predictive value: true negatives/all who test negative, i.e. the probability that a subject who tests negative is truly negative: $d/(c+d)$

	Disease positive	Disease negative	Totals
Test positive	*a*	*b*	*a+b*
Test negative	*c*	*d*	*c+d*
Totals	*a+c*	*b+d*	*a+b+c+d*

Sensitivity = $a/(a+c)$
Specificity = $d/(d+b)$
Positive predictive value = $a/(a+b)$
Negative predictive value = $d/(c+d)$
Odds ratio = $(ad)/(bc)$

Error

- Same assessor – intra-observer
- Different assessor – inter-observer

Correlation and regression

Correlation coefficient (r): measures the degree of association between two parameters and varies from complete association (=+1 or –1) to no association at all (=0).

- Pearson's correlation coefficient – a measure of linear (parametric) association
- If one parameter increases as the other does, then the correlation is positive (and vice versa)
- If a curved line is needed to express the relationship then more complicated measures of correlation must be used, specifically Spearman's rank for non-parametric data

Regression: once correlation is established, regression is the line drawn over the scatter plot, using the regression equation $y = a+bx$; regression coefficient = direction coefficient of the regression line.

- Interpolation – measurements made on slope within data range
- Extrapolation – if the line is continued beyond the data range and the relationship inferred

Probability: possible occurrences of x/total number of possible occurrences, e.g. one possible occurrence of 6 on a die/6 possible occurrences when the die is thrown = 0.17. Therefore, there is a 17% probability of throwing a 6.

KAPPA analysis: involves adjusting the observed proportion of agreement in relation to the proportion of agreement expected by chance:

- 1 indicates complete agreement
- 0 indicates agreement can be expected purely by chance
- A negative value suggests systematic disagreement

Data collection

Study type

- Case study
- Case series
- Case–control study
- Cross-sectional study
- Cohort study
- Randomized controlled trial (RCT)

- Equivalence study
- Sequential analysis

Case series

The outcomes of a group are reported, but there is no comparison group. Weak.

Case–control study

Retrospective form of a cohort study. Patients with an outcome of interest and a control group are followed backwards from some point in time to ascertain whether some early treatment or other exposure had a relationship to that outcome.

Cohort (longitudinal)

A cohort is a group of patients. In a cohort study, two groups, one of which has undergone an intervention or treatment, are followed up over time in order to compare outcomes such as onset of disease or adverse events.

Cross-sectional studies

Patients or events examined at one point in time.

Randomized controlled trial

Gold standard. Groups of patients are randomized to receive or not receive an intervention or treatment, and the outcomes are compared in a prospective manner. The aim of the study and the hypothesis to be tested are clearly stated. Important features of RCTs include the following:

- **Randomization:** avoids bias. Ensure that all prognostic variables, both known and unknown, will be distributed equally among the treatment groups. Types include
  - **Simple:** treatment allocations assigned by computer-generated tables
  - **Block:** treatment is allocated by blocks of set size. This ensures that equal numbers of patients are assigned to each treatment

- **Stratified:** ensures prognostic variables which are extremely important are equally distributed between the treatment groups
- **Inclusion/exclusion criteria**
- **Outcome measure:** measures of outcome should be valid, reproducible and responsive to change
- **Bias:** this refers to a flaw in impartiality that introduces systematic error into the methodology and results of a study
  - **Experimenter bias:** during either selection or treatment
  - **Patient bias**
  - **Observational/experimental bias:** errors in the measurement or classification of disease
  - **Publication bias**
- **Power analysis**
- **Ethical approval**
- **Informed consent**
- **Collection of data** and **results**
- **Analysis**
- **Conclusions**
- **Publication:** important to know where (if!) the study will be published
- **Clinical significance versus statistical significance**
- **Masking/blinding:** this protects against bias. Can be single (patient) or double (patient, investigator)
- **Distorting influences**
  - Extraneous treatment
  - Contamination
  - Changes over time
  - Confounding factors: these are independent variables that interfere with the drawing of statistically valid conclusions from a study
- **Sequential analysis:** performed if there is a very important outcome, e.g. cancer. Two modalities are compared, power is determined, analysis is performed at predetermined points and the trial is stopped when statistical significance is reached
- **Equivalence study:** opposite to the null hypothesis. RCT where we expect two treatments to have the same outcome. Hypothesis is that there is a difference

Appraising a paper – the standard questions

- Study design
  - Appropriate to objectives?
- Study sample
  - Representative – study population, target population?
- Control group acceptable?
- Sampling methods
  - Random and unbiased?
- Quality measurements and outcomes
- Completeness – compliance, drop outs, deaths, missing data
- Distorting influences – extraneous treatment, contamination, changes over time, confounding factors

Survival analysis

Advantages

- Allows for variable dates of entry into study
- Patients can be followed for different lengths of time
- Can be analysed continuously (actuarial life table) or at times of failure (Kaplan–Meier)
- Provides a graphical comparison of the survival (or failure to survive) of different groups over time

Disadvantages – must be careful in how

- Failure is defined
- Loss to follow-up and death are treated
- Cohort effect (how introducing a change may affect survival, e.g. introducing a new cement)
- Must include confidence intervals
- Tail end imprecision occurs due to small numbers of survivors

Life table

- Survival probability is calculated at (yearly) intervals. Withdrawn patients are "censored" whilst patients who fail are "uncensored"
- The graph can be recognized as it is *stepped*

- Best- and worst-case scenarios should be given (with respect to loss to follow-up)

Kaplan–Meier

- aka Product limit analysis
- Survival is calculated from patient to patient with the rank of a patient's survival
- The graph can be recognized as it is *smooth*
- You must be able to read off 5-year and median (i.e. when 50% have failed) survival rates from such graphs!

Censorship

In most survival studies, some surviving subjects are not followed for the entire span of the curve:

- Some subjects are still alive at the end of the study but were not followed for the entire span of the curve
- Some drop out of the study early. Perhaps they moved to a different city
- In either case, you know that the subject survived up to a certain time but have no useful information about what happened after that
- Information about these patients is said to be censored. Before the censored time, you know they were alive and following the experimental protocol, so these subjects contribute useful information. After they are censored, you cannot use any information on the subjects

---

Examination corner

Basic science oral 1

Scatter plot: regression analysis, linear versus non-linear relationship, skewing of the curve

Basic science oral 2

- Survivorship analysis in joint replacement
- Kaplan–Meier curve: draw one and explain the *x* and *y* axes
- Confidence intervals and their importance

Examiner: You can see each death as a downward step in the curve. These steps get bigger as you go along the graph. Does that mean the data are more accurate?

Candidate: No. There are fewer patients in the study and therefore when one dies the step is bigger.

Examiner: You mean that the data are less accurate?

Candidate: Yes.

Examiner: What happens to patients who are followed up for say five years but then move to a different part of the country and are not followed up? Should we include these data?

Candidate: You are talking about censorship.

Before the censored time, you know they were alive and following the experimental protocol, so these subjects contribute useful information. After they are censored, you can't use any information on the subjects.

Basic science oral 3

- Normal distribution curve, standard deviation
- Null hypothesis, *p* values, Type I and II errors, power of a study

Basic science oral 4

- Sensitivity
- Specificity
- Drawing of the 2×2 contingency table with an example to simplify the answer (practise this beforehand)
- Positive predictive value and negative predictive value

Basic science oral 5

Examiner: Your consultant asks you to review the results of their first 1000 THR. How would you go about this?

Candidate: I would perform a survivorship analysis curve.

Examiner: What are the types of survival analysis curves that can be performed?

Examiner: What are the advantages of Kaplan–Meier over the actuarial method?

Examiner: How do you account for loss to follow up and then how do you calculate it within your survivorship curve?

Examiner: What about mortality?

Examiner: What is a confidence interval?

Basic science oral 6

Examiner: What will you do if you get five infections in close succession in your joint replacements?

Candidate: I burbled and blabbered on about audit, etc.

Examiner: How do you know that this is not a random occurrence and is probably due to system failure?

Candidate: I wasn't sure. The examiner prompted me – what about the organisms. I didn't get it. He answered for me. What if you get all five hips infected by the same organism. Only then did I see his reasoning.

Basic science oral 7

- How would you plan to start using a different type of knee arthroplasty?
- Survival analysis – details, methods, Kaplan–Meier curve
- Draw a survival analysis curve and describe it
- Confidence intervals

Basic science oral 8

Ten minutes of the basic science oral was spent on statistics. Topics covered included:
- Mean
- Median
- Mode
- Theory of central tendency
- Variance
- Standard deviation
- Correlation coefficient
- Regression analysis
- ANOVA

Basic science oral 9

- I was asked to draw the normal distribution curve and comment on it
- What is standard deviation?
- Setting up a study: discussion on null hypothesis, *p* values, type I and II errors, power, etc.

Basic science oral 10

- What information do you need to know in order to perform a statistical power calculation?

Basic science oral 11

- Define what a *p* value of 0.005 means

Basic science oral 12

Examiner: What types of studies exist?

Candidate: I mentioned several but the examiner didn't seem impressed.

Examiner: Your boss wants you to review 10 years worth of results of the THA that they use.

How do you go about it?

What type of study would it be?

Candidate: I hesitated with a fairly long pause but recovered. However I barely got started before the examiner started to lose interest in my answer and switched to another topic.

Examiner: You don't seem to know a great deal on this topic let's move on to another one.

Candidate: I hadn't anticipated this type of question and just was not sharp enough with the answer. You can't predict every question you will get asked.

[Fail]

Candidate: I spent a lot of time studying statistics and I was not asked particularly much about it in the examination. I wish I had spent less time on it because it was wasted effort.

Much as we have been trying to steer you into topics that tend to be asked in the FRCS Orth exam, one cannot entirely predict what the examiners will ask any particular candidate at any particular time.

Resign yourself to the fact that some "dead certain" topics learnt will not be asked. Accept it, don't dwell on it and move on to the next topic.

Ethics and orthopaedics

This somewhat "soft" topic is easily ignored in the rush for the facts, yet it's easy to come unstuck if you forget the principles ...

Duties of care

The "core" document to refer to is *Good Medical Practice*, published by the General Medical Council. This document sets out the duties and responsibilities of a doctor. It is available on the web in pdf format at the GMC website – http://www.gmc-uk.org.

The underlying principle of this document is:

All patients are entitled to good standards of practice and care from their doctors. Essential elements of this are professional competence; good relationships with patients and colleagues; and observance of professional ethical obligations.

Consent

The reference document for issues relating to informed consent is *Consent: Patients and Doctors Making Decisions Together*, June 2008. Again, this is available on the GMC website.

The basic information that should be communicated includes:

- Details of the diagnosis, and prognosis, and the likely prognosis if the condition is left untreated
- Uncertainties about the diagnosis including options for further investigation prior to treatment
- Options for treatment or management of the condition, including the option not to treat
- The purpose of a proposed investigation or treatment; details of the procedures or therapies involved, including subsidiary treatment such as methods of pain relief; how the patient should prepare for the procedure; and details of what the patient might experience during or after the procedure including common and serious side-effects
- For each option, explanations of the likely benefits and the probabilities of success; and discussion of any serious or frequently occurring risks, and of any lifestyle changes which may be caused by, or necessitated by, the treatment
- Advice about whether a proposed treatment is experimental

- How and when the patient's condition and any side-effects will be monitored or re-assessed
- The name of the doctor who will have overall responsibility for the treatment and, where appropriate, names of the senior members of his or her team
- Whether doctors in training will be involved, and the extent to which students may be involved in an investigation or treatment
- A reminder that patients can change their minds about a decision at any time
- A reminder that patients have a right to seek a second opinion
- Where applicable, details of costs or charges which the patient may have to meet

You should be able to explain how you would proceed with a patient of suspected mental incapacity with an orthopaedic injury (a common example might be an elderly patient with dementia who has sustained a fractured femoral neck).

Medical negligence

You need to have an understanding of this at two levels:

1. Your own competence and efforts you make to maintain and monitor it – education and training, educational supervision, logbook, the role of the Postgraduate Dean, audit.
2. Your approach to concerns regarding the competency of others in the workplace.
   - Your prime objective is to protect patients from harm
   - This might include reference to a senior clinician/manager
   - Local policies followed within the legal framework set out by the GMC
   - Where local system fails the issue can be referred to the GMC

Bone neoplasia

This section carries key facts associated with the main tumours that are likely to be encountered in the exam – however you are strongly advised to read this topic up more widely, and to be familiar with the radiographic appearances of bone tumours.

Metastatic bone disease

Best managed as a multidisciplinary team.[27]

Epidemiology

- Prostate, breast, renal, lung and thyroid carcinoma are the "big five"
- An estimated 20000+ patients develop bony metastases per annum in the UK

Preoperative assessment

- Standard history and examination
- NB Bone profile blood test
- Staging – full length radiographs, consider bone scan. CT/MRI as clinically indicated

Biopsy

- Where diagnosis is in doubt
- Consider especially in solitary lesions
- Should only be undertaken on discussion with bone tumour service
- Solitary renal metastases – may behave as a primary neoplasm and should be referred to the bone tumour service

Prophylactic internal fixation

- Assess fracture risk using Mirel's score[28]:
  - Site: upper limb (1), lower limb (2), intertrochanteric (3)
  - Pain: mild (1), moderate (2), limits function (3)

[27] Key reference – *Metastatic Bone Disease: A Guide to Good Practice*. London: British Orthopaedics Association. This is available on the BOA website: www.boa.ac.uk.
[28] Mirels H (1989) Metastatic disease in long bones. A proposed scoring system for diagnosing impending pathologic fractures. *Clin Orthop Relat Res* **249**: 256–64.

- Lesion: blastic (1), mixed (2), lytic (3)
- Size (maximal cortical destruction): <1/3 (1), 1/3–2/3 (2), >2/3 (3)
- Add scores: ≥8 are high fracture risk, require ORIF before radiotherapy
- Stabilize all lesions in a given bone
- Adjuvant radiotherapy is usually palliative, given in a single fraction. It may prevent fracture

Stabilization of pathological fractures

Aim for:
- Immediate stability
- Immediate weight bearing
- Radiotherapy may impede fracture healing but prolong the patient's life
- Assume non-union will occur; therefore fixation is for "lifetime"

Decompression ±stabilization of spine

- Present with pain/neurological deficit
- Consider possibility of unstable spine
- MRI to assess extent of involvement – whole spine, chest X-ray, chest CT, liver ultrasound or CT, bone scan
- Biopsy only on advice of spinal centre
- Radiotherapy if no instability, it is a radiosensitive tumour, multi-level, stable neurology, or as adjuvant postoperatively
- Surgery if unstable, progressive neurological deficit

Chemotherapy, bisphosphonates and hormonal manipulation may all have a role in the management of metastatic bone disease.

Benign bone tumours

Simple bone cyst

- aka "unicameral bone cyst"
- Affect children/young adults
- Usually asymptomatic unless they undergo pathological fracture

- Arrange follow-up radiographs or investigate where there is diagnostic uncertainty – CT, needle biopsy
- Management – may resolve after fracture, steroid injection or curette and graft

Aneurysmal bone cyst

- May undergo pathological fracture
- Often treated by curettage and/or radiotherapy. Cured by excision
- May recur in younger patients

Enchondroma

- 60% in hands/feet
- Early adulthood
- May undergo pathological fracture
- Treated by curettage and grafting
- In Ollier's disease there are multiple enchondromas, with a 30% chance of malignant transformation. Need skeletal survey and ongoing surveillance
- In Maffucci's syndrome there are multiple enchondromas with haemangiomas. Prone to low-grade chondrosarcomatous transformation. Need surveillance

Osteochondroma

- aka "cartilage capped exostosis"
- Usually a metaphyseal lesion due to a growth defect at epiphysis
- Commonly distal femur/proximal tibia
- Rarely undergoes malignant transformation (said to be <1%)
- Can be multiple in *diaphyseal aclasis* (aka multiple hereditary exostoses) – increased risk of malignancy

Fibrous dysplasia

- Presents in children under 10
- Can cause bowing of bones: "Shepherds crook femoral neck"

- "Ground glass" appearance on radiographs
- Occur multiply with precocious puberty in Albright's syndrome

Osteoid osteoma

- Lesion 1 cm or less in diameter in diaphysis or posterior elements of spine
- Pain incessant, often worse at night, relieved by NSAIDs
- Have radiolucent "nidus" on radiographs with sclerotic surrounding bone
- Hot on bone scan, may be missed on CT if cuts are too thick
- Treated by excision or thermocoagulation

Chondroblastoma

- Occurs in young adults in metaphyses, usually femur or tibia
- *Recur* after incomplete excision
- Benign lung metastases occur

Osteoblastoma

- Rare, may affect long bones or spine
- *Recur* after incomplete excision

Eosinophilic granuloma

- Affect children's skull, mandible, rib, long bone or vertebra (where they cause collapse as "vertebra plana")
- "Punched-out lesion"
- May resolve spontaneously or require curette and graft
- May form part of Hand–Schüller–Christian disease (aka histiocytosis X or Langerhans cell histiocytosis)

Giant cell tumour

- Account for 20% of benign bone tumours
- Present in second and third decade

- Management can include curettage and phenolization, or block resection. Embolization and radiotherapy have a limited role
- 5% transform to osteosarcoma

Primary bone neoplasia

Is rare and accounts for only 0.5% of cancer deaths.

Staging – Enneking

Benign
Latent/active/aggressive

Malignant
I   Low grade, no metastases
     (A) Intracompartment
     (B) Extracompartment
II   High grade, no metastases
     (A) Intracompartment
     (B) Extracompartment
III Low or high grade, metastasess
     (A) Intracompartment
     (B) Extracompartment

Investigations

CT of the lung and region of interest, bone scan, MRI, biopsy (by or with permission from the tumour surgeon).

Surgical – histological margins

- Intracapsular – within the lesion, implies incomplete excision
- Marginal – extracapsular but within the zone of reactive tissue
- Wide – normal tissue margin completely surrounds excised lesion
- Radical – extracompartmental

Multiple myeloma

- The commonest primary neoplasia of bone
- Due to plasma cell monoclonal proliferation, can be isolated or diffuse

- Usually >40 years old
- Features include normocytic anaemia, Bence Jones proteins, bone marrow infiltrated with plasma cells, severe bone pain

Osteosarcoma

- Young adult presentation, more common in Paget's and fibrous dysplasia
- Distal femur, proximal tibia, proximal humerus
- Chemotherapy and prosthetic limb salvage or en-bloc resection
- 95% 5-year survival with optimal management if grade 4 (i.e. complete) histological necrosis of tumour cells
Variants
- Central
- Surface
- Parosteal – 80% affect distal/posterior femur. Do not respond to chemotherapy or DXT

Chondrosarcoma

- Presents in middle to old age. Slow growing pelvic tumours
- Require wide resection. Chemotherapy and radiotherapy are not useful as primary management
- 50% 10-year survival
Variants:
- Central – low grade
- Periosteal
- Dedifferentiated – aggressive, poor prognosis
- Clear cell – reasonable prognosis
- Mesenchymal – poor prognosis
- Secondary, e.g. to an osteochondroma

Ewing's sarcoma

- Childhood and early adulthood presentation
- Fever and malaise, raised inflammatory markers
- Chemotherapy then en-bloc resection or limb salvage surgery. Postoperative radiotherapy with respect to margin of resection
- 70% 5-year survival

Fibrosarcoma

- An aggressive tumour, de novo or 20% secondary to previous radiotherapy
- Presents in middle age
- Long bones, especially femur, involved
- Preoperative chemotherapy, wide resection ±reconstruction
- 30% 5-year survival

Malignant fibrous histiocytoma (MFH)

- 30% secondary with fibrous dysplasia or bony infarcts or radiotherapy
- Femur, tibia, pelvis and humerus
- Presents in middle to old age
- Management as for osteosarcoma
- 70% 5-year survival

Chordoma

- Forms from notochord remnants
- Presents in middle to old age
- 50% in sacral/coccygeal region
- Pain and neurological deficits
- Survival with respect to excision – about 50% at 5 years

Soft-tissue tumours

There are soft-tissue versions of MFH, fibrosarcoma.

Liposarcoma

- Soft-tissue tumour. Not limited to "fatty tissues"
- Typical, atypical, round cell, myxoid, pleomorphic
- Surgery ±radiotherapy
- 50% 5-year survival in extremities, reduced if lesion is in the torso

Leiomyosarcoma

- Rare
- 50% retroperitoneal

- Wide resection ±radiotherapy
- 60% 5-year survival for extremity lesions

Synovial sarcoma

- Presents in young adults
- Locally aggressive, pulmonary metastases may not preclude survival
- Wide excision ±radiotherapy
- 68% 5-year survival

Rhabdomyosarcoma

- Childhood presentation
- 30% affect extremities/torso
- Chemotherapy and surgery
- Survival with respect to stage, from 20% to 90% 5-year survival rates

---

Examination corner

Basic science oral 1

Shown radiograph demonstrating lytic lesion in the greater trochanter femur. Asked to describe management, investigations and likely diagnosis. Discussed Mirel's scoring system.

Basic science oral 2

Describe this tumour (prop-based question usually using a plain radiograph occasionally other imaging modalities).

Basic science oral 3

Radiograph of osteosarcoma of the femur. Describe the X-ray appearance
   Principles of tumour staging and biopsy

Examiner: You are the tumour surgeon and how are you going to stage this tumour and manage it?

Basic science oral 4

Radiograph of a lytic lesion midshaft humerus in an elderly woman. Describe the X-ray and differential diagnosis. Diagnosis was myleloma. Other areas of bony involvement. Where else do you get myeloma deposits? How do you confirm diagnosis? Management of the lytic lesion.

Basic science oral 5

Radiograph of a fibrous cortical defect in distal tibia with pathological fracture. Differential diagnosis and management. How do you manage the fracture? How do you confirm the diagnosis?

Venous thromboembolism

Epidemiology

- DVT occurs in 1/1000 of the general population but in up to 50% of lower limb arthroplasty patients without prophylaxis, but is usually asymptomatic
- Asymptomatic DVT is diagnosed by ultrasound, ^{125}I fibrinogen or venography (the "gold standard")
- Symptomatic DVT involves leg swelling and pain
- Pulmonary embolism is due to DVT in 90% of cases but is a rare complication of DVT. Risk is increased 10× by surgery or trauma
- Post-thrombotic syndrome (ulceration, dermatitis, chronic swelling) occurs in up to 10% of DVT patients within 10 years
- Routine prophylaxis is used to reduce the morbidity and mortality of thromboembolism, however treatment of asymptomatic DVT is not shown to be effective
- Aspirin is not as effective as heparins at reducing the risk of asymptomatic DVT. *But* remember – fatal pulmonary embolism is catastrophic and therefore the most relevant end-point
- Aspirin or heparins both reduce the overall absolute risk of a fatal pulmonary embolism in a surgical patient from 0.6% to 0.2% with equal efficacy

- Aspirin carries a lower relative risk of bleeding than the heparins (1.24 and 1.75 respectively)

Risk factors

- Age – exponential increase in risk
- Obesity – 3× risk
- Varicose veins – 1.5× risk
- Prior venous thromboembolism – 5% recurrence per annum increased by surgery
- Thrombophilias – e.g. factor V Leiden, antiphospholipid syndrome
- "Thrombotic states" – neoplasia (7× risk), cardiac failure, recent myocardial infarction or cerebrovascular accident, infection, polycythemia
- Combined oral contraceptive pill, hormone replacement therapy, high-dose progestogens
- Pregnancy – 10× risk
- Immobility – bed rest for more than 3 days can increase risk by 10×
- Hospitalization – 10× risk
- Anaesthesia – risk associated with GA is twice the risk associated with a spinal

Types of prophylaxis

General

- Mobilization/leg exercises
- Adequate hydration

Mechanical

- Graduated elastic compression stockings (reduce the risk of asymptomatic DVT in active patients but there is poor evidence for below knee and it is contraindicated in up to 20% by oedema, peripheral arterial disease or neuropathy, deformity or dermatitis). Evidence for synergy with chemoprophylaxis
- Intermittent pneumatic compression (calf/foot pumps) is effective in decreasing rates of asymptomatic DVT
- Contraindicated in patients who have a high risk of limb ischaemia

Chemoprophylaxis

- Aspirin – shown to reduce asymptomatic DVT, PE and fatal PE. PE prevention trial[29] randomized hip fractures and elective hip arthroplasty to 1 month of 160 mg daily aspirin or placebo plus "other measures thought necessary". Results showed increased bleeding, no overall reduction in mortality but a significant reduction in fatal PEs. Contraindicated in those with bleeding disorders and peptic ulcer disease
- Low-molecular-weight heparin (LMWH) – has a longer half-life than unfractionated heparin and is therefore taken once daily. Causes more bleeding than aspirin, reduces fatal PEs but does not reduce overall mortality. NB Risk of thrombocytopaenia, prolonged use associated with osteoporosis
- Pentasaccharides, e.g. fondaparinux, inhibit factor Xa, lower the risk of DVT more effectively than LMWH
- Warfarin – contraindicated in bleeding disorders, pregnancy, spinal/epidural anaesthesia. Requires monitoring of INR. May be suitable for long-term patients with a target INR of 2–2.5
- Dextrans – require IV administration, are cumbersome and can cause anaphylaxis
- Evidence is convincing for either mechanical and/or chemoprophylaxis in elective orthopaedic lower limb surgery. The position of prophylaxis in trauma remains less certain. The SIGN guideline[30] states "there is no evidence that any prophylactic method reduces the risk of clinical VTE or mortality in trauma patients." In April 2007, NICE published guidelines aimed at reducing the risk of thromboembolism after surgery

[29] Pulmonary Embolism Prevention Trial Collaboration Group (2000) Prevention of fatal post operative pulmonary embolism and deep vein thrombosis with low dose aspirin. Pulmonary Embolism Prevention (PEP) Trial. *Lancet* **355**: 1295–302.

[30] Scottish Intercollegiate Guidelines Network (2002) *Prophylaxis of Venous Thromboembolism*. SIGN guideline no. 62 (Oct 2002, review 2005). Edinburgh: SIGN.

Miscellaneous topics

25. Candidates' accounts of the examination 569

Paul A. Banaszkiewicz and Niall Munro

26. Examination failure 587

Paul A. Banaszkiewicz

Candidates' accounts of the examination

Paul A. Banaszkiewicz and Niall Munro

The exam has changed and evolved since these candidate accounts were first made. In particular, the short notes in the written paper have been superseded by the MCQ and EMI papers, but have been included here for completeness.

There are numerous candidate accounts of the examination floating around out in the orthopaedic domain. It is easy to get hold of them with a bit of detective work. When I sat the FRCS Orth examination these were very difficult to obtain. Initially these were secretly passed down from one trainee to another with many favours owed (a great deal of begging required) to obtain them and sworn secrecy not to pass them on to other candidates.

This moved up a level as these papers began to circulate amongst groups of trainees from various regions sitting the exam using them as a frame of reference for revision. After the group sat the exam they were then passed down to the trainees below them preparing to sit the examination.

These papers began to find their way on to the Internet and now BOTA has a dedicated examination site, which contains numerous past papers of candidates.

These candidate accounts can go on and on and miss the point. They give the candidate a much better guide as to which areas to concentrate revision on than the official syllabus (which can be somewhat vague in places). They are however just a frame of reference, albeit a very useful revision tool. Be aware of over reliance on them to get you through the examination. The examination is not just about regurgitation of facts; it indirectly assesses the processing of information, and the application of skills, knowledge and experience to complex clinical scenarios. More subjectively it assesses professionalism and attitudes. A mature professional approach to patient care and safety is of paramount importance for the examiners to identify amongst candidates sitting the exam in order to successfully pass them.

Notes on the FRCS (Tr & Orth) Exam 1

Written paper 1

Short answers and MCQs

In this paper you will encounter five short questions, worth six marks each.
1. Neonate with congenital absence of the fibula
   - What are the expected clinical findings?
   - What are the expected X-ray findings?
   - What are the treatment options available?
   - What problems are peculiar to limb lengthening in congenital longitudinal fibula deficiency (CLFD)?
2. A 25-year-old male, who has been rugby tackled, has a varus knee, with no pulse and has decreased sensation in common peroneal nerve (CPN) distribution. X-rays show posterior cruciate ligament avulsion, and fracture of the fibular head
   - What is your management?

Postgraduate Orthopaedics: The Candidate's Guide to the FRCS (Tr & Orth) Examination, Ed. Paul A. Banaszkiewicz,
Deiary F. Kader, Nicola Maffulli. Published by Cambridge University Press. © Cambridge University Press 2009.

3. A 25-year-old male with a healing abrasion over the little finger metacarpophalangeal (MCP) joint with pus seen over the abrasion. He says he accidentally banged into a wall
   • What is your management?

4. A 35-year-old labourer who has had a unilateral painful hip for 4 years – 30° fixed flexion deformity, gross osteoarthritis including acetabular changes, and no history to suggest avascular necrosis
   • What is your management?

5. Drawing of stress/strain curve
   • Mark points – yield, ultimate tensile strength, plastic and elastic phases
   • Endurance limit
   • Work hardening
   • Toughness of material

Interpretation of a paper

Paper from *Journal of Bone and Joint Surgery* (Wigderowitz CA, Rowley DI, Mole PA, Paterson CR, Abel EW (2000) Bone mineral density of the radius in patients with Colles' fracture. *J Bone Joint Surg Br* **82-B**: 87–89), from Dundee, looking at BMD in young and elderly patients with distal radial fractures.

There were 5 questions, each with 4 stems, based on this – total 20 marks, marked negatively. About 7 questions were very easy. Roughly 8 tested basic statistical knowledge (*p* values, tests of significance, etc.). The rest seemed to be laborious tests of English grammar – double negatives, three-line sentences, etc.

Clinicals

Long case

An 81-year-old male with bilateral varus osteoarthritis of the knees – gross deformity, with associated fixed flexion contractures of about 15° in each knee, some symptoms suggestive of spinal stenosis, good pulses, no internal rotation in the left hip, painful extension with lumbar spine movement, and good pulses.

• Thorough history, including social and recreation, etc.

• Demonstration of valgus/varus laxity
• Demonstration of anterior drawer and Lachman's tests
• Theory behind the pivot shift test
• Demonstration of hip rotations in flexion and extension
• Usual questions on possible spinal/vascular/hip aetiology for anterior knee pain
• Take informed consent for TKA
• Shown the radiographs – what type of TKA would you do for this gentleman?
• What problems do you anticipate – patellar eversion, rectus snip, etc.?
• How do you sequentially release the medial structures?
• How do you correct fixed flexion contracture intraoperatively?
• How do you re-create the joint line in TKA?

Short cases

1. Bilateral pes cavovarus due to diastematomyelia
   • Take a short history
   • Ideally I should have asked:
     • Congenital, or, if acquired, when did it develop?
     • Family history
     • Sensory involvement
     • Urinary problems
     • Spinal problems
   • Assessment of gait
   • Examination of motor power and sensation to locate the level
   • Demonstration of knee reflexes and ankle clonus
   • Scar of Jones transfer. What is this scar suggestive of? Why is the operation done?

2. Ankle pain in an elderly woman
   • Why are you making her stand on her toes?
     • Assessment of tibialis posterior function
     • Demonstration of the ankle's range of movement – active and passive
     • Demonstration of subtalar range of movement

3. Massive rotator cuff tear in an elderly gentleman

- Ask for a short history – age, dominance, pain/stiffness/weakness?
- Inspect and examine range of movement – why is he unable to initiate abduction but able to maintain it?

4. Dupuytren's contracture
   - Asked to talk about the condition for a few minutes
     - What are the various cords and what are the bands contributing to each?
     - Various finger incisions
     - Role of the open-palm technique
     - Diathesis
     - Recurrence rate

5. Scaphoid non-union advanced collapse
   - Examine range of movement in the wrist – active first and then passive
   - Kirk Watson's test – theory and principles
   - X-ray – what are DISI and VISI?

6. Hallux rigidus
   - Demonstrate range of movements in the joints
   - Management options, including MTP arthrodesis – position of arthrodesis

7. Post HTO scar
   - What do you think this scar is due to?
   - What are the indications for HTO?
   - Do you think the operation works?! (The examiner wanted me to say yes)

Orals

In the orals you will encounter 4 sessions of 25 min each.

Basic sciences

- Fracture healing – mechanisms of bone healing and role of local cytokines
- Bone scans – principles of technetium and indium scanning
- Inheritance patterns of disease – including Duchenne muscular dystrophy
- Discussion on dystrophin deficiency

- Achondroplasia – inheritance patterns – what zone in the growth plate does it affect?
- Draw the growth plate
- Cell maturation, etc. in the growth plate
- Effects of various hormones on the growth plate
- Location of various disease processes, e.g. SUFE, rickets, in the growth plate
- Osteoporosis and osteomalacia – presenting symptoms, difference in pathology and blood tests in each condition
- MRSA epidemiology – general discussion
- Antibiotic prophylaxis – rationales and doses
- Survivorship analysis in joint replacement surgery
- Kaplan–Meier curve – draw one and explain the x and y axes
- Confidence intervals and their importance
- General discussion on DVT prophylaxis and management

Adult elective orthopaedics

1. Osteochondroma of proximal humerus
   - Possible presenting symptoms – complications
   - Approach to the proximal humerus – deltopectoral – basics only

2. Lytic lesion in the femoral head
   - Differential diagnosis

3. Cut section of femoral head showing subchondral collapse
   - Radiographic findings in AVN
   - Grading of AVN
   - Management for this grade – role of fibular grafts, decompression
   - Very superficial discussions throughout

4. Pathogenesis of osteoarthritis
   - Grading of osteoarthritis (Outerbridge)
   - Differences in radiographs between osteoarthritis and rheumatoid arthritis

5. Radiograph of massive subsidence after impaction grafting
   - What is impaction grafting?
   - Complications of impaction grafting, etc. (The examiner was getting bored at this stage)

6. Radiograph of a lytic lesion with a thin sclerotic margin in the lower femoral metaphysis
   - Probably a Brodie's abscess – management
   - Role of CT and MRI in defining cortical/medullary lesions
7. Preoperative evaluation in patients with rheumatoid arthritis
   - Cervical spinal involvement in RA, including values of the atlas–dens interval, space available for the cord
8. Radiograph of an infected TKA – investigations, aspiration, two-stage re-implantation, spacers, Prostalac® prosthesis
9. Draw the AP view of the L5 nerve root and its relevant anatomy in relation to the foramina and pedicles

Trauma

1. AP view of dislocated shoulder
   - Management in Casualty, reduction techniques, postoperative physiotherapy, recurrence rate. What is a Bankart lesion?
2. Un-united lateral condylar fracture
   - Draw the Milch I and II fractures. Why are lateral condylar fractures prone to non-union whilst supracondylar fractures unite? How would you fix it? What is tardy ulnar nerve palsy? What structures can compress the ulnar nerve around the elbow? What is the cubital tunnel? What is Osborne's ligament ?
3. Wrist radiograph – scaphoid fracture
   - Usual questions on Mayfield's progression up to lunate dislocation
4. Fractured neck of femur
   - Elderly female, undisplaced intracapsular fractured neck of femur
   - Garden classification. Inter- and intra-observer error – paper from Peterborough,[1] management options, including risks of AVN and non-union for displaced/undisplaced fractures

---

[1] Parker MJ (1993) Garden grading of intracapsular fractures: meaningful or misleading? *Injury* **24**(**4**): 241–2.

Examiner: What would you do for this patient?
Candidate: I would perform a hemiarthroplasty.
Examiner: Why?
Candidate: Because I think the risk of AVN is too high in an elderly patient. Why not just do a hemiarthroplasty and treat her definitively?
Examiner: Well in fact a two-hole DHS was performed. This is her radiograph at 6 months.
Candidate: It shows AVN.
Examiner: We should have done what you originally suggested and avoided this problem.

5. Isolated medial malleolus fracture
   - Lauge-Hansen classification
   - How would you fix this particular fracture?

Hands and paediatrics

1. Trigger finger – presentation, types and treatment (injection)
2. Picture of swollen hand – compartment syndrome. How do you achieve decompression?
3. Picture of laceration across the base of the finger – how do you check digital nerve function?
   - End result of zone 2 repair
   - Rehabilitation protocols after flexor tendon repair – pros and cons of each
4. What structures are at risk when doing a trapeziectomy – superficial radial nerve, radial artery and FCR
5. Principles of treatment of traumatic neuromas
6. Amputation just distal to DIPJ in a young musician – how would you manage?

Saved by the bell

1. Pronator quadratus type of distal radial fracture – how would you reduce it and would you fix it? If so, how and why?
2. Accessory navicular bone
3. Radiograph followed by discussion of disc space infection in children – treatment principles
4. Unstable and gross SUFE – treatment, including AVN rates, corrective osteotomy
5. Supracondylar fracture of humerus – nerve injury patterns, and method of management including K-wiring technique
6. DDH

- Late presentation
- Role of arthrogram
- Economics of preoperative traction before open reduction

Notes on the FRCS (Tr & Orth) Exam 2

Written paper

MCQ paper

A paper[2] on a comparison between the use and non-use of surgical drains in a group of 70 patients following fixation of fractured neck of femur, 35 patients in each group. Negative marking for incorrect answers.

Typical questions included:
- This is a cohort study
- This is a randomized prospective clinical trial
- This is a paired study
- The surgeon was blinded during fixation of the fracture
- This was a single blinded trial
- There was a statistically significant difference in wound infection between the two groups
- The results of this paper are in general agreement with the two articles mentioned in the introduction

There were about 12 fairly easy questions, the remaining questions being a bit tricky or ambiguous. I answered the majority of questions leaving only two or so unanswered that would have been complete guesses.

Short questions

1. Discuss the factors that influence the choice of whether to perform an above- or below-knee amputation [2]
    What is the ideal length of a below-knee stump and why? [2]

[2] Cobb JP (1990) Why use drains? *J Bone Joint Surg Br* **72-B:** 993–5.

What are the components of a below-knee prosthesis? [2]

2. You are called to see a 48-hour-old baby on the paediatric ward who has a suspected brachial plexus injury
    Discuss your assessment of the situation
    Are there any other possibilities? [3]
    How will you manage the condition? [1]
    What will you tell the parents as regards the prognosis? [1]
    When would you refer on for consideration of surgical exploration? [1]

3. A rheumatoid patient is noticed to have an extensor lag in her little and ring fingers. Discuss the possible causes and your management of the condition. (Extensor tendon rupture, subluxed MCP joints, subluxation of the extensor tendons, posterior interosseous nerve palsy, trigger fingers)

4. A previously well 70-year-old man is seen in the outpatient clinic with a 5-week history of increasingly severe low back pain with no sciatic symptoms. His radiographs show collapse of 50% of vertebral body height with no history of trauma. Discuss your management of the case

5. A 29-year-old gentleman is seen with a proximal humeral non-union. Discuss the radiographic findings that will influence your method of treatment
    What type of bone graft will you use and why?
    Are there any alternative bone grafts you would consider using?
    Discuss osteoinduction and osteoconduction

Clinicals

Long case

History
    A 59-year-old male with longstanding rheumatoid arthritis
    Current problems are severe pain and restriction of activities of daily living in the right shoulder and left wrist
    Awaiting right shoulder hemiarthroplasty and left wrist fusion

Previous bilateral knee replacements

Previous medical history: asthma, osteoporosis, hypertension

On methotrexate

Examination

I essentially performed a full shoulder, wrist and hand examination in front of the examiners talking as I went along.

Discussion about the functional assessment of hand (tip-to-tip, key grip, monkey grip, power grip, etc.).

I also briefly examined both knees and both hips although I was not asked to demonstrate any findings by the examiners. I examined his neck movements. The patient volunteered that various doctors in the past had got very excited about his reflexes: he demonstrated hyperreflexia and signs of a cervical myelopathy (Hoffman's sign, etc.) and I was specifically asked by the examiners to test his reflexes.

Discussion

Discussion about whether to stop methotrexate before surgery and evidence in the literature to support this (none).

General discussion about increasing the dose of prednisolone after surgery.

Principles of assessment of the rheumatoid patient (lower limbs before upper limbs; proximal before distal).

I was asked whether I would do shoulder arthroplasty or wrist fusion first and the reasons why. I was shown his wrist radiographs and asked to describe them (gross rheumatoid wrist with carpal collapse). I was shown an MRI of his shoulder and asked to describe it (gross supraspinatus discontinuity).

I was asked whether I would perform a total or a hemi shoulder replacement and the reasons for my decision.

Asked to describe the deltopectoral approach to the shoulder.

Discussion of the rheumatoid neck: atlanto-axial subluxation, subaxial subluxation and basilar invagination.

Discussion about Chamberlain, McGregor and McRae lines.

I was asked when it was appropriate to order new radiographs of the cervical spine in a rheumatoid patient due to have a general anaesthetic.

Short cases

1. Ulnar claw hand, low lesion, pathology at Guyon's canal, no sensory changes

Examiner: Would you like to examine this gentleman's right hand and tell me what you see?

Candidate: Various well-healed traumatic and surgical scars over the dorsal surface of the wrist, gross interosseous muscle wasting and gross clawing of the hand. On the volar surface of the wrist there is a recent longitudinal scar over Guyon's canal.

I examined for sensory deficit but to my surprise found none.

Examiner: What difference would you expect to find in sensation between a high and low ulnar nerve lesion?

Would you care to examine the motor function of the ulnar nerve?

Candidate: The patient had a positive Froment's test. The FDP of the little finger was working (I explained, therefore, that there was a low ulnar nerve lesion at Guyon's canal affecting motor but not sensory function).

2. Examination of a hip

I performed a Thomas test of the patient's hip.

Range of movement: stiff hip, no fixed flexion deformity, no internal or external rotation in flexion, no abduction, 20° adduction.

I was shown radiographs of the pelvis and asked to comment: central dislocation of the hip. Postoperative radiographs showed the acetabular fracture had been fixed with pelvis reconstruction plates and there was gross AVN of the hip. I was asked to discuss management.

Candidate: He has a stiff hip but no pain. There is no reason at this stage to do anything; I would follow him up in clinic, and if he develops pain then I would perform a total hip replacement.

Examiner: That is absolutely correct. In the absence of hip pain nothing further needs to be done at this stage but I would continue to review him on a regular basis in clinic.

3. I was asked to examine a shoulder

The patient was an elderly lady, with gross muscle wastage of the deltoid and pectoralis major; she had a old cleavage line incision scar over the front of the joint.

I carried out inspection and palpation only – the examiner did not want me to examine the range of movement, power of rotator cuff muscles, etc.

4. ACL-deficient knee and probable repair of the PCL

On examination I noted a recent anterior midline longitudinal scar, slight loss of full extension and gross restriction of knee flexion. (I missed a large scar posteriorly.)

I was asked how I could test for the patient's PCL function with only 30° flexion (I mentioned the quadriceps active contracture test).

5. Radioulnar synostosis

The patient was a young child in a chair with her mother. The examiner asked me to examine her elbow. The diagnosis was immediately obvious because of the lack of elbow supination.

I missed a 5° fixed flexion deformity of the elbow.

I was shown radiographs and asked to describe them.

I was asked about how I would manage the condition (conservatively).

6. Diaphyseal aclasis

I was asked to examine the back of a young boy.

I noted a large exostosis of the scapula.

(I missed rib exostosis more anteriorly.)

I was asked about possible causes of multiple bony swellings in a child.

7. Mild hallux valgus deformity of a right foot in a young female, 25 years old

The patient was sitting on a chair.

I was asked to examine her right foot.

I carried out inspection, palpation, assessment of range of movement, etc.

The deformity was fully correctable, and there was minimal pain with minimal symptoms.

I was asked about management (conservative)

Surgical management was not discussed.

(Apparently they were short of good short cases that day.)

8. Severe Dupuytren's disease

I was asked to examine the patient's hand – inspection only.

There then followed discussion about aetiological factors.

(The bell went.)

Orals

Hands and paediatrics

1. Mallet finger
    • Classification
    • Indications for operative treatment
    • Results and complications from operative intervention
2. Rheumatoid swan-neck deformity
    • Nalebuff's and Millender's classifications
    • How do you treat a Nalebuff type 2 swan-neck deformity?
3. Photograph of a palm laceration over the ulnar nerve territory with clawing of the hand
    • Discussion about results of ulnar nerve repair compared to median and radial nerve repair
    • What functional deficit will you have? (Loss of pinch grip between thumb and index finger and ulnar claw hand)
    • Discussion of tendon transfers for this condition (EIP to first dorsal interossei, FDS split transfer to the middle finger, the Zancolli lasso technique for the clawing hand)
4. Undisplaced waist scaphoid fracture
    • What are the pros and cons of conservative versus operative management?
    • Management of established non-union, avascular necrosis of the scaphoid, etc.
5. Management of an electrical burn to the fingertip

    I burbled a bit on this one and did not answer the question particularly well. The whole finger needs to be opened up, thoroughly debrided and then left open.
6. Clinical photo of Galeazzi's sign

    Discussion of the causes of leg length inequality.
7. Ultrasound scan of the hip of a newborn child

I was asked to point out various anatomical structures on the ultrasound scan. I was completely stuck on this one, as this was a subject that I had not revised at all! Discussion about Graf angles.

8. Radiograph of DDH

   Obvious diagnosis:

   • Describe the radiograph

   • Discuss the structures that prevent closed reduction

9. Pavlik harness

   • Complications

10. Severe SUFE

    • Classification of slips, Southwick angle, Loder

    • Incidence

    • Management

    • Do you know any papers published in the last year about SUFE?

11. Perthes disease

    Describe the radiograph

    • Gage's head-at-risk signs

    • Clinical prognostic indicators of poor outcome

    • Herring's, Catterall's and Salter–Thomson's classifications

Basic science

1. General discussion about tourniquets

   • Maintenance

   • Tourniquet pressures in the upper and lower limbs

   • Complications of tourniquet use

   • Safe tourniquet time

2. General discussion about nerve conduction studies

   • Features, principles, etc.

   • Where do you stick your electrodes?

   • What do you tell your patients about the procedure?

   • Why do you use two electrodes – to take into account the neuromuscular junction, which delays conduction

3. Stress/strain curve

   • Discussion about everything!

4. Growth plate

   • Shown a photograph of a growth plate and asked to point out relevant features

5. Survival curves

   • Asked to draw one

   • Type I and type II errors, power analysis

6. Vitamin D metabolism

   • Pass/fail question

7. Osteoclasts

   • Histological features, receptors, function

8. Genetics: types of inheritance

Adult elective orthopaedics

1. Chronic ankle instability

   Shown a varus stress radiograph with obvious tibiotalar diastasis. Discussion about treatment: anatomical versus non-anatomical reconstruction ±augmentation

2. Radiograph of chondrosarcoma of the proximal humerus

   Go through the whole set talk about staging of tumours. Site of biopsy (anterior because you are going to perform an extensile deltopectoral approach to resect the lesion)

3. How does an MRI scanner work?

4. AVN hip

   Shown an MRI scan and asked to describe its features, aetiology, the Ficat classification system, treatment of Ficat 1 and Ficat 4 disease. Discussion about metal-on-metal hip replacements

5. Shown a radiograph of a broken femoral prosthesis (Gruen type 4 failure), followed by discussion about Gruen modes of failure of femoral stems, DeLee and Charnley acetabular loosening zones and bony acetabular defects

Trauma

1. Radiograph of a hip broken just below a previously sited cannulated screw for fixation of the hip

   The fracture was due to stress riser – I was asked about management (removal of the screw plus four-hole DHS)

2. Open book pelvis

   Questions on the following: resuscitation; Judet views; inlet/outlet views. I was shown a photograph of an external fixator applied to but not correcting the diastasis and was asked what I would do now.

3. Open intra-articular distal femoral fracture with no distal pulse in a young patient who has had an RTA

   Discussion about various treatment options – call the vascular surgeons!

4. Colles' fracture

   Management and complications

   Outcome

   Discussed the use of K-wires versus MUA and literature supporting the use of K-wires over simple MUA alone

5. RSD types 1 and 2

   Management

   Prognosis

6. Radiograph of a fracture dislocation of the ankle

   Initial treatment

7. Displaced middle-third clavicle fracture

   What are the complications from this injury?

   What are the indications for surgical fixation?

8. Lateral radiograph and CT of the cervical spine

   Odontoid peg fracture

   What is the initial management?

Saved by bell

Notes on the FRCS (Tr & Orth) Exam 3

Clinicals

Long case

   A 36-year-old female, who has been suffering from JCA since the age of 18 months

   Current problems: Pain, stiffness, clicking and locking of both elbows

   History and examination, with demonstration of various signs, etc.

   There then followed a discussion of JCA: classification, pathology, diagnosis, differential diagnosis with acute arthritis, management, various

joints and systemic involvement, cervical spine involvement in RA, atlantoaxial instability and cranial migration

Short cases

I was shown seven cases. The average was about five.

1. PCL-deficient knee

   Signs, examination

2. Patient with intramedullary tibial nail and fasciotomy scars

   Identify, compartment syndrome, monitoring, fasciotomy, claw toes (why do such patients get claw toes?)

3. Ankle osteoarthritis

   Diagnosis and management

4. Ulnar tunnel syndrome following non-union of a medial epicondylar fracture

   Diagnosis and management

5. Hallux rigidus with dorsal osteophytes and skin changes

   Diagnosis and management

6. Posterior interosseous and ulnar nerve palsy

   Diagnosis, demonstration of signs, differentiation between high and low radial lesions

7. Hallux valgus

   Examination and plan of management

   Patient had severe deformities – the examiner wanted to hear basal osteotomy

Orals

Paediatrics

1. Brodie's abscess. Diagnosis, differential diagnosis, further tests, management options, surgical management including types of incision and techniques. The examiner wanted to know what kind of material is seen at curettage!

2. Cerebral palsy. Clinical photograph: description, diagnosis, classification, definition, treatment for the hip problems in CP

3. Radiograph of femoral shaft fracture. Description, management, outline of the acceptable position

for conservative management, operative management, complications

Hands

1. Rheumatoid hand. Description, classification of thumb deformities, management, pathology of deformities
2. Extensor tendon rupture. Associated with RA. Diagnosis of sudden loss of extension of the fingers, causes, management, and Mannerfelt syndrome
3. Enchondroma of the hand. Diagnosis, differential diagnosis and management options. What type of bone graft is needed and from where and why?
4. Scaphoid non-union. Describe the X-ray, blood supply of scaphoid, non-union rate, treatment of acute fracture and established non-union, SNAC wrist

Basic sciences

1. Scatter plot: regression analysis, value of the coefficient, linear versus non-linear relationship, skewing of the curve
2. DEXA scan: comment on the findings and whether they are osteoporotic or osteopenic. Definition of osteoporosis (try remembering the WHO definition as well). What is standard deviation?
3. Posterior approach of lumbar sacral spine: layer by layer down to bone; specific anatomical location of the exiting and traversing nerve root; which root is affected in a given disc lesion; Bateson's venous plexus, anatomy, surgical importance, direction of flow
4. Classification of nerve injury: Seddon and Sunderland, recovery times of each
5. Posterior thigh (the examiner had a photocopy of the whole of the posterior thigh from an atlas). I had to identify all the muscles, giving their attachments and nerve supply; I had to identify and describe the surface anatomy of the sciatic nerve

6. Popliteal fossa: anatomy, approaches, neurovascular structure, anatomy arrangement
7. Posterior approach to the hip: structures going above the piriformis and below it; anatomy of the superior and inferior gluteal nerves and arteries, pudendal nerve; safe zones for acetabular screws; femoral head blood supply
8. MRI of the lumbar spine. What is an MRI scan? What are T_1- and T_2-weighted images? How are they produced? Distinguish between infection and tumour, discitis, pyogenic/granulomatous
9. AVN: diagnosis, classification

Trauma

1. Tibial fracture: pathoanatomy of a mid-shaft fracture; management of acute injury; postoperative management; compartment syndrome; pathophysiology; diagnosis/management; whether to fix the fracture first or decompress the compartments; monitoring; tibial compartments with approaches for decompression; Gustilo classification; Cierne classification of soft-tissue injury; non-union
2. Reaming complications; reamed versus unreamed nails; blood supply of a long bone
3. Biomechanics of intramedullary nails: area moment and polar moment; working length of a nail; effect of reaming on the working length
4. Acetabular fractures: classification and broad outline of management
5. Pelvic fractures: classification and management of open book fracture; haemodynamics; external fixator; whether to fix in A/E or in the theatre. General discussion!
6. Plates: types, uses, differences, strength, effect of making holes on the bone, stress risers, oval versus square hole, principle of tension band

Adult elective orthopaedics

1. Osteochondroma of the proximal femur, differential diagnosis, approach, management
2. Ewing's: differential diagnosis, management

3. AVN (again!): classification, management, causes
4. Distal radial fracture: classification, management
5. DVT: pathology; what is "your" preference in THA?
6. Subtalar arthritis: triple arthrodesis, joints involved, approaches to subtalar joint. Blood supply of talus, attachments of lateral ligament complex and peroneal tendons
7. Kohler's disease: classification, management
8. SLAC wrist: Mayfield classification, management

Notes on the FRCS (Tr and Orth) Exam 4

Although this is constructed from notes made at the time, the whole thing does tend to become a bit of a blur and undoubtedly I have missed out some questions, and perhaps even translated some questions from one oral to another. It may, however, give some idea as to the flavour of the whole procedure.

Written paper

- The written paper lasted 2 hours – not a generous amount of time, but adequate (unless your knowledge is encyclopaedic!)
- The structure was five "short notes" questions for six marks each, along the following lines

1. Clinical governance. A scenario was presented whereby 4 weeks after starting as a consultant, your unit had a 5% mortality rate for joint replacement. Questions asked for a definition of clinical governance, with whom the responsibility of clinical governance rests, what should be done in this scenario, and what should be done if the reason is found to rest with the surgeon involved
2. Scenario of a patient in their 40s presenting with a painful varus knee. Questions asked about indications for osteotomy and the surgical principles of wedge osteotomy. I was asked for definitions of mechanical and anatomical axes of lower limb, and their angular relationship to the vertical axis

3. Describe the anterolateral approach to the cervical spine for a C5/6 discectomy, paying attention to the various structures that may be injured in this approach
4. Question about a female infant being referred from the neonatal unit with a possibly unstable hip. I was asked to describe my management over the first 6 months of life
5. Trauma scenario, with a female motorcycle pillion passenger in her 20s being brought into A&E. She was stable and had undergone initial ATLS survey and resuscitation, but had a posterior fracture dislocation of her hip, an ipsilateral femoral shaft fracture and an ipsilateral non-intra-articular tibial fracture. Questions asked about the timing of the management of her injuries, and what might be reasonably done after midnight, assuming an adequately staffed theatre and facilities. Question asking for two causes of her developing low blood pressure and hypoxia in the anaesthetic room (presumably fat embolism and hypovolaemia)

Paper interpretation

This was a short (two-page) paper from *The Knee* about a non-randomized study looking at arthroscopy wound complications when portals were either closed with Steristrips or left open. There were 5 true/false stems with 4 questions each. It was fairly similar to the specimen paper. Questions included the following:

This study was an example of: cohort study, cross-sectional survey, randomized controlled study, etc.

Power

Interpretation of the quoted p value

Valid conclusions that can be drawn from the study

Which tests could have been used to analyse the data (chi-squared, t-test, Kruskal–Wallis, etc.)

Types of bias that the authors attempted to reduce in the study

I found it helpful to answer the MCQs first, and then I could adjust my short notes according to how much time I had left. For the paper interpretation section, we were advised to read the questions before the paper, which was good advice.

Clinicals

Short cases

Each short case session lasted 25 min, half with each of two examiners. Approximately 20 patients were placed around the periphery of the room. The examiners are directed to take candidates around at least six cases, and most take you round more. There is not time to undertake a complete examination of each area in question along the lines given in a clinical examination book. Do exactly what the examiners tell you: if they tell you to examine the movement in someone's shoulder, don't spend 5 min inspecting, palpating and examining their cervical spine as a preliminary.

Short cases that I saw included:

1. Patient in his 30s with hip disarticulation and prosthesis. I was asked to observe and describe his gait. After this I was informed that he had hip disarticulation for necrotizing fasciitis. I was asked about the design of a socket for a hip disarticulation prosthesis, about methods of suspension and about the different types of knee components with their pros and cons

2. Diaphyseal aclasis. I was introduced to father and son, both with prominent lumps. I was asked to examine, describe and give a diagnosis. I was asked about what additional problems osteochondromata could give in the forearm (supination/pronation). I was then asked to examine supination and pronation, which were markedly decreased on the left arm. I was asked about inheritance and other complications (malignancy, and incidence)

3. Frozen shoulder. Asked to examine the right shoulder of a lady in her 40s. I moved fairly quickly on through inspection and palpation and was then asked to specifically examine movements. Abduction and especially external rotation were very limited, being the clues to diagnosis

4. Surgical fusion of the hip. I was asked to examine the hip of a man in his 30s, who was lying in bed. On inspection I noted a scar over his left hip. I was then asked specifically to check the Thomas test (25° FFD) and then to check other movements, of which there were none. I was asked what had been done. I was shown a radiograph and asked to comment (Cobra plate and good fusion). I was asked about the reasons for trying to preserve the abductors and ways of doing this (trochanteric osteotomy, anterior approach, etc.)

5. Dislocating DRUJ after trauma. Asked to examine the wrist. There were various scars and the patient could easily demonstrate dislocation. I was asked for a diagnosis and to discuss treatment. Soft-tissue procedures had previously failed, so options included Sauve–Kapandji and Bowers

6. 16-year-old FDP and FDS injury (unrepaired) in a man in his 40s. I was asked to examine his hand: he had a small scar in his palm and an inability to flex his little finger. (He also had a camptodactyly.) I was asked about treatment options

7. Holstein–Lewis fracture. I was asked to examine a man with a scar on his posterior humerus and wrist drop. I was asked what muscles were affected by radial nerve injury, and to demonstrate weakness. I was shown X-rays and asked about treatment options and recovery times for nerves. I was asked how the scar would differ if it were from fixation of an intra-articular elbow fracture, and the approach that I would use for this

8. Ilizarov frame on tibia. I was asked what the frame was and to comment on it and the reasons it might have been applied. There was a sling to keep the foot in neutral, etc. I was shown the patient's radiographs of a comminuted pilon fracture. I was asked about treatment options and the timing of surgery after injury

9. Equinus foot after trauma (motorcyclist who had had severe bony and soft-tissue injuries of the lower limb). I was asked about the scars on his foot (from tendon transfer, probably tibialis posterior)

Long case

Retired farmer of 62 with a 10-year history of increasing right hip pain. Basically a fairly classical presentation of hip OA, who was due to be admitted the following week for THA. He had had a CVA and MI 10 years previously, with good recovery. The only pitfall was that if you specifically asked, he had some tingling in the dorsum of his foot, and some pain below the knee. It might have been problematic if you had not picked this up, but otherwise it was very straightforward for a long case. You have approximately 25 min to perform a history and relevant examination.

There were two examiners, each given 15 min. The first took me to the patient and asked me to present the history. On beginning to present my examination findings I was stopped and asked to demonstrate specific signs. I was asked to demonstrate the Thomas test and the Trendelenburg test and to describe the patient's gait. I was asked to examine movement, make leg length measurements and to test sensation in the lower limb. I was also asked about alternative sensory modalities that can be tested and following on from this how I would demonstrate proprioception (a nice easy way to use up a few minutes of time!).

After the bell we left the patient and went to sit down at a table, when the second examiner took over. I was asked to describe the patient's pelvic X-ray (classical hip OA) and spinal radiograph (quite a severe degenerative scoliosis). I was asked to look at a few specific sagittal MRI pictures and was asked what they were (T_1-weighted MRI spinal images) and what they showed (I think we all agreed that these pictures did not reveal much beyond what you could see on the radiographs).

I was asked about the risks of THA specifically relating to this patient (with his previous CVA and MI plus he was overweight), whether I would defer surgery until he had lost weight, and whether telling patients to lose weight has much effect. I was asked about the risk of DVT and what my choice of DVT prophylaxis would be, and why. I was asked what broad type of implant I would use. The examiner

asked in some detail how long I would tell the patient that the THA would be likely to last, and what evidence I had from the literature that the implants I would use would do so.[3]

NB This is the old style long case as now the examiners are with candidates throughout the initial history taking and examination.

Orals

These are held in a large room with probably about 20 numbered tables and 2 examiners at each one (and sometimes a future examiner who is merely observing). Each oral lasts 25 min, split into two sections, and in the 5 min between orals you come out of the room and are given the table number for your next one. It's very well organized, and although it sounds like a recipe for chaos, it's almost impossible to get lost. The four orals are back to back, although they will always be split at some point by a coffee break or lunch break. This time round, the second half of the alphabet had their orals on the Tuesday and the first half on the Wednesday.

Trauma

1. Shown two screws: one a titanium cortical screw, and one a cancellous stainless steel screw. I was asked about the indications for each, to describe the differences between them (material, pitch, core diameter), to define pitch, and when I would use titanium and when I would use stainless steel (and relative costs between the two)

2. Shown a DHS. I was asked to describe its principles, the purpose of the compression device and whether I usually used it, the indications for a DHS and ways of minimizing failure (correct placement, etc.)

3. Radiograph of a Salter Harris Type II fracture of the distal femur in a teenager. Asked about management (conservative, operative methods, type

---

[3] Williams HD, Browne G, Gie GA, Ling RS, Timperley AJ, Wendover NA (2002) The Exeter universal cemented femoral component at 8 to 12 years. A study of the first 325 hips. *J Bone Joint Surg Br* **84(3):** 324–34.

of plaster) and complications (angular deformity, limb shortening, neurovascular)

4. Shown a radiograph of an intra-articular Y-shaped fracture of the distal humerus. Asked to describe the fracture, management and what kit I would ask theatre to get out before starting, etc. Asked whether I had done any such operations and what they were like to do (i.e. not easy!)

5. Asked about a volar Barton's fracture in 30-year-old concert pianist (no radiograph or prop), who also had median nerve tingling. Asked about management, whether I would put screws in the distal part of the buttress plate (and in what situations I might do so), the advantages of the newer plates (I had said I would use a traditional small fragment T-plate), postoperative regime (plaster or otherwise, mobilization, return to work, etc.), how long nerve symptoms are likely to take to resolve and types of nerve injury (neurapraxia, etc. – and how to spell it!)

Hands

This is one-half of the combined paediatrics/hand oral.

1. Photograph showing volar wrist ganglion with overlying scar. Asked about diagnosis, what causes a ganglion, what lines the inside of a ganglion, treatment options (discussed recurrence rates with different treatments) and whether I would do any investigations before treatment (i.e. radiographs)

2. Radiograph of fourth and fifth metacarpal shaft fractures with anterior angulation in a patient who had punched a wall. Asked how I would treat it (discussed manipulation, plating and my preferred technique of K-wiring). Asked how I would insert K-wires

3. Picture of drop wrist after humeral fracture. Asked about the types of splint one might use, about EMG and electromyographic findings and how they might differentiate between different types of nerve injury (struggling here!) and when to explore

4. Picture of an open wound over volar thumb IP joint with divided tendon, digital nerves and skin loss. Asked about how I would obtain skin cover (flap/skin graft) and which I would use

5. Photograph of rheumatoid wrist with synovial swelling and dropped fingers. Bell went before I was asked any questions!

Paediatrics

This is the other half of the combined paediatrics/hand oral.

1. Shown a radiograph of two AP knees in a 12-year-old child with left knee pain, which had allegedly been sent to you by the patient's GP for advice. Asked to describe the radiograph. There was some periosteal reaction in the femur which was just visible at the edge of the film, and which took me some time to detect. Asked about the characteristics of the periosteal reaction (apparently it was meant to show layering or onion skinning, although this was difficult to see even with the eye of faith!). I was told that when the child was seen in clinic, he had a hot, tender swelling in the thigh. Asked differential diagnosis (tumour: Ewing's, osteosarcoma; or possibly infection). Asked about management: history, examination, blood tests, local staging (MRI) and distal staging (bone scan, CT chest and abdomen). Asked about principles of biopsy (excise tract, etc.)

2. Photograph of a child with intoeing. Asked how I would do a rotational profile. I described the foot progression angle (asked about its significance: non-specific measure of intoeing), the heel bisection angle, the foot thigh angle and assessment of femoral anteversion (asked to draw what angle you measure)

3. Radiographs of child with an anterior (Bado I) Monteggia fracture. Asked what classification system I use, and to describe it. I was asked how I would treat it and in what position I would immobilize it

Basic science

1. Compartment syndrome. Asked about diagnosis, and particularly diagnosis using pressure monitoring: how and where I would insert the probe, what threshold for diagnosing compartment syndrome I would use, etc. Shown cross-sectional diagram of the leg and asked to identify compartments and to describe how I would do a fasciotomy. Asked about the nerve at risk from an anterolateral approach (superficial peroneal)
2. Genetics. Asked to draw a diagram to show autosomal inheritance patterns. Asked about the percentage of offspring who would inherit a dominant and recessive pattern
3. Asked about neurofibromatosis: diagnostic criteria and inheritance. Asked on which chromosome the defect is found (17)
4. Brachial plexus. Shown a diagram of the brachial plexus. Asked to identify a specific nerve (long thoracic), what it does and where it runs. Asked then to identify the other branches
5. Asked what the compensatory mechanisms for OA hip are (looking for antalgic gait and Trendelenburg gait with the centre of gravity shifted over and above the osteoarthritic side, not for compensations for specific deformities). Shown a free body diagram of the hip and asked to explain with reference to the diagram how these would be affected by physiotherapy (increasing the strength of abductors as shown on diagram), decreasing weight, using a stick and the Trendelenburg lurch
6. Shown a survival curve. Asked about different methods of calculating survival curves (Kaplan–Meier, actuarial). Asked how data should be presented if patients are lost to follow-up (different presentations as recommended by Murray *et al.*,[4] including worst case scenario, etc.). Asked about appropriate end points (discussed use of revision, patient satisfaction). Asked about "censorship"

7. Asked about measures that can be taken in theatre to reduce the risk of infection
8. Asked about the types of metals used in orthopaedics. Asked about the contents of 316L stainless steel. Asked to name the different possible methods of corrosion, and which commonly occurred in orthopaedics
9. Asked to list the criteria for a successful tendon transfer

Adult elective orthopaedics

I was told to consider myself as being at an orthopaedic clinic, with the following patients presenting:
1. Picture of hallux valgus. Asked to describe the patient's condition, and asked about radiographs and angles that can be measured (and their values). Asked about management options, and specifically when I would do a proximal osteotomy
2. Radiograph of a rheumatoid foot. Asked to describe the patient's condition and to give a diagnosis. Asked about the macroscopic appearance of a rheumatoid joint at surgery. Asked to "comment if I could" on some histology slides, which apparently showed pannus (they weren't too bothered that I didn't work that out!). Asked what pannus is
3. Radiograph of a femur in a patient in their 70s with Paget's disease. It showed bowing. A scenario was given whereby the patient had pain and limb shortening. Asked for diagnosis, to describe the pathophysiology (blastic/clastic phases, etc.), theories of causation, medical therapies and mechanisms of action of calcitonin and bisphosphonates. Asked what I would do if problems persisted despite medical treatment, and what surgery could be done. Asked about problems with surgery (blood loss, hypercalcaemia, etc.). Asked whether the pain came from the clastic or blastic phase (apparently it is from the former)
4. Asked about an 18-year-old fast bowler who came to clinic with low back pain. Asked about

[4] Murray DW, Carr AJ, Bulstrode C (1993) Survival analysis of joint replacements. *J Bone Joint Surg Br* **75**(5): 697–704.

the most likely diagnosis (spondylolysis). Asked how to treat it

5. Asked about a patient in their 40s presenting with pain on the lateral aspect of their elbow with activity and the most likely diagnosis (tennis elbow). Asked about pathophysiology, treatment, clinical findings (provocative tests, etc.)

6. Asked about a patient in their 20s presenting with medial knee pain after a twisting injury and the likely diagnosis (medial meniscal tear). Asked about examination findings and treatment

7. Sciatica. Asked about the commonest cause of sciatica (disc prolapse). Asked to describe the pathophysiology of disc prolapse and to draw an axial diagram of how this causes nerve impingement. Asked what nerve root would usually be affected by L4/5 prolapse, and to explain how L4 signs could arise from an L4/5 prolapse (far lateral prolapse). Asked about other causes of sciatic pain (stenosis; vertebral collapse or pressure from fracture, tumour, neurofibromatosis, infection; intra-abdominal pathology from tumour, aneurysm, diverticulitis, etc.; peripheral entrapment, e.g. piriformis syndrome, although I think we all agreed that piriformis syndrome probably doesn't exist!)

8. Picture of a swollen infected knee replacement in a 70-year-old diabetic 2 weeks after surgery, with some skin necrosis. Asked about investigation and management, and other specialties that it would be useful to involve

The results

The chairman of examiners tells you to come back at a specific time for the results (1730 hours in our case). There is a separate examiners' meeting after each day of orals, so if your orals are on the Tuesday you don't need to wait until the whole exam is over before you hear. They have tried to do away with the institutional humiliation inherent in announcing results in the FRCS exam (results aren't called out; all the envelopes are the same size, etc.). You are given an envelope according to your candidate number and this contains a piece of paper offering either congratulations or commiserations. If you are successful, you are invited to join the examiners for a drink. It's actually a very informal and sociable occasion, and it is interesting meeting the examiners in a much more relaxed context. They generally seem by this stage to have forgotten all the ludicrous things you said in the heat of the exam (although one examiner did comment that he was intrigued by how many candidates found a full range of motion in the hip fusion patient!).

Sources

There is no shortage of sources for studying, but equally there is no perfect source. I found it reasonable advice to use one as a "core" (most people use Miller[5]) but to use a number of different short sources. Personally I didn't find reading major chapters from "definitive" books such as the *Oxford Textbook*[6] much use (I did try it), and found advice to use lots of smaller sources more helpful.

1. "Key topics" books on trauma and elective orthopaedics (the former is the better of the two). I used these as a basic introduction right at the start of my revision. They are fairly basic, but they do cover some things you otherwise wouldn't think to read up on, and they can be absorbed in small amounts if your studying is fairly "low level"

2. Miller. Most people use this as a core text, and I did likewise. It is very broad ranging, but it does have limitations in that it has few illustrations (especially clinical pictures) and numerous printing errors, and while there is great deal of information on some topics there is very little on others. However, I suppose it is "tried and tested" so I'm a little reluctant to suggest throwing it in the bin!

3. Orthoteers.[7] I didn't like this when I originally looked right at the beginning of revision, but

[5] Miller MD (2008) *Review of Orthopaedics*, 5th edn. New York: Saunders.

[6] Bulstrode C, Buckwalter J, Carr A, *et al.* (eds.) (2001) *Oxford Textbook of Orthopedics and Trauma.* Oxford: Oxford University Press.

[7] See www.orthoteers.com

found it very useful in the last few weeks. I had decided that if I failed the exam I would probably base my studying "second time round" on Orthoteers, as it is possibly better approached with some knowledge already. It is much better illustrated than Miller, and is quite good on classifications. There are some deficient areas, and the "purpose written" notes are better than some of the links they have

4. *Journal of the American Academy of Orthopaedic Surgeons*. I found the CD version very useful for reading up on topics I knew nothing about, midway through revision. Their articles are very well edited, and it is difficult to find a bad one. They give good and amply sufficient detail, but are still comprehensible. Some of the articles are now ageing a little however, and could do with being revisited by the journal

5. Clinical examination. I suspect Reider's book[8] may be the best, although I didn't actually use it (you need to order it early if you want it!). Remember that the clinicals are 40% of the exam, and the one part you need to pass, so plenty of practice at ward rounds, etc. is invaluable rather than just reading books

6. Statistics. I used the last chapter in Miller, two or three selected chapters from the BMA publication *How to Read a Paper*[9] and two of the sections from Orthoteers on "how to choose a statistical test" and survivorship analysis

7. Basic sciences. The Oswestry notes[10] are very useful: I used these and Miller. The Oswestry notes do not themselves cover biomechanics, although this is to some extent covered by booklets from ORLAU in Oswestry[11]

8. Anatomy/surgical approaches. This is a significant part of the exam, and comes up in the written paper and orals. I used Tubiana's volumes on upper[12] and lower[13] limb surgical approaches (personally I prefer them to Hoppeneld[14]), and plugged gaps with Crawford Adams' book,[15] and (very) occasionally Campbell's[16]

9. *Journal of Bone and Joint Surgery*. I went through the last 2 years, and made very brief summaries of the most important papers in each volume (not in detail). You thus have a brief summary which can be "crammed" in the week before the exam. Most people's experience is that they are not asked vast amounts about the literature, but invariably you are asked a bit

10. Classifications. Again, these do come up, although not as often as you might think. The only classification I was asked about in detail was the Bado classification (although knowing it probably salvaged a hitherto dubious Paeds oral). I found keeping a list of classifications that could be revised periodically was helpful

11. Courses. These are of limited value. Most people do a basic sciences course. The annual Durham University one (in Stockton) is a one-week course taught fairly didactically, and was reasonable. The Oswestry one is supposed to be good, but interactive and "high stress" and is probably therefore best done just before the exam. Most people who did 2-day basic sciences courses seem to have found them too short to be of much use. In terms of hand courses, there are ones in Nottingham in the autumn and Edinburgh around Easter, and both are

[8] Reider B (2005) *The Orthopaedic Physical Examination*, 2nd edn. New York: Saunders.

[9] Greenhalgh T (2000) *How to Read a Paper*. London: BMJ Publishing Group.

[10] Cassar-Pullicino VN, Richardson JB (2007) *Basic Science for FRCS (Trauma and Orthopaedics)*. Oswestry: Institute of Orthopaedics (Oswestry) Publishing Group.

[11] ORLAU is the Orthotic Research and Locomotor Assessment Unit based at the Robert Jones & Agnes Hunt Orthopaedic & District Hospital NHS Trust in Oswestry.

[12] Tubiana R, McCullough CJ, Masquelet AC (1990) *An Atlas of Surgical Exposures of the Upper Extremity*. London: Lippincott Williams and Wilkins.

[13] Masquelet AC, McCullough CJ, Tubiana R *et al.* (1993) *An Atlas of Surgical Exposures of the Lower Extremity*. London: Lippincott Williams and Wilkins.

[14] Hoppenfeld S, Deboer P (2003) *Surgical Exposures in Orthopaedics: The Anatomic Approach*. London: Lippincott Williams and Wilkins.

[15] Crawford Adams J (1976) *Standard Orthopaedic Operations: A Guide for the Junior Surgeon*. London: Churchill Livingstone.

[16] Canale ST, Beaty JH (2007) *Campbell's Operative Orthopaedics*, 11th edn. New York: Mosby.

supposed to be quite good. They fill up quickly (Edinburgh in particular I think was full before it was advertised in 2007) so book very early. There is a paediatric course in Nottingham close to the time of the hand course and also one in Liverpool. I did one in Dublin, which was reasonable (the oral practice was the most useful part). There are also general courses for the FRCS Orth in Oswestry and Oxford. I know people who did the latter found it OK, but expensive for what it was. I think it was partly a case of doing practice orals: if there are people who will do this for you locally that is perhaps as good

12. Locally, going to teaching ward rounds for 3 or 4 months before the exam is a very useful and time-honoured institution. Various consultants will do orals/tutorials, which is useful

General observations

1. The examiners now are given specific instructions about how to examine. This involves not trying to "catch out" or distract candidates from a correct course, but trying to guide them towards how much they do know. Examiners are assessed, and will not be asked back if they deviate from this. Ergo, if in the middle of a short case or oral you are asked "are you sure?" the correct answer is invariably "no" (although your abrupt change of direction can be made to sound a little more subtle, with the appropriate skills)

2. The pass rate does appear to be increasing. It was 77% on the day I did it

3. The whole process is far from pleasant, but it is exceptionally well organized, and the administrators, chairman of examiners, and most of the examiners do go out of their way to minimize your nerves. The chairman (currently James Hutchison) is not an examiner himself, and is available to discuss any concerns or worries of any nature

4. You are as likely, or indeed more likely, to be asked about simple things than rarities. Don't read only about proximal focal femoral deficiency, Morquio syndrome and Gaucher's disease, and attend the exam knowing nothing about ganglia, tibial fractures and tennis elbow (see above)

5. Abiding memory: a group of candidates discussing the different methods of obturator dislocation at lunchtime before their final oral. This rather misses the point: most of us will gain far more marks from keeping calm and thinking clearly than from an extra 10 min of cramming. Having said that, some subjects do lend themselves to revision in the last few days. Re-learning the brachial plexus a couple of days before stood me in good stead

6. In the exam, most topics start with a prompt such a radiograph, clinical photograph or (in the clinicals) a patient. It's a different way of approaching things to the standard textbook way (aetiology, pathology, epidemiology, presentation, treatment, prognosis), so get into the way of things with plenty of oral practice, and use some picture atlases of "classical cases". Miller's in particular has a problem with this, because there is little in the way of illustration, especially clinical pictures/X-rays, etc.

26

Examination failure

Paul A. Banaszkiewicz

By the law of averages some candidates will inevitably fail.

Introduction

We are informed that the FRCS Orth is not a competitive examination and that the pass rate is not set and will vary from examination to examination depending on the standard achieved. In recent years, the rate has varied between 55% and 78%. It may be stating the obvious, but the pass mark means that some candidates are going to fail. There has been an unconfirmed view from recent candidates that because of the changes of "*3 attempts only in the clinicals and you are back at the beginning*" the pass mark has gone up. "*It is not in the examiners' interests to fail candidates unnecessarily.*" The examiners, however, have a duty to protect the public and if there is any doubt whatsoever about a candidate, they are failed.

Prevention is better than cure

In our "candidates' accounts" section we offer many dialogues when the candidate knew they had performed badly and had blown it. This is to alert you to be on your guard for various pitfalls and hopefully avoid them.

That said during the examination do not under any circumstances assume that you have failed and give up – you have failed only when you have that piece of paper in your hand confirming this to be the case.

There is always going to be a small number of candidates who perform so poorly in the clinicals that they instinctively know they have failed. Go to the orals and give it your best shot if only for the experience, as it will be much easier next time in the orals knowing what to expect. There are too many stories recounted of candidates who did not turn up for the orals after the clinicals because they were convinced they had failed only to find out later that they had in fact passed well.

A common mistake is to dwell too much on a perceived poor performance in one section of the examination, allowing this to affect the performance of the remaining examination.

The trauma oral went very badly and I let it affect me in the other orals particularly the paeds/hands oral as it followed straight on afterwards. In fact I passed the trauma oral very well (and also the other two orals), but failed the paeds/hands oral – the trauma oral completely unnerved me.

During the duration of the examination, it is mentioned by the chairman of examiners that each examiner is instructed not to discuss any individual candidate's performance with any other unrelated examiner; in other words one should not be hearing that a particular candidate was poor. Genuine grievances during the course of the examination can be taken up with various secretarial staff present or the chairman of examiners.

One example was when a candidate straight after his general adult and pathology oral overheard an

Postgraduate Orthopaedics: The Candidate's Guide to the FRCS (Tr & Orth) Examination, Ed. Paul A. Banaszkiewicz, Deiary F. Kader, Nicola Maffulli. Published by Cambridge University Press. © Cambridge University Press 2009.

examiner say he had performed poorly and would have to make "*A hell of an effort with the other orals to scrape through*". The candidate felt that the comment was unhelpful and although it did not put him off the remainder of the examination it may have done so in other circumstances (he in fact passed).

With candidates who fail, there is a cooling off period after the examination in which they are actively discouraged from questioning the examiners on the reasons for failure. The assumption is that emotions are running high at this point and that in the heat of the moment things could be said that both candidate and examiner may have cause to regret later.

The results

The examiners meet in the evening to go through the results of each candidate. It is claimed that they try to get as many candidates as they can through the examination. In the past if a candidate had failed the long case, then they could not be passed and that was that. This has changed so that in theory you can fail your long case and still pass the examination but it is difficult to get through in any other way apart from a minor fail. Some candidates may have had a borderline performance, and a poor performance in one area may be compensated for by an above-average performance elsewhere.

It is claimed that the examiners do not like to fail anybody and although it is terrible for candidates to fail, it is just as bad a feeling for examiners to fail a candidate! The borderline candidates or (if you're lucky) distinction candidates presumably take up most of the discussion. If you have failed or passed outright, there is very little to discuss.

Examiners are now scrutinized much more than in the past. Their pass rate is compared to the average along with whether the candidates they pass or fail were in general agreement with the other examiners' assessments. Again it is claimed that if an examiner is failing too many candidates, especially in an erratic manner, he or she may be pulled in and called to task. Examiners are now expected to be much more candidate friendly and politically correct in their approach.

One of the most annoying parts of the examination is the hanging around afterwards for the results. The buzz generated by 100 or so 30-somethings waiting around for what seems like forever is quite something. Invariably, there is always a delay, which can be as long as an hour. If candidates are unable to wait they can phone a special telephone number later in the evening for their results. In practice the majority of candidates do wait around for the results.

You are given your result in a plain white envelope, with no distinguishing features to identify beforehand whether you have passed or failed. There are always going to be candidates who have passed who jump up and down with excitement, kneeling and kissing the floor with sheer joy – this is not particularly pleasant if you are one of the unfortunate ones who happen to have failed. If you have serious reservations about whether you have passed and do not want to be a part of this scene, leave at the end of the exam and phone up afterwards. If you cannot bear to wait for the result get your envelope and disappear into a quiet corner, away from everybody where you can open it up in peace.

If you have been successful, you will be invited to share a drink with the examiners – go to this, as it is an immensely enjoyable experience. Drink as much champagne and sherry as possible – you deserve it – you have indirectly paid for all of this with your exam fees.

The post mortem

There is no nice way to put it, but quite simply if you fail it will be a crushing blow and a huge disappointment. One will end up dwelling on many things, not least what part of the examination went wrong. Have a few drinks that evening and try to put things behind you. Do not ruminate alone in a hotel room.

Most colleagues are sympathetic to you after failure: "*It could happen to anybody*", "*Hard luck*", "*I would fail it if I had to sit it now*", etc. Most will be curious as to what went wrong. Probably the best option is to be honest with them and try not to talk around it. Do not keep going on with stories of how the examiners were merciless and how hard done by you feel, as even if this is true it will quickly bore people. Say simply that you are not sure, that you think it might have been the orals or the short cases and that you will not know until you get the official report.

The official confidential white paper summary of performance takes between 3 and 4 weeks to arrive. This is sent directly to the candidate, a further copy is sent to the candidate's head of training and the chairman of examiners keeps a copy. This in theory should offer feedback to candidates on their overall performance and deficiencies – essentially why you failed. The vast majority of candidates I have talked to find it at best "unhelpful" and at worst it reopens wounds that were just about beginning to heal. Sometimes with the official report there are no surprises, but for most candidates it can be a shock to find out where exactly they came unstuck and usually this is not where they had originally predicted.

Generally speaking, try to be ahead of the game and informally discuss your failure with your head of training a couple of days or so after the exam. They should have some idea from feedback from the examiners where you went wrong. It is a long time to wait for feedback from the official report. Although a matter of personal preference, I would suggest ringing up the Royal College a week or so after the exam and ask informally about what you slipped up on. The college is not obliged to divulge this information, but is generally very helpful. One candidate I knew did this and found out that his performance had not been that bad and that he had marginally failed two orals but passed everything else reasonably well – he was able then to sleep properly at night.

Without doubt one of the biggest headaches will be that your head of training will want to formally speak with you about your examination failure. They will probably wait until your formal summary of performance has been received.

This is a very important meeting so treat it very seriously and do not be too casual about it. Analyse where you went wrong and, more importantly, show that you have thought about where you went wrong and offer suggestions on how you are going to rectify things and pass next time. You should be positive and explain why you think you failed and what you are going to do about it. Your head of training will in all probability offer some advice, but take the initiative yourself. Maybe we are painting a bleak picture of events and the meeting will go very smoothly without any unforeseen problems, but it is best to be prepared for a possible hard time. At the end of the day, you are on your own – passing the examination is your own responsibility and only you can do it.

Your head of training may recommend that on your performance you should prepare for a longer period of time and miss the next diet of examinations. This is a very difficult thing to stomach, but, on balance, you should probably go along with this unless there are exceptional circumstances.

The next time

You will need to re-focus and re-motivate yourself for the next attempt. Several candidates at their second attempt claimed they had put in a minimal amount of work and it all went very smoothly. It is certainly an advantage the second time around knowing what to expect. However, in some respects this is a double-edged sword, as no doubt nervousness and exam fatigue will play a much more significant role second time round. One small crumb of comfort of sitting the examination the second time is that, as the material is already vaguely familiar, it is a lot easier to relearn rather than to learn.

Another potential advantage is that, when you do pass it, you will have learnt your orthopaedics to a much better standard than the first time round and this will undoubtedly be of benefit in your long-term clinical practice.

Repeated failure

If this occurs, and it can happen, it is a time for holding your own counsel, not saying too much but quietly thinking about your next step. Something is not happening with the exam. Is it just bad luck, deficiencies in the training programme, your own deficiencies or a combination of everything all together?

The third time sitting the examination is much harder than either the first or second attempt. It is claimed that each time a candidate sits the examination, the slate is wiped clean and this is a fresh attempt with no prejudices carried forward from previous attempts. My own subjective opinion is that this is probably not the case. At the third attempt, the examiners would want to make absolutely sure the candidate is safe to allow through to practise independently as a consultant and has not just fluked it on the day.

The situation will need to be discussed with your head of training and some sort of action plan sorted out, whether it be a period of intensive coaching, a deferred sitting or a temporary move to another training programme.

And finally an alternative view of the FRCS Orth Exam

The inter-collegiate speciality examination consists of an archaic process of poorly managed stress interviews or orals.

What exactly is being examined? Misdirected examiners link success in the examination to competence in independent elective and emergency practice. But neither knowledge nor competence is tested – rather the candidate's ability to develop rapport under unrealistic duress not encountered in normal working practice.

Experts in interpersonal communication agree that:

- 7% relates to words
- 38% relates to voice tonality
- 55% depends on physiology or "state"

Candidates fail the inter-collegiate speciality examination primarily because of their physiological state and consequent discordant rapport with examiners and not because of poor preparation or lack of knowledge.

For candidates who fail, careers can stall, substantive jobs are lost and family life can be severely affected.

The onus rests on the candidate to develop an instant rapport with the examiners, something that can be enhanced by the matching of physiologies, voice tonalities and even choice of words. Not only can the two examiners display dissimilar and inappropriate incongruent states, varying from uninterested to disdainful, but rapport building can also be severely compromised by the candidate's stress response.

Many examiners recognize this and encourage rapport but some lack basic communication skills. Examiners' poor interviewing techniques can induce a highly unresourceful state in many candidates. The FRCS Orth examines not competence, but rapport in a rare physiological state.

Index

AAOS classifications, 184–5

abduction test, subacromial impingement, 52

abductor digiti minimi (ADM), examination, 30

abductor pollicis brevis (APB), 37, 38, 39

abrasion arthroplasty, 480

abrasive wear (ploughing), 507

abscess, 263, 346, 392–3

acetabular component/cup, 182, 184, 509, 513

acetabular dysplasia, 360

acetabular fractures, 430–2, 434

acetabular labral injuries, traumatic hip
    dislocation, 434

acetabular safe zones, 178

acetabular socket design, confined/constrained,
    169

acetabulum, 431

  in dysplastic hip, 162

  lining, augmentation, PLAD, 169

  loosening, 179

  preparation for THA, 165

  travelling/wandering, 100

acetabulum labrum, DDH, 362

Achilles tendon, 382, 388, 447–8

Achterman and Kalamchi classification, 397

acid phosphatase, tartrate-resistant, 465

acromioclavicular joint (ACJ), 138

  arthritis, 51, 138–9

  degenerative changes, 409

  dislocation, 408–10

  pain, 51, 138, 409

acromion, 51, 406

acromioplasty, 140, 141

actin, 484–5

adhesive capsulitis, 55, 144–5, 580

adhesive wear, 507

adolescent idiopathic scoliosis, 243–4

general orthopaedics and pathology oral, 137
   candidates' accounts, 571–2, 576, 578–9, 583–4
   general guidance, 135–7
   see also oral examinations; *individual*
      core topics/joints
adynamic lesion of bone, 525
ageing, cartilage, *vs* osteoarthritis, 479
air, clean, in theatre, 551
Allen's test, 22, 26, 302
allergy, metal, 183, 500–1
Allis and Bigelow technique, 435
allografts, 203, 210–11, 474, 475
alumina ceramic, femoral head, 512
aluminium toxicity, 525
ALVAR, after metal-on-metal hip resurfacing, 183
ambulation abduction bracing, 75, 373
amputation, 173–4, 331–2, 397, 398
amyoplasia (arthrogryposis multiple congenita), 391
analgesia, 88, 463
anatomical snuffbox, 277–8, 306
aneurysmal bone cyst, 561
anisotropic, definition, 490
ankle
   acute inversion injury, 219
   anatomy, 219
   arthritis, 216–19
   arthrodesis *see* arthrodesis, ankle
   arthroplasty *see* arthroplasty, ankle
   arthroscopy, 215–16
   biomechanics, 215
   cerebral palsy, 382–3
   chronic instability, 219–23, 576
   clinical cases, 16, 110–25
   congenital talipes equinovarus, 387
   debridement, 217
   equinus, in CP, 382
   forced inversion injury, 219
   fractures, 445–7
   fusion, and position for, 119
   loose body, 220
   nerve supply, 232–3
   oral core topics, 215–36
   osteoarthritis, 118–19
   pain, 119, 220, 221, 570
   short case list, 16
   sprains, 219, 221
   stability testing, 118
   syllabus on, 215
   unstable injuries, 219

ankle/brachial index, 225
ankle dorsiflexors, paralysis, 65
ankle-foot orthosis (AFO), 552
ankylosing hyperostosis, 541
ankylosing spondylitis, 540–2
   cervical fracture, 254
   hip (clinical case), 71–2
   spine, 64, 254, 260, 540–1
annealing, metal, 500
annulus fibrosus, normal, 240–1
anterior apprehension test, 146
anterior cruciate ligament (ACL)
   anatomy, 202
   deficiency, 105
   injury, 202–5
   repair/reconstruction, 203, 204
   rupture, trauma long case, 457
anterior drawer test, 56, 146, 219
anterior interosseous artery, 41
anterior interosseous nerve injuries, 421
anterior interosseous syndrome, 286
anterior plating technique, hip arthrodesis, 186
anterior talar shift stress test, 219
anterior tarsal tunnel syndrome, 236
antibiotics/antibacterials, 172, 174, 550
antibiotic spacer, infected THA, 173
anti-shock garment, 429
antituberculous drugs, 192
ape-thumb deformity, 37, 39
arcade of Struthers, 31, 287, 288
artery of ligamentum teres, 155
arthritis *see individual joints*
arthritis mutilans, 315
arthrodesis
   ankle, 111, 122, 218–19
   AVN of femoral head, 158
   Beak triple, 386
   distal interphalangeal joint, 44
   elbow, in osteoarthritis, 149
   finger, 317
   Grice, 383
   in hallux rigidus, 115–16, 226
   hip *see* hip, arthrodesis
   ischiofemoral, 192
   knee, 208–9
   proximal interphalangeal joint, 44
   in rheumatoid arthritis, 91, 351
   shoulder, 57–8, 142
   subtalar, 391

thumb base, 306
  in tibial plafond fractures, 444
  triple, 383, 386, 391
  tuberculosis of hip, 102
  wrist, 300, 309–10, 350–1
arthrofibrosis, 518–19
arthrography, hip, 363
  DDH, 363, 367
  infected THA, 171
  painful THA, 97
  Perthes disease, 374
arthrogryposis, 20
arthrogrypotic syndromes, 391–2
arthroplasty, 511–16
  abrasion, 480
  ankle, 217–18
  basic science oral, 516
  bone cement *see* cement
  complications, 153–4, 166–7, 534
  elbow, 149, 154
  excision, tuberculosis of hip, 102
  extracapsular femoral neck fractures, 438
  hemiresurfacing, AVN of femoral head, 158
  hip, 169, 172–3, 511–13
    resurfacing *see below*
    total/revision *see* total hip arthroplasty (THA)
  Keller's excision, 116
  knee
    total, 90, 194–8, 584
    unicompartmental, 199
  MCP, 310
  metatarsophalangeal joint, 226, 235
  patellofemoral joint, 201
  proximal interphalangeal joint, 44
  resection, 143, 169, 173
  resurfacing, hip, 158, 183–4, 513
  resurfacing, patella, 197–8
  resurfacing, shoulder, 153
  shelf, Perthes disease, 373
  shoulder, 142, 153–4
  thumb, 306
  wear debris *see* wear debris
  wrist, 310
arthroscopic procedures, 61, 138, 140, 145,
    149, 217, 409
arthroscopy
  ankle, 215–16
  carpal instability, 326
  shoulder and elbow, 152–3

aseptic loosening, 154, 177
  hip *see* total hip arthroplasty (THA)
  wear debris *see* wear debris
aspirin, DVT prevention, 564–5
atlanto-axial joint injuries/instability, 242, 250–1
atlas (C1), 241–2, 251
atlas (C2) fractures, 251–2
autografts, 179–180, 203, 475
avascular necrosis (AVN), 532–4
  acetabular fractures, 432
  hip arthroplasty and, 534
  hip/femoral head, 93–5, 156–61, 534, 542
    exam questions, 94, 158–9, 160–1, 576
  intracapsular femoral neck fractures, 439
  lunate *see* Kienböck's disease
  osteotomy complication in SUFE, 369
  proximal humeral fractures, 415
  scaphoid non-union, 321, 322
  shoulder, 143
  talar fracture, 452
  traumatic hip dislocation, 434
avulsion injuries, 330, 332–3
axilla, radial nerve palsy causes, 34
axillary artery damage, 415
axis, injuries/fractures, 250, 251–2
axonotmesis, 487

Baciu and Filibiu technique, 218
Bado's classification, Monteggia fracture, 425, 582
Baker's procedure, 382
ballistics, 496–7
Bankart lesion, 146, 412
Bankart procedure/repair, 146, 412
Barton's fracture, 582
basic science oral, 461–565
  candidates' accounts, 571, 576, 578, 583
  information resources, 585
  "top ten" (must know) topics, 461–2
basilar impression, 241
basilar neck fractures, 438
belly press test, 53, 141
bending (biomechanics), 489
Benediction hand (sign), 32, 37, 39, 41
Bennett's fracture, 355
biceps, 57, 60
biceps tendinopathy, 139
bilateral pars (hangman's) fracture, 252
biofilms, 550
biomaterials, 498–504, 511

biomechanics, 215, 452–6, 466, 489–94, 498
  stress/strain curve, 484, 490–1, 494
biopsy, 172, 560
bisphosphonates, 81, 468, 521, 530
Blair technique, ankle arthrodesis, 218
Blatt capsulodesis, 326
Blauth's classification, thumb hypoplasia, 343
blood flow, bone, 469
Blount's disease (tibia vara), 395, 396
bone, 464–8
  cancellous (spongy/trabecular), 466, 475
  cells, 465
  cortical (compact), 465–6, 470, 475
  density, 162
  erosion, tuberculosis of hip, 101
  formation, 465, 467, 469
  growth plate see growth plate/physis
  ligament–bone junction, 486
  matrix, demineralized, 476
  pain, 526, 529
  resorption, 180, 465, 467, 524
  resorption–formation coupling, 470
  subchondral, 212, 478–9
  surgical growth arrest, 47, 373, 378
  tendon insertion, 482
  thermal necrosis, 516
  woven, 466
bone age, determinants, 378
bone banking, 476
bone cement, 174, 440, 514–16
bone cysts, 384, 397, 561
bone graft/grafting, 103, 260, 320, 473–7, 534
  allografts, 474
  autografts, 179–80, 203, 475
  impacting, 179, 180
  vascularised, 157–8, 300, 320, 475–6
bone lining cells, 465, 470
bone marrow, 476
bone marrow oedema syndrome, 533
bone patella tendon bone (BPTB) grafts, 204
bone scan, 95–6, 97, 156, 171, 544–5
bone-specific proteins, 464
bone tumours, 243, 246, 560–3
bony ankylosis, rheumatoid arthritis, 311
Bosworth screw (coracoclavicular screw), 407, 409
Bouchard's nodes, 307
boundary lubrication, 505, 506
boutonnière deformity, 316–17
boutonnière-like deformity thumb, 315

Boyd's classification, 396–7
brachial artery injury, 41, 61
brachial plexus, 31, 32, 40, 337, 583
  injury, 58–61, 337, 338, 340
brachioradialis, testing, 34
bracing, 75, 373, 498
breech presentation, DDH and, 360
Brittain's ischiofemoral arthrodesis, 192
brittle, definition, 490
brittleness, ceramics, 501
Brodie's abscess, 392–3, 577
Brooker classification, heterotopic calcification, 187
Brostrom–Gould repair, 221, 223
Brostrom–Karlsson repair, 221
Brostrom repair, 221, 223
brown tumours, 524, 525
Brunner's incision, 296–7
Bryant's triangle test, 72, 79, 90, 93, 99, 100
Buck–Gramcko classification, thumb hypoplasia, 342–3
Buechel-Pappas™ ankle arthroplasty, 218
bullets, expandable, injuries, 497
burns, full-thickness, compartment syndrome, 451
bursa, 140, 347
bursitis, olecranon, 151–2
burst fractures, 253, 255–6, 257
Butler procedure, 131

C1 (atlas) fractures, 251
C2 fractures, injuries, 250, 251–2
C3 to C7 injuries, 252–4
cadence (steps/minute), 496
Caisson's disease, 94, 533
calcaneal navicular coalition, 123, 390
calcaneal osteotomy, 386
calcaneal sensory nerve branches, 232
calcaneocavus deformity, 120
calcaneonavicular (C-N) coalition, 123, 390
calcaneus, 110, 387
Calcar pivot, 178
calcification, 143, 187, 526, 532
  see also heterotopic ossification (HO)
calcific tendinopathy, 143–4
calcitonin, 468, 472, 521, 523–4, 530
calcium homeostasis/ metabolism, 522, 523, 524
calcium channel blockers, 464
calcium stearate, 502
calcium supplements, osteoporosis, 521
calf/foot pumps, 565
callotasis, 470

camptodactyly, 343, 345
canaliculi, cortical bone, 466
candidates' accounts of examination, 569–86, 587–8
Capener splint, 316, 353
capital physeal femoral neck angle, 369
capitate shortening, 300
capitellum fractures, 419
capitolunate angle, 328
capsulitis, adhesive *see* frozen shoulder
capsulodesis, 32, 326, 335
capsulotomy, elbow osteoarthritis, 149
caput ulnae syndrome, 308
Carney's classification, SUFE, 368
carpal height ratio, 45, 328
carpal injury adaptive (CIA), 324–5
carpal instability, 323–7
carpal instability complex (CIC), 324
carpal instability dissociative (CID), 324
carpal instability non-dissociative (CIND), 324
carpal tunnel, 280–2, 283, 284, 312
carpal tunnel syndrome, 35–7, 282–5, 291
    in rheumatoid arthritis, 24, 308, 312
carpal tunnel syndrome of foot, 236
carpectomy, proximal row, 300
carpometacarpal joint, 303–4, 315
carpus anatomy/ kinematics, 323–4
cartilage, 477–81
    ageing *vs* osteoarthritis, 479
    injury and healing, 213–14, 479–80
"cartilage capped exostosis," 561
casting (metal processing), 500
casting/casts, 498
Catterall's classification, Perthes disease, 372
Catterall's head-at-risk signs, 372, 375
cauda equina syndrome, 247, 265
causalgia, 351–2, 519
cavovarus deformity, 120, 121
cement (bone cement), 174, 440, 514–16
cemented implants
    fractures, 175–7, 183
    rheumatoid arthritis, 92
    in THA, 92, 158, 159, 175, 177–8, 182, 512
cement mantle, 512, 516
cement reaction, 516
cement spacers, antibiotic, 173
central slip extensor tendon, examination, 22
ceramics, 476, 501, 512
cerebral palsy (CP), 126, 379–84, 496, 577
    foot and ankle, 382–3

hands, 383
hip, 381
scoliosis, 245, 381
spine, 381
cervical myelopathy, 68–9, 258–9
cervical radiculopathy, 68–9, 258
cervical rib, 70
cervical spine, 241
    ankylosing spondylitis, 260
    congenital disorders, 241
    degenerative conditions, 258–60
    developmental problems, 242–3
    disc calcification, 242
    facet joint injuries, 252–3
    flexion deformity, 260
    fractures, 252, 253–4
    hyperextension injury, 254
    immobilization, 248, 250
    infections, 260
    instability, 102
    kyphosis, 242
    osteomyelitis, 260
    paediatric pathology, 102, 241–3
    rheumatoid arthritis, 102, 242, 259
    sprains/strains, 254
    surgical approaches, 237
    trauma, 248–54
    tumours, 243, 260
cervical spondylosis, 258
cervical spondylotic myelopathy, 258–9
Charcot foot, 111–12, 233–4
Charcot Marie Tooth disease, 112–13
Charnley approach, 164, 167, 498
Charnley's 'Law of Closed Treatment,' 498
Charnley's technique, cementing, 515
cheilectomy, hallux rigidus, 115, 226
cheiralgia paraesthetica, 293
chemonucleolysis, 268
Chiari osteotomy, 75, 366, 373
chin-on-chest deformity, 260, 540
chondroblastoma, 562
chondrocytes, 471, 477, 479, 480–1, 517
chondrodiastasis, 379
chondroid, 526
chondrolysis, 369, 432, 435
chondromalacia, 478
chondrosarcoma, 563, 576
chordoma, 563
Chrisman–Snook repair, 221

chromosomes, 488
chymopapain, 268
Cincinnati incision, 388
circulation, bone, 468–9
claudication, neurogenic, 265, 266
clavicle
    congenital pseudoarthrosis, 127–8
    distal, resection, 407
    fractures, 406–8
clavicular hook plate, 409
claw hand, 32
    intrinsic minus, 40–1
    ulnar nerve lesion, 32, 40, 291, 574
claw toes, 112, 113–14, 224, 234
clay shoveler's fracture, 252
clean air, theatres, 551
Cleland's ligament, 278
clinical cases
    ankle, 110–25
    candidates' accounts, 570–1, 573–5, 577, 580–1
    elbow, 20, 51–63
    foot, 110–25
    hand, 20–50
    hip, 71–104
    knee, 105–9
    paediatric, 126–31
    shoulder, 20, 51–63
    spine, 64–70
    wrist, 20–50
    see also long cases; short cases; individual topics
clinodactyly, 343–4
clubfoot, 386–9
cobalt chromium, 500
Cobb's angle, 67
Cobra head plate technique, 186
Codman's divisions of proximal humerus, 413
cohort (longitudinal) study, 556
cold working, metals, 500
Coleman block test, 112, 120, 385
collagen, 464, 468, 478, 482, 483
collars, hip arthroplasty, 512
Colles' fracture, 39, 428
Colton's classification, olecranon fractures, 423
column theory, wrist, 324
compartment pressure, normal fascial, 450, 549
compartment syndrome, 450–1, 548–9
    exam questions, 451, 583
    forearm, 424, 426, 451, 549
    hand, 334, 451

lower leg/foot, 450–1, 549
complex regional pain syndrome (CRPS), 284, 351–3, 518, 519–20
compound muscle action potential (CMAP), 487
compression force, 490
compression stockings, 565
computed tomography (CT), 543–4
congenital discoid menisci, 211–12
congenital muscular torticollis, 242
congenital pseudoarthrosis, 127–28, 396–7
congenital radial head dislocation, 128–9
congenital scoliosis, 243
congenital talipes equinovarus (CTEV), 386–9
consent see informed consent
contractures
    brachial plexus injury, 59
    cerebral palsy, 380, 381, 383
    congenital talipes equinovarus, 387
    Dupuytren's see Dupuytren's contracture
    MCP PIP joints, 26, 27
    quadriceps, 382
    soft-tissue, arthrogrypotic syndromes, 391
    Volkmann's see Volkmann's ischaemic contracture
coracoclavicular cerclage, 409
coracoclavicular screw (Bosworth screw), 407, 409
coronoid process fractures, 423
corpectomy, 238
corraline xenograft, 476
correlation coefficient (r), 555
corrosion, 507, 510–11
corticosteroids, 102–3, 145, 249, 336, 464, 472, 521
costotransversectomy, 238
Coventry and Johnson classification, 397
coxa plana see Perthes disease
coxa vara, 375–6
crack propagation, 500
Crankshaft phenomenon, 244
crank test, 43, 304
creep, 490, 508, 515
crevice corrosion, 510
critical analysis, papers, 557
cross body (horizontal) adduction test, 51
cross-sectional study, 556
Crowe classification, dysplastic hip, 162, 163
cubital tunnel, 31, 288
cubital tunnel syndrome, 31, 288–9
cubital valgus, 62
cubitus varus deformity, 32
cuff tear arthropathy, 142

curly toes, 114, 389–90
cyst(s) *see individual cysts*
cysteine proteases, 465
cytokines, 294, 465, 468

dactylitis, 348
Darrach's procedure, 309, 310
data collection, 555–6
data interpretation, 554
De Bastiani Orthofix, 379
Decompression *see individual conditions*
deep flexor-pronator aponeurosis, 31
deep palmar arch, 278
deep peroneal nerve, 233
deep vein thrombosis (DVT), 92, 432, 564–5
deformation, definition, 490, 491
Dellon's sign, 293
delta phalanx, 344
deltoid, testing, 60
dendrites, 486
Denham pin, 498
Denis's three-column theory, 255
dens, fractures, 251–2
dental treatment, prophylactic antibiotics, 174
de Quervain's disease, 355
dermofasciectomy, Dupuytren's disease, 296
dermoid cyst, subungual inclusion, 354
developmental dysplasia of hip (DDH), 68, 71–2,
    86, 360–7
DEXA, osteoporosis, 520
diabetic foot, 114–15, 223–5, 233
diabetic neuropathy, foot, 223–4
diaphyseal aclasis, 561, 575, 580
diaphyseal lengthening/osteotomy, 379
diastematomyelia, 121, 570
digital fascia, 295
1,25-dihydroxycholecalciferol, 467–8, 523
Dimeglio classification, 387–8
dimple sign, knee dislocation, 206
discitis, 263
discography, 266
distal interphalangeal joint (DIP), 44, 313, 316
distal radioulnar joint (DRUJ), 21, 424, 426, 580
distraction osteogenesis, 470
dorsal intercalated segment instability (DISI), 326
dorsal interossei, 30, 62, 277
drapes, theatre, 551
Drennan's (metaphyseal-diaphyseal) angle, 395
drills, screw insertion, 453

drop foot gait (steppage gait), 65
dropped fingers, 23, 25, 311, 314
dual energy X-ray absorptiometry (DEXA), 520
Duchenne's muscular dystrophy, 245
dumb bell tumour, 384
Duncan and Masri classification, 175–6
Dupuytren's contracture, 294, 295, 571
Dupuytren's diathesis, 294
Dupuytren's disease (DD), 26–9, 294–9
    exam questions, 27–9, 295, 298–9, 575
    surgery/management, 26, 295, 296, 298
Durkin's test, 36, 283
duties of care, 559
dwarfism, 246

Eastwood and Cole method, 378
Eaton and Littler classification, 43, 304–5
Ehlers–Danlos syndrome, 363
elastohydrodynamic lubrication, 505
elbow
    arthritis, 148–9
    arthrodesis, 149
    arthrogrypotic syndromes, 392
    arthroplasty, 149, 154
    arthroscopy, 152–3
    aseptic loosening at, 154
    clinical cases, 15, 20, 51–63
    coronoid process fractures, 423
    cubital valgus, 62
    dislocation, 421–2
    flexion test, 289
    fracture dislocation, 422
    golfer's, 151
    injuries, radial head fractures, 422–3
    instability/stability, 150
    joint debridement, 149
    lateral resurfacing procedure, 149
    medial condylar avulsion, 422
    oral core topics, 138–54
    osteoarthritis, 148–9
    pathological conditions, 150–2
    prostheses, 154
    radial nerve palsy causes, 34
    rheumatoid arthritis, 62, 149
    stiff, 61
    tendon transfers at, 335
    tennis, 62–3, 150–1
    ulnar nerve palsy, 31
electrical stimulation, AVN of femoral head, 157

electromyography (EMG), 266–7, 487
electrosurgery, 549–50
embryology, 462–3
"empty can" (Jobe's) test, 53, 56, 141
enchondral ossification, 371, 375, 469
enchondroma, 340, 561
endoneurium, 486
endorphins, 463
Enneking's classification, tumours, 562
enthesopathy, ankylosing spondylitis, 541
eosinophilic granuloma, 562
epicondylectomy, medial, decompression with, 288
epicondylitis
    lateral (tennis elbow), 62–3, 150–1
    medial (golfer's elbow), 151
epidermal inclusion cyst, 340
epineurium, 486, 488
epiphysiodesis, 47, 373, 378
eponychia, 346
Epstein classification, hip dislocation, 433
equinovalgus/equinovarus deformity, 383
equinus deformity, 110, 382, 580
Erb's palsy, 33
erythrocyte sedimentation rate (ESR), 95, 171
ethics, in orthopaedics, 559–60
ethylene oxide, PE sterilization, 503
Evans' classification, 437
Evans procedure, ankle reconstruction, 220–1
Ewing's sarcoma, 563
examinations see FRCS Orth examination
Exeter prosthesis, 89, 182–3, 512
exsanguination, 547
Extended Matching Item (EMI) questions, 5, 9
extensor carpi radialis longus (ECRL), 9, 60–1
extensor digitorum communis, 61, 278
extensor pollicis longus (EPL), 33, 39–40, 428
extensor tendons, hand/wrist, 277, 312–14
extensor tenosynovitis, in RA, 308, 312–14
external fixators, 449

facet syndrome, 267
Fanconi's syndrome, 341, 526
fascial compartment pressure, 450, 549
fascicles, 485, 486, 488
fasciectomy, 26–7, 27–8, 296
fasciotomy, 296, 549
fat emboli, 167, 448
fatigue
    bone cement, 515

metal, 511
fatigue failure, definition, 490, 500
fatigue wear, 507
fat pad, 518
felon, 346
Felty's syndrome, 536
femoral canal, 81, 516
femoral component, 181–2, 184–5
    see also femoral head; femoral stem
femoral epiphysis, ischaemic episodes, 370, 371
femoral fractures
    distal, 441–3
    complications, 442, 443, 456
    trauma long case/oral, 456, 581–2
    neck, 175, 183, 434,
        436–8, 439–41
    periprosthetic, 175–7, 183
    shaft, 432, 434, 577–8
femoral head
    arthroplasty, 181–2, 512–13
    AVN see avascular necrosis (AVN)
    blood supply to, 155, 155, 439
    DDH, 362
    dislocation, 430
    fractures, 434, 435–6
    non-inflammatory idiopathic AVN, 74–7, 370–5
    penetration into acetabular cup, 509
    preparation for THA, 165
    retroversion, 367
    size, wear, 508
femoral neck fractures, 175, 183, 434, 436–8, 439–41
femoral neck line, 369
femoral neck–shaft angle, 511–12
femoral offset, THA, 165, 181
femoral osteotomy see proximal femoral osteotomy
femoral roll-back, 194
femoral shaft fractures, 432, 434, 577–8
femoral stem, 165, 177, 178, 512
    adult and general pathology oral, 179–80
    cemented, 177–8, 182, 512
    cementless, 512
    collar, 512
    design features, 181
    fixation, 512
    fractures around, 175–6
    impaction grafting, subsidence after, 179–80
    loosening, 177–8, 179, 180
    monoblock, 512
    taper polished, 512, 513

femur, 511
  fractures *see* femoral fractures
  in TKA, 196
  in dysplastic hip, 162
Ferguson's approach, hip, 364–5
fibrosarcoma, 563
fibrous ankylosis, hip, 86–7
fibrous dysplasia, 561–2
fibula, absent/dysplastic, 397
fibula hemimelia, 397
fibular grafts, free vascularized, 157–8
Ficat classification, 157, 158–9, 160, 533
finger(s), 278
  abscess, 346
  arthrodesis, 317
  avulsion injuries, 332–3
  boutonnière deformity, 316–17
  contractures, in CP, 383
  dropped, in rheumatoid arthritis, 23, 25
  extensors, 33
  flexion, tendon transfer, 38
  lateral plane deformity, 343–4
  mallet, 333
  osteomyelitis, 347
  rugger jersey, 355
  squamous cell carcinoma, 340
  trigger, 48–9, 335–7
fingertip injuries, 333, 355
Fisk graft, 320
Fitton's operation, 221
fixation
  ACJ dislocation, 409
  antegrade locked intramedullary nails, 416
  biomechanics of implants, 452–6
  bone screws, 442, 452–4, 581
  cancellous screws, 453
  clavicle fractures, 407
  compression plate/screws, 416
  condylar blade plate, 442
  condylar buttress plate, distal femoral
     fractures, 442
  coracoclavicular screw (Bosworth screw), 407, 409
  distal humeral fractures, 419–20
  distal radius fractures, 427
  dynamic hip screw (DHS), 581
  external, 209, 407, 417, 425, 429, 442, 444, 449–50
  femoral neck fractures, 437–8, 439–40
  forearm fractures, 425
  hook systems, thoracolumbar spine injuries, 258

humeral shaft fracture, 417, 416–17
internal, 254, 416–17, 419–20, 442, 560–1
intramedullary implants, 448
intramedullary nailing, 209, 407, 416–17, 425, 448–9,
  455–6
K-wires, contraindication, 409
LISS plate, distal femoral fractures, 442
locking screws, intramedullary, 448
nailing *see* fixation, intramedullary nailing
non-reamed locked intramedullary nails, 417
ORIF
  acetabular fractures, 431–2
  carpal instability, 327
  clavicle fractures, 407
  intracapsular femoral neck fractures, 440
  proximal humeral fractures, 414
  scaphoid fractures, 319–20
  tibial plafond fractures, 444
pedicle screw systems, 258
pelvic ring fractures, 429
plates, 209, 407, 442, 454–5
proximal humeral fractures, 414
retrograde intramedullary nails, 417, 442
scaphoid fractures, 319–20
screws, 442, 452–4, 581
sliding hip screw-plate system, 437–8
Steinmann pin, 351, 409, 498
tibial plafond fractures, 444
transarticular sliding hip screw, 186
wrist arthrodesis, 351
fixators, 449
flexion contractures, 336, 382
flexion deformity, congenital (camptodactyly),
  343, 345
flexor carpi ulnaris (FCU), 30, 31
flexor contractures, causes, 336
flexor digitorum profundus (FDP), 22, 30, 280, 330, 580
flexor digitorum superficialis (FDS), 22, 278, 280
  injury, short case, 580
  paralysis, 39
  tenodesis, 318
  testing, 38
flexor pollicis longus (FPL), 22, 38, 39
flexor pulleys, fingers and thumb, 276
flexor retinaculum, 280
flexor sheath infections, 347
flexor tendon(s)
  hand/wrist, 22, 284, 312–14, 330
  injuries, 312–14, 329, 330–1

flexor tenosynovitis, 308, 312, 314
floating shoulder, 408
fluid film lubrication, 505, 506
foot
  arthrogrypotic syndromes, 392
  biomechanics, 215
  cerebral palsy, 382–3
  Charcot, 111–12, 233–4
  clinical cases, 16, 110–25
  compartment syndrome, 451, 549
  deformities, 110
  diabetic, 114–15, 223–5
  equinus deformity, 110, 382, 580
  everted, 110
  gout, 539
  inverted, 110
  Lisfranc injury, trauma long case, 456–7
  movement testing, 67–8
  nerve supply, 232–3
  neuropathic, in diabetes, 115, 223–4
  oral core topics, 215–36
  prosthetic, 553
  rheumatoid arthritis, 121–2, 234–5, 583
  syllabus on, 215
  talipes equinovarus, 386–9
  valgus/varus deformity, 110, 112
  see also forefoot; hindfoot; toe
foot progression angle (FPA), 399
foot thigh angle (FTA), 395, 400
forearm
  compartment syndrome, 450–1, 548–9
  fractures, 424–7
  surgical approaches, 425, 426
forefoot
  rheumatoid arthritis, 90, 235
Forestier's disease (ankylosing hyperostosis), 541
forging, metal, 500
"fracture of necessity," 426
fractures
  avoidance in plate removal, 454
  healing, blood flow role, 469
  malunion, 407–8, 415, 449
  non-operative management, 497–8
  non-union, 407, 417, 426, 439, 449
  pathological, 525, 527, 561
  *see also individual fractures and types
    of fractures*
Frankel grading system, 248
FRCS Orth examination, 3

alternative view of, 590
candidates' accounts, 569–86, 587–8
clinical cases *see* clinical cases
failure, 587–90
general guidance, 3–6
  hand oral, 274
  long cases, 17–18
  orals, 135–7
  paediatrics oral, 359
  short cases, 13–14
  written paper, 9–10
general observations, 586
information sources, 584–6
marking *see* marking of examination
new format (2007), 5, 9–10, 13–14, 17–18
orals *see* oral examinations
pass mark, 587, 588
repeating/new attempt, 589
results, 584, 587–8
syllabus, 215, 273–4, 461
written *see* written examination
free body diagrams, 492, 494
free radicals, 294, 503, 504
fretting corrosion, 510
fretting wear, 507
friction/ frictional force, 504
Froment's sign/test, 30, 289
frozen sections, infected THA, 172
frozen shoulder, 55, 144–5, 580
Frykman classification, 427

Gage's prerequisites, normal gait, 496
Gage's sign, 372, 375
gait, 494–6
  antalgic, 72, 76, 93, 115
  cerebral palsy, 380, 382, 383
  cervical myelopathy, 68
  equinus, 65
  genu varum, 395
  normal, Gage's prerequisites, 496
  Perthes disease, 76, 371
  Steppage (drop foot), 65, 112
  Trendelenburg, 66
  tuberculosis of hip, 101
  waddling, DDH, 361
Galeazzi fracture, 426
Galeazzi's sign, 78, 99, 361, 366
Galeazzi's test, 72, 90, 93, 100
gallium-67 citrate scan, 171, 545

galvanic corrosion, 510
gamekeeper's thumb, 315
gamma sterilization, 503
ganglion, 49–50, 302, 303, 582
Ganz osteotomy, 366
Garden classification, femoral neck fractures, 439
Garrod's pads, 27, 294
gate theory of pain, 463
Gaucher's disease, 533
Gauvain's sign, 100
gene(s)/genetics, 488
genetic disorders, types, 489
gentamicin, 516
genu valgum, 66, 393–4
genu varum, 394–6
Gerber's lift off test, 53, 141
giant cell response, wear debris after THA, 177
giant cell tumours, 5, 340, 562
gigantism, 396
Gilula's lines, 325, 327
glenohumeral joint, 55–6, 142, 411, 412–13
glenoid fossa fracture, 406
glenoid fracture, 146, 406, 412
gliding zone, cartilage, 478
glomus tumour, 340, 354
gluteus maximus, testing, 67
glycosaminoglycans (GAGs), 478
golfer's elbow, 151
gout, 46, 537–9
Graf hip angle measurement, 361, 361–2
grafts
    ACL injury management, 203, 204
    bone *see* bone graft/grafting
    hamstring/quadriceps, 204
granulation tissue, 144, 392
granuloma, 183, 562
Grayson's ligament, 278, 295
greater trochanter, 169, 373
Green–Anderson tables, 377
Grice arthrodesis, 383
grind test, 20, 43, 304
groove of Ranvier, 471
ground reaction/reactive force, 492, 496
growth factors, 462, 465, 472–3
growth plate/physis, 276, 469, 470–3
Guhl arthroscopic classification, 213
Guyon's canal, 287, 289, 290
Guyon's canal compression syndrome,
    31–2, 289–91

haemarthrosis, acute, ACL injury *vs*, 203
haematoma, THA complication, 166
haemochromatosis, arthritis, 307
haemophilia, 534
haemorrhage, 429, 166
haemorrhagic phase, tendon healing, 483
hallux rigidus, 115–16, 225–7, 571
hallux valgus, 116–17, 227–30
    exam questions, 117–18, 234, 229–30, 575, 577, 583
halo vest, complications, 260
hammer toe, 234
hamstrings, 67, 204, 382, 441
hand(s), 276
    arthrogrypotic syndromes, 392
    bands/cords, 27, 277, 295
    blood supply, 278–9
    cerebral palsy, 383
    clinical cases, 20–50
    compartment syndrome, 334, 451
    congenital deformities, 341–5
    examination, 3, 21–2
    exam questions, 15–16, 21, 273, 274, 293
    gout, 46, 539
    human bites, 347–8
    infections, 345–8
    intrinsic minus, 40–1
    intrinsic positive, 41
    ligaments, 277, 278
    muscles, 22, 276–7
    oral core topics, 276–355
    osteoarthritis, 44
    paediatrics, 274
    pigmented villonodular synovitis, 353–4
    rheumatoid arthritis *see* rheumatoid arthritis
    scars, 21
    SLE, 543
    small muscle wasting, 41, 112, 287
    splinting, 353
    surgery, training, 273
    swelling, 354
    trauma, 42, 274
    tumours, 21, 340
hand oral, 40, 42, 271–355
    candidates' accounts, 572–3, 575–6, 578, 582
    core topics, 276–355
    general guidance, 274
    syllabus, 273–4
hand washing, 552
Hangman's fracture, 252

Harrington rods, 244, 257, 261

Harris classification, of loosening, 98

Harrold and Walker classification, 388

Hawkins' classification, talar fractures, 452

Hawkin's sign, 139, 452

healing, biology, 329, 469, 479–80, 483

Heberden's nodes, 43, 44, 307, 517

Heikel's classification, 341

hemiarthroplasty

    femoral head/neck, 158, 438, 439, 440

    shoulder, 142, 153, 153–4, 414

Herring lateral pillar classification, 372

heterotopic ossification (HO), 92, 167, 187–8, 432, 435, 532

Heuter–Volkmann law (of growth plate), 470

high-pressure injection injuries, 334

high tibial osteotomy (HTO), 108, 207–8, 571

Hilgenreiner's epiphyseal angle (HEA), 376

Hill model, 485

Hill-Sachs lesion, 146, 147, 412

hindfoot, 234, 235, 387, 389

hip, 155–6

    angle measurement (Graf), 361–2

    arthrodesed, 84–7

    arthrodesis, 102, 173, 185–7, 192

    arthrogrypotic syndromes, 392

    arthroplasty *see* total hip arthroplasty (THA)

    aspiration, 96, 97, 171

    AVN *see* avascular necrosis (AVN)

    in cerebral palsy, 381

    clinical cases, 71–104

    disarticulation, short case, 580

    dislocation, 433–6, 457

    dysplastic, 162–3, 362

        see also development dysplasia of hip (DDH)

    examination, short case, 574

    fibrous ankylosis, 86–7

    free body diagram, 492

    infections/sepsis, 78, 79

    instability, 78, 98

    migration index, 381

    movements, measuring, 67, 84–5

    oral core topics, 155–93

    osteoarthritis, 87–9, 185, 581, 583

    osteotomy, 188–90

    outcome measurements, 193

    pain, 75, 77–8, 79, 80, 87, 96–7, 191

        referred, 76, 78

    post-traumatic OA, 82–4, 435

pseudoarthrosis, 85

PVNS, 190–1

reduction, of DDH, 364

resurfacing articulations, 143, 169, 173, 158, 183–4

revision surgery, 77–80

rheumatoid arthritis, 25, 307, 535–7

rotation, range (Staheli), 399

screw in joint, checking, 369

sensation testing, 79

short case list, 16

stiffness, 78, 88, 89

surgical approaches, 186, 364–5

surgical fusion, short case, 580

total arthroplasty *see* total hip arthroplasty (THA)

traumatic dislocation, 433–6, 457

tuberculosis, 85, 99–102, 191–2

valgus/varus, 493

windswept, 381–2

hip joint capsule, 435

    DDH, 362

    fractures within, 435

hip ratio measurement, 361

hip screw, 186, 437–8, 581

    history-taking, 17–18

HIV infection, 533

HLA-B27, 540

Hoffer classification, ambulation potential, 380

Hoffman–Tinel sign, 487

Holstein–Lewis fracture, 291, 416, 580

hook systems, thoracolumbar spine injuries, 258

hormone(s), effects on growth plate, 472–3

hormone replacement therapy (HRT), 521

hot pressing, metal, 500

Hueston's tabletop test, 27, 295

human bites, hand, 347–8

humeral head, 412, 413

humeral shaft fracture, 291, 415–1

humerus, distal, fractures, 418–21, 582

humerus, proximal, 413, 414

    fractures, 413–15

hydrodynamic lubrication, 505, 506

hydrostatic lubrication, 506

hydrostatic pressure theory, Perthes disease, 371

hyperbaric oxygen therapy, 157

hypercalcaemia, 522

hyperextension injury, cervical spine, 254

hyperparathyroidism, 524, 525

hypersensitivity, metal, 183, 500–1

hypertrophic zone, growth plate, 471, 472

hypocalcaemia, 522–3
hypophosphataemia, 527–8
hypophosphatasia, 526, 528
hypovolaemic shock, 248
hysteresis, 490

iliopsoas tendon, 67, 362
Ilizarov fixator, 217, 218, 389
Ilizarov frame (circular), 379, 580
immunoglobulin G indium scan, infected THA, 171
impaction grafting, 179–80
impingement, definition, 52
impingement syndrome, 55, 139
impingement tests, 52
implants, 452–6, 511
incidence, definition, 555
inclusion corrosion, 511
indium-111-labelled white cell scan, 171, 545
infantile and juvenile scoliosis, 244–5
infections, 551
    acetabular fractures, 432
    control, 550–1, 551–2
    forearm fracture, 426
    intramedullary fixation complication, 448
    leg length discrepancy, 377
    rheumatoid arthritis, 92
    THA, 95–6, 166, 169–75
information resources, 584–6
informed consent for surgery, 559–60
    Dupuytren's disease surgery, 295–6
    hip arthrodesis, 187
    interdigital neuroma, 232
    partial fasciectomy, 26–7, 27–8
    total hip arthroplasty, 89, 164
infraspinatus tendon/muscle, 53, 60,141
inheritance, mechanisms, 489
innominate osteotomy, 75, 365–6, 373
instruments, sterilization, 551
insulin, 473
interdigital neuroma, 231–2
intergranular corrosion, 511
intermembranous ossification, 469
interosseous muscles, 29, 277
interphalangeal (IP) joints, osteoarthritis, 44
intertrochanteric fractures, 436
intervertebral disc, 240–1
    calcification, cervical spine, 242
    degenerative disease, 240–1, 268
    prolapse, 246–7, 258, 264, 265

replacement, 267
    spinal stenosis due to, 268
intoeing, 394, 399, 400, 582
intramedullary nailing *see under* fixation
ischaemic ulcer, diabetic foot, 115, 224, 225
ischiofemoral arthrodesis, 192
isokinetic/isometric contraction, muscles, 485
isostatic moulding, UHMWPE, 502–3
isotonic contraction, muscles, 485

Jackson's classification, cartilage degeneration, 479
Jeanne's sign, 289
Jobe's ("empty can") test, 53, 56, 141
Johansson classification, 175
joint levelling procedures, 300
joint reaction force (JRF), 492–3
Jones classification, tibia hemimelia, 398
Jones procedure, 113, 386
Jones transfer (tendon transfer), 34
juvenile chronic arthritis, 577
juvenile rheumatoid arthritis, 102–3, 242

Kalamchi classification, tibia hemimelia, 398
Kanavel's cardinal signs, 347
Kaplan–Meier survival analysis, 557
Kaplan's cardinal line, 278, 281
KAPPA analysis, 555
Keller's excision arthroplasty, 116, 226
Kienböck's disease, 44–5, 299–302, 531
Kirk Watson's test, 21, 45, 325, 327
Kirner's deformity, 344
kite's talocalcaneal angle, 388
Kleinman shear test, 325
Kline's line, 368
Klippel–Feil syndrome, 128, 242
Klumpke's palsy, 33, 40
knee
    arthritis, 86, 108, 194
    arthrodesis, 208–9
    arthrogrypotic syndromes, 392
    articular cartilage injury, 213–14
    clinical cases, 16, 105–9
    clinical examination, 214
    dislocation, 206–7
    extension/flexion, testing, 67
    fixed flexion deformity, 197, 392
    flexion contracture, cerebral palsy, 382
    fracture/subluxation, 214
    free body diagram, 493, 494

knee (*cont.*)
  knock-knee deformity
  oral core topics, 194–214
  osteoarthritis, 105–7, 570
  pain, 90, 582
  pigmented villonodular synovitis, 108
  previous high tibial osteotomy, 108
  rheumatoid arthritis, 108
  stiffness after femoral fracture, 441, 443
  total arthroplasty, 90, 194–8, 584
  unicompartmental replacement, 199
  valgus, 108, 198–9, 208
  varus, medial release, 197
Kocher–Langenbeck approach, extended, 432
KT 1000, ACL reconstruction, 204
K-wires, contraindication, 409
kyphosis, 242, 243, 259, 262

Lachman's test, 202
lacunae, cortical bone, 466
lag screws, 442, 453
lag sign tests, rotator cuff tears, 53
lambda value, 505
lamellae, bone, 466, 470
laminar flow, theatre, 551
Langenskiold's classification, tibia vara, 395
lateral column procedure, elbow osteoarthritis, 149
lateral mass compression fracture, 252, 254
lateral patella compression syndrome, 202
lateral plantar nerve, 232
Lauenstein view, SUFE, 369
Lauge-Hansen classification, ankle fractures, 445
leaching corrosion, 511
Leffert classification, 337, 338
Legg-Calvé-Perthes disease, 370
leg length discrepancy, 376–9
  DDH, 72, 361
  hip needing revision surgery, 78–9
  Perthes disease, 74
  post-traumatic OA of hip, 83
  protrusio acetabulum, 99
  SUFE, 90
  THA complication, 166
leg lengthening procedures, 379, 470
leiomyosarcoma, 563–4
Letournel and Judet classification, 431
leucocyte scan, 171, 545
Lichtman classification, 299, 301

life table, 557
ligament(s), 486
  ankle, 219
  carpal, 323
  contractures, CTEV, 387
  hand, 277, 278
  stress/strain curve, 484
  thumb, 304
  wrist, 323
  see also individual ligaments
ligament–bone junction, 486
ligamentous laxity, DDH aetiology, 360
ligament reconstruction/tendon interposition, 305–6
ligamentum teres, DDH, 362
limb
  embryology, 462
  ischaemia, 339
  length discrepancy *see* leg length discrepancy
  lengthening, 379, 470
limp, 88, 99, 361, 368, 376
linear wear, 508
lipoma, forearm, 293
liposarcoma, 563
Lisfranc injuries, trauma long case, 456–7
LISS plate, 442
Littler procedure, 317
load/deformation, definition, 491
Loder classification, SUFE, 368
long cases, 17–18
  candidates' accounts, 570, 573–4, 577, 581
  list (possible cases), 19
  marking, 4
  old *vs* new format, 17, 77
  pass mark, 4, 588
longitudinal (cohort) study, 556
loose body, ankle, 220
Looser's zones, 526, 528
lordosis, loss, 259
low-back pain, 264
lower limb, 19
  arthrogrypotic syndromes, 391
  compartment syndrome, 450–1, 549
  motor and sensory testing, 67–8
low-molecular-weight heparin (LMWH), 565
lubrication, 504–7
lumbar spinal stenosis, 265–7
lumbar spine, 264
lumbrical muscles, anatomy, 276

lunate
  avascular necrosis *see* Kienböck's disease
  dislocation, 324, 327
lunotriquetral ligament (LTL), 21, 326
luxatio, 411, 412

Madelung's deformity, 46–8, 50
Maffucci's syndrome, 561
magnetic resonance imaging (MRI), 546
main-en-griffe *see* claw hand
Maisonneuve fracture, 445
malignant fibrous histiocytoma (MFH), 563
malleoli, 394, 445–6
mallet finger, 333
malunion of fractures, 407–8, 415, 449
manipulation (under anaesthesia), 145, 226, 250
Mannerfelt lesion, 23
Mannerfelt–Norman syndrome, 286, 314
marble bone disease (osteopetrosis), 531
Marfan's syndrome, 245
marking of examination, 4, 9
Mason's classification, 422
Matev procedure, 317
matrix metalloproteinases (MMPs), 294, 517
Mayfield classification, 324, 327
McCash open technique, 297
McDaniel's rule of thirds, 203
McMurray test, 212
medial plantar nerve, 232
median nerve, 279–80
  decompression, 283
  entrapment, 285, 487
    see also carpal tunnel syndrome
  injuries, 421–2, 427
  lesions, irritation, testing, 36, 37–9
  palsy, causes, 39
  tendon transfer, 335
median nerve compression test, 36, 283
medical negligence, 560
melanoma, amelanotic, 354
Mendelian inheritance, 489
meniscus, 209–12
metabolic bone diseases, 522
metacarpophalangeal (MCP) joints
  boutonnière-like deformity, 315
  contracture, measurement, 26, 27
  hyperextension, 40, 306, 315
  replacement, 310
  rheumatoid arthritis, 23, 24, 310

metal
  allergy/hypersensitivity, 183, 500–1
  corrosion/fatigue, 510–11
  particles, 183, 509
  processing, 500
metal-on-metal hip resurfacing, 183–4
metal-on-metal prosthetic implantation, 501
metaphyseal blanch sign of Steel, 368
metaphyseal-diaphyseal angle, genu varum, 395
metaphyseal–epiphyseal system, 468
metastatic bone disease, 560–1
metatarsophalangeal joint (MTP), 234, 235
  degenerative arthritis, 115–116, 225–7, 571
  lateral deviation *see* hallux valgus
Meyerding classification, 247
microelastohydrodynamic lubrication, 506
microfracture, cartilage defect management, 480
midcarpal instability assessment, 21
middle finger extension test, 63, 292
midhumerus, radial nerve palsy causes, 34
Milch classification, distal humeral fractures, 419
mithramycin, Paget's disease, 530
moment (force), 492
monoclonal antibodies, radiolabelled, 545
monosodium urate crystals, 537, 538, 539
Monteggia fracture, 425, 582
mosaicism, 489
mosaicplasty, 480
Moseley straight line method, 377
motor nerve testing, 22, 30, 67–8, 487
moulding, UHMWPE, 502
mucin, 49, 302
mucous cyst, 303
multiple choice questions (MCQs), 9, 10, 274
  FRCS (Tr & Orth) Exam, 569–70, 573
multiple myeloma, 562–3
muscle(s), 484
  contraction, 485
  ischaemia, tourniquet-induced, 548
  spasm, 85, 100
  transfers, 409, 486
muscle relaxants, 464
muscle–tendon junction, 485–6
myelodysplasia, scoliosis, 245
myelography, 249, 266
myofibroblast, Dupuytren's disease, 294, 295
myonephropathic metabolic syndrome, 548
myositis ossificans, 420, 532
myositis ossificans progressiva, 532

nail, 278
   infections, 346
nail bed, pigmented lesion, 354
Nalebuff and Millender classification, 316
Nalebuff's classification, 315, 318
neck stiffness, ankylosing spondylitis, 64
needle biopsy, infected THA, 171
Neer's classifications, 140, 406, 413
Neer's impingement test, 139
Neer's sign/test, 52, 139
negative predictive value, 555
neocapsule tissue reaction, 183
neoplasia *see* tumours
nerve(s), 486–8
   injuries, 166, 412, 414–15, 421–2, 426, 429 487–8
   supply, ankle and foot, 232–3
nerve blocks, 464
nerve roots, 58, 279, 286, 288
neural trauma, cervical spine, 249
neurapraxia, 487
neurofibromatosis, 245, 384–5
neurogenic claudication, 265, 266
neurological examination, hand, 22
neuroma, interdigital, 231–2
neuromuscular scoliosis, 245
neuropathic arthropathy, Charcot foot, 111–12
neuropathic foot, diabetes, 115, 223–4
neuropathic foot disease, 111–12, 233–4
neuropathic ulcer, 115, 224, 225
neuropathy, 115, 488
neurotmesis, 488
neurovascular compromise/injuries, 408, 449
Newton's laws, 492
nickel sensitization, 501
nightstick fracture, 425–6
non-parametric tests, 553
non-steroidal anti-inflammatory drugs
    (NSAIDs), 463
Noyes' rule of thirds, ACL injury, 203

oblique retinacular ligament (ORL), 277
occipital condyle fractures, 250
occiput, injuries, 250
odontoid anomalies, 242
oestrogen therapy, osteoporosis, 521
olecranon bursitis, 151–2
olecranon fractures, 423
olecranon groove, ulnar nerve compression, 31
Ollier's disease, 561

operating theatre, design and practice, 551–2
oral core topics
   foot and ankle, 215–36
   hand, 276–355
   hip, 155–93
   knee, 194–214
   shoulder and elbow, 138–54
oral examinations, 135–7
   adult *see* general orthopaedics and pathology oral
   basic science *see* basic science oral
   candidates' accounts, 571–3, 575–9, 581–4
   format, 581
   hands *see* hand oral
   marking, 4
   paediatric *see* paediatrics oral
   specialist questions, 137
   trauma *see* trauma oral
ORIF *see under* fixation
orthopaedic diseases, long case list, 19
orthoroentgenogram, 378
orthoses, 552
Ortolani's test, 361, 367
ossification, 465, 467, 469
   enchondral, 371, 375, 469
   heterotopic *see* heterotopic ossification (HO)
osteoarthritis, 432, 479, 516–18
   ankle, 118–19
   base of thumb, 42–3, 303–7
   elbow, 148–9
   glenohumeral, 55–6
   hand, 44
   hip, 87–89, 185, 581, 583
   knee, 105–7, 570
   post-trauma *see* post-traumatic osteoarthritis
   shoulder, clavicle fractures, 408
   small joint, 307
osteoblastoma, 562
osteoblasts, 465, 466, 467, 470
osteochondral plugs, 480
osteochondritis *see* osteochondroses
osteochondritis dissecans (OCD), 212–14, 531
osteochondroma, 561
osteochondroses, 531–2
osteoclasts, 465, 467, 470, 528, 531
osteoconductive properties, bone graft, 474
osteocytes, 465, 533
osteogenesis imperfecta, 246
osteoid, 465, 526
osteoid osteoma, 562

osteoinductive properties, bone graft, 474
osteoligamentous trauma, 249, 250
osteoma, osteoid, 562
osteomalacia, 521, 526
osteomyelitis, 246, 260, 347
osteonecrosis *see* avascular necrosis (AVN)
osteopetrosis, 531
osteophytes, 88, 118
osteoporosis, 191, 520–1
osteoprogenitor cells, 465
osteoprotegerin (OPG), 470
osteosarcoma, 563
osteosclerosis, 525
osteotomy, 188–90
  base of thumb, 305
  calcaneal, 386
  Chiari, 75, 366, 373
  closed wedge HTO, 208
  closing wedge, proximal phalanx, 115, 226
  diaphyseal, 379
  dysplastic hip, 162
  Ganz, 366
  high tibial, 108, 207–8, 571
  hip, 188–90
  innominate, 75, 365–6, 373
  intertrochanteric (Kramer), 369
  open wedge HTO, 207–8
  pelvic, 188, 189, 365–6
  Pemberton, 365
  proximal femoral *see* proximal femoral
      osteotomy
  radial, 300
  rheumatoid arthritis, 91
  rotational, radio-ulnar synostosis, 130
  Salter innominate, 365
  Steel triple innominate, 365–6
  in SUFE, 369, 370
  trochanteric, 81, 103, 164
  valgus, 75, 189–90, 373
  varus, 75, 189, 208
Otto's pelvis (idiopathic protrusio), 162
outcome measures/measurements, 193, 553
Outerbridge-Kashiwagi (OK) procedure, 149
outtoeing, causes, 399
over-riding fifth toe, 131

paediatric clinical cases, 126–31
paediatric orthopaedics
  hand, 274

long case list, 19
short case list, 16
spine, pathology, 240–1
paediatrics oral, 359–400
  candidates' accounts, 572–3, 575–6,
      577–8, 582
Paget's disease, 80–2, 528–30
pain, 463–4
  back, 264
  bone, 526, 529
  compartment syndrome, 450, 549
palmar erythema, in rheumatoid arthritis, 25
palmar interossei, 30, 277
palmar space infections, 347
Panton-Valentine leukocidin (PVL), 551
Pappas classification, 213
paralysis, orthoses, 552
parametric tests, 553
parathyroid hormone (PTH), 467–8, 472, 523
  recombinant (teriparatide), 521
parathyroid-related peptide, 471
paronychia, 346
passivation, 500, 510
patella
  anterior displacement, after TKA, 197
  fractures, traumatic hip dislocation with, 434
  instability, 200–2
  malalignment, 200
  realignment, 201
  resurfacing, 197–8
patella baja, 198
patellectomy, 202
patellofemoral joint (PFJ), 197, 200–2
patient-based measures outcome, 193
Pauwels' classification, 439
Pavlik harness, 363–4
pedicle screw systems, 258
pelvic obliquity, 66, 72, 84, 100
pelvic osteotomy, 188, 189, 365–6
pelvic ring fractures, 428–30
Pemberton osteotomy, 365
"pencil in cup" deformity, 307, 540
perichondral ring of Lacroix, 471
perilunate dislocation, acute, 326–7
periosteal release, 379
periosteal system, bone circulation, 468–9
periosteum, 466
peripheral nerves, 487
  injuries, 33, 488

peripheral neuropathy, causes, 115
periprosthetic femoral fractures, 175–7, 183
Perkins traction, 499
peroneal nerve palsy/injury, 65
Perthes disease, 74–7, 370–5
pes cavovarus, 570
pes cavus, 110, 119–21, 385–6
pes planus, 110
PET (positron emission tomography), 545
Peyronie's disease, 26, 27, 294
Phalen's sign, 36, 283
phosphate, 522
phosphate diabetes, 526, 527
physeal distraction, 379
physeal injuries, 471
physeal line, 369
physeal–metaphyseal junction, 471
physiotherapy, 145, 147, 391
physis, 276, 469, 470–3
piano key sign test, 21, 308
pigmented villonodular synovitis (PVNS), 108, 190
    hand, 353–4
    hip, 190–1
pillar pain, 284
pilon fractures, tibial, 443–4, 446
pinch test, 313
Pipkin classification, hip dislocation, 433
Pirani scoring system, 387
piriformis syndrome/test, 76
pistoning behaviour, 177–8
pitting, corrosion, 510
pivot shift test, ACL, 203
plantar release, in pes cavus, 386
plaster slabs, 498
platelet-derived growth factor (PDGF), 474
plates/plating, 209, 407, 442, 454–5
PMMA, 514, 516
polio, 65–6
Pollock's test, 287, 289
polyethylene, 502, 503, 504
polymethyl methacrylate, 514, 516
Ponseti casting technique, 388
popliteal cyst, 399
positive predictive value, 555
positron emission tomography (PET), 545
posterior apprehension test, 146
posterior cruciate ligament (PCL), 205
    injury, 107–8, 205–6
    in knee arthroplasty, 194, 195

    reconstruction/repair, 205–6, 575
posterior drawer test, 146, 205
posterior interosseous nerve (PIN), 291–2
    palsy, 23, 25, 34, 426, 577
posterior lip augmentation device (PLAD), 169, 513
posterior tibial nerve, 232
postlaminectomy deformity, 262
post-tourniquet syndrome, 548
post-traumatic kyphosis, 262
post-traumatic osteoarthritis
    ankle, 216
    elbow, 149
    hip, 82–4, 435
    knee, 107
pre-axial polydactyly (thumb duplication), 342, 344
pre-ganglionic injury, 338
press fit designs, femoral component, 182
prevalence, definition, 555
probability (statistical), 555
proliferative zone, growth plate, 471, 472
pronator syndrome, 285
pronator teres, testing, 38
pronator teres syndrome, 39
prostheses, 498–504, 553
proteoglycans, 464, 478
protrusio acetabulum, 81, 92, 98–9, 161–2
proximal femoral osteotomy, 158, 188, 189, 190
    THA after, 190
    types, 189–90
    valgus, 75, 189–90
    varus, 75, 189, 365, 373
proximal humeral fractures, 413–15
proximal interphalangeal (PIP) joint
    arthrodesis/arthoplasty, 44
    boutonnière deformity, 316
    contracture, incomplete correction, 27
    Dupuytren's disease, 295, 297–9
proximal tibial osteotomy (HTO), 108, 207–8, 571
pseudoarthrosis, 85, 127–8
pseudogout, 539
pseudostability test, 21, 325
pseudotumours, 183
psoriatic arthropathy, 25, 94, 307, 540
pulses, 22, 25, 387

Q angle, 201, 494
quadriceps, 67, 382, 398
quadriceps active drawer sign/test, 107, 205
quadriceps graft, 204

quadrigia effect, hand, 22, 40

radial artery, 278–9, 306
radial bursa, infections, 347
radial club hand, 341, 345
radial head
  congenital dislocation, 128–9
  excision, elbow RA, 149
  fractures, 422–3
radial hemimelia, 341
radial nerve
  compression, 291, 293, 487
  injuries, 291, 415, 417, 418, 421–2
  palsy, 32–5
  tendon transfers, 335
radial side wrist pain (RSWP), 20
radial tunnel syndrome, 151, 292–3
radial ulnar synostosis, 426
radiography, 6, 543
radiology, 543–7
radionuclides, 544
radionuclide scans, 95–6, 97, 156, 171, 544–5
radio-ulnar joint instability, RA, 308
radio-ulnar synostosis, 129–31
radius
  fractures, 39, 422–4, 426, 427–8
  growth plate, epiphysiodesis, 47
ram extrusion, 502
randomized controlled trials (RCT), 556
range (statistics), 49, 554
Reagan's ballottement, 21, 325
reflex sympathetic dystrophy (RSD), 519
Regan and Morrey classification, 423
regression (statistics), 555
renal metastases, 263
renal osteodystrophy, 525–6
resection synostosis, radio-ulnar synostosis, 130
reserve zone, growth plate, 471, 472
resisted active supination test, 292
resisted wrist extension test, 63
resurfacing arthroplasty see arthroplasty
retinacular ligaments, 277
revision arthroplasty, hip see total hip
    arthroplasty (THA)
rhabdomyosarcoma, 564
rheumatoid arthritis, 25, 307, 535–7
  ankle, 216–19
  bony ankylosis, 311
  carpal tunnel syndrome, 24, 308, 312

cervical spine, 259
differential diagnosis, 537
elbow, 62, 149
foot, 90, 121–2, 234–5
hand and wrist, 22–5, 307–12
  boutonnière deformity, 314, 316–17
  exam questions, 24, 311–12, 314, 537
  flexor/extensor tendons, 312–14
  swan-neck deformity, 315, 317–18
  syllabus, 274
  thumb, 314–316
  trigger finger, 24, 49
hip, 90–2
history, 308
juvenile, 102–3, 242
knee, 108
long case, 573–4
posterior interosseous nerve palsy, 25
short case question, 25, 537
shoulder, 143
thumb, 314–16
rheumatoid factor, 536
rheumatoid nodules, 308
rhomboids, testing, 60
rickets, 521, 526–8
ring avulsion injuries, 332–3
ring sign, 325, 328
Riseborough and Radin classification, 419
Rockwood classification, 408
rotational profile, assessment, 399–400
rotator cuff muscles, 406, 413, 415
rotator cuff tears, 52–5, 139, 140–2, 142–3, 412
  short cases, 54–5, 570–1
row theory, wrist, 324
Rüedi and Allgöwer classification, 443
rugger jersey finger, 355
rule of thirds, ACL injury, 203
Russe graft, 320
Russell traction, 499
Ryder method, femoral anteversion, 399–400

sacroiliac joint, 428, 541, 542
sagittal band, 277
Salter's innominate osteotomy, 365
Salter–Thomas classification, Perthes disease, 372
saphenous nerve, 232
Sarmiento functional bracing, 416, 498
Sauve–Kapandji procedure, 310
scanograms, leg length discrepancy, 378

scaphoid, blood supply, 318–19
scaphoid fractures, 318–22
scaphoid non-union advanced collapse (SNAC) wrist, 45, 320, 322–3
scaphoid shift test *see* Kirk Watson's test
scapholunate advanced collapse wrist, 45–6, 325, 327–8
scapholunate angle, 328
scapholunate instability, 21, 325
scapholunate ligament injury, 324, 326
scapula, fractures, 405–6
scars, 21, 480
Scheuermann's disease, 247–8
sciatica, 76, 264–5, 584
sciatic nerve, 85, 432, 434
scoliosis, 66–7, 243
    adolescent idiopathic, 243–4
    adult, 261–2
    arthrogrypotic syndromes, 392
    cerebral palsy, 245, 381
    congenital, 243
    dystrophic/non-dystrophic, 384, 385
    idiopathic, 261
    infantile and juvenile (early onset), 244–5
    neurofibromatosis, 241, 384
    neuromuscular, 245, 261
    secondary, 245–6
screening tests, 554–5
screws, 442, 452–4, 581
scurvy (vitamin C deficiency), 535
Seddon's classification, nerve injuries, 33, 487–8
Seinsheimer's classification, 437
selective oestrogen receptor modulators, 521
Semmes–Weinstein hairs, 225, 487
sensation/sensory testing, 486–7
    Dupuytren's disease (DD), 26–7
    hand examination, 22, 24
    hip needing revision surgery, 79
    lower leg, 67–8
    upper limb, 30
sensitivity, test, 555
sensory-evoked potentials (SEPs), 265, 267
sensory nerve action potential (SNAP), 487
septic loosening, hip, 78
serratus anterior, testing, 60
shear stress, 491–2
sheet compression moulding, 502
shock, 248
short cases, 13–14
    candidates' accounts, 570–1, 574–5, 577, 580

list (possible cases), 15–16
Short Clinical Case examination, 4, 5–6
shortening (height), 78, 101
shoulder/shoulder joint
    arthritis and osteonecrosis, 143
    arthrodesis, 57–5, 142
    arthroplasty, 142, 153–4
    arthroscopy, 152
    asymmetry, 56
    clinical cases, 20, 51–63
    dislocations, 57, 411–13
    floating, 408
    frozen, 55, 144–45, 580
    hemiarthroplasty, 142, 153–4, 414
    instability, 56–7, 145–8
    oral core topics, 138–54
    pain, 51, 54, 138, 139
    radiographs, 138, 139, 141, 146
    rheumatoid arthritis, 143
    short cases, 15, 56–7, 575
    stiffness, after proximal humeral fractures, 415
sickle cell disease, 348, 533, 535
Silastic implant/spacer, 116, 226, 306
Single Best Answer questions, 9
single photon emission computed tomography, 545
sintering, 500
"six S's" classification, 408
skeletal dysplasia syndromes, 377, 394, 531
skin flora, 550
skull, diseases affecting, 527, 529
SLAC wrist, 45–6, 325, 327–8
SLAP lesions, 148
slipped upper femoral epiphysis (SUFE), 84, 89–90, 367–70
Smith–Peterson approach, 186, 365
Smith–Robinson approach, cervical spine, 237
SNAC wrist, 45, 320, 322–3, 571
soft tissue, in fractures, 498
    soft tissue tumours, 563–4
soft-tissue release, stiff elbow, 61
somatosensory-evoked potentials, 487
Sommerfield number, 505
Southwick angle, 369
spastic crouch contracture, cerebral palsy, 382
specificity, test, 555
spica cast, DDH, 364
spinal cord
    compression, cervical, 258–9
    injury, 245–6, 249
    monitoring, 264

spinal fusion, 267
spinal muscular atrophy, 245
spinal shock, 248
spinal stenosis, 265–7, 268–9
spina ventosa (tuberculous dactylitis), 348
spine, 240–1
    age-related changes, 240–1
    ankylosing spondylitis, 64, 254, 260, 540–2
    arthrogrypotic syndromes, 391, 392
    cerebral palsy, 381
    clinical cases, 16, 19, 64–70
    congenital disorders, 241
    developmental problems, 242–3
    embryology, 462–3
    fractures, 541
    infections, 263–4
    oral core topics, 237–69
    paediatric pathology, 241–8
    Paget's disease, 80, 529
    stabilization, in metastatic disease, 561
    surgical approaches, 237–40
    trauma, 248–28
    tumours, 243, 262–3
spinous process avulsion, thoracolumbar, 256
spinous process fracture, 252
splinting, 353, 416
split tibialis tendon transfers, 382, 389
spondylolisthesis, 69–70, 247, 252
spondylolysis, 247
spongiosa, 471, 472
squamous cell carcinoma, 340
squeeze film, 506
Staheli's range of hip rotation, 399
Staheli's shelf procedure, 366
stainless steel 316L, 498–9, 583
standard deviation, 554
standard error mean, 554
Staphylococcus, hip infection, 79
Staphylococcus aureus, 151, 246, 346, 550, 551
Staphylococcus epidermidis, 550
STAR (Scandinavian total ankle replacement), 218
statistical analysis paper, 9
statistics, 553–9
Steel's metaphyseal blanch sign, 368
Steel triple innominate osteotomy, 365–6
Steindler flexorplasty, 339
Steinmann pin fixation, 351, 409, 498
step length, definition, 496
sterilization

instruments, 551
    UHMWPE, 503–4
sternoclavicular joint dislocation, 410–11
stiffness, 455, 491
Stimson technique, 435
srain/strain energy, 491
stress, definition, 491
stress corrosion, 511
stress fractures, 530
stress relaxation, 490, 515
stress/strain curve, 483, 484, 490–1, 494
stride length, definition, 496
Stulberg's rating system at maturity, 373–4
subacromial impingement, 51–2, 139–40
subchondral bone, 212, 478–9
subchondral cysts, 88
subcoracoid impingement, 139
subscapularis tendon, 53, 144, 413
subtrochanteric fracture, 369, 436, 437, 438
subungual exostosis, 354
Sudeck's atrophy, 519
SUFE, 84, 89–90, 367–70
Sunderland's classification, nerve injuries, 488
superficial palmar arch, 278
superficial peroneal nerve, 233
supinator muscle, testing, 33, 61
supinator tunnel, radial nerve palsy, 34
supracondylar fracture, femoral, 176, 441, 443
supraspinatus tendon, 54, 60
    tear, 53, 54, 140
    testing (Jobe's test), 53, 56, 141
sural (medial) nerve, 233
survival analysis, 557, 583
swan-neck deformity, 315, 317–18
Swanson's classification, 341, 342
syllabus *see* FRCS Orth examination
syndactyly, 345
synovectomy, 91
    Darrach's procedure with, 309, 310
    elbow, 149
    hand/wrist, 309, 313–14
synovial fluid, 504, 505, 506
synovial joints, lubrication mechanisms, 506
synovial sarcoma, 564
synovitis, 101, 313–14
systemic lupus erythematosus (SLE), 307, 542–3

talar fracture, 452
talar tilt (angle), 446

talar tilting, 219, 222–3
talar tilt stress test, 219–20
talipes equinovarus, congenital, 386–9
talocalcaneal coalition, 123, 390, 391
talocrural angle, 446
tarsal coalition, 122–3, 390
tarsal tunnel syndrome, 232, 234, 236
teardrop fracture-dislocation, cervical spine, 253–4
technetium-99m scan, 171, 544, 545
teleroentgenogram (grid films), 66, 378
tendinous mallet finger, 333
tendon(s), 481–3, 486
    healing, 329, 483
    repair, 314
    ruptures, 447–8
tendon sheath, 482
tendon transfers, 334–5
    median nerve lesions, 38–9, 335
    radial nerve, 34, 335
    ulnar nerve (low lesion), 31–2, 335
tennis elbow, 62–3, 150–1
tenodesis, 318, 326
tenodesis test, 22
tenosynovectomy, 313
tenosynovitis
    extensor, 308, 312–14
    flexor, 308, 312, 314
    stenosing (trigger), 48–9, 335–7
tenovaginitis, digital (trigger finger), 48–9, 335–7
tensile force, 490
teres minor, assessment, 53
teriparatide, 521
textbooks and information resources, 584–6
theatre, operating, 551–2
thenar muscle wasting, 35, 36, 37
Thiemann's disease, 532
thigh foot angle, 395, 400
third body abrasive wear, 507
Thomas splint, 191, 499
Thomas test, 80, 83, 90, 99
Thompson and Epstein classification, 433
Thompson approach, to forearm, 425
thoracic spine
    disc prolapse, 264
    surgical approaches, 238–9
thoracolumbar spine
    developmental problems, 243–8
    dislocations, 256, 257
    extension injuries, 256, 257

flexion distraction injuries, 256, 257
fracture dislocations, 256, 257
fractures, 255–8
infections, 246, 263–4
kyphosis, 243, 259, 262
osteomyelitis, 246
postlaminectomy deformity, 262
reconstruction, 260–262
scoliosis see scoliosis
spinous process avulsion, 256
surgical approaches, 239–40
trauma, 254–8
tuberculosis, 246, 263, 264
tumours, 243, 262–3
thromboembolism, 92, 432, 564–5
thumb, 277, 303–4
    amputation, 331–2
    base, osteoarthritis, 42–3, 303–7
    deformities, 315
    CMC subluxation, 315
    duplication, 342, 344
    gamekeeper's, 315
    hypoplasia, 342–3
    reconstruction, 343
    rheumatoid arthritis, 314–16
    skier's, 355
thyroxine, 472
tibia
    absent, 398
    bowing, causes, 81, 82
    congenital pseudoarthrosis, 396–7
    cut, TKA, 196
    fractures, 397, 456, 578
    sabre, 80, 82
tibia hemimelia, 398
tibial components, mobile bearing in TKA, 195–7
tibialis anterior tendon, transfer, split, 382, 389
tibialis posterior tendon, 123–5, 382
tibial plafond (pilon) fractures, 443–4, 446
tibial torsion, 394, 395
tibia vara (Blount's disease), 395, 396
tibiofemoral angle, genu varum, 395
tibiofibular syndesmosis, rupture, 445, 446
tibiotalar tilt, 222–223
tidemark, cartilage zone, 478
Tile classification, pelvic ring fractures, 428
Tinel's sign, 36, 39, 283, 293
titanium alloys, 499–500
toe

claw, 112, 113–14, 224, 234
curly, 114, 389–90
fifth, over-riding, 131
gout, 46
hammer, 117–18, 234
tomography, cervical spine trauma, 249
tophi, 538, 539
torque, 489
torticollis, congenital muscular, 242
total ankle arthroplasty (TAR), 217, 218
total hip arthroplasty (THA), 164–8
  acetabular safe zones, 178
  after previous osteotomy, 190
  age limit, 439
  ankylosing spondylitis, 71–2
  antibiotic spacer use, 173
  arthrodesis conversion to, 185
  aseptic loosening, 77, 96, 166, 177–81
    after impaction grafting, 179, 180
    cemented femoral stem modes, 177–8
    metal-on-metal articulation use, 183–4
    modes of wear, 177
    oral exam questions, 179–80, 181
    osteolysis, 177
    radiography, 178, 179, 180
    surgical approach, 179
    technical problems contributing, 178
    wear debris see wear debris
    zones, 179
  AVN see avascular necrosis (AVN) of hip/femoral head
  basic science oral, 166
  cemented implants, 92, 158, 159, 175
  complications, 166–7, 534
  contraindications, 164
  debridement and antibiotics, 172
  design features, 181–3
  difficulties, in SUFE, 90
  dislocation, 103–4, 169
  dysplastic hip, 162, 163
  Exeter prosthesis, 182–3, 426–7
  femoral head see femoral head
  femoral prosthesis break, 180
  femoral stem see femoral stem
  heterotopic ossification after, 167, 187–8
  hybrid, 182
  infected/infection, 95–6, 166, 169–75
  informed consent, 89, 164
  long case, 581
  osteoarthritis of hip, 89

outcome measurements, 193
Paget's disease, 530
painful, 96–8
periprosthetic femoral fractures, 175–7, 183
Perthes disease, 75, 77
post-operative plan, 516
recurrent dislocation, 103–4
revision, 3, 77–80, 85, 184–5
  dislocation of THA, 168
  femoral fractures, 175
  impaction grafting and autografts, 179–180
  infected THA, 172–3
  stages, 172–3
rheumatoid arthritis, 91–2, 103
salvage, 173
septic loosening, 78
surgical approach, 164–5, 167
technical tips, 165
tuberculosis of hip, 102, 191–2
uncemented implants, femoral fractures, 175
wear, 177, 508–9
see also arthroplasty, resurfacing
total knee arthroplasty (TKA), 90, 194–8, 584
total shoulder replacement, 142, 153–4
toughness, definition, 490
tourniquet(s), 547–8
tourniquet-induced skeletal muscle ischaemia, 548
tourniquet paralysis syndrome, 547
traction, 250, 498, 499
training, operative hand surgery, 273
transarticular sliding hip screw, 186
transformation, non-parametric data, 553
transgluteal Hardinge approach, to THA, 164
transmalleolar-thigh angle, 400
trapdoor procedure, 158
trapeziectomy, 305, 306
trapeziometacarpal joint, 303–4, 305
trapezius, testing, 60
trauma
  biomechanics of implants, 452–6
  leg length discrepancy, 377
  long cases, 403, 456–7
  see also individual anatomical structures
trauma oral, 403–40
  candidates' accounts, 572, 576–7, 578, 581–2
  hand, 42
  miscellaneous questions, 457–8
  styles, 403, 404
  topics, 403–40

Trendelenburg test, 76, 80, 83
triangular fibrocartilage complex (TFCC), 21, 349
    lesions, 348, 349, 350, 351
tribology, 504–10
triceps, testing, 34, 60
trigger finger, 24, 48–9, 335–7
trochanteric advancement, 75
trochanteric fractures, 175, 436, 438
tuberculosis, 192
    dactylitis, 348
    hip, 85, 99–102, 191–2
    spinal, 192, 246
tumours, 19
    bone, 43, 246, 560–3
    soft-tissue, 563–4

UHMWPE, 502–4
ulna
    distal, excision, 47
    fractures, 422–4, 425–6
ulna claw hand, 32, 40, 291, 574
ulna paradox, 32
ulnar bursa, infections, 347
ulnar club hand, 342
ulnar head replacement, 310
ulnar nerve, 286–7
    anterior transposition, 288–9
    compression, 31, 287, 487
    decompression, 288, 291
    lesion(s), 29–32, 291, 335
ulnar nerve palsy, 31, 32, 288, 290, 577
ulnar paradox, 287
ulnar side wrist pain (USWP), 20
ulnar subluxed extensor tendons, 23
ulnar tunnel syndrome, 31–2, 289–91
ultra high molecular weight polyethylene, 502–4
ultrasound, 141, 361–2, 520, 546–7
unicompartmental knee replacement (UKR), 199
"universal precautions," 552
unmyelinated nerve fibres, 486
upper limb, 60, 391
    common/long cases, 19, 20

valgus deformity
    foot, 110
    knee, 108, 198–9, 208
    MTP see hallux valgus
Vancouver classification (Duncan and Masri),
        175–6

variance, statistical, 554
varus deformity, foot, 110, 112
vascular injuries, 167, 339, 412, 417, 421, 426, 427
Vaughan Jackson syndrome, 23, 308, 314
venous thromboembolism, 92, 422, 564–5
vertebrae
    block, 243
    "cod fish," 526, 527
    fractures, evaluation in osteoporosis, 521
    sandwich, 531
vertebral body, 262, 384, 529, 541
Vince and Miller's classification, 426
vinculae, 276, 482
viscoelastic materials/properties, 490
vitamin C deficiency, 535
vitamin D, 473, 523, 524
    deficiency, 521, 526
    supplements, 521
volar intercalated segment instability (VISI), 326
volar ulnar decompression, 451, 549
Volkmann's ischaemic contracture, 41–2
volumetric wear, 508
von Recklinghausen's disease, 384
von Willebrand's disease, 534

Waldenstrom's radiographic staging, 371–2
walking
    Hoffer classification, ambulation potential, 380
    osteoarthritis of hip, 87
    see also gait
Wallerian degeneration, 488
Wartenberg's sign, 31, 289
Wartenberg's syndrome, 293
Wassel classification (thumb duplication), 342
water, content of cartilage, 477
Watson classification, SLAC wrist, 328
Watson Jones approach, THA, 165
Watson Jones tenodesis (ankle), 220
Watson test see Kirk Watson's test
wear (implants), 507–8, 509–10
wear debris, 177, 183, 508, 509
Weber classification, ankle fractures, 446
web space infection, 346–7
weeping lubrication, 506
Weinstein classification, coxa vara, 375
wettability, 506
wheelchair, 91, 552–3
White–Menelaus rule of thumb, 377–8
Wilson's severity of slip, SUFE, 368

Windlass mechanism, 215
Wolff's law, 470
work hardening, 491
Wrisberg's variant, congenital discoid
    menisci, 212
wrist, 323–4
    arthrodesis, 300, 309–10, 350–1
    arthrogrypotic syndromes, 392
    arthroplasty, 310
    clinical cases, 20–50
    dorsal extensor compartments, 277
    drop, 582
    examination/tests, 20–1
    pain, 20, 304
    partial fusion, 300
    radial side wrist pain (RSWP), 20, 304
    rheumatoid arthritis *see* rheumatoid arthritis
    rickets, 528
    short case list, 15–16
    splinting, 353
    synovectomy, 309
    tendon transfers at, 335
    ulnar nerve palsy, 31

    ulnar side wrist pain (USWP), 20
    see also hand
wrist extension test, resisted, 63
wrist extensors, examination, 33
written examination, 3, 9–10
    candidates' accounts, 569–70, 573, 579–80
    MCQs *see* multiple choice questions (MCQs)
    new exam, 5
    paper interpretation, 570, 579
    short questions, 573

xenograft, corraline, 476
X-rays, 6, 543

Young and Burgess classification, 428
Young's modulus of elasticity, 491, 517

Zancolli capsulodesis, 32, 335
Zdravkovic–Damholt classification, 405
zirconia, 501
Z-lengthening, Achilles tendon, 382
zone of polarizing activity (ZPA), 462
z-plasty, Dupuytren's disease, 297